9/11: Mental Health in the Wake of Terrorist Attacks

"This is a great and exciting book; a volume filled with stories of endeavour, achievement, appraisal and learning; stories of heroism, challenge and hope. It will become a handbook for all who would research the impact of disaster and terrorism on mental health and well-being."

Beverley Raphael

Does terrorism have a unique and significant emotional and behavioral impact among adults and children?

In what way does the impact of terrorism exceed the individual level and affect communities and specific professional groups, and test different leadership styles?

How were professional communities of mental health clinicians, policy makers, and researchers mobilized to respond to the emerging needs post-disaster?

What are the lessons learned from the work conducted after 9/11, and the implications for future disaster mental health work and preparedness efforts?

Yuval Neria and his team are uniquely placed to answer these questions having been involved in modifying ongoing trials and setting up new ones in New York to address these issues straight after the attacks. No psychiatrist, mental health professional or policy-maker should be without this book.

Yuval Neria is Associate Clinical Professor of Medical Psychology at the Department of Psychiatry at the College of Physicians and Surgeons, Columbia University; and the Department of Epidemiology, Joseph L. Mailman School of Public Health; and Associate Director of Trauma Studies and Services at The New York State Psychiatric Institute.

Raz Gross is Assistant Professor of Epidemiology and Psychiatry, Department of Epidemiology, Joseph L. Mailman School of Public Health; and Department of Psychiatry, College of Physicians and Surgeons, Columbia University.

Randall D. Marshall is Director of Trauma Studies and Services, New York State Psychiatric Institute; Associate Director, Anxiety Disorders Clinic, New York State Psychiatric Institute, and Associate Professor of Clinical Psychiatry, Columbia University College of Physicians and Surgeons.

Ezra Susser is Professor of Epidemiology and Psychiatry at the College of Physicians and Surgeons, Columbia University; Chair of the Department of Epidemiology at the Joseph L. Mailman School of Public Health, Columbia University; and Head of the Department of Epidemiology of Brain Disorders at the New York State Psychiatric Institute.

This book is dedicated to those killed in the attacks of September 11, 2001; and is written for those who survived them, and mourned, and to all who have suffered because of what they saw and feared and felt, and lost.

Yuval Neria: For Mariana, Michal, Oren and Maya, who shared this journey and created the safe space which enabled its fulfillment; and for my dear parents and sister with love.

Raz Gross: For Natalie, Roy, Elie, and Daria; for my dear parents; and for my brother Aeyal and my sister Vardit, with great love.

Randall Marshall: For Tessa, Rory and Thalia, and my parents and brother Rodney, who are my teachers on the nature of love; and for Reece Marshal (1971–2001), who would have understood.

9/11: Mental Health in the Wake of Terrorist Attacks

Edited by

Yuval Neria

Raz Gross

Randall D. Marshall

Guest Editor

Ezra S. Susser

With a foreword by
Beverley Raphael

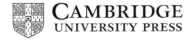

CAMBRIDGE
UNIVERSITY PRESS

CAMBRIDGE UNIVERSITY PRESS
Cambridge, New York, Melbourne, Madrid, Cape Town, Singapore, São Paulo

CAMBRIDGE UNIVERSITY PRESS
The Edinburgh Building, Cambridge CB2 2RU, UK

Published in the United States of America by Cambridge University Press, New York

www.cambridge.org
Information on this title: www.cambridge.org/9780521831918

First published 2006

Printed in the United Kingdom at the University Press, Cambridge

A catalogue record for this publication is available from the British Library

Library of Congress Cataloguing in Publication data

ISBN-13 978-0-521-83191-8 hardback
ISBN-10 0-521-83191-1 hardback

Every effort has been made in preparing this publication to provide accurate and up-to-date information which is in accord with accepted standards and practice at the time of publication. Although case histories are drawn from actual cases, every effort has been made to disguise the identities of the individuals involved. Nevertheless, the authors, editors and publishers can make no warranties that the information contained herein is totally free from error, not least because clinical standards are constantly changing through research and regulation. The authors, editors and publishers therefore disclaim all liability for direct or consequential damages resulting from the use of material contained in this publication. Readers are strongly advised to pay careful attention to information provided by the manufacturer of any drugs or equipment that they plan to use.

Contents

Part I   Introduction

Part II   The psychological aftermath of 9/11

Acknowledgments

The editors thank the dedicated staff of Trauma Studies and Services at The New York State Psychiatric Institute and Columbia University, College of Physicians and Surgeons who have devoted themselves to our 9/11 work from the very beginning: Eun Jung Suh, Larry Amsel, Donna Vermes, Steve Rudin, Gretchen Seirmarco, Helena Rosenfeld-Alvarez, Kimesha Thompson, Arturo Sánchez-Lacay, Smit Sinha, and Jaime Cárcamo, together with Franklin Schneier, Blair Simpson and Michael Liebowitz and the late Sharon Davies of the Anxiety Disorders Clinic.

The editors thank Helena Rosenfeld-Alvarez, the editorial coordinator in New York City; and also thank Alana Balaban for her editorial assistance.

Support for this book and for our work described herein has been provided in part from the National Institute of Mental Health (Neria, Marshall); The New York Times Neediest Fund (Marshall, Neria); Spunk Fund, Inc. (Neria); the New York Community Trust (Marshall); Project Liberty (Marshall); The Atlantic Philanthropies (Marshall); The September 11th Fund (Neria, Marshall); and The Robin Hood Foundation (Marshall).

Editors brief bio

Yuval Neria, PhD

Dr. Neria is Associate Professor of Clinical Psychology at the Departments of Psychiatry and Epidemiology at Columbia University and Associate Director of Trauma Studies and Services at The New York State Psychiatric Institute. He received his doctorate in Psychology from Haifa University, Israel, in 1994, and subsequently served on the faculty of Tel Aviv University until his recruitment to Columbia University in New York City after the attacks of 9/11. He has been working in the area of trauma, loss and post-traumatic stress disorder (PTSD) both in research and in treatment over the last 15 years. His trauma research is inspired by his extensive combat experience. He was injured in the Yom Kippur 1973 War where he was awarded *Itur Hagevura*, the highest medal for bravery that is awarded in Israel. He has authored numerous publications in the area of PTSD and resilience and his projects have been funded by the National Institute of Mental Health (NIMH), National Alliance for Research on Schizophrenia and Depression (NARSAD) and multiple charity organizations. He is currently leading a number of research projects related to the aftermath of 9/11 including a nationwide survey on traumatic grief and a longitudinal study among low income minority, primary care patients affected by the 9/11 attacks. Together with Dr. Randall D. Marshall, he has founded The Center for the Study of Trauma and Resilience, aiming to conduct research, training, and educational projects; enhance preparedness for terrorism and mass violence-related trauma; to promote resilient coping with adversities; and to improve the medical and psychological treatment of individuals affected by trauma of all kinds, including terrorist attacks and major disasters.

Raz Gross, MD, MPH

Dr. Gross received his MD degree from Tel Aviv University. After serving as a physician in the Israeli Defense Forces he trained in medicine and then in psychiatry. He moved to New York where he completed a 3-year Post-Doctoral Fellowship in

Psychiatric Epidemiology at Columbia University. He received his Masters degree in Public Health at the Mailman School of Public Health of Columbia University. Dr. Gross is currently Assistant Professor of Epidemiology and Psychiatry at Columbia University. He is involved in studies of workers who participated in the clean up and recovery effort at Ground Zero after September 11, and of the mental health consequences of 9/11 on primary care patients in Northern Manhattan. Dr. Gross is also a member of the core research team conducting a web-based survey on the psychological effects of losing a loved one on 9/11. His other areas of research include studies examining the relationship between psychiatric and medical conditions, prenatal and early life risk factors for major psychiatric disorders, and clinical trials.

Randall D. Marshall, MD

Dr. Marshall is Director of Trauma Studies and Services at the New York State Psychiatric Institute and Associate Professor of Clinical Psychiatry at Columbia University. He received his degree in Medicine from Johns Hopkins University in 1989, and subsequently trained as a resident and research fellow at the New York State Psychiatric Institute, Columbia University. He has published over 100 articles, case reports, chapters, and editorials, and received numerous research grants funded by the National Institute of Mental Health (NIMH), private industry, and multiple philanthropic sources. He is currently conducting a NIMH-funded treatment study of persons with PTSD related to the 9/11 attacks. His research related to psychological trauma has encompassed the role of trauma and dissociation in the anxiety disorders, nosology of trauma-related diagnoses, pharmacotherapy, cognitive–behavioral therapy, dissemination of evidence based treatments, the biology of treatment response in PTSD, and most recently, the study of serious mental health complications in bereaved persons. Most recently, he and Dr. Yuval Neria have founded The Center for the Study of Trauma and Resilience, which aims to conduct state-of-the-art research, training, and educational projects to enhance preparedness for terrorism, and mass violence-related trauma; promote resilient coping with adversity; and improve the medical and psychological treatment of individuals affected by trauma of all kinds, including terrorist attacks and major disasters.

Ezra Susser, MD, DrPH

Ezra Susser is the Anna Cheskis Gelman and Murray Charles Gelman Professor and Chair of the Department of Epidemiology at the Mailman School of Public Health of Columbia University, and Head of the Department of Epidemiology of Brain Disorders at the New York State Psychiatric Institute. Much of his research focuses on the developmental origins of health and disease throughout the life course. He heads the Center for Developmental Origins of Health, a collaborative birth cohort research program in which epidemiologists seek to uncover the causes of a broad range of disease and health outcomes, including psychiatric and neurodevelopmental disorders, obesity, cardiovascular disease, reproductive performance, and breast and ovarian cancers. Elsewhere in his research, he has taken an active role in using epidemiology to better understand social inequalities of health by focusing in the health of inner city populations. He has studied the interrelationships between homelessness, HIV, and psychotic disorders and was formerly director of the Center for Urban Epidemiologic Studies at the New York Academy of Medicine. Following September 11, 2001, he worked in close partnership with the New York State Office of Mental Health and the New York City Department of Health and Mental Hygiene to coordinate the research and services response of the public and academic sectors. He lead the preparation of a broad needs assessment submitted by New York State to the federal government estimating the scope and costs of mental health needs arising from the terror attacks. He also received funding for and implemented a free and confidential mental health services program, A Common Ground, for the union workers who participated in the World Trade Center (WTC) rescue and recovery effort. This program provided psycho-education, outreach, and group, family and individual counseling and psychiatric services to thousands of union members and their families.

List of contributors

Jennifer Ahern, MPH
Senior Research Analyst
Center for Urban Epidemiologic
Studies
New York Academy of Medicine
1216 Fifth Avenue, Room 553
New York, NY 10029, USA
Tel: +212-822-7297
Fax: +212-876-6220
E-mail: Jahern@nyam.org

Lawrence V. Amsel, MD, MPH
Assistant Professor of Clinical
Psychiatry
Columbia University College of
Physicians and Surgeons
Director of Dissemination Research for
Trauma Studies and Services
New York State Psychiatric Institute
Associate for Medical Education
Hasting Center for Bioethics
245 West 107th Street, Suite 14-F
New York, NY 10025-3064, USA
Tel: +212-592-3804
Fax: +212-678-6752
E-mail: lva@columbia.edu

Diana Bilimoria, PhD
Associate Professor
Department of Organizational Behavior
Weatherhead School of Management
Case Western Reserve University
10900 Euclid Avenue
Cleveland, OH 44106-7235, USA
Tel: +216-368-2115
Fax: +216-368-6228
E-mail. dxb12@po.cwru.edu

Richard E. Boyatzis, PhD
Professor and Chair
Department of Organizational Behavior
Case Western Reserve University
10900 Euclid Avenue
Cleveland, OH 44106-7235, USA
Tel: +216-368-2055
Fax: +216-368-4785
E-mail: reb2@weatherhead.cwru.edu

Naomi Breslau, PhD
Professor
Department of Epidemiology
Michigan State University
B645 West Fee Hall

East Lansing, MI 48824, USA
Tel: +517-353-8623, ex. 170
Fax: +517-432-1130
E-mail: breslau@epi.msu.edu

Evelyn J. Bromet, PhD
Professor of Psychiatry and Preventive
Medicine
School of Medicine
SUNY at Stony Brook
Putnam Hall-South Campus
Stony Brook, NY 11794-8790, USA
Tel: +631-632-8853
Fax: +631-632-9433
E-mail: ebromet@notes.cc.sunysb.edu

Shawn P. Cahill, PhD
University of Pennsylvania
3535 Market Street, Suite 600 N.
Philadelphia, PA 19104, USA
Tel: +215-746-3327
Fax: +215-746-3311
E-mail: scahill@mail.med.upenn.edu

Marylene Cloitre, PhD
Cathy and Stephen Graham Professor
of Child and Adolescent Psychiatry
Director, Institute for Trauma and Stress
Child Study Center
New York University School of Medicine
215 Lexington Avenue 16th Floor
New York, NY 10016, USA
Tel: +212-263-2471
Fax: +212-263-2476
E-mail: marylene.cloitre@med.nyu.edu

Susan W. Coates, PhD
Clinical Professor of
Psychology in Psychiatry
College of Physicians & Surgeons
Columbia University
Teaching Faculty

Columbia Center for Psychoanalytic
Training & Research
205 West 89th Street
New York, New York, 10024, USA
Tel: +212-580-1423
Fax: +212-580-1423
E-mail: swcl@columbia.edu

Roxane Cohen Silver, PhD
Professor, Department of Psychology
and Social Behavior
Professor, Department of Medicine
3340 Social Ecology II
University of California, Irvine
Irvine, CA 92697-7085
Tel: +949-824-2192
Fax: +949-824-3002
E-mail: rsilver@uci.edu

Amar Das, MD, PhD
Assistant Professor
Stanford Medical Informatics
Departments of Medicine and of
Psychiatry and Behavioral Sciences
Stanford University School of Medicine
MSOB X-233
251 Campus Drive Stanford, CA
94305, USA
Tel: +650-736-1632
Fax: +650-725-7944
E-mail: akd@SMI.stanford.edu

Joanne L. Davis, PhD
Assistant Professor
Department of Psychology
University of Tulsa
600 South College
308C Lorton Hall
Tulsa, OK 74104, USA
Tel: +918-631-2875
Fax: +918-631-2833
E-mail: Joanne-Davis@utulsa.edu

Lori Davis, Psy. D
107 West 82nd Street, Suite P106
New York, NY, USA 10024
Tel: +212-580-0271
Fax: +212-292-8945
E-mail: loridavis@nyc.rr.com

JoAnn Difede, PhD
Associate Professor of Psychology in
Psychiatry
Director, Program for Anxiety and
Traumatic Stress Studies
Payne Whitney Clinic, Department of
Psychiatry
Weill/Cornell Medical College
New York Presbyterian Hospital
New York, NY, USA
Tel: +212-746-3079
Fax: +212-746-5418
E-mail: jdifede@med.cornell.edu

Sheila Donahue, MA
Director, Bureau of Data Analysis and
Performance Measurement
Center for Information Technology
and Evaluation Research
New York State Office of Mental Health
44 Holland Avenue
Albany, New York, USA 12229
E-mail: coevsad@omh.state.ny.us

John Draper, PhD
Director of Public Education and the
LifeNet Hotline Network
Mental Health Association of
New York City, Inc.
666 Broadway, Suite 405
New York, NY 10012, USA
Tel: +212-614-6309 (direct/voice mail)
     +212-614-6357
     +1-800-543-3638 (LifeNet hotline)
E-mail: jdraper@mhaofnyc.org

Cristiane S. Duarte, PhD
Assistant Professor of Clinical
Psychology in Psychiatry
Division of Child Psychiatry
Columbia University
1051 Riverside Drive, Unit 43
New York, NY 10032, USA
Tel: +212-543-5688, 212-543-5725
Fax: +212-781-6050
E-mail: duartec@child.cpmc.
columbia.edu

Spencer Eth, MD
Professor and Vice Chairman
Department of Psychiatry and
Behavioral Sciences
New York Medical College
Medical Director and Senior
Vice President
Behavioral Health Services
Saint Vincent Catholic Medical Centers
144 West 12th Street
New York, NY 10011, USA
Tel: +212-604-8195
Fax: +212-604-8197
E-mail: seth@svcmcny.org

Adriana Feder, MD
Assistant Professor
Department of Psychiatry
Mount Sinai School of Medicine
One Gustave L. Levy Place, Box 1218
New York, NY, USA 10029
Tel: +212-241-1563
Fax: +212-824-2302
E-mail: Adriana.feder@mssm.edu

Chip J. Felton, MSW
Senior Deputy Commissioner and
Chief Information Officer Center for

Information Technology and
Evaluation Research
New York State Office of Mental
Health
44 Holland Avenue
Albany, NY 12229, USA
Tel: +518-474-7359
E-mail: cfelton@omh.state.ny.us

Edna B. Foa, PhD
Professor of Clinical Psychology in
Psychiatry
University of Pennsylvania
3535 Market Street, Suite 600 N.
Philadelphia, PA 19104, USA
Tel: +215-746-3327
Fax: +215-746-3311
E-mail: foa@mail.med.upenn.edu

Mindy Thompson Fullilove, MD
Professor of Clinical Psychiatry and
Public Health
New York State Psychiatric Institute,
Unit 29
1051 Riverside Drive
New York, NY 10032, USA
Tel: +212-740-7292
Fax: +212-795-4222
E-mail: mf29@columbia.edu

Sandro Galea, MD, DrPH
Associate Professor
Department of Epidemiology,
University of Michigan School of
Public Health
1214 South University, Room 243
Ann Arbor, MI 48104-2548
Tel: +734-647-9741 (direct)
    +917-930-6923 (cell)
Fax: 734 998 0006
E-mail: sgalea@umich.edu

Marc J. Gameroff, PhD
Research Scientist
Department of Clinical and Genetic
Epidemiology,
New York State Psychiatric Institute
1051 Riverside Drive / Unit 24
New York, NY, USA 10032
Tel: +212-543-5849
Fax: +212-568-3534
E-mail: gameroff@childpsych.
columbia.edu

Virginia Gil-Rivas, PhD
Assistant Professor
Department of Psychology
University of North Carolina, Charlotte
9201 University Boulevard
Charlotte, NC 28223 0001, USA

Vincent Giordano, PhD
New York Academy of Medicine,
Office School Health Programs,
Senior Consultant National Center for
School Crisis and Bereavement,
Advisory Board Member
Denizen Consulting, Partner
Association for Supervision and
Curriculum Development
37 Mount Tom Road
New Rochelle, New York, NY 10805 USA
Tel: +914-654-8897
Fax: +914-654-8897
Cell: +914-393-4541
E-mail: vgiordano@verizon.net

Lindsey Godwin, Doctoral Candidate
Department of Organizational
Behavior
Weatherhead School of Management
Case Western Reserve University
324 E. 310 Street

Willowick OH, USA 44095
Tel: +440-537-0971
E-mail: lng2@case.edu

Raz Gross, MD, MPH
Assistant Professor
Department of Epidemiology,
Mailman School of Public Health,
Columbia University
Department of Psychiatry,
College of Physicians & Surgeons,
Columbia University
722 West 168th Street
New York, NY 10032, USA
Tel. l 212-304-6591
Fax: +212-544-4221
E-mail: rg547@columbia.edu

Sandra Hanish
Psychiatric Clinical Nurse Specialist
Walter Reed Army Medical Center
Pentagon/Operation Solace

Johan M. Havenaar, PhD
Managing Director of Adult Psychiatry
Buitenamstel Institute of Mental
Health Care; Department of Psychiatry
Vrije Universiteit Amsterdam
Amsterdam, The Netherlands
Tel: +31-30-2308686
Fax: +31-30-2308885
E-mail: j.havenaar@altrecht.nl

Elizabeth A. Hembree, PhD
Assistant Professor of Clinical
Psychology in Psychiatry
University of Pennsylvania
3535 Market Street, Suite 600 N.
Philadelphia, PA 19104, USA
Tel: +215-746-3327
Fax: +215-746-3311
E-mail: hembree@mail.med.upenn.edu

Robin Herbert, MD
Associate Professor
Department of Community and
Preventive Medicine
Mount Sinai School of Medicine
New York, NY 10029, USA
E-mail: robin.herbert@mssm.edu

Kimberly Hoagwood, PhD
Professor of Clinical Psychology and
Psychiatry
Center Director for Child and
Adolescent Services, Research
Division of Child and Adolescent
Psychiatry
Columbia University
1051 Riverside Drive, Box 78
New York, NY 10032, USA
Tel: +212-543-6131
Fax: +212-543-5966
E-mail: Hoagwood@childpsych.
columbia.edu

Stevan E. Hobfoll, PhD
Distinguished Professor and Director
Applied Psychology Center
Kent State University
Director
Center for the Treatment and Study of
Traumatic Stress
Summa Health System and Kent State
University
Kent, OH 44242, USA
E-mail: shobfoll@kent.edu

E. Alison Holman, FNP, PhD
Health Policy and Research
University of California, Irvine
100 Theory, Suite 110
Irvine, CA 92697-5800, USA
Tel: +949-824-6849

Fax: +949-824-3002
E-mail: aholman@uci.edu

Barry A. Hong, PhD, FAACP
Professor of Psychiatry
Washington University School of
Medicine
600 S. Euclid Ave., Campus Box 8134
St. Louis, MO 63110
Tel: +314-362-4270
Fax: +314-362-4857
E-mail: hongb@psychiatry.wustl.edu

Margaret M. Hopkins, PhD
Case Western Reserve University
Weatherhead School of Management
Department of Organizational
Behavior
Cleveland, OH 44106, USA
Tel: +216-651-2414
Fax: +216-651-3796
E-mail: mxh9@po.cwru.edu

Lourdes Hernández-Cordero, DrPH
Assistant Professor of Clinical
Sociomedical Sciences
Community Liaison
Columbia University Center for Youth
Violence Prevention
Community Research Group
Mailman School of Public Health
513 West 166th Street, 3rd floor
New York, NY, USA 10032
Tel: +212-740-7292
Fax: +212-795-4222
E-mail: ljh19@columbia.edu

Christina W. Hoven, DrPH
Child Psychiatric Epidemiologist
Department of Epidemiology
Mailman School of Public Health
Columbia University

Research Scientist
Division of Child Psychiatry
New York State Psychiatric Institute
1051 Riverside Drive, Unit 43
New York, NY 10032, USA
Tel: +212-543-5688
Fax: +212-781-6050
E-mail: HOVEN@childpsych.
columbia.edu

Nimali Jayasinghe, PhD
Instructor of Psychology in Psychiatry
Department of Psychiatry
Weill/Cornell Medical College
New York Presbyterian Hospital
525 East 68th Street, Box 200
New York, NY 10021, USA
Tel: +212-821-0728
Fax: +212-821-0994
E-mail: nij2001@med.cornell.edu

Peter S. Jensen, MD
Ruane Professor of Child Psychiatry
and Director
Center for the Advancement of
Children's Mental Health
Department of Child Psychiatry
Columbia University/New York State
Psychiatric Institute
1051 Riverside Drive, Unit No. 78
New York, NY 10032, USA
Tel: +212-543-5334
Fax: +212-543-5260
E-mail: pj131@columbia.edu

Krzysztof Kaniasty, PhD
Professor
Department of Psychology
Uhler Hall, 1020 Oakland Avenue
Indiana University of Pennsylvania
Indiana, PA 15705-1068, USA

Department of Psychology
Opole University, Poland
Tel: +724-357-5559/2426 (office)
Fax: +724-357-2214
E-mail: kaniasty@iup.edu

John Kastan, PhD
Vice President, Behavioral Health
Services
Saint Vincent Catholic Medical Centers
Assistant Professor
Department of Psychiatry and
Behavioral Sciences,
New York Medical College
203 West 12th Street, Rm. 603
New York, NY, USA 10011
Tel: +212-604-1571
Fax: +212-604-8794
E-mail: jkastan@svcmcny.org

Craig L. Katz, MD
Clinical Assistant Professor of
Psychiatry,
Mount Sinai School of Medicine
President, Disaster Psychiatry Outreach
1100 Park Ave., Suite 1B
New York, NY 10128, USA
Tel: +212-860-8665
E-mail: craig.katz@mssm.edu

Shawn M. Kennedy, PhD
The University of Tulsa
Department of Psychology
600 S. College Avenue 74104
Tulsa, OK, USA
Tel: +918-631-2031
E-mail: shawn-kennedy@utulsa.edu

Rafael Lantigua, MD
Professor of Clinical Medicine
Director, General Medicine Outpatient
Services

Director, Columbia Center for the
Active Life of Minority Elders (CALME)
Columbia University Medical Center
622 West 168th Street, VC2-205
New York, NY, USA 10032
Tel: +212-305-6262
Fax: +212-305-6279
E-mail: ral4@columbia.edu

Carol Barth Lanzara, MS, JD
Research Scientist
Center for Information and Evaluation
Research
Evaluation Research Branch
NYS Office of Mental Health
44 Holland Avenue
Albany, New York, USA 12229
Tel: +518-408-2042
Fax: +518-474-7361
E-mail: clanzara@omh.state.ny.us

Willis Todd Leavitt, MD
LTC, MC, USA
Psychiatry Consultant, Great Plains
Regional Medical Command
Combat/Operational Stress Control
Program Manager
Tel: +210-221-8235
Fax: +210-221-7235
E-mail: Willis.Leavitt@cen.amedd.
army.mil

Pam Leck, PhD
Instructor of Psychology in Psychiatry
Department of Psychiatry
Weill/Cornell Medical College
New York Presbyterian Hospital
New York, NY, USA
Tel: +212-746-0554
Fax: +212-746-8552
E-mail: pal2002@med.cornell.edu

Stephen M. Levin, MD
Associate Professor
Department of Community and
Preventive Medicine
Mount Sinai School of Medicine
New York, NY 10029, USA
E-mail: stephen.levin@mssm.edu

Tony Lingham, PhD
Case Western Reserve University
Weatherhead School of Management
Department of Organizational Behavior
2040 Stearns Road, Apartment No. 1
Cleveland, OH 44106, USA
Tel: +216-496-8816
E-mail: TXL28@po.cwru.edu

Brett T. Litz, PhD
Professor, Departments of Psychology
and Psychiatry,
Boston University
Associate Director,
National Center for Posttraumatic
Stress Disorder / Behavioral Science
Division (116-B5)
Boston Department of Veterans
Affairs Medical Center
150 South Huntington Avenue
Boston, MA 02130, USA
Tel: +617-232-9500 ext: 4131, 6198,
6191
Fax: +617-264-6523 or 617-278-4501
E-mail: brett.litz@va.gov

Shira Maguen, PhD
San Francisco Veterans' Administration
Medical Center
University of California San Francisco
PTSD Program (116P)
4150 Clement St., Building 8,
Room 206
San Francisco, CA 94121, USA
Tel: +415-221-4810 ext. 2511
E-mail: shira.maguen@va.gov

Donald J. Mandell, PhD
Professor, State University of New York
Research Scientist, New York State
Psychiatric Institute
1051 Riverside Drive, Unit 43
New York, NY 10032, USA
Tel: +212-543-5688 (main)
E-mail: mandell@child.cpmc.
columbia.edu

Randall D. Marshall, MD
Associate Professor of Clinical Psychiatry,
Columbia University College of
Physicians & Surgeons
Director of Trauma Studies & Services,
New York State Psychiatric Institute,
New York Office of Mental Health
Co-Director, Center for the Study of
Trauma & Resilience,
New York State Psychiatric Insitute
and Columbia University
Associate Director, Anxiety Disorders
Clinic,
New York State Psychiatric Institute
1051 Riverside Drive, Unit 69
New York, NY 10032, USA
Tel: +212-543-5454
Fax: +212-543-6515
E-mail: Randall@nyspi.cpmc.
columbia.edu

Gerald McCleery PhD
Associate Executive Director
Mental Health Association of
New York City
666 Broadway, 2nd floor
New York, NY 10012, USA

Tel: +212-614-6305
Fax: +646-654-0593
E-mail: GMcCleery@mhaofnyc.org

Daniel N. McIntosh, PhD
Associate Professor of Psychology
Department of Psychology
University of Denver
2155 S. Race Street
Denver, CO 80208, USA
Tel: +303-871-3712
Fax: +303-871-4747
E-mail: dmcintos@du.edu

Richard J. McNally, PhD
Professor
Department of Psychology
Harvard University
33 Kirkland Street
Cambridge, MA 02138, USA
Tel: +617-495-3853
Fax: +617-495-3728
E-mail: rjm@wjh.harvard.edu

Stephen S. Morse, PhD
Associate Professor
Columbia University
Mailman School of Public Health
Center for Public Health Preparedness
722 West 168th Street, Suite 522C
New York, NY 10032, USA
Fax: +212-543-8793
E-mail: ssm20@columbia.edu

Laura Murray, PhD
Center for the Advancement of Children
Columbia University/New York State
Psychiatric Institute
1051 Riverside Drive, Unit 78
New York, NY 10032, USA
Tel: +212-543-5428
Fax: +212-543-5966

E-mail: MurrayL@childpsych.
columbia.edu

Yuval Neria, PhD
Associate Professor of Clinical
Psychology
Department of Psychiatry,
College of Physicians & Surgeons
Department of Epidemiology
Mailman School of Public Health
Columbia University
Associate Director, Trauma Studies
and Services
New York State Psychiatric Institute
1051 Riverside Drive / Unit 69
New York, NY USA 10032
Tel: +212-543-6061
Fax: +212-543-6515
E-mail: ny126@columbia.edu

Elana Newman, PhD
Associate Professor
Department of Psychology, Lorton Hall
University of Tulsa
600 South College Avenue
Tulsa, OK 74104-3189, USA
Tel: +918-631-2836
Fax: +918-631-2822
E-mail: elana-newman@utulsa.edu

Fran H. Norris, PhD
Research Professor
Department of Psychiatry,
Dartmouth Medical School and
National Center for PTSD
Veterans' Administration Medical
Center 116D
215 North Main Street
White River Junction, VT 05009, USA
Tel: +802-296-5132
Fax: +802-296-5135
E-mail: fran.norris@dartmouth.edu

Carol S. North, MD, MPE
Professor of Psychiatry
Nancy and Ray L. Hunt Chair in Crisis
Psychiatry
UT Southwestern Medical Center
Department of Psychiatry
6363 Forest Park Rd.
Dallas, TX, USA 75390-8828
Tel: +214-648-5381
Fax: +214-648-5376
E-mail: carol.north@southwestern.edu

Mark Olfson, MD, MPH
Professor of Clinical Psychiatry
Columbia University and New York
State Psychiatric Institute
New York, NY, USA
Tel: +212-543-5293
E-mail: mo49@columbia.edu

Elizabeth A. Pease, RN, MS
New York State Office of Mental
Health (NYSOMH)
44 Holland Avenue
Albany, New York, USA 12229
Tel: + 518-402-2411
Fax: + 518-474-7361
E-mail: Coeveap@omh.state.ny.us

Betty Pfefferbaum, MD, JD
Chairman, Department of Psychiatry
and Behavioral Sciences
Director, Terrorism and Disaster
Center of the National Child
Traumatic Stress Network
University of Oklahoma Health
Sciences Center
Tel: +405-271-5121
Fax: +405-271-8775
E-mail: betty-pfefferbaum@
ouhsc.edu

Judith Pizarro, MA
University of California, Irvine
E-mail: jpizarro@uci.edu

Michael Poulin, PhD
Department of Psychology and Social
Behavior
University of California, Irvine
3400 Social Ecology II
Irvine, CA 92697, USA
Tel: +949-824-6849
Fax: +949-824-3002

**Beverley Raphael, AM, MBBS, MD,
FRANZCP, FRCPsych., FASSA,
Hon. MD (Newcastle, NSW)**
Professor Population Mental Health
and Disasters
University of Western Sydney
Parramatta Campus
Locked Bag 1797
Penrith South, NSW DC 1797
AUSTRALIA
Tel: +61-2-9685-9575
Fax: +61-2-9685-9554
E-mail: b.Raphael@usw.edu.au
and
Professor of Psychological Medicine
Australian National University

Irwin Redlener, MD
National Center for Disaster
Preparedness
Mailman School of Public Health,
Columbia University
722 West 168th Street, 10th Floor
New York, NY 10032, USA
Tel: +212-342-5161

Heidi Resnick, PhD
Professor
National Crime Victims Research and
Treatment Center

Department of Psychiatry and
Behavioral Sciences
Medical University of South Carolina
165 Cannon Street, PO Box 250852
Charleston, SC 29425, USA
Tel: +843-792-2947
E-mail: resnickh@musc.edu

Elspeth Cameron Ritchie, MD, MPH
COL, USA
Psychiatry Consultant to the US Army
Surgeon General
Skyline 6, Suite 684
5109 Leesburg Pike
Falls Church, VA, USA 22041-3258
Tel: +703-681-1975
Fax: +703-681-3163
E-mail: Elspeth.Ritchie@amedd.
army.mil

Jennifer Roberts, PhD
Assistant Professor of Psychology in
Psychiatry
Department of Psychiatry
Weill/Cornell Medical College
New York Presbyterian Hospital
Tel: +212-746-6167
Fax: +212-746-5418
E-mail: jroberts@med.cornell.edu

Jim Rodriguez, MSW, PhD
Research Scientist, Department of
Child Psychiatry, Columbia
University and New York
State Office of Mental Health
Columbia University
Child and Adolescent Psychiatry
1755 Broadway, Suite 715
New York, NY 10019, USA
Tel: +646-328-4417
Fax: +646-443-8191
E-mail: rodriguija@childpsych.
columbia.edu

Jack Rosenthal
President
The New York Times Company
Foundation
229 West 43rd Street
New York, NY, USA 10036
Tel: +212-556-1091
Fax: +212-556-4450
E-mail: rosebud@nytimes.com

Jack Saul, PhD
Assistant Professor of Clinical
Population and Family Health
Director, International Trauma
Studies Program
Mailman School of Public Health
Columbia University
155 Avenue of the Americas, 4th Floor
New York, NY 10013, USA
Tel: +212-691-6499
Fax: +212-807-1809
E-mail: js2920@columbia.edu

Richard Schaedle, DSW
The Mental Health Association of
New York City
666 Broadway, 4th Floor
New York, NY 10012, USA
Director of the Crisis Resource Center
at LifeNet
Work: 212-614-6345
Home: 718-834-6061
E-mail: rschaedle@mhaofnyc.org

Daniel S. Schechter, MD
Assistant Professor of Clinical Psychiatry
in Pediatrics, College of Physicians
and Surgeons, Columbia University
New York, NY, USA
Tel: +1-212-543-6920
Fax: +1-212-463-0702
E-mail: dss11@columbia.edu

Gila Schwarzbaum, MBA
Mount Sinai School of Medicine
Bronx Veterans Affairs
130 West Kingsbridge Road
526 Office of Mental Health PTSD 116/A
Bronx, NY 10468, USA

Arieh Y. Shalev, MD
Professor of Psychiatry,
Head, Department of Psychiatry
Hadassah University Hospital,
PO Box 12000
Kiriat Hadassah, 91120
Jerusalem, Israel
Tel: +972-2-6777184
Fax: +972-2-6413642
E-mail: ashalev@cc.huji.ac.il

Steven Shea, MD
Hamilton Southworth Professor of
Medicine and Professor of Epidemiology
Chief, Division of General Medicine
Vice Dean of the Faculty of Medicine
and Senior Associate Dean for Clinical
Affairs
Columbia University
622 West 168th Street
PH 9 East, Rm. 105
New York, NY, 10032
Tel: +212-305-9379
Fax: +212-305-9349
E-mail: ss35@columbia.edu

Rebecca P. Smith, MD
Assistant Professor of Psychiatry
Mount Sinai Hospital and Medical
School
Staff Psychiatrist, Disaster Psychiatry
Outreach
World Trade Center Volunteer, Rescue
and Salvage Worker Screening Program

1200 Fifth Avenue, First Floor
New York, NY 10128, USA
Tel: +212-241-9057
E-mail: Rebecca.smith@mssm.edu

Eun Jung Suh, PhD
Instructor in Clinical Psychology
Department of Psychiatry
Columbia University College of
Physicians and Surgeons
New York State Psychiatric Institute
1051 Riverside Drive, Unit 69
New York, NY 10032, USA
E-mail: ejs161@columbia.edu

Ezra S. Susser, MD, DrPH
Anna Cheskis Gelman and
Murray Charles Gelman Professor
and Chair
Department of Epidemiology
Mailman School of Public Health,
Columbia University
Professor of Psychiatry and
Department Head,
Epidemiology of Brain Disorders
New York State Psychiatric Institute
722 West 168th Street, Room 1508
New York, NY, USA 10032
Tel: +212-342-2133
Fax: +212-342-2286
E-mail: ess8@columbia.edu

David Vlahov, PhD
Director
Center for Urban Epidemiologic studies
Professor Department of Epidemiology
Mailman School of Public Health,
Columbia University
Center for Urban Epidemiologic
Studies

New York Academy of Medicine
1216 Fifth Avenue
New York, NY 10029, USA
Tel: +212-822-7382
E-mail: dvlahov@nyam.org

Myrna M. Weissman, PhD
Professor of Epidemiology in Psychiatry
Columbia University College of
Physicians & Surgeons
1051 Riverside Drive Unit 24
New York, NY, 10032
Tel: +212-543-5880
E-mail: weissman@childpsych.
columbia.edu

Simon Wessely, PhD
Director, King's Centre for Military
Health Research
King's College London
Weston Education Centre
Cutcombe Road
London
SE5 9 RJ, UK
Tel: +0044-207-848-0448
Fax: +0044-207-848-5408
E-mail: s.wessely@iop.kcl.ac.uk

Ping Wu, PhD
Assistant Professor of Clinical Public
Health in Psychiatry
Departments of Psychiatry and
Epidemiology
Columbia University
1051 Riverside Drive, Unit 43
New York, NY 10032, USA
Tel: +212-543-5688 (main),
212-543-5190
Fax: +212-781-6050
E-mail:
wup@child.cpmc.columbia.edu

Rachel Yehuda, PhD
Professor of Psychiatry
Mount Sinai School of
Medicine/Bronx Veterans Affairs
130 West Kingsbridge Road
526 Office of Mental Health PTSD
116/A
Bronx, NY 10468, USA
Tel: +718-584-9000; ext: 6964 or 6677
Fax: +718-741-4773
E-mail: Rachel.yehuda@med.va.gov

Foreword

This is a great and exciting book; a volume filled with stories of endeavor, achievement, appraisal and learning; stories of heroism, challenge and hope. It will become a handbook for all who would research the impact of disaster and terrorism on mental health and well-being. It is a courageous contribution to the science of this field in giving testimony to the research that was done to assess need, to study reactions over time, and to provide and evaluate the best possible care. It is also courageous in that the research is presented openly, with its challenges, its successes, its imperfections, and with critical appraisal provided by "outside" experts. It is all the more powerful for this. It is the most comprehensive drawing together of the wide range of initiatives that followed a specific incident, initiatives that were implemented in the times of chaos and uncertainty. It was instigated by researchers and clinicians who were, at the time, themselves also experiencing the multiple, acute and subsequent stressors of the attack and its aftermath. It is a further contribution in terms of the universal wish to make meaning of what has happened. As mental health professionals and scientists, this surely, is one of our ways of making meaning.

A number of themes thread their way through this book: The enormity, unexpectedness and uniqueness of what happened; not only was America assaulted, but the world saw, and felt what happened. Courage, the "democracy" of distress, resolve, resilience – the coming together of peoples: ranging from the comforts of strangers, to the convergence of those who would provide help, all attested to the wish to repair, to undo the damage, to make the world right and safe again, to heal. There is the acknowledgment and measurement of the research reported: the psychological injuries experienced by many, and, as well, the stressors that arose subsequently and made further burdens for those fighting to recover. There is a suffering revealed vividly when we listen to the words of those most directly affected. Recognition of the extent of the catastrophe, and its possible effects, the "global distress", as well as the individual pathology, has led most contributors to talk of the public health issues. There is documentation of need for the "population injury" to be dealt with, as well as the clinical psychological injury; and many of the diverse concepts, initiatives and research mobilized to address these, including those of powerful community driven responses. This recognition also demonstrated the need for a coherent population health framework for such an approach for mental health, including the importance of core baseline data and surveillance programs (Commonwealth of Australia, 2000). There is also the pluralism which is so essentially American; the multiplicity of approaches which has been creative and productive – yet the need for consistency and coordination of response – all most obvious is the convergence of agencies, ideas and methodologies, which demonstrate the need for the reassurance of governance, coordination and structure in the face of chaos and uncertainty.

Researchers and commentators highlight the vital importance of evaluation, not only of individual treatments, but also of organizational response of the public health as well as the clinical initiatives. The aims to provide the "highest quality evidence-based practice" and "rigorous outcome evaluations" are important but extremely difficult to achieve at most times, let alone in the face of catastrophe. Further research questions are also seen as relevant; for instance, what are the exposures of "terrorism" and its aftermath; what is resilience; how are interventions to be really targeted to those with greatest need related to their experience of this incident; what is the nature of "psychological trauma" and "collective trauma" and how can we better deconstruct these scientifically to research their etiological significance; and how can excessive "trauma expectations" be avoided? There is also the need for better scientific appraisal of ethno-cultural "trauma" impacts.

Sophisticated science for "ecological assessment" to inform learning from these responses; for instance, how positive dynamics can be supported and negative changes mitigated is also important. Changes such as those associated with social network damage, splitting, fear and rejection of those who are different, perhaps in terms of ethno-cultural distinctions, need to be better understood. This should include an understanding and tracking of what happens to the anger and rage in such settings and the complex social consequences, the coming to terms with the "darker side of human nature" – both in our attackers and ourselves.

What are the effects of no clear end points to an event, and more specifically of ongoing terrorism "threat" – what changes occur socially, personally, and individually and politically as a consequence? How do individual and collective perceptions and realities interact? How can beliefs that have attached to models of response, for instance, debriefing and screening, be changed by evidence and how can evidence inform the realities of care in such circumstances? How do individuals and communities live with, prepare for a threat, with individual and community plans, that will be of wider value, that will promote well-being, even if the event does not occur, while preparing for effective response if it does?

All these are important questions for future research. But such research should learn from the rich contributions of this volume and the further work to come, from what Yuval Neria, Raz Gross, Randall D. Marshall have so powerfully drawn together, and from all the excellent contributions that comprise this work. The reviews of previous research, the science and actualities of response so comprehensively documented and the unflinching critiques provide a valuable resource. We will all learn from it in terms of research, but also in policy and planning ahead: much of what has been learned can also enrich planning and research agendae world wide, including those such as WHO–AIMS–E, (WHO, 2005) and other guidelines. The need for core minimum data sets is critical for future research so that the knowledge base can be built (Consensus Conference December 2005 Sydney, Australia), so that we can compare what we do; and share and learn from others, including other cultures and worlds. This book is a foundation stone for such future endeavors.

With this volume, and with the story of 9/11, there are other powerful themes that shadow response. One is the theme of grief, grief for the multiple losses, the terrible deaths, but also the consequent losses of the sense of invulnerability, trust in safe, controllable worlds. Grief is touched upon for instance in describing Guliano's leadership, symbolized by how he "turned the grief and shock into action and compassion" (this volume, p. 193). It is noted in the risk associated with the loss of a loved one, the loss of social network, place of work, the loss of community, "of a place to collectively mourn" (this volume, p. 343). As suggested in the contribution about the Pentagon, those in the services, and Americans generally, had to prepare for war, and indeed there is the documentation of the many subsequent challenges of the anthrax attacks, wars in Afghanistan and Iraq, terrorist attacks elsewhere, and of course more recently by international and national natural disasters of catastrophic proportions, the Tsunami, Katrina, Pakistan earthquake to name a few. The shadows of grief, the sadness of lost pasts, and future fears reflect changed worlds. That such challenges will be courageously met is attested to by this volume, but is not easy, it is sad, sadness, that is a human grief requiring recognition, comfort, memorialization and commitment to value our loved ones and to make strong compassionate futures for our worlds.

As is so well evidenced by this magnificent work: "to come to terms with catastrophe must reinforce human values of family and society, of love and hope, and of passionate commitment to life, its value, and its preservation" (Raphael, 1986, p. 311).

Beverley Raphael

REFERENCES

Commonwealth of Australia (2000). *Population Mental Health*, ed. B. Raphael. Canberra: AGS.
Raphael, B. (1986). *When Disaster Strikes*, New York: Basic Books.
World Health Organisation (2005). *WHO Assessment Instrument for Mental Health Services – Emergency (draft)*. Geneva: The World Health Organization.

Part I

Introduction

Mental health in the wake of terrorism: making sense of mass casualty trauma

Yuval Neria, Raz Gross and Randall D. Marshall

On the morning of September 11, 2001, with the attacks on the World Trade Center (WTC) and the Pentagon, the world that many of us thought we knew, was altered. While thousands of people were directly exposed to or witnessed the attacks from close proximity, millions around the globe watched the events in real time or repeatedly over time on news channels. The attacks of 9/11 will likely be the most witnessed terrorist acts in modern history.

The events that unfolded on and after 9/11, and the subsequent terrorism around the globe have created a climate of fear and anxiety. These are the psychological outcomes that terrorists seek to inflict. Terror can only be effective if it leaves lingering concerns about safety; if it disrupts the most basic ways citizens manage and control their lives.

The overall goal of this volume is to document and critically examine the comprehensive and wide ranging mental health response after 9/11. Specifically, this volume aims to examine:

(1) Whether the research on the psychological consequences of 9/11 suggest a unique and substantial emotional and behavioral impact among adults and children.

(2) In what way the impact of these attacks exceeded the individual level, affected communities and specific professional groups, and tested different leadership styles.

(3) How professional communities of mental health clinicians, policy makers and researchers were mobilized to respond to the emerging needs post-disaster.

(4) What are the lessons learned from the work conducted after 9/11, and the implications for future disaster mental health work and preparedness efforts.

Contemporary terrorism: a psychological warfare

While early definitions of disasters typically implied a single "event" that affected a single "social group" and was usually limited to a specific point of "time" or "location" (see Quarantelli, 1998; Lopez-Ibor, 2005), the scale of the 9/11 events, occurring simultaneously in two major urban centers, challenges early concepts of disasters. The unfolding series of post-9/11 al-Qaeda assaults (e.g., March 11, 2004 in Madrid; July 7, 2005 in London) has impacted enormous numbers of people sending a clear message that terrorism is primarily psychological warfare rather than conventional military warfare, aimed at causing fear and disarray in large populations.

More than 25 years ago, before suicide terrorism had become a worldwide concern, Mengel (1977) distinguished between terrorism that seeks to discriminate its target selection and terrorism that involves random acts. While the first type of terrorism has a political agenda and uses bargaining to maximize its political power, the second type, rooted in an extreme ideology, aims to create global conflicts, and to maximize the destruction of its "enemy". In the pre-9/11 era terrorist activities targeted mostly narrow and specific objectives, were limited to specific geographical areas (e.g., Israel, Lebanon, Indonesia), and the terrorists benefited from relatively limited media coverage. Contemporary terror campaigns, however, target major metropolitan areas with vast geopolitical and economic significance, threatening large masses, relying on wide media coverage, and benefit from worldwide attention to accomplish their agenda.

9/11 and the following stream of terrorist attacks demonstrate that contemporary terrorism has an extremely effective capacity to impact the psychological and social well-being of citizens in places never before disrupted by security problems. Large urban cities are especially vulnerable to terrorist assaults because they are open, easy to infiltrate, and easy to hit.

More than seven decades ago, Carr (1932) conceptualized a disaster not only as an "event" but rather as the collapse of a community's "cultural protections". Accordingly, large-scale, unanticipated, incidents such as the orchestrated attacks of 9/11, or for that matter any large-scale unpredicted disaster, has the potential to intimidate large communities causing them to doubt whether they are able to effectively defend themselves and to guarantee their own existence.

As previously discussed elsewhere (Neria *et al.*, 2005) a major aim of contemporary terrorism, especially in its suicidal form, is to ignite a worldwide clash between ideological and religious groups: to create a division between "good" and "evil", between "true believers" and "infidels" and to stigmatize people who don't believe in a certain divinity as sinners doomed to be rebuked and eventually exterminated from the earth.

Continuous exposure to this sort of stress might result in a wide range of behavioral changes. In several urban centers around the globe, citizens are voluntarily limiting their actions, avoiding public transportation, changing social habits such as entertainment in crowded spaces. In Jerusalem, for example, many people have developed the so-called "security zones", where they can socialize freely, creating the illusion of security or invulnerability. In other cities (e.g., New York City), citizens are being monitored, their bags checked, and they are being questioned and asked to show identification papers more and more often.

Sadly, these are the calculated consequences of terrorism as warfare (see Levy & Sidel, 2003; Post, 2003; Susser *et al.*, 2002; Yehuda & Hyman, 2005). Terrorism's objective is emotional and behavioral modification of entire populations through widespread dissemination of fear and psychological distress (Velez, 2005). Terrorists accomplish their goals by inducing instability and distress, violating the underpinnings of daily life (Fullerton *et al.*, 2003) and inflicting changes to the ordinary routines of the general population (Holloway & Fullerton, 1994). Although typically, terrorism does not pose existential danger to nations due to its lack of significant military impact, it is effective in attacking the public's morale, reducing trust in democratic processes, and eventually eroding resilience in continuously exposed communities.

Individual and community sequelae of disaster trauma: vulnerability and resilience

Terrorism is often perceived as a "pervasive generator" of psychopathology (Fullerton *et al.*, 2003; p. 4 Holloway *et al.*, 1997; North *et al.*, 1999; North & Pfefferbaum, 2002). However, research on the mental health consequences of terrorism, with the exception of the Oklahoma City bombing (e.g., North *et al.*, 1999; Pfefferbaum, 1999), has been relatively scant.

In the immediate aftermath of a disaster, affiliative, attachment-motivated behaviors such as bonding, caring, and collaborating were suggested to be common among victims and rescue forces (Mawson, 2005; Raphael, 2005). Indeed the extreme experiences of disasters often bring people together with altruistic intent to help victims, directly, or indirectly (e.g., making or raising donations). These types of behaviors may be common in the first and the second post-disaster phases referred to respectively as the "rescue" and the "honeymoon" phases (Raphael, 2005). However, when the hard facts about the toll of the disaster sink in (e.g., scale of loss and destruction), and penetrate the "denial shield" typical to the immediate aftermath of the disaster, a "disillusionment" phase often takes place, and fatigue and bereavement take over.

Previous research has underscored the role that immediate responses to trauma play in the long-term adjustment of the exposed individuals, suggesting that uncontrolled behaviors are powerful predictors of chronic post-traumatic stress disorder (PTSD; e.g., Neria *et al.*, 2000a). Similarly, 9/11 studies have shown that the experience of panic during the attacks is strongly associated with PTSD in people exposed to the WTC attacks (Galea *et al.*, 2002).

The nature and the impact of the immediate response of the public to disasters are yet to be understood and so far the findings are not conclusive (see Mawson,

2005; Raphael, 2005). Early reports on Londoners in the aftermath of the attacks during the summer of 2005 suggest that panic was uncommon in the immediate aftermath of the attacks (Wessley, 2005). However, images of people running from the WTC site during the morning of the 9/11 attacks suggest that many people experienced acute and intense fear and horror. The images recently received from Hurricane Katrina sites (September 2005) similarly suggest intense anger and panic-type responses in neglected neighborhoods, rescue sites and temporary shelters especially among people caught in extreme conditions waiting for rescue and help that are late to come. Dysfunctional behaviors (e.g., people who engaged in aim-less, dissociative and stunned behaviors) have also been observed when disasters strike (Tyhurst, 1951; Weisath, 1989), and it has been suggested that bio-terrorist events may further escalate fears of chemical or biological agents (see Ursano *et al.*, 2004). Differences in the collective, immediate responses in affected populations might be accounted for by specific characteristics of the exposure (e.g., whether the way out of a building is cleared), availability of help, and social support and cultural differences.

Research on the long-term effects of extreme traumatic events has provided use-ful information, enabling disaster clinicians and policy makers to make inferences about risk and vulnerability among affected populations. Traumatic events are common (Kessler *et al.*, 1995) and most of the individuals exposed to trauma effectively cope with such events, even if they experience significant adversities (Bonanno, 2005; Bonanno, *et al.*, 2005; Neria *et al.*, 1998, 2000b). At the same time, disaster research has systematically documented that a significant minority will experience functionally impairing distress, especially in the immediate aftermath; some are likely to manifest behavioral and cognitive changes; and others will develop long-term trauma-related psychiatric disorders such as PTSD, trauma-related depression and substance abuse (e.g., Norris *et al.*, 2002a&b).

The severity of a post-disaster psychopathology is associated with various risk and protective factors including type, intensity and duration of exposure, level of resource loss, social support, sense of community and meaning making (e.g., Norris *et al.*, 2002a). Sociodemographic factors such as previous trauma history, mental health problems, age, gender and education might also play a role in onset and per-sistence of psychiatric symptoms (Brewin *et al.*, 2000). The interaction of human loss and trauma exposure may be particularly powerful in post-traumatic adapta-tion (Neria & Litz, 2004; Neria *et al.*, this volume). At the same time, traumatic experiences may serve as an opportunity for positive growth, an enhanced sense of purpose, and an opportunity to reprioritize everyday life goals. Persons who are able to draw positive appraisals of their adversities were found to grow personally from traumatic experiences, as compared to those who do not, even if they suffer symptoms of PTSD (Dohrenwend *et al.*, 2004).

To date, the effects of large-scale disasters on communities and individuals have been focused almost entirely on natural disasters (Norris *et al.*, 2002a&b). However, when a community is struck by terrorism, the experience is likely to differ from that of a natural disaster. Natural disasters (Kaniasty, this volume; Kaniasty & Norris, 2004; Norris, this volume) are usually limited to time and space, are often expected (e.g., hurricanes) and their pace usually enables some coordination of rescue efforts, sheltering and deployment of medical services. Terrorism, however, usually occurs randomly and unexpectedly with regard to place and time. Accordingly, the psychological impact is likely to be accumulative, wide, non-specific and enduring, affecting how whole communities cope with subsequent threats and demands (Shalev, 2005; Maguen & Litz, this volume).

Indirect exposure and post-disaster psychopathology

The nature of the psychological effect of disasters, especially man made, may exceed the scope of the particular epicenter where the impact occurred (see Schlenger *et al.*, 2002; Galea *et al.*, this volume; Silver *et al.*, this volume). The magnitude of this kind of exposure might not be necessarily limited to the well-documented dose response associations of trauma and effect. The studies presented in this volume provide a rare opportunity to address this topic. For example, while Neria *et al.* in their study of primary care patients exposed to the 9/11 attacks in Northern Manhattan did not find indirect exposure to WTC attacks by itself to be related to PTSD (Neria *et al.*, this volume), other studies conducted in national samples after 9/11 (Schlenger *et al.*, 2002; Silver *et al.*, 2002; Stein *et al.*, 2004; Silver *et al.*, this volume) or in distant population areas after the Oklahoma City bombing (Pfefferbaum *et al.*, 2000) or in Israel after the 1991 Scud missile attacks (Bleich *et al.*, 1992) provide some evidence for probable relationships of indirect exposure and PTSD. These kinds of findings may challenge the core definition of PTSD. They lead to the question whether a person who was not directly exposed to trauma, witnessed it, or lost a loved one, might be traumatized by this type of exposure and would be eligible for a positive Diagnostic and Statistical Manual for Mental Disorders (DSM) Criteria A of PTSD.

Instead of direct exposure to the attacks of 9/11 most of the persons interviewed in post-9/11 national surveys reported indirect exposure (e.g., watching live and retransmitted coverage on TV). The inclusion of this type of exposure is certainly new to the discipline of trauma research and brought experts to doubt its reasoning and validity (e.g., Southwick & Charney, 2002; McNally, 2003; Breslau & McNally, this volume). The events of 9/11, the subsequent wars in Afghanistan and Iraq, and terrorist events in Europe and recent major natural disasters provide a further opportunity to examine whether direct exposure to trauma is a necessary condition for PTSD, or alternatively an interaction between a "sufficient" level of exposure and certain risk factors (e.g., genetic susceptibility) can result in post-exposure psychopathology even via indirect exposure.

Post-disaster outreach and intervention

It was suggested that most of the people exposed to 9/11 attacks did not seek mental health care (e.g., Stein *et al.*, 2004). The degree to what other sorts of care (e.g., from friends, colleagues, employers or clergy), often mentioned in the media, are utilized in the face of disasters is not clear and has never been systematically studied. Indeed, people exposed to traumatic experiences often remain in isolation due to shame and guilt associated with the trauma, stigma associated with treatment of mental health problems, and the social context (Litz, 2004). However, when trauma has occurred in the public domain (e.g., national disasters) and is associated with a public emergency, large and varied groups of professionals are likely to intervene at the disaster sites in attempts to aid affected populations during, immediately or soon after the incident. Most early responders (e.g., firefighters, police officers, medical teams, National Guard, Red Cross) are not qualified or trained to provide mental health care. They are focused on providing for the safety and basic needs of victims and evacuees. However, some first responders may also be required to address the mental health needs of victims, especially in the acute phase when fear and terror are prevalent. It is especially important to address immediate interventions aimed at high-risk groups such as the injured children and the elderly (Litz, 2004). To date little is known about the emotional care, screening or triage conducted in the immediate phase after impact. Schechter and Coates (this volume) provide a rare opportunity to learn about immediate intervention provided to children in the immediate aftermath of the WTC attacks.

Despite emerging evidence that did not provide any support for the effectiveness of psychological debriefing post-exposure (Bisson *et al.*, 1997, 2000; Mayou *et al.*, 2000; Rose *et al.*, 2002), this type of intervention was still common among people involved in 9/11 rescue and recovery efforts (http://edition.cnn.com/2002/US/07/20/wtc.police/?related). Randomized clinical trials conducted in the last decade consistently support the use of cognitive behavioral treatment (CBT) post-exposure (Foa & Cahill, this volume). The differences between these two modalities are substantial. Psychological debriefing was originally conceptualized to be implemented by non-clinicians, immediately but not only after the exposure, consisting of a single and long meeting, and without a clinical evaluation either before or after the intervention. On the other hand, CBT programs are initiated at least 2 weeks after the exposure, implemented only by clinicians, usually consist of 4–12 sessions, and entail a systematic pre- and post-intervention evaluation. While the efficacy and effectiveness of CBT was consistently proven (Foa & Cahill, this volume), debriefing was found to be either not effective in preventing PTSD (Bisson *et al.*, 2000; Rose *et al.*, 2002) or delayed recovery (Bisson *et al.*, 1997; Mayou *et al.*, 2000). Several explanations were suggested to explain the poor performance of debriefing (e.g., for a review see Friedman *et al.*, 2004) such as that debriefing interferes with habituation and cognitive changes that are beneficial for recovery (Foa & Cahill, this volume); that a focus on acute post-traumatic symptoms may foster negative cognitions about oneself and the world (McNally, 2003); and that the timing of the intervention in psychological debriefing is too early and impedes normal remission and normal recovery (Ehlers & Clark, 2003).

The terrorist attacks of 9/11 had an enormous impact on the mobilization of the professional community in the New York area (Marshall *et al.*, this volume; Felton *et al.*, this volume). Large-scale training programs aiming at dissemination of knowledge of trauma treatment were offered to clinicians (Amsel *et al.*, this volume); treatment programs for adults (Katz *et al.*, this volume; Difede *et al.*, this volume; Marshall *et al.*, this volume) and children (Hoven *et al.*, this volume; Murray *et al.*, this volume; Schechter & Coates, this volume) were developed; and statewide out-reach (Draper *et al.*, this volume) and counseling programs (Felton *et al.*, this volume) were rapidly developed and employed.

Drawing quality lessons from horrific experiences such as 9/11 attacks is central to the future work mental health professionals will conduct before (e.g., prepared-ness), during (e.g., management and triage), and after (e.g., long-term care; training and dissemination) the next mass casualty trauma. This volume was created to facilitate this learning process. Clinicians, researchers and policy makers who are involved in this work devote their best intellectual and emotional resources. Effective and meaningful disaster research relies on reliable observations and the ability to update the questions asked, and the tools selected to answer them (Galea *et al.*, this volume). We hope that this volume will contribute to all domains of dis-aster and terrorism-related mental health knowledge.

REFERENCES

Amsel, L.V., Neria, Y., Suh, E.J. & Marshall, R.D. (this volume). Mental health community response to 9/11: training therapists to practice evidence-based psychotherapy. In *9/11: Mental Health in the Wake of Terrorist Attacks*, eds. Y. Neria, R. Gross & R. Marshall. Cambridge, UK: Cambridge University Press.

Bisson, J.I., Jenkins, P.L., Alexander, J. & Bannister, C. (1997). Randomized controlled trial of psychological debriefing for victims of acute burn trauma. *British Journal of Psychiatry*, **777**, 78–81.

Bisson, J.L., McFarlane, A.C. & Rose, S. (2000). Psychological Debriefing. In *Effective Treatments for PTSD: Practice guidelines from the International Society for Traumatic Stress Studies*, pp. 39–59, eds. E.B. Foa, T.M. Keane, & M.J. Friedman. New York, NY: Guilford.

Bleich, A., Dycian, A., Koslowsky, M., Solomon, Z. & Wiener, M. (1992). Psychiatric implications of missile attacks on a civilian population. Israeli lessons from the Persian Gulf War. *Journal of the American Medical Association*, **268**(5), 613–615.

Bonanno, G. (2005). Loss, trauma, and human resilience – have we underestimated the human capacity to thrive after extremely aversive events? *American Psychologist*, **59**, 20–28.

Bonanno, A.G., Rennicke, C. & Dekel, S. (2005). Self enhancement among high exposure survivors of the September 11th terrorist attack: resilience or social maladjustment? *Journal of Personality and Social Psychology*, **88**, 984–998.

Breslau, N. & McNally, R. (this volume). The epidemiology of 9/11: technical advances and conceptual conundrums. In *9/11: Mental Health in the Wake of Terrorist Attacks*, eds. Y. Neria, R. Gross & R.D. Marshall. Cambridge, UK: Cambridge University Press.

Brewin, C.R., Andrews, B. & Valentine, J.D. (2000). Meta-analysis of risk factors for posttraumatic stress disorder in trauma-exposed adults. *Journal of Consulting and Clinical Psychology*, **68**(5), 748–766.

Carr, L. (1932). Disasters and the sequence-pattern concept of social change. *American Journal of Sociology*, **38**, 207–218.

Difede, J., Roberts, J., Jaysinghe, N. & Leck, P. (this volume). Evaluation and treatment of firefighters and utility workers following the World Trade Center attacks. In *9/11: Mental Health in the Wake of Terrorist Attacks*, eds. Y. Neria, R. Gross & R.D. Marshall. Cambridge, UK: Cambridge University Press.

Dohrenwend, B.P., Neria, Y., Turner, J.B., Turse, N., Marshall, R.D., Lewis-Fernandez, R. & Koenen, K.C. (2004). Positive tertiary appraisals and posttraumatic stress disorder in U.S. male veterans of the war in Vietnam: the roles of positive affirmation, positive reformulation, and defensive denial. *Journal of Consulting and Clinical Psychology*, **72**(3), 417–433.

Draper, J., McCleery, G. & Schaedle, R. (this volume). Mental health services support in response to September 11th: the central role of the Mental Health Association of New York City. In *9/11: Mental Health in the Wake of Terrorist Attacks*, eds. Y. Neria, R. Gross & R.D. Marshall. Cambridge, UK: Cambridge University Press.

Foa, E.B. & Cahill, S.P. (this volume). Psychological treatments for PTSD: an overview. In *9/11: Mental Health in the Wake of Terrorist Attacks*, eds. Y. Neria, R. Gross & R.D. Marshall. Cambridge, UK: Cambridge University Press.

Friedman, M.J., Hamblen, J.L, Foa, E.B. & Charney, D.S. (2004). Commentary on "A National Longitudinal Study of the Psychological Consequences of the September 11, 2001, Terrorist Attacks: Reactions, Impairment, and Help-Seeking"; Fighting the Psychological War on Terrorism. *Psyciatry*, **67**(2), 123–137.

Fullerton, C.S., Ursano, R.J. & Norwood, A.E. (2003). Planning for the psychological effects of bioterrorism. In *Bioterrorism: Psychological and Public Health Interventions*, eds. R.J. Ursano, C.S. Fullerton & A.E. Norwood. London, UK: Cambridge University Press.

Galea, S. (this volume). Mental health research in the aftermath of disasters: using the right methods to ask the right questions. In *9/11: Mental Health in the wake of Terrorist Attacks*, eds. Y. Neria, R. Gross, & R.D. Marshall. Cambridge, UK: Cambridge University Press.

Galea, S., Ahern, J., Resnick, H., Kilpatrick, D., Bucuvalas, M., Gold, J. & Vlahov, D. (2002). Psychological sequelae of the September 11 attacks in Manhattan, New York City. *New England Journal of Medicine*, **346**, 982–987.

Ginzburg, K., Solomon, Z., Dekel, R. & Neria, Y. (2003). Battlefield functioning and chronic PTSD: associations with perceived self-efficacy and causal attribution. *Personality and Individual Differences*, **34**, 463–476.

Holloway, H.C. & Fullerton, C.S. (1994). The psychology of terror and its aftermath. In *Individual and Community Responses to Trauma and Disaster: The Structure of Human Chaos*, eds. R.J. Ursano, B.G. McCaughey & C.S. Fullerton. New York: Cambridge University Press, pp. 31–45.

Holloway, H.C., Norwood, A.E., Fullerton, C.S., Engel, C.C. & Ursano, R.J. (1997). The threat of biological weapons: prophylaxis and mitigation of psychological and social consequences. *Journal of the American Medical Association*, **278**(5), 425–427.

Hoven, C.S., Mandell, D.J., Duarte, C.S., Wu, P. & Giordano, V. (this volume). An epidemiological response to disaster: the New York City Board of Education's Post 9/11 Needs Assessment. In *9/11: Mental Health in the Wake of Terrorist Attacks*, eds. Y. Neria, R. Gross & R.D. Marshall. Cambridge, UK: Cambridge University Press.

Kaniasty, K. & Norris, F.H. (2004). Social support in the aftermath of disasters, catastrophes, and acts of terrorism: altruistic, overwhelmed, uncertain, antagonistic, and patriotic communities. In *Bioterrorism: Psychological and Public Health Interventions*, eds. R. Ursano, A. Norwood & C. Fullerton. Cambridge, UK: Cambridge University Press.

Katz, C.L., Smith, R., Herbert, R., Levin, S. & Gross, R. (this volume). The World Trade Center Worker/Volunteer Mental Health Screening Program. In *9/11: Mental Health in the Wake of Terrorist Attacks*, eds. Y. Neria, R. Gross & R.D. Marshall. Cambridge, UK: Cambridge University Press.

Kessler, R.C., Sonnega, A., Bromet, E., Hughes, M., & Nelson, C.B. (1995). Posttraumatic stress disorder in the National Comorbidity Survey. *Archives of General Psychiatry*, **52**(12), 1048–1060.

Levy, B.S. & Sidel, V.W. (2003). *Terrorism and Public Health*, eds. B.S. Levy & V.W. Sidel. New York: Oxford University Press.

Litz, B.T. (2004). *Early Intervention for Trauma and Traumatic Loss*, ed. B.T. Litz. New York: Guilford Publications.

Lopez-Ibor, J. (2005). What is a disaster? In *Disasters and Mental Health*, ed. J. Lopez-Ibor, New York: Willey.

Maguen, S. & Litz, B. (this volume). Coping with the threat of terrorism. In *9/11: Mental Health in the Wake of Terrorist Attacks*, eds. Y. Neria, R.Gross & R.D. Marshall. Cambridge, UK: Cambridge University Press.

Marshall, R.D., Neria, Y., Suh, E.J., Amsel, L.V., Kastan, J., Eth, S., Davis, L., Cloitre, M., Schwarzbaum, G., Yehuda, R. & Rosenthal, J. (this volume) The New York Consortium for Effective Trauma Treatment. In 9/11: Mental Health in the Wake of Terrorist Attacks, eds. Y. Neria, R. Gross, R.D. Marshall. Cambridge, UK: Cambridge University Press.

Mawson, R.A. (2005). Understanding mass panic and other collective responses to threat and disaster. *Psychiatry*, **68**(2), 95–113.

Mayou, R.A., Ehlers, A. & Hobbs, M. (2000). A three-year follow-up of psychological debriefing for road traffic accident victims. *British Journal of Psychiatry*, **176**, 589–593.

McNally, R.J. (2003). *Remembering Trauma*. Cambridge, MA: Belknap Press of Harvard University Press.

Mengel, R.W. (1977). Terrorism and new technologies of destruction. An overview of the potential risk. In *Disorder and Terrorism: Report of the Task Force on Disorders and Terrorism*, US National Advisory Committee on Criminal Justice Standards and Goals. Washington, DC: US Government Printing Office, pp. 443–473.

Murray, L., Rodriguez, J., Hoagwood, K. & Jensen, P. (this volume). Child and adolescent trauma treatments and services after September 11: implementing evidence-based practices into complex child services systems. In *9/11: Mental Health in the Wake of Terrorist Attacks*, eds. Y. Neria, R. Gross & R.D. Marshall. Cambridge, UK: Cambridge University Press.

Neria, Y. & Litz, B.T. (2004). Bereavement by traumatic means: the complex synergy of trauma and grief. *Journal of Loss and Trauma*, **9**, 73–87.

Neria, Y. Soloman, R. & Dekel, R. (1998). Eighteen-year follow up of Israeli prisoners of war and combat veterans. *The Journal of Nervous and Mental Disease*, **186**, 174–182.

Neria, Y., Solomon, R. & Dekel, R. (2000a). Adjustment to the stress of war captivity: the role of sociodemographic background, trauma severity and coping in prison in the long-term mental health of Israeli ex-POWs. *Anxiety, Stress, and Coping*, **13**, 229–246.

Neria Y., Solomon, Z., Ginzburg, K., Dekel, R., Enoch, D. & Ohry, A. (2000b). Posttraumatic residues of captivity: a follow-up of Israeli ex-prisoners of war. *Journal of Clinical Psychiatry*, **61**(1), 39–46.

Neria, Y., Roe, D., Beit-Hallahmi, B., Mneimneh, H., Balaban, A. & Marshall, R.D. (2005). The Al Qaeda 9/11 instructions: a study in the construction of religious martyrdom. *Religion*, **35/1**, 1–11.

Neria, Y., Gross, R., Olfson, M., Gameroff, M.J., Das, A., Feder, A., Lantigua, R., Shea, S. & Weissman, M.M. (this volume). Screening for PTSD in low-income, predominantly Hispanic, primary care patients in New York City one year after 9/11 attacks. In *9/11: Mental Health in the Wake of Terrorist Attacks*, eds. Y. Neria, R. Gross & R.D. Marshall. Cambridge, UK: Cambridge University Press.

Norris, F.H., Friedman, M.J., Watson, P.J., Byrne, C.M., Diaz, E. & Kaniasty, K.Z. (2002a). 60,000 disaster victims speak: Part I: An empirical review of the empirical literature, 1981–2001. *Psychiatry*, **65**, 207–239.

Norris, F.H., Friedman, M.J. & Watson, P.J. (2002b). 60,000 disaster victims speak: Part II: Summary and implications of the disaster mental health research. *Psychiatry*, **65**, 240–260.

North, C.S. & Pfefferbaum, B. (2002). Research on the mental health effects of terrorism. *Journal of the American Medical Association*, **288**, 633–636.

North, C.S., Nixon, S.J., Shariat, S., Mallonee, S., McMillen, J.C., Spitznagel, E.L. & Smith, E.M. (1999). Psychiatric disorders among survivors of the Oklahoma City bombing. *Journal of the American Medical Association*, **282**(8), 755–762.

North, C.S., Tivis, L., McMillen, J.C., Pfefferbaum, B., Cox, J., Spitznagel, E.L., Bunch, K., Schorr, J. & Smith, E.M. (2002). Coping, functioning, and adjustment of rescue workers after the Oklahoma City bombing. *Journal of Traumatic Stress*, **15**(3), 171–175.

Pfefferbaum, B. (1999). Posttraumatic stress responses in bereaved children after the Oklahoma City bombing. *Journal of American Academy of Child and Adolescent Psychiatry*, **38**, 1372–1379.

Pfefferbaum, B., Seale, T.W., McDonald, N.B., Brandt, E.N., Rainwater, S.M., Maynard, B.T., Meierhoefer, B. & Miller, P.D. (2000). Posttraumatic stress two years after the Oklahoma City bombing in youths geographically distant from the explosion. Phychiatry, **634**, 358–370.

Post, J.M. (2003). Prospects for chemical/biological terrorism: psychological incentives and constraints. In *Bioterrorism: Psychological and Public Health Interventions*, eds. R.J. Ursano, C.S. Fullerton & A.E. Norwood. London, UK: Cambridge University Press.

Quarantelli, E.L. (ed.) (1998). *What is a Disaster: Perspectives on the Question*. London/New York: Routledge.

Raphael, B. (2005). Crowds and other collectives: complexities of human behaviors in mass emergencies. *Psychiatry*, **68**, 2.

Rose, S., Bisson, J. & Wessely, S. (2002). Psychological Debriefing for Preventing Posttraumatic Stress Disorder (PTSD) (Cochrane review). In *The Cochrane Library*, Issue 2, Oxford, UK: Update Software.

Schechter, D. & Coates, S.W. (this volume). Relationally and developmentally focused interventions with young children and their caregivers in the wake of terrorism and other violent experiences. In *9/11: Mental Health in the Wake of Terrorist Attacks*, eds. Y. Neria, R. Gross & R.D. Marshall. Cambridge, UK: Cambridge University Press.

Schlenger, W.E., Caddell, J.M., Ebert, L., Jordan, B.K.M., Wilson, D., Thalji, L., Dennis, J.M., Fairbank, J.A. & Kulka, R.A. (2002). Psychological reactions to terrorist attacks: findings from the National Study of Americans' Reactions to September 11. *Journal of the American Medical Association*, **288**, 581–588.

Shalev, A. (2005). The Israeli experience of continuous terrorism (2000–2004). In *Disasters and Mental Health*, eds. J.J. Lopez-Ibor, G. Christodoulou, M. Maj, N. Sartorius & A. Okasha. New York: Willey.

Silver, R.C., Holman, E.A., McIntosh, D.M., Poulin, M. & Gil-Rivas, V. (2002). Nationwide longitudinal study of psychological responses to September 11. *Journal of the American Medical Association*, **288**, 1235–1244.

Silver, R.C., Holman, E.A., McIntosh, D.N., Poulin, M., Gil-Rivas, V. & Pizarro, J. (this volume). Coping with a national trauma: a nationwide longitudinal study of responses to the terrorist attacks of September 11th. In *9/11: Mental Health in the Wake of Terrorist Attacks*, eds. Y. Neria, R. Gross & R.D. Marshall. Cambridge, UK: Cambridge University Press.

Southwick, S. & Charney, D.S. (2002). Response to trauma: normal reactions or pathological symptoms. *Psychiatry*, **67**(2), 170–173.

Stein, B.D., Elliott, M.N., Jaycox, L.H., Collins, R., Berry, S., Klein, D.J. & Shuster, M.A. (2004). A national longitudinal study of the psychological consequences of the September 11, 2001, terrorist attacks: reactions, impairment, and help seeking. *Psychiatry*, **67**(92), 105–117.

Susser, S.E., Herman, D.B. & Aaron, B. (2002). Combating the terror of terrorism. *Scientific American*, **287**(2), 70–77.

Tyhurst, J.S. (1951). Individual reactions to community disaster. *American Journal of Psychiatry*, **107**, 764–769.

Ursano, R.J., Fullerton, C.S. & Norwood, A.E. (eds.) (2004). *Bioterrorism: Psychological and Public Health Interventions*. London, UK: Cambridge University Press.

Velez, T. (2005). Personal communication to Yuval Neria.

Weisath, L. (1989). A study of behavioral responses to an industrial disaster. *Acta Psychiatrica Scandinavica Supplementum*, **355**(80), 13–24.

Wessley, S. (2005). The London attacks aftermath: victimhood and resilience. *New England Journal of Medicine*, **353**, 6.

Yehuda, R. & Hyman, S.E. (2005). The impact of terrorism on brain, and behavior: what we know and what we need to know. *Neuropsychopharmacology*, **30**, 1773–1780.

Part II

The psychological aftermath of 9/11

Preface

Ezra S. Susser, Yuval Neria, Raz Gross and Randall D. Marshall

The visibility and the political import of the collapse of the World Trade Center Towers made it an extraordinary event even in a world replete with disasters and wars. These massive buildings symbolized the financial center of the world. Their dramatic collapse was witnessed directly by millions of people in New York City, and indirectly on television by countless others around the globe. Thousands died, tens of thousands narrowly escaped death, and the effects rippled across communities of a wide region.

The chapters in this part of the book are concerned with the way in which this event affected the mental health of people in New York City and elsewhere in the USA. The authors of three key studies of the mental health effects describe the way in which their research was conceived and executed, and some of their most striking results. Leading psychiatric epidemiologists were invited to critique these studies, and comment more generally on the nature of research on mental health effects of disasters. In addition, one of the study authors was invited to respond to the critiques. We are indebted to all of the authors for their contributions.

By design, therefore, the chapters present divergent viewpoints about the nature and the magnitude of the mental health effects of September 11th. This approach results in a lively exchange, and enables readers to appreciate the ongoing debate and form their own opinions about it. But readers also have a right to know what the editors perceive to be the main lessons of this work. We will highlight five which have clear implications for future studies of the mental health effects of large scale terrorist attacks and other disasters.

First, the mental health impact could not be captured only in the effects on the "direct" victims who were present at the scene. The event precipitated symptoms of mental disorder in large numbers of adults and children in New York who were very far from the buildings themselves. Indeed, some psychological symptoms were reported by people across the entire USA.

Second, the mental health impact on this broader population could not be captured only in the occurrence of post-traumatic stress disorder. The mental health effects extended over a fairly wide range, including not only post-traumatic stress disorder, but also symptoms of depression, panic, substance use, agoraphobia in children, and probably medically unexplained symptoms. Not all of these manifestations should be considered as psychopathology, but some of them might be.

Third, the impact was dependent on the social context as well as the experience of the event *per se*. For example, the effects were substantially greater for those who lost jobs. The social context tends to receive too little attention, and therefore, we dedicate a full part of this book to it (Part III). Social tensions across groups might have been important, as well as social ties within groups. One might imagine that the effects of September 11 were greater in communities that suffered discrimination and stigma in its aftermath, notably Muslim communities, but we have no data to bear on this point.

Fourth, advance preparation is required for rigorous studies of the effects of disasters. The preparation should extend to studies of interventions to promote resilience. Some of the interventions we have been using to support individuals in the immediate aftermath of a disaster, such as psychological debriefing, do not appear to work. Nor can we say with any surety what kind of political leadership or other actions make a whole community more resilient in the aftermath. We need to find out, and the only way to do so is to be ready at the time of the disaster, with an intervention and a research design to test it. This should be an integral part of disaster preparedness, and requires substantial organization beforehand, including collaborative arrangements among service providers and researchers, procedures for expediting ethical reviews, and carefully developed guidelines for conducting evaluations that balance feasibility with scientific rigor.

Finally, we need to strike a balance between a local and a global view of this event. It is never appropriate to be dismissive of human suffering on the grounds that there is greater suffering elsewhere. The tragedy of September 11 stands as a watershed event in the history of New York City and merits the attention it has received. At the same time, it is important for us to keep in mind that even the thousands of deaths and the massive destruction of September 11 pale in comparison to disasters that occur every year in other parts of the globe. Our response should be to heighten our awareness of these events and their effects on other peoples, and to look for ways to prevent their occurrence, as well as to mitigate their impact in the aftermath.

3

Post-traumatic stress symptoms in the general population after a disaster: implications for public health

Sandro Galea, Jennifer Ahern, Heidi Resnick and David Vlahov

Introduction

Post-traumatic stress after disasters and after September 11, 2001

Major disasters are associated with increased rates of psychological distress and morbidity among survivors (Norris et al., 2002a, b; Galea et al., 2005). The vast majority of post-disaster research has focused on the groups that are typically considered to be most affected by disasters and a substantial literature has documented the burden of psychopathology faced by survivors of disasters (North et al., 1999; Salcioglu et al., 2003) persons who are involved in the post-disaster recovery efforts (North et al., 2002), and family and friends of persons who are killed or seriously injured in disasters (Stoppelbein & Greening, 2000). Post-traumatic stress disorder (PTSD) is the most commonly studied, and likely the most prevalent mental health problem in these groups after disasters (Green & Lindy, 1994; Galea et al., 2005), although other mental health problems including depression (Kuo et al., 2003), generalized anxiety disorder (Smith et al., 1990), and non-specific psychological stress (Carr et al., 1997) have been studied.

In the aftermath of the September 11 attacks there was every reason to believe that the impact of the attacks among the survivors of the attacks would be comparable to that among survivors of other major disasters. For example, in the aftermath of the bombing of the Murrah Federal Building in Oklahoma City, North and colleagues reported that 34.3% of adult survivors of the bombing who were either in the building at the time of the bombing or in close proximity had symptoms consistent with a diagnosis of PTSD in the first 6 months after the bombing (North et al., 1999). Official estimates of the number of persons who were survivors of the September 11 attacks vary. A report commissioned by the New York City (NYC) Mayor's Office and conducted by a private consulting company estimated that there were 9–12,000 family members of the deceased, up to 3000 persons injured by the attacks and 12,000 residents of the immediate area around the World Trade

Center (WTC) (south of Canal Street) (NYC Fire Department, 2002). Although this was a larger number of survivors (who are traditionally both the subject of research and the focus of much of the public health attention in the aftermath of disasters) than after most other previous US disasters, this number represented a very small proportion of the total residents of the NYC metropolitan area.

A number of factors also suggested that the September 11, 2001, terrorist attacks would have substantial mental health consequences in the NYC metropolitan area that extended beyond those direct victims of the attacks. The NYC metropolitan area is the largest and the most densely populated metropolitan areas in the US (Bureau of the Census, 2000). Although estimates of population size vary, depending on the areas selected as boundaries of the metropolitan area, approximately 15 million people live in the vicinity of NYC in the tri-state area of New York State, New Jersey, and Connecticut. The attacks on the WTC were perceived as an attack on the US (Kennedy, 2001). During the day of September 11, "fog of war" rumors had many in the NYC metropolitan area afraid for their lives. Early rumors of more planes being hijacked and aimed for other NYC and national targets were rife. As round-the-clock, real-time television coverage of the attacks saturated the airwaves, millions in the area saw images of people waving for help from the towers of the WTC, and subsequently saw the towers fall. Meanwhile, countless residents of the tri-state area knew someone or were related to someone who was working in the WTC. Disrupted communications systems meant that many were uncertain about the fate of family or friends for most of the day of September 11 and, in many cases, for days after.

Therefore, in the aftermath of September 11, we developed a study to assess the potential mental health consequences of the September 11 attacks in the general population of the NYC metropolitan area (Galea *et al.*, 2002a). Underlying this work was the premise that all residents of the NYC metropolitan area were potentially exposed to the September 11 attacks, and could plausibly develop post-traumatic stress symptoms related to the attacks. There were three key research questions guiding this work. First, it was considered of paramount importance to determine the burden of post-traumatic stress in the general population a month after the September 11 attacks; this could both contribute to public mental health planning and also add new insight to the literature where there were no peer-reviewed papers documenting the early prevalence of PTSD in the general population. Second, it was considered equally important to document the course of PTSD in the general population in the months after September 11. Third, we wanted to identify specific groups that were at high risk of post-traumatic stress symptoms in the general population after the terrorist attacks and who would, as such, benefit from targeted public mental health interventions. This research group conducted a number of studies to address these questions in NYC metropolitan area. We discuss here the rationale behind the studies conducted and the study design chosen, evidence about post-traumatic stress in the general population in the first 6 months after September 11, and the implications of this work for public health planning after major disasters in densely populated urban areas.

Study history and motivation

In the immediate aftermath of the attacks, there was a rapid mobilization of health care personnel in NYC to provide care to those injured and affected by the attacks. Mental health clinicians began assisting families of the deceased and rescue personnel who were working at the disaster site and, eventually, to residents of NYC at large. In concert with the provision of mental health services there was also clear need for assessments that could determine the scope of mental health need both among persons who were directly affected by the terrorist attacks as well as in the general population at large. In that context, The New York State Psychiatric Institute (NYSPI) began working with the Substance Abuse and Mental Health Services Administration (SAMHSA) to prepare a mental health needs assessment that could be used as part of an application for Federal Emergency Management Agency (FEMA) funding for mental health services (Herman *et al.*, 2002). In its early stages the assessment began to draw on published research. However, although previous research provided estimates of the prevalence of post-disaster mental health problems, published data had limited applicability to the NYC context. The studies that had been carried out provided estimates of the prevalence of mental health problems in the general population ranging from 2.0% to 18.3% (Hanson *et al.*, 1995, Carr *et al.*, 1997). Thus, it became clear that a primary role for public health researchers in NYC would be to characterize the mental health consequences of the attacks in NYC, both among those directly affected by the attacks, and in the NYC population at large.

The Center for Urban Epidemiologic Studies (CUES), the institution primarily responsible for the research discussed here, is a division of the New York Academy of Medicine (NYAM). CUES is a research institute comprised of epidemiologists and physicians with an interest in the health of urban populations. CUES research is funded by the Centers for Disease Control and Prevention, the National Institutes of Health (NIH), and by private foundations. CUES was explicitly founded as an unaffiliated center that could work through collaborations with other academics in NYC and throughout the country. Throughout its history CUES had worked collaboratively with a number of universities in NYC and in other parts of the country. Also, prior to September 11, the epidemiology of emergent conditions, including the epidemiology of mental health after severe trauma was one of the research interests at CUES. As such, investigators at CUES had both an *a priori* interest in the questions that were rapidly emerging in the aftermath of the attacks and were well positioned to develop a project which would require the collaboration of researchers and practitioners at multiple institutions. Approximately a week after September 11, in consultation with the New York Department of Health and Mental Hygiene (NYDOHMH), NYSPI, and SAMSHA, CUES investigators started work on designing, and implementing, research that could estimate the prevalence of mental health problems in the general population and identify groups who were particularly at risk of psychopathology and who could benefit from acute mental health intervention.

In deciding to develop an assessment to document the mental health consequences of the September 11 attacks in the NYC population at large, CUES investigators sought to collaborate with other investigators and institutions with specific experience in post-disaster research. The National Crime Victims Research and Treatment Center (NCVC) is a division of the Department of Psychiatry and Behavioral Sciences at the Medical University of South Carolina in Charleston, South Carolina. The primary focus of NCVC investigators is to understand the impact of violence on adults, children, and their families. In more recent years, NCVC research efforts have expanded to include an examination of the mental health impact of natural disasters and urban violence. NCVC studies have been sponsored by agencies and organizations such as the NIH and the National Institute of Justice. NCVC researchers are often involved in providing consultation to other researchers and agencies interested in pursuing work related to the psychological consequences of severe trauma and disasters.

One of the major projects carried out by NCVC was the National Women's Study (NWS), a large epidemiological research project that involved the assessment of national household probability samples of adult women about a variety of topics including history of traumatic events, PTSD, and major depression (Resnick *et al.*, 1993; Kilpatrick *et al.*, 1997). These assessments happened via telephone over a 3-year period between 1989 and 1993. As part of this project, NCVC researchers had developed and validated modified diagnostic measures for PTSD and depression that were particularly relevant to the work that CUES investigators were considering in NYC. The NWS PTSD module probably represents the most widely used telephone instrument for lay-assessment of PTSD that is currently extant and as such lent itself particularly well to the planned assessment of the burden of psychopathology in the general population that was being planned by investigators at CUES.

In addition to looking for content expertise in a collaboration with NCVC, CUES investigators also sought to collaborate with an institution with expertise, and a track record in rapid implementation of population representative surveys. CUES had previously collaborated with Schulman, Ronca, & Bucuvalas Inc. (SRBI), a global research firm based in NYC, in conducting the Harlem Social Environment Study (Galea *et al.*, 2001). SRBI specializes in public policy and opinion surveys, health care, and communications and has a long track record collaborating with academic institutions. Coincidentally, SRBI also had been responsible for implementing the NWS in collaboration with NCVC investigators making a CUES–NCVC–SRBI collaboration natural to guide the planned research. Ultimately, all three parties involved in organizing this research were committed to its rapid and rigorous execution. CUES' status as an unaffiliated small institution, relatively unencumbered by much of the bureaucracy that is often endemic in larger institutions and with a history of carrying out rapid epidemiological studies was a catalyst for moving quickly on implementing the post-September 11 research described here. NCVC and SRBI both understood the importance of implementing research rapidly and the three teams worked around the clock in the first few weeks after September 11 to implement the first phases of this research.

Choosing a research design

There were several considerations that guided the choice of research design at project inception. Principal among these was the necessity for a rapid assessment that could contribute data to the ongoing NYSPI and SAMSHA mental health needs assessment. Recognizing that the extant literature that had studied the prevalence of PTSD in the general population provided a broad range of possible estimates, and that previous studies had been conducted at least 6 months after disasters, implementing an intervention that could assess the burden of post-traumatic stress in the general population 1 month after the September 11 attacks was considered of paramount importance. Two principal study designs and three primary sampling methods were considered.

The first decision that had to be made was the specific study design to be employed. Given our interest in documenting both the baseline burden and the course of post-traumatic stress in the general population, we first sought to implement a prospective cohort study whereby participants could be recruited 1 month after the September 11 attacks and subsequently followed up over the coming years. However, there were two factors that precluded the implementation of a cohort study in this context. The first limitation was one of human subjects protection. In the aftermath of September 11, given the widespread consequences of the attacks throughout NYC, coordination of committee meetings and space for quiet discussion were difficult to come by. In consultation with the Institutional Review Board (IRB) at NYAM, it was apparent that it would not be feasible to fully review a cohort study and the necessary attendant human subjects precautions in the month after the attacks. As such, it was decided that the first wave of this research should be anonymous; that is, that no identifying data would be collected about any respondent enrolled in the study. With this decision in place, NYAM IRB provided expedited approval of the study protocols on October 2, 2001. This precluded longitudinal follow-up of respondents or collection of any potentially identifying data such as addresses (the intersection closest to respondents' residence was instead collected as a means of determining distance from the WTC site). We then opted to implement a serial cross-sectional study design in order to permit assessment of the course of post-traumatic stress symptoms after the September 11 attacks while obtaining only anonymous data. The serial cross-sectional study implemented was designed to mimic a natural history study, whereby persons recruited in each subsequent cross-section were persons who were living in NYC on September 11, 2001, and as such persons who would have been eligible for each of the survey waves. The second factor that precluded the implementation of a cohort study was financial. Although, as described below, funding was eventually obtained to permit the implementation of three cross-sectional surveys, at the time these studies were being designed there was no assurance of funding availability nor that funds would become available in time to implement what was recognized to be a time sensitive project. As such, a serial cross-sectional design that could add survey waves as funding became available was considered optimal and was the eventual study design implemented.

With respect to sampling method to implement in this study design, the investigators first considered the possibility of carrying out in-person interviews. However, in the first weeks after the disaster, security measures throughout NYC prevented movement south of 14th Street (the area closest to the WTC) making door-to-door contact with an important portion of NYC residents difficult. In addition, experience at SRBI suggests that door-to-door interviews in NYC is particularly difficult given the high prevalence of high rises with doormen preventing access to a random sampling of households. Second, was the possibility of carrying out a phone survey with a complex, stratified, phone sampling technique that would selectively over-sample persons who were directly affected by the event (e.g., families of victims, persons who were in the WTC during the attacks) for comparison with the general population. This option was considered not feasible due to the cost that would be associated with screening for these subgroups specifically. Although the September 11 attacks affected a large number of persons, screening for those directly affected in NYC at large would require an estimated 50 screening interviews for every target person interviewed making the cost associated with such a project prohibitive. The third option and the option eventually chosen by the research group, was a simple area probability random digit dial (RDD) survey of residents of NYC. This option was considered feasible, and would provide the research team with estimates of mental health problems in the general NYC population that could guide the ongoing needs assessment.

There were a number of reasons why it was considered optimal to carry out RDD telephone survey sampling in this context. First, telephone survey methods have been shown to be an efficient method for collecting information from large representative samples of respondents at a relatively low cost with non-significant response bias or detection of critical variables of interest as compared to in-person interview approaches (Weeks *et al.*, 1983; Simon *et al.*, 1993). In addition, studies suggest that telephone assessments of psychiatric conditions produce results that are comparable to those obtained through in-person assessments. For example, one study compared telephone and in-person assessment of *Diagnostic and Statistical Manual for Mental Disorders, Third Edition* (DSM-III) Axis I disorders, including anxiety disorders, affective disorders, alcoholism, and no mental disorder using a structured diagnostic interview. Kappas ranging from 0.69 to 0.84 were obtained, even with a delay between in-person and telephone methods of 12–19 months (Paulsen *et al.*, 1988). RDD telephone survey method has been gaining in importance in public health research and surveillance in the past decade and is currently used routinely in important national projects such as the Centers for Disease Control Behavioral Risk Factor Surveillance System (BRFSS) which assesses risk behaviors within the adult population.

In addition to these decisions about study design and sampling methodology, other decisions had to be made about sampling area, languages to use in the surveying, and several other design details that would ultimately have bearing on the final results documented. Although there was a strong interest in carrying out the initial assessment of all of NYC and in a variety of languages, uncertainty about funding that would be available for this project suggested that a more limited sampling frame would have to be selected at least for the first stages of the project. After some discussion it was decided that the first survey wave would sample residents of Manhattan living south of 110th Street for three primary reasons. First, this was the area of Manhattan closest to the WTC site of the September 11 attacks. Second, given finite resources, a broader geographic focus would have diluted the representation of those directly affected. Third, a substantial proportion of residents of Manhattan's Upper West and Upper East sides worked in southern Manhattan and were thus more likely to witness the attacks or to be affected directly (through loss of relatives or colleagues) or indirectly (through loss of employment) by the attacks. Time considerations limited this first assessment to English and Spanish. The survey was translated and back translated into Spanish and surveying was carried out in English and Spanish using bilingual interviewers. Funding for both the first assessment and for subsequent surveying became available about a week before the first assessment started. As such, subsequent surveys were conducted in all of NYC and in the NYC metropolitan and included other languages in the assessments.

Funding

One of the primary difficulties faced by the research group in carrying out this work was obtaining funding, or assurance of funding, to carry out this research. Although early on all the investigators were donating their time to the project in-kind, financial resources were needed to fund the data collection. It was clear early on that if the assessment was to be implemented early after September 11, preparations for the research would have to be made in the absence of assurances of funding. In the early weeks after the September 11 attacks, several NYC foundations were formed with the explicit intent of funding post-September 11 relief efforts. However, the vast majority of these resources were earmarked for clinical relief services. In the weeks after September 11, the investigative team approached private foundations and federal funding agencies for resources to carry out the assessment. Although the majority of the requests were unsuccessful, assurances of funding eventually were obtained from the National Institute on Drug Abuse (in the form of an administrative supplement to an ongoing research project) and from The New York Community Trust/United Way Consortium that had been formed to administer donations received for post-September 11 work. Assurances of funding were received about a week before the start of data collection. Eventually funding was also obtained from the National Institute on Mental Health that permitted the subsequent survey waves.

Methods

Sample

Overall, three serial cross-sectional RDD household surveys were conducted. The first survey ($n = 988$) was conducted between October 16 and November 15, 2001, the second survey ($n = 2001$) was between January 15 and February 21, 2002, and the third survey ($n = 2752$) was between March 25 and June 25, 2002. The sampling frame for survey 1 included adult residents (18 years of age or older) of Manhattan living south of 110th Street. The sampling frame for survey 2 included all adults in NYC with an over-sampling of residents of Manhattan living south of 110th Street to permit comparison between surveys. The sampling frame for survey three included all adults in the NYC metropolitan area with over-sampling of residents of Manhattan south of 110th Street and of NYC to permit comparison among surveys. Further detail about these surveys is available in other work published by the authors (Galea *et al.*, 2002a, b, c; Galea *et al.*, 2003; Vlahov *et al.*, 2002; Vlahov *et al.*, 2004). Here, we present results from survey 3. The sampling frame for this survey included all adults in the following contiguous geographic areas: NYC and Nassau, Westchester, Suffolk, and Rockland counties in New York State, Hudson, Essex, Bergen, Passaic, Union, Middlesex, Monmouth, Morris, and Somerset counties in New Jersey, and Lower Fairfield county in Connecticut. The counties in New York State, New Jersey, and Connecticut chosen were those closest to the WTC site of the attacks and with a high proportion of residents who commuted to NYC. The adult population of this region was 15,802,925 in the 2000 US Census (Bureau of the Census, 2000). The sampling frame was divided into four zones, radiating concentrically from the WTC sites with over-sampling of the zones closest to the site. All interviews were conducted by trained interviewers using a computer-assisted telephone interview system. Interviews were conducted in English, Spanish, and Chinese. Native English, Spanish, Mandarin, and Cantonese speakers administered the interviews (using translated questionnaires) in their respective languages. Surveys were approximately 35 minutes long and the measures used were consistent between surveys to allow for comparison. The overall cooperation rate was 56% and the response rate was 34%. Sampling weights were developed and applied to our data to account for the number of household telephones, persons in the household, and over-sampling. Further discussions of the methods and results from these surveys can also be found elsewhere (Galea *et al.*, 2002b, c; Vlahov *et al.*, 2002).

Survey instrument

Respondents were asked questions using a structured interview which assessed the mental health consequences of disasters (Freedy *et al.*, 1993). We asked questions about demographic characteristics (age, race/ethnicity, gender, yearly household income, education, and marital status), assessed proximity to the disaster site (south of 14th Street in this analysis; the WTC complex is in the south end of the borough of Manhattan and the area south of 14th Street is the area closest to the complex within NYC), and asked about September 11 event experiences including: if the respondent was in the WTC complex, was injured during the attacks, witnessed the attacks of September 11, was afraid for her/his life during the attacks, was displaced from home as a result of the attacks, if the respondent was involved in the rescue efforts, lost a job or possessions as a result of the September 11 attacks, and if friends or relatives were killed during the attacks. For the purposes of these analyses we combined the event exposure variables into a composite variable (referred to as being "directly affected" by the attacks) including: being in the WTC complex during the attacks, injured in the WTC attacks, having a friend or relative killed, losing possessions during the attacks, losing a job as a result of the attacks, or being involved in the post-disaster rescue effort (e.g., construction workers, doctors). We also assessed if the respondent reported experiencing symptoms consistent with a panic attack in the first few hours after hearing about the September 11 attacks. Symptoms of a peri-event panic attack were consistent with DSM-IV symptoms for panic attacks (American Psychiatric Association, 1994).

We used the NWS PTSD module to assess PTSD symptoms. The NWS was a large epidemiological research project carried out by the National Crime Victims' Research and Treatment Center (NCVC) at the Medical University of South Carolina that involved the assessment of national household probability samples of adult women about a variety of topics including history of traumatic events,

PTSD, major depression, and drug and alcohol use (Resnick *et al.*, 1993; Kilpatrick *et al.*, 1997). These assessments were made by telephone interviews over a 3-year period between 1989 and 1993. As part of this project, NCVC researchers developed and validated a diagnostic measure for PTSD and that was used in this work. The NWS PTSD module was validated in a field trial against the PTSD module of the Structured Clinical Interview for DSM-III-R (SCID; Spitzer *et al.*, 1992) administered by mental health professionals. The NWS PTSD module has been used in a number of RDD studies throughout the US (Hanson *et al.*, 1995; Kilpatrick *et al.*, 1997). In the field trial, inter-rater kappa coefficients for SCID based diagnoses were 0.85 and 0.86 for diagnoses of lifetime and current PTSD, respectively. In terms of comparison between the NWS PTSD module and the SCID, the kappa coefficient of the NWS PTSD module with SCID diagnosis of PTSD was 0.77 for lifetime PTSD and 0.71 for current PTSD. Instrument sensitivity was 99% and specificity was 79% when compared to SCID diagnosis (Resnick *et al.*, 1993; Kilpatrick *et al.*, 1998). Previous research using this measure among persons with a history of specific potentially traumatic events (e.g., rape, physical assault, or crime more generally) has shown that associations of these covariates with the PTSD were highly consistent with those reported in other epidemiological studies that carefully assessed both history of events and PTSD (Kilpatrick *et al.*, 1998), suggesting good construct validity for the NWS PTSD module.

The NWS PTSD module is a measure of PTSD that assesses the presence of Criterion B, C, and D symptoms and determines content for content-specific symptoms (e.g., content of dreams or nightmares) if symptom presence is endorsed. We measured PTSD symptoms and probable PTSD related to the September 11 attacks. We assessed probable PTSD since September 11 and current probable PTSD at the time of the survey based on prevalence of necessary PTSD Criterion B, C, and D symptoms since September 11 and within the previous 30 days, respectively. All re-experiencing symptoms (Criterion B) and all content-specific (e.g., avoidance of thoughts or feelings) avoidance symptoms (Criterion C) were required to be related to the September 11 attacks. Specifically, for each relevant content related PTSD symptom endorsed as being present for 2 weeks or more in the relevant time period, respondents were asked: "Was this related to the WTC disaster or to something else?" A subset of avoidance symptoms and all the arousal symptoms (Criterion D) could only be linked to the attacks by time frame (occurrence since September 11 or within the past 30 days). Participants were then required to report at least one re-experiencing symptom specific to the attack, at least three avoidance symptoms, and two arousal symptoms for a diagnosis of probable PTSD related to the September 11 attacks. Those reporting the combination of symptoms since September 11 or in the past 30 days were classified as having probable PTSD in the relevant time period.

Data presentation in this chapter

We present here prevalences of current probable PTSD and probable PTSD since September 11 as measured 6 months after September 11 for each of the key geographic areas in the NYC metropolitan area. These areas were: the boroughs of NYC (Manhattan, Brooklyn, Bronx, Queens, and Staten Island), the rest of New York State (NYS) (excluding NYC), New Jersey (NJ), and Connecticut (CT). We present the prevalence of each of the 17 DSM-IV PTSD symptoms and the prevalence of persons having sufficient symptoms to meet Criteria B, C, or D in the diagnosis of PTSD for the overall sample. We also present key bivariate relations between covariates assessed and the prevalence of probable PTSD since the September 11 attacks in the population sampled. We present variables that were significantly associated ($p < 0.05$) with probable PTSD since September 11 in two-tailed Chi-square testing. We used bivariate logistic regression analyses to determine odds ratios (OR) describing the relations between key covariate levels and probable PTSD.

Results

Characteristics of sample

Table 3.1 shows the demographic characteristics of the respondents interviewed for the entire sample and for the NYC subsample together with comparable data from the 2000 US Census to show similarity between the demographic estimates. Both the overall sample and the NYC subsample are statistically comparable to the population estimates from the US Census and do not suggest appreciable differences between the survey sampled and the underlying population.

Prevalence of probable PTSD in the NYC metropolitan area

The prevalences of probable PTSD in the different geographic regions of interest are shown in Table 3.2. Overall, 5.8% of respondents met criteria for probable PTSD in the aftermath of the September 11 attacks and 0.9% of respondents met criteria for current probable PTSD 6 months after September 11. The prevalence of probable PTSD after September 11 was highest in the NYC boroughs of Bronx, Brooklyn, and Staten Island (9.0% each for Bronx and Brooklyn, and 8.5% for Staten Island, compared to Manhattan prevalence of 7.7%). The prevalence of probable PTSD in these boroughs remained higher than that of other boroughs 6 months after September 11 (2.6% in Bronx, 2.4% in Brooklyn, 1.9% in Staten Island compared to 0.7% in Manhattan). The overall prevalence of probable PTSD since September 11 in NYC was 7.4% and the current prevalence 6 months after September 11 was 1.5%. The prevalence of probable PTSD in NYC was higher than that in the rest of NYS, NJ, or CT. In these three areas, the prevalence of probable PTSD since September 11 was 4.6% (NYS), 5.3% (NJ), and 1.1% (CT); current prevalence was 0.1% (NYS),

Table 3.1. Demographic characteristics of respondents surveyed 6 months after September 11 in the NYC metropolitan area compared to anticipated demographic characteristics based on the 2000 US Census (*n* = 2752)

Characteristics	NYC (*n* = 1530)			NYC metropolitan area (*n* = 2752)		
	Weighted percent from sample	Percent from 2000 US Census	Chi-square *p*-value	Weighted percent from sample	Percent from 2000 US Census	Chi-square *p*-value
Age						
18–24	14.7	13.2	0.58	13.6	11.7	0.69
25–34	27.0	22.5		23.7	20.4	
35–44	19.6	20.8		20.6	21.9	
45–54	18.3	16.7		19.0	17.7	
55–64	11.2	11.3		12.3	11.8	
65+	9.2	15.5		10.7	16.5	
Gender						
Male	44.1	46.2	0.67	46.3	46.9	0.90
Female	55.9	53.8		53.7	53.1	
Race						
White	35.8	38.7	0.51	55.4	54.8	0.80
African-American	23.7	23.0		15.8	16.5	
Asian	6.3	10.1		5.2	7.7	
Hispanic	28.7	24.7		19.6	18.5	
Other	5.5	3.6		4.0	2.6	

Table 3.2. Prevalence of probable PTSD in the NYC metropolitan area after September 11

	Probable PTSD after September 11	Current probable PTSD 6 months after September 11
Overall	5.8	0.9
Bronx	9.0	2.6
Brooklyn	9.0	2.4
Manhattan	7.7	0.7
Queens	4.6	0.3
Staten Island	8.5	1.9
NYC overall	7.4	1.5
New York State[a]	4.6	0.1
New Jersey	5.3	1.0
Connecticut	1.1	0.0

[a] New York State not including NYC.

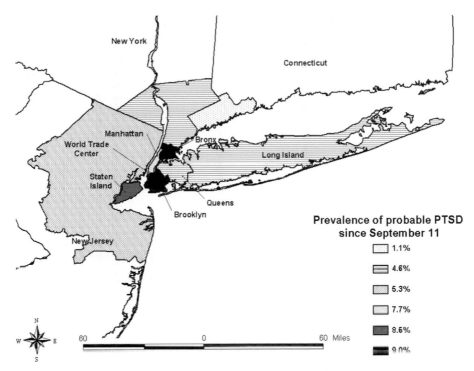

Figure 3.1   Geographic distribution of probable PTSD in the NYC metropolitan area.

1.0% (NJ), and 0.0% (CT) 6 months after September 11. Figure 3.1 illustrates the geographic distribution of the prevalence of probable PTSD since September 11.

Symptoms of PTSD in the overall sample

Twenty point four percent (20.4%) of respondents met re-experiencing symptom criteria (Criterion B), 9.9% of respondents met avoidance symptom criteria (Criterion C), and 20.7% met hyper-arousal symptom criteria (Criterion D) after the September 11 attacks. These prevalences had decreased to 8.9%, 3.9%, and 9.2%, respectively 6 months after the attacks. The most commonly reported symptoms after the September 11 attacks were insomnia (20.7%), irritability (17.4%), and intrusive memories (16.0%), and the most commonly reported symptoms 6 months after the attacks were insomnia (13.2%) intrusive memories (11.8%), and irritability (6.3%). Prevalences of PTSD symptoms since the September 11 attacks and 6 months after the attacks are shown in Figure 3.2.

Bivariate relations between demographic and event-exposure covariates and probable PTSD in the aftermath of the September 11 attacks in the NYC metropolitan area

Figure 3.3 shows socio-demographic variables that in bivariate analyses were significantly associated with the likelihood of probable PTSD since September 11 among

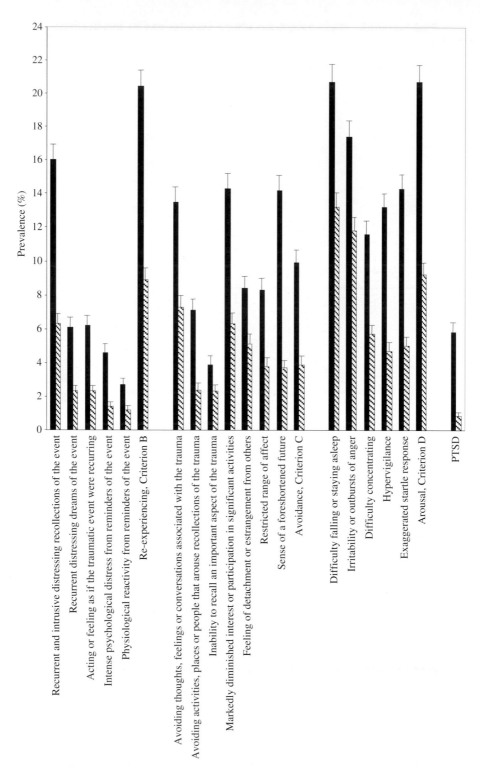

Figure 3.2   Prevalence of post-traumatic stress symptoms and of symptom criteria assessed in the NYC metropolitan area. Solid bars represent prevalence of symptoms since September 11 and the cross-hatched bars represent current symptoms, both measured 6 months after September 11.

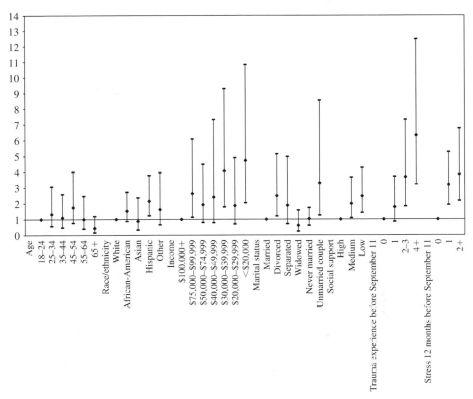

Figure 3.3   Odds Ratios describing the relations between key socio demographic variables and probable PTSD in residents of the general population of the NYC metropolitan area assessed 6 months after September 11 (n = 2752)

residents of the NYC metropolitan area. Some of the variables that were associated with a higher likelihood of probable PTSD in the aftermath of September 11 in the NYC metropolitan area were: being Hispanic (OR = 2.15 vs. white referent), income (OR = 2.62 for annual income of $75,000–$99,999; OR = 4.06 for annual income of $30,000–$39,999; OR = 4.71 for annual income less than $20,000; all compared to referent annual income of more than $100,000), marital status (OR = 2.48 for persons who were divorced; OR = 3.27 for members of unmarried couples; both compared to married persons as referent), social support (OR = 1.99 for medium; OR = 2.46 for low social support; both compared to high social support as referent), lifetime traumatic event experience prior to September 11 (OR = 3.65 for previous experience of 2–3 traumatic events; OR = 6.30 for previous experience of four or more traumatic events; both compared to no prior traumatic event experience), and stressors in the 12 months prior to September 11 (OR = 3.16 for persons who experienced one stressor and OR = 3.82 for persons who experienced two stressors; both compared to persons with no stressors in the

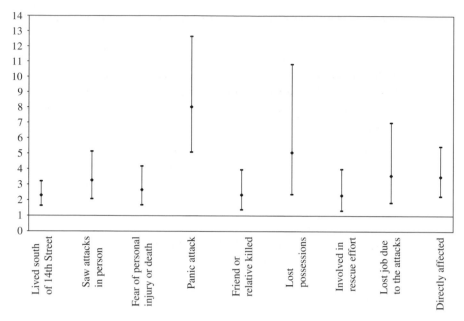

Figure 3.4   Odds Ratios describing the relations between event exposures and probable PTSD among residents of the NYC metropolitan area assessed 6 months after September 11 (*n* = 2752).

12 months prior to September 11). Figure 3.4 shows event exposure variables that in bivariate analyses were significantly associated with the likelihood of probable PTSD since September 11 among residents of the NYC metropolitan area. Event exposure variables that were associated with a higher likelihood of probable PTSD were living south of 14th Street, that is, in close proximity to the WTC (OR = 2.30), seeing the attacks in person (OR = 3.27); having been afraid of personal injury or death (OR = 2.66), experiencing a peri-event panic attack (OR = 8.03); losing possessions during the attacks (OR = 5.07), having been involved in the rescue efforts (OR = 2.31), and losing a job due to the attacks (OR = 3.59). Persons who were directly affected by the attacks (28.1% of overall sample) had 3.51 times greater odds of reporting symptoms consistent with probable PSD since September 11.

Discussion

In the aftermath of a large man-made disaster in a densely populated urban area our work showed that there are symptoms of post-traumatic stress in the general population beyond those who are typically considered to be victims of such disasters. Consistent with previous work, we showed that persons who were more exposed to the disaster (e.g., persons who lived closer to the WTC complex, persons who had a friend or relative killed in the attacks) were more likely to have symptoms consistent with PTSD after September 11. Overall, we estimated that persons directly affected by the attacks were 3.5 times more likely to have probable PTSD after the attacks than persons who were not directly affected by the attacks. However, we also showed that persons in the NYC metropolitan area who were not directly affected by the attacks also reported post-traumatic stress symptoms.

It is difficult to compare the absolute prevalence of probable PTSD documented here with prior research given both the uniqueness of the September 11 attacks and our focus on the general population. However, the preponderance of hyperarousal symptoms and of intrusive memories documented here are consistent with other post-disaster work (North *et al.*, 1999; McMillen *et al.*, 2000) and confirm our previous findings after this disaster (Galea *et al.*, 2002b). The geographic distribution of the prevalence of probable PTSD documented in this study was somewhat surprising, and an important reminder of the fact that multiple factors beyond proximity to the event determine the likelihood of psychopathology at the population level. We found that although Manhattan residents who lived closest to the WTC complex were more likely to develop probable PTSD after September 11, in the overall population, the prevalence of probable PTSD was highest in the boroughs of Brooklyn, Bronx, and Staten Island. This was true both for the development of probable PTSD since September 11 and for the current prevalence of PTSD as measured 6 months after the attacks. We conducted our earlier studies of PTSD after September 11 only in Manhattan due to our *a priori* assumption that the highest prevalence of PTSD would be in the borough where the WTC was located (Galea *et al.*, 2002a, b). However, this study showed that other factors beyond proximity are probably important in determining population prevalence of post-disaster psychopathology. It is likely that different factors contributed to the high prevalence of PTSD in Brooklyn, Bronx, and Staten Island. The former borough is to the east of Manhattan and residents of Brooklyn had probably the best views of the WTC complex from the attacks to the collapse of the towers. Also, Brooklyn is a predominantly commuter borough with residents of Brooklyn traveling to Manhattan for work on a daily basis. It is plausible that a combination of directly witnessing the event and being afraid of having friends or relatives killed in the attacks contributed to the high PTSD prevalence in Brooklyn. Staten Island is also a commuter borough and home to many of the rescue workers employed by the city police and fire departments. In contrast, the Bronx is a borough in northern NYC, further away from the WTC. However, the Bronx is predominantly Hispanic and our work has consistently shown Hispanicity to be a risk factor for the development of PTSD. Although it is likely a combination of factors that contribute to the higher prevalence of PTSD in these two boroughs compared to Manhattan, this observation serves to highlight the contribution of a complex set of variables to overall population prevalence in the aftermath of a disaster.

This relation between the individual risk of psychopathology and the population prevalence of psychopathology is interesting in this context, and has implications for public mental health planning in the aftermath of disasters. In this study, we estimated that 28.1% of respondents to this survey were, in some way, directly affected by the September 11 attacks. For the purposes of this analysis we used a very liberal definition of persons who might have been directly affected, with an eye to identifying as broad a range of persons as possible who may be conventionally referred to as "victims" of the disaster in one way or another. This group had odds 3.5 times higher than the rest of the respondents surveyed of developing probable PTSD related to the attacks. In the NYC metropolitan area that was the sampling frame for our work, we estimate approximately 4,440,000 persons directly affected by the attacks and 11,400,000 persons not directly affected by the attacks (Bureau of the Census, 2000). The net burden of probable PTSD in the former group would then be expected to be 500,000 and in the latter group 300,000 persons. While this calculation is meant to be merely illustrative and not a definite assessment of the number of people who had psychopathology, it demonstrates that the net burden of psychopathology in the aftermath of a disaster in a densely populated urban area may be at least as high among persons who are not directly affected by the disaster as it is among those who are. Calculations using different definitions about what constituted being directly affected by the attacks (e.g., different combinations of whether respondents saw events in person, lost relatives or friends, etc.) yield similar results. This discussion of the population burden of psychopathology is premised on two primary observations. First, although persons who are more exposed to an event are substantially more likely to have post-disaster psychopathology, this group is small relative to the general population. Second, the prevalence of post-traumatic stress symptoms in the general population of persons not directly affected by an event is not zero. As the general population is substantially larger than the group of persons who are directly affected, there is a substantial contribution from the general population to overall psychopathology. While the first of these observations is uncontroversial, the second is quite controversial. The DSM-IV diagnostic definition of PTSD requires that a person "experienced, witnessed, or was confronted with an event or events that involved … a threat to the physical integrity of self or others" (Criterion A1) and that the person have a subjective experience of "fear, helplessness, or horror" (Criterion A2). (American Psychiatric Association, 1995). On September 11 and during the difficult days afterwards there were many reasons for residents of the NYC metropolitan area to fear that their personal safety and that of others was under threat, to be confronted by the attacks, and to experience helplessness or horror, even if they were not directly affected on the morning of September 11. In the context of the September 11 attacks, persons who were not directly affected by the attacks may have been aware of the attacks through media, word-of-mouth, and communication with friends or family who were present for the attacks and who subsequently suffered post-traumatic stress symptoms. Our results argue that these exposures, albeit indirect, may have been sufficient for "indirectly affected" residents of the NYC metropolitan to experience the attacks and to subsequently suffer substantial post-traumatic psychopathology.

We have previously documented the progression of probable PTSD in the NYC subsample of this survey. The progression of probable PTSD in the NYC metropolitan area reflects that in the larger area, as in the City, a substantial proportion of symptoms resolve spontaneously in the first 6 months after the event (Galea *et al.*, 2003). This is consistent with other work. For example, the National Comorbidity Survey showed a steep decline in PTSD symptoms in the first year after a traumatic event and remission of approximately two thirds of PTSD cases (Kessler *et al.*, 1995). Longer-term studies of the longitudinal course of PTSD, particularly among Vietnam veterans, also suggest that only a third of PTSD cases persist chronically (Kulka *et al.*, 1990; O'Toole *et al.*, 1996) and prospective studies of patients hospitalized due to a traumatic event, female rape victims, and persons who were affected by motor vehicle accidents have shown that more than half of the cases of PTSD remit in the first 3–6 months after onset (Shalev *et al.*, 1988; Rothbaum *et al.*, 1992; Blanchard *et al.*, 1996). However, of particular interest to the public health community are the persons who have persistent PTSD in the long-term. Extant research suggests that a substantial proportion of persons who continue to have PTSD 6 months after an event will have symptoms in the long term (Kessler *et al.*, 1995). Further longitudinal work is required to assess this after September 11. It is worth noting that the overall prevalence of probable PTSD documented here 6 months after September 11 was 0.9%. Although this prevalence is low, in the general population of the NYC metropolitan area this is equivalent to approximately 142,000 persons (and to 92,000 persons in NYC proper), a substantial proportion of whom may be expected to have long-term symptoms. This further highlights the long-term ramifications of disasters in densely populated areas.

We have previously commented on the role of specific covariates in relation to the development of probable PTSD in the aftermath of September 11 in Manhattan and in NYC (Galea *et al.*, 2002b, c). The observations reported here are largely consistent with those earlier findings and with the current literature. For example, our observation that marital status and social support were predictors of PTSD onset after September 11 is consistent with findings from other research (Boscarino, 1995; Bromet *et al.*, 1998; Brewin *et al.*, 2000) and suggests that in the general population specific groups may be at particular risk of psychological consequences of disasters and may warrant more focused screening. Our finding that peri-event emotional reactions may be an important predictor of PTSD suggests that early interventions to address these emotional reactions may have the potential to reduce the incidence of PTSD after disasters (Resnick *et al.*, 1993). The importance of job loss highlights the complex relations between individual experiences (i.e., the job loss itself) and features of the recovery environment (i.e., the availability of jobs) and suggests that societal factors may be important determinants of symptom development after a disaster. The association of post-traumatic stress symptoms, substance use, and television viewing in this population are beyond the scope of this report and has been addressed elsewhere (Ahern *et al.*, 2002; Vlahov *et al.*, 2002; Vlahov *et al.*, in press).

Limitations

There are a number of limitations to this work in general and to this analysis in particular. Many of these limitations have been discussed in previous publications by this research team (Galea *et al.*, 2002a, b, c). We discuss briefly here some of the primary limitations of this work. Given the phone survey methodology and the lay-administered PTSD ascertainment instrument employed, case ascertainment and sampling bias are the two primary concerns with this work. With respect to the former, it is possible that since the NWS PTSD module is linked to event content only for content-specific symptoms, our probable PTSD prevalence is an overestimate of the true burden of psychopathology. There are two reasons why we think this is unlikely to be the case: (a) we have reported substantially lower prevalence of probable PTSD in the general population 1 month after September 11 than did the only other published representative population sample estimates of PTSD in NYC during the same time frame (Galea *et al.*, 2002b; Schlenger *et al.*, 2002); (b) a comparison between probable PTSD prevalence assessed using the PTSD Symptom Check List (PCL) and the NWS PTSD module, conducted on a subsample of 229 participants in survey 2, suggested that the NWS PTSD module provides a conservative estimate of the prevalence of probable PTSD compared to the PCL (Galea *et al.*, 2002d, Ruggiero *et al.*, in press). However, case ascertainment remains the primary limitation of assessments such as ours.

With respect to sampling bias, it is possible that our telephone sampling selectively sampled persons who were different than the rest of the population. Comparison of our sample to census demographic and socio-economic characteristics provides some reassurance in this regard. We note, however, that the response rate obtained in our study suggest that most people contacted in fact did not agree to participate in the survey. This is a problem endemic to all telephone surveys, irrespective of investigators' careful efforts to maximize response rates. There have been a number of recent observations that provide reassurance about the extent of sampling bias introduced in telephone surveys. Specifically, the RDD telephone survey method has also been routinely used to complete the CDC BRFSS which assesses risk behaviors in adults. A recent analysis of BRFSS data suggests that with changing response rates over the past 20–30 years have introduced minimal bias in data accuracy (Mariolis,

2001; Mariolis, 2002). Also, other work has shown that making extraordinary effort to reduce non-response in telephone efforts can in fact introduce bias in samples (due to the inclusion of respondents who are different than other non-responders) and that there are very few significant differences in key covariates over a range of reasonable response rates (Keeter *et al.*, 2000). In our surveys we were able to replicate our estimates of event exposure prevalence and symptom prevalence in each of the three surveys suggesting that only systematic sampling bias present in all three surveys is plausible. However, the potential for sampling bias remains. It is possible that persons with post-traumatic stress symptoms were less likely to participate in our surveys; this would suggest that our reported prevalence is an underestimate of the true burden of psychopathology in the general population. Conversely, if persons burdened by post-traumatic stress symptoms were more eager to talk on the phone it is possible that estimates presented here of probable PTSD represent overestimates.

Ultimately, it is worth noting that generalizability is a concern with this work. Although one of the prime motivations of this work was to provide reliable estimates of the population prevalence of PTSD after a disaster, the September 11 terrorist attacks in many ways were unique. Future terrorist attacks in the US are unlikely to be as unexpected as were the September 11 attacks. In addition, the September 11 attacks were accompanied by other ongoing events (e.g., the anthrax threats) that make the post-September 11 context unique. At best the burden of psychopathology estimated here can then serve as a guide as to what may be expected after other disasters in densely populated urban areas.

Directions for future research

This work encourages research in four areas. First, this research has been among the few to study PTSD in the general population starting immediately after a disaster. Soon after we published the first assessment of PTSD in the general population after September 11 (Galea *et al.*, 2002b), other authors (Cohen Silver *et al.*, 2002; Schlenger *et al.*, 2002) published work premised on similar assumptions to the ones we made and discuss here (although methods used, particularly by Cohen Silver and colleagues were substantially different than ours). Results, particularly from Schlenger and colleagues' study (Schlenger *et al.*, 2002) were similar to ours, providing further credence to some of the issues that we raise here about the implications of our observations for public health and for our conceptualization of PTSD. Therefore, a primary area of research that is encouraged by this work is the study of the impact of large-scale disasters in densely populated urban areas on the general population. As discussed above, this has substantial implications for public health practice and for our understanding of the burden of PTSD in a population. In addition, better understanding of the differences in the nature of PTSD between persons who are heavily, and less heavily affected by a disaster may also shed insight into the biology of PTSD.

Second, this research points the way to more focused work to explore the longitudinal course of PTSD in the general population after disasters. Although, as discussed in this chapter, the research implemented through the NYAM studies made use of a serial cross-sectional design to study the course of PTSD in the general population, a more explicit exploration of many of the observations that are emerging from this work (Galea *et al.* 2003b) is only possible through longitudinal studies. In addition, longitudinal studies can assess the course of PTSD in the general population in the longer term, and whether the currently accepted dogma that most cases of PTSD after disaster arise in the immediate short term is valid in a study of the general population.

Third, this work points to the need for further research about peri-event emotional reactions, and the extent to which interventions that target these emotional reactions (particularly among different racial/ethnic groups) may be effective in reducing incident PTSD. We showed in this chapter and in other work (Galea *et al.*, 2002b, c) that peri-event panic attacks were among the most important predictors of probable PTSD onset and that these emotional reactions may be differently important for persons of different ethnicities (Galea *et al.*, unpublished data). These observation point to the importance of a better understanding of the determinants of PTSD and highlights our current paucity of understanding of PTSD cross-culturally and cross-nationally. Future research on PTSD must include cross-national and cross-cultural comparisons that have the potential both to illuminate the true global burden of PTSD and also to suggest differences in pathophysiology that can lead to greater biological understanding and the potential for preventive interventions.

Fourth, our work suggests the need for further research that considers the implications of the range of possible exposures to disaster both for the diagnosis of PTSD and for public mental health interventions in the general population. With respect to the diagnosis of PTSD, further work is needed to understand the range of exposures in the general population of densely populated urban areas after disasters, and to corroborate our observations about the importance of PTSD in the general population in the aftermath of disasters. Future studies need to consider the range of services that are needed in the general population after a disaster, especially among specific subgroups (e.g., Hispanics) within the general population that may be particularly vulnerable to the development of PTSD.

Implications for mental health intervention in the post-disaster setting

In the aftermath of disasters limited resources for research and care have resulted in a focus on persons who are at highest risk of developing psychopathology. This study, like others before it, identified persons who were directly affected by the event as being at greater individual risk of PTSD. Here, we also confirm our earlier reports that Hispanicity and the presence of a peri-event emotional response are important determinants of PTSD that must be considered in conjunction with other, better established risk factors such as prior life stressors. However, studying the general population of the NYC metropolitan area shows the complex relation between individual risks and the ultimate population burden of psychopathology post-disaster. Clearly, public health practice must concern itself not only with persons who are high risk, but also with the larger population of persons who may be at low risk but may still develop post-traumatic symptoms. In the aftermath of a major disaster in a densely populated urban area it is possible that there may be more persons in the low-risk group who require attention than there are in the high-risk group. Unfortunately, this does not make public health intervention in the aftermath of a disaster easier. In many ways, it is easier to target persons who are directly affected for intervention (e.g., relatives of family members who die in a disaster are likely to be involved in support groups) than persons in the general population who otherwise share few risk factors. This highlights the importance of extensive general population outreach to people not otherwise connected to the post-disaster infrastructure. Recent work showing the difficulty in reaching persons through public health announcements (Rudenstine et al., 2003) and the scope of unmet mental health need (Kessler et al., 2001) suggests that this is not easily done. In that light, innovative early post-disaster interventions that may be easily accessed by the general population may be particularly important after future disasters.

REFERENCES

American Psychiatric Association (1994). *Diagnostic and Statistical Manual of Mental Disorders* (4th ed.). Washington, DC: American Psychiatric Press.

Ahern, J., Galea, S., Resnick, H., Kilpatrick, D., Bucuvalas, M., Gold, J. & Vlahov, D. (2002). Television images and psychological symptoms after the September 11th terrorist attacks. *Psychiatry*, **65**(4), 289–300.

Blanchard, E.B., Jones-Alexander, J., Buckley, T.C. & Forneris, C.A. (1996). Psychometric properties of the PTSD checklist. *Behavioral Research and Therapy*, **34**(8), 669–673.

Boscarino, J.A. (1995). Post-traumatic stress and associated disorders among Vietnam veterans: the significance of combat exposure and social support. *Journal of Traumatic Stress*, **8**(2), 317–35.

Brewin, C.R., Andrews, B. & Valentine, J.D. (2000). Meta-analysis of risk factors for posttraumatic stress disorder in trauma-exposed adults. *Journal of Consulting and Clinical Psychology*, **68**(5), 746–766.

Bromet, E., Sonnega, A. & Kessler, R.C. (1998). Risk factors for DSM-III-R posttraumatic stress disorder: findings from the National Comorbidity Survey. *American Journal of Epidemiology*, **147**(4), 353–361.

Bureau of the Census (2000). *Census Summary Tape, File 3A (STF 3A)*. Washington, DC: US Department of Commerce.

Carr, V.J., Lewin, T.J., Webster, R.A. & Kenardy, J.A. (1997). A synthesis of the findings from the Quake Impact Study: a two-year investigation of the psychosocial sequelae of the 1989 Newcastle earthquake. *Social Psychiatry and Psychiatric Epidemiology*, **32**(3), 123–136.

Cohen Silver, R., Holman, E.A., McIntosh, D.N., Poulin, M. & Gil-Rivas, V. (2002). Nationwide longitudinal study of psychological response to September 11. *Journal of the American Medical Association*, **288**, 1235–1244.

Freedy, J.R., Kilpatrick, D.G. & Resnick, H.S. (1993). Natural disasters and mental health: theory, assessment, and intervention. In *Handbook of Post-disaster Interventions* [special issue]. *Journal of Sociological Behavior and Personality*, **8**(5), 49–103.

Galea, S., Nandi, A. & Vlahov, D. (2005). The epidemiology of post-traumatic stress disorder after disasters. *Epidemiologic Reviews*, **27**, 78–91.

Galea, S., Ahern, J., Fuller, C., Freudenberg, N. & Vlahov, D. (2001). Needle exchange programs and experience of violence in an inner-city neighborhood. *Journal of AIDS,* **28**(3), 282–288.

Galea, S., Vlahov, D., Resnick, H., Kilpatrick, D., Bucuvalas, M. & Morgan, M. (2002a). An investigation of the psychological effects of the September 11th attacks on NYC: developing, and implementing research in the acute post-disaster period. *CNS Spectrums*, **7**(8), 593–596.

Galea, S., Ahern, J., Resnick, H., Kilpatrick, D., Bucuvalas, M., Gold, J. & Vlahov, D. (2002b). Psychological sequelae of the September 11th attacks in Manhattan, NYC. *New England Journal of Medicine*, **346**(13), 982–987.

Galea, S., Resnick, H., Ahern, J., Gold, J., Bucuvalas, M., Kilpatrick, D., Vlahov, D. (2002c). Posttraumatic stress disorder in Manhattan, NYC, after the September 11th terrorist attacks. *Journal of Urban Health*, **79**(3), 340–353.

Galea, S., Boscarino, J., Resnick, H. & Vlahov, D. (2002d). Mental health in New York City after the September 11 terrorist attacks: Results from two population surveys. Chapter 7. In *Mental Health, United States, 2001*, eds. R.W. Manderscheid & M.J. Henderson. Washington, DC: Supt of Docs, US Govt Print Office.

Galea, S., Vlahov, D., Resnick, H., Ahern, J., Susser, E., Gold, J., Bucuvalas, M. & Kilpatrick, D. (2003). Trends in the prevalence of probable posttraumatic stress disorder in NYC after the September 11 terrorist attacks. *American Journal of Epidemiology*, **158**(6), 514–524.

Green, B.L. & Lindy, J.D. (1994). Post-traumatic stress disorder in victims of disasters. *Psychiatric Clinics of North America*, **17**(2), 301–309.

Hanson, R.F., Kilpatrick, D.G., Freedy, R. & Saunders, B.E. (1995). Los Angeles County after the 1992 civil disturbances: degree of exposure and impact on mental health. *Journal of Consulting and Clinical Psychology*, **63**(6), 987–996.

Herman, D., Susser, E. & Felton, C. (2002). Rates and treatment costs of mental disorders stemming from the World Trade Center terrorist attacks: an initial needs assessment. The Center for Mental Health Services, Substance Abuse and Mental health Services Administration.

Keeter, S., Miller, C., Kohut, A., Groves, R.M. & Presser, S. (2000). Consequences of reducing nonresponse in a national telephone survey. *Public Opinion Research Quarterly*, **64**, 125–148.

Kennedy, R. (2001). With city transit shut down, New Yorkers take to eerily empty streets. *The New York Times*, September 12, 2001, Sect A: 8 (col. 1).

Kessler, R.C., Sonnega, A., Bromet, E., Hughes, M. & Nelson, C.B. (1995). Posttraumatic stress disorder in the National Comorbidity Survey. *Archives of General Psychiatry*, **52**, 1048–1060.

Kessler, R.C., Berglund, P.A., Bruce, M.L., Koch, J.R., Laska, E.M. & Leaf, P.J. (2001). The prevalence and correlates of untreated serious mental illness. *Health Services Research*, **36**(6) Part 1, 987–1007.

Kilpatrick, D.G., Acierno, R., Resnick, H.S., Saunders, B.E. & Best, C.L. (1997). A two year longitudinal analysis of the relationship between violent assault and alcohol and drug use in women. *Journal of Consulting and Clinical Psychology*, **65**(5), 834–847.

Kilpatrick, D.G., Resnick, H.S., Freedy, J.R., Pelcovitz, D., Resick, P.A., Roth, S. & van der Kolk, B. (1998). The posttraumatic stress disorder field trial: evaluation of the PTSD construct – criteria A through E. In *DSM-IV Sourcebook*, Vol. 4, eds. T.A. Widiger, A.J. Frances, H.A. Pincus, M.B. First, R. Ross & W. Davis. Washington, DC: American Psychiatric Association Press, pp. 803–844.

Kulka, R.A., Schlenger, W.E., Fairbank, J.A., Hough, R.L., Jordan, B.K., Marmar, C.R. & Weiss, D.S. (1990). *Trauma and the Vietnam War Generation: report of findings from The National Vietnam Veterans Readjustment Study*. New York: Brunner/Mazel.

Kuo, C.J., Tang, H.S., Tsay, C.J., Lin, S.K., Hu, W.H. & Chen, C.C. (2003). Prevalence of psychiatric disorders among bereaved survivors of a disastrous earthquake in Taiwan. *Psychiatric Services*, **54**(2), 249–251.

Mariolis, P. (2001). Data accuracy: how good are our usual indicators? *Proceedings of Statistics Canada Symposium 2001. Achieving Data Quality in a Statistical Agency: A Methodologic Perspective*, Ottawa, CA.

Mariolis, P. (2002). Response rates and data accuracy. *American Association of Public Opinion Research* [Oral Presentation]. Nashville, TN, May 2002.

McMillen, J.C., North, C.S. & Smith, E.M. (2000). What parts of PTSD are normal: intrusion, avoidance, or arousal? Data from the Northridge, California, earthquake. *Journal of Traumatic Stress*, **13**(1), 57–75.

NYC Fire Department (2002). McKinsey Report. Retrieved 28 May 2003, from http://www. nyc.gov/html/fdny/html/mck_report/exhibits.html

Norris, F.H., Friedman, M.J., Watson, P.J., Byrne, C.M., Diaz, E. & Kaniasty, K. (2002a). 60,000 disaster victims speak. Part I: An empirical review of the empirical literature, 1981–2001. *Psychiatry*, **65**(3), 207–239.

Norris, F.H., Friedman, M.J. & Watson, P.J. (2002b). 60,000 disaster victims speak. Part II: Summary and implications of the disaster mental health research. *Psychiatry*, **65**(3), 240–260.

North, C.S., Nixon, S.J., Shariat, S., Mallonee, S., McMillen, J.C., Spitznagel, E.L. & Smith, E.M. (1999). Psychiatric disorders among survivors of the Oklahoma City bombing. *Journal of the American Medical Association*, **282**(8), 755–762.

North, C.S., Tivis, L., McMillen, J.C., Pfefferbaum, B., Spitznagel, E.L., Cox, J., Nixon, S., Bunch, K.P. & Smith, E.M. (2002). Psychiatric disorders in rescue workers after the Oklahoma City bombing. *American Journal of Psychiatry*, **159**(5), 857–859.

O'Toole, B.I., Marshall, R.P., Grayson, D.A., Schureck, R.J., Dobson, M., French, M., *et al.* (1996). The Australian Vietnam Veterans Health Study, III: psychological health of Australian Vietnam veterans and its relationship to combat. *International Journal of Epidemiology*, **25**, 331–340.

Paulsen, A.S., Crowe, R.R., Noyes, R. & Pfohl, B. (1988). Reliability of the telephone interview in diagnosing anxiety disorders. *Archives of General Psychiatry*, **45**, 62–63.

Resnick, H.S., Kilpatrick, D.G., Dansky, B.S., Saunders, B.E. & Best, C.L. (1993). Prevalence of civilian trauma and PTSD in a representative national sample of women. *Journal of Consulting and Clinical Psychology*, **61**(6), 984–991.

Rothbaum, B.O., Foa, E.B., Riggs, D.S., Murdock, T. & Walsh, W. (1992). A prospective evaluation of post-traumatic stress disorder in rape victims. *Journal of Traumatic Stress*, **5**, 455–475.

Rudenstine, S., Galea, S., Ahern, J., Felton, C. & Vlahov, D. (2003). Awareness and perceptions of a community-wide mental health program 4–5 months after the September 11 terrorist attacks in NYC. *Psychiatric Services*, **54**(10), 1404–1406.

Ruggiero, K., Rheingold, A.A., Resnick, H., Kilpatrick, D.G. & Galea, S. (in press). Comparison between two widely-used PTSD screening instruments: implications for public mental health planning, *Journal of Traumatic Stress*.

Salcioglu, E., Basoglu, M. & Livanou, M. (2003). Long-term psychological outcome for non-treatment-seeking earthquake survivors in Turkey. *Journal of Nervous and Mental Disease*, **191**(3), 154–160.

Schlenger, W.E., Caddell, J.M., Ebert, L., Jordan, K., Rourke, K.M., Wilson, D., Thalji, L., Dennis, J.M., Fairbank, J.A. & Kulka, R.A. (2002). Psychological reactions to terrorist attacks: findings from the National Study of Americans' Reactions to September 11. *Journal of the American Medical Association*, **288**(5), 581–588.

Shalev, A.Y., Freedman, S., Peri, T., Brandes, D., Sahar, T., Orr, S.P., *et al.* (1988). Prospective study of posttraumatic stress disorder and depression following trauma. *American Journal of Psychiatry*, **155**(5), 630–637.

Simon, G.E., Revicki, D. & VonKorff, M. (1993). Telephone assessment of depression severity. *Journal of Psychiatric Research*, **27**(3), 247–252.

Smith, E.M., North, C.S., McCool, R.E. & Shea, J.M. (1990). Acute postdisaster psychiatric disorders: identification of persons at risk. *American Journal of Psychiatry*, **147**(2), 202–206.

Spitzer, R.L., Williams, J.B., Gibbon, M. & First, M.B. (1992). The structural clinical interview for DSM-III-R (SCID), I: history, rationale, and description. *Archive of General Psychiatry*, **49**(8), 624–629.

Stoppelbein, L. & Greening, L. (2000). Posttraumatic stress symptoms in parentally bereaved children and adolescents. *Journal of the American Academy of Child and Adolescent Psychiatry*, **39**(9), 1112–1119.

Vlahov, D., Galea, S., Resnick, H., Ahern, J., Boscarino, J.A., Bucuvalas, M., *et al.* (2002). Increased use of cigarettes, alcohol, and marijuana among Manhattan Residents after the September 11th terrorist attacks. *American Journal of Epidemiology*, **155**(11), 988–996.

Vlahov, D., Galea, S., Ahern, J., Resnick, H. & Kilpatrick, D. (in press). Sustained increased consumption of cigarettes, alcohol and marijuana among Manhattan residents following the events of September 11, 2001. *American Journal of Public Health*.

Weeks, M.F., Kulka, R.A., Lessler, J.T. & Whitmore, R.W. (1983). Personal versus telephone surveys for collecting household health data at the local level. *American Journal of Public Health*, **73**(12), 1389–1394.

4

Coping with a national trauma: a nationwide longitudinal study of responses to the terrorist attacks of September 11

Roxane Cohen Silver, E. Alison Holman, Daniel N. McIntosh, Michael Poulin, Virginia Gil-Rivas and Judith Pizarro

The terrorist attacks of September 11, 2001, exposed every person in the USA to an experience that, in recent decades, was unprecedented in its scope and traumatic impact. Perhaps over 100,000 individuals directly witnessed these events, and many others viewed the attacks and their aftermath via the media (Yehuda, 2002). It has been argued that this national trauma "influenced and will continue to influence the clinical presentation of patients seeking health care services" in the USA (Yehuda, 2002, p. 108).

A wide range of responses can be expected following traumatic life events. Research conducted after the Oklahoma City, OK, bombing indicates that responses to a terrorist attack are likely to be highly variable (North *et al.*, 1999). Research in the broader field of stress and coping has also demonstrated considerable variability in emotional and cognitive responses to stressful experiences (Silver & Wortman, 1980; Wortman & Silver, 1989, 2001). Despite advances in understanding reactions to traumatic events, our understanding of responses to community-level events in general, and terror attacks in particular, is limited. Progress in understanding the social and psychological process following such occurrences requires examination of how responses to a variety of stressful events are similar and different at both the group and individual level. Research has matured to the point that large-scale, prospective, longitudinal studies with the scope to examine mediators and moderators of adjustment processes are not only possible, but also necessary (North & Pfefferbaum, 2002). Moreover, the threat of future terrorist attacks demands that a higher level of urgency and research sophistication be directed not only at understanding the effects of such attacks, but also at the individual and social variables that predict psychological outcomes to such events over time.

The purpose of our research has been to document the variability in acute and ongoing responses to the largest community-based trauma in recent US history across a nationally representative sample of individuals. Specifically, we have sought to understand psychological responses to the September 11th attacks and their aftermath across the USA, and identify specific personal, social, and psychological factors that predict differences in outcomes over time. Our work is informed by decades of research on stress and coping that suggests a dynamic process in which responses to events are influenced by both individual and social variables (McCann & Pearlman, 1990; Kaniasty & Norris, 1995; Lepore *et al.*, 1996; McFarlane & Yehuda, 1996; van der Kolk, 1996; King *et al.*, 1999). The accumulated data in the stress and coping field present a wide variety of relations among psychological responses and psychiatric symptoms (e.g., distress, positive affect, depression, posttraumatic stress disorder (PTSD)), social and psychological variables (e.g., social support, world views), and behaviors (e.g., coping strategies) (Janoff-Bulman, 1992; Norris & Kaniasty, 1996; Taylor *et al.*, 2000; North *et al.*, 2001). However, integrating these findings has been hindered by the lack of methodological consistency across studies that examine adjustment to different events, using different measures, and sampling different populations. This prior work has nonetheless provided empirical and theoretical foundations for a comprehensive and rigorous examination of adjustment processes in a social context.

Since September 2001, we have conducted a longitudinal panel study of responses to the terrorist attacks of September 11 in a national probability sample of Americans. The national scale of the terrorist attacks allowed us to examine the emotional, cognitive, and social impact of a single event within a representative sample of individuals. Early results indicated substantial variability in response (Silver *et al.*, 2002). One goal of our ongoing research is to examine factors that may account for this variability, and to identify early predictors of long-term adjustment to this traumatic event. Tracking the interplay of social and psychological factors in responses to the terrorist attacks over time will provide baseline data for understanding reactions to other community disasters.

As noted by others (North *et al.*, 2001; Norris *et al.*, 2002a), empirical evidence concerning the adjustment process can aid clinicians by identifying potential risks, and may facilitate the design of interventions for individuals coping with stressful life events (e.g., Chemtob *et al.*, 1997). As potentially harmful myths of coping remain prevalent in both lay and professional communities (Wortman & Silver, 2001), rigorous examination of various paths for adjustment among a representative sample of individuals allows us to address and challenge these myths directly.

Overcoming limitations in the study of adjustment to stressful events

As research on adjustment to stressful events has evolved, increasingly sophisticated methods have become necessary to advance our understanding of the coping process. Adjustment is likely to be influenced by interactions among intrapersonal and interpersonal factors (Pritchard & McIntosh, 2003; Holman & Zimbardo, submitted). As yet, little is known about the development of, and interactions between, cognitive, social, and emotional responses to trauma. Most traumatic events (both natural and human-made) occur locally, and most studies use samples too small to examine these interactions thoroughly. The field has reached the point at which a major effort is needed to explicate the adjustment process in its complexity.

Our project has sought not only to document variability in responses to a community trauma, but also to address several important questions derived from the research literature. The nationwide impact of the attacks has offered us the opportunity to examine adjustment processes unhindered by a number of methodological limitations typical to this research area. Our study also addresses several weaknesses noted in recent reviews of coping research (Compas *et al.*, 2001; Norris *et al.*, 2002b). First, with few exceptions (Shalev *et al.*, 1996; Koopman *et al.*, 1997; North *et al.*, 1997; Holman & Silver, 1998), researchers have yet to study the long term progression of cognitive, social, and emotional responses to trauma starting with early baseline responses. Only longitudinal research allows identification of plausible causal pathways and detection of patterns over time. As levels of distress do not change linearly over time (Wortman & Silver, 1989; Norris *et al.*, 2002b), their association with coping responses may vary with time since the event. Among survivors of a mass murder incident, for example, active outreach coping was negatively associated with disorders at 3–4 months and 3 years, but not 1-year post-event; acceptance/reconciliation was negatively associated with outcomes at 3-years post-event, but not at 3–4 months or 1-year post-event (North *et al.*, 2001). Thus, longitudinal studies with low attrition rates are required to document possible patterns of adjustment and identify the paths through which traumatic events impact individuals and the processes by which they adjust.

Second, data collection rarely begins early enough. Due to the difficulties inherent in identifying "at-risk" populations, few studies have been able to collect pre-trauma information, or to use data collected before a stressful event occurs (for exceptions, see Harlow *et al.*, 1991; Mendes de Leon *et al.*, 1994; Carnelley *et al.*, 1999; Reifman *et al.*, 2000). Without information on pre-event functioning, it is very difficult to disambiguate the effects of the trauma on later outcomes. It is perhaps even more difficult to collect data in the immediate aftermath of a traumatic event, and few studies provide clear data on acute responses to such experiences (Shalev *et al.*, 1996; Holman & Silver, 1998). Because some disaster survivors later report having never had symptoms that they reported closer to the time of the event (North *et al.*, 1997), only data collected shortly after a trauma allow for comparisons of adjustment over time. As noted by North and Pfefferbaum, "Delay in initiating data collection limits opportunities to obtain early information needed to understand mental health effects of disasters. If researchers cannot act quickly, important data may be lost forever" (North & Pfefferbaum, 2002, p. 634).

Third, although most longitudinal studies complete data collection within 12 months of the event (Norris *et al.*, 2002b), longer follow-ups are necessary to assess long-term consequences of traumatic experiences (Tait & Silver, 1989; Wortman & Silver, 2001). For example, Murphy found disaster victims showed higher symptom levels than controls, even 3-years post-event (Murphy, 1984, 1985; see also Lehman *et al.*, 1987, for a similar result 4–6 years after loss of a spouse or child in a motor vehicle accident). Because many studies fail to follow individuals for several years after a stressful event, limited information is available about the long-term effects of responses seen in the trauma's immediate aftermath. In fact, although several studies have provided snapshots of early reactions to the September 11th attacks (Schuster *et al.*, 2001; Galea *et al.*, 2002; Schlenger *et al.*, 2002), the long-term implications of these early distress responses and psychiatric symptoms are unknown (North & Pfefferbaum, 2002).

Fourth, too few studies include assessments of the ongoing occurrence of stressful events. Recent research demonstrates that negative events and other stressors that occur post-disaster are strong predictors of mental health outcomes, including PTSD (Norris *et al.*, 1999; Maes *et al.*, 2001). Thus, information on ongoing events is critical in tracking patterns and processes of adjustment. Without information on the occurrence of stressful events following an initial trauma, it is impossible to know whether specific factors such as low SES are tied to long-term negative adjustment because they are related to higher initial impact, to fewer resources, or to greater frequency of negative events over time.

Fifth, the sample size and composition of most studies precludes comparisons of responses across demographic groups (e.g., SES, geographic region, ethnicity), as well as across groups of individuals with certain psychosocial characteristics (e.g., substance use to cope). The median sample size for studies of adjustment following disaster is 149 (Norris *et al.*, 2002b). Given that the vast majority of current research is conducted on non-minority, middle-class respondents (Compas *et al.*, 2001; Norris *et al.*, 2002b), little is known about how demographic groups may differ in processes associated with adjustment. Studies that include minority participants tend to find that the impact of events differs across ethnic groups (Norris *et al.*, 2002b) and may depend, in part, on prior lifetime exposure to trauma (Holman *et al.*, 2000). However, studies typically do not have enough respondents to allow analysis of low-frequency groups (based on demographic or other individual difference variables), events (e.g., traumatic events that occur between waves of data collection), or behaviors (e.g., atypical coping strategies), or to examine their interactive effects with emotional, cognitive, or social responses.

Sixth, far too few methodologically rigorous studies conducted in the aftermath of a traumatic event pay adequate attention to mechanisms underlying the variability that has been identified in response to trauma (Wortman & Silver, 1989, 2001).

In fact, it is critical to identify important intervening variables that may mediate the relations between trauma and mental and physical health outcomes. For example, work by members of our research team has highlighted the importance of several cognitive processes in adaptation to traumatic experiences. We have found that the extent to which individuals continue to focus attention on their past experiences, in part by engaging in attributional searches (Downey *et al.*, 1990), counterfactual thinking (Davis *et al.*, 1996), or the search for meaning (Silver *et al.*, 1983; McIntosh *et al.*, 1993), appears to be associated with long-term psychosocial difficulties. In fact, global ratings of the extent to which individuals remain focused on their past have been associated with both negative mental health outcomes and higher rates of social conflict 2 years after the event in our prior studies on coping with trauma (Holman & Silver, 1998; Holman & Zimbardo, submitted).

Finally, the impact of the social environment on coping with traumatic events remains poorly understood. We know that social network responses to an individual's attempts to come to terms with a traumatic event are likely to have a direct impact on long-term psychosocial adjustment (Silver & Wortman, 1980; Tait & Silver, 1989; Holman & Silver, 1996). In fact, research has demonstrated that having the opportunity to discuss one's traumatic life experiences with a supportive audience can facilitate long-term adjustment (Pennebaker, 1989; Lepore *et al.*, 1996), whereas an unsupportive environment may exacerbate the maladaptive tendency to focus one's attention on the past (*cf.* Tait & Silver, 1989; Holman & Silver, 1996; Lepore *et al.*, 1996; Holman & Zimbardo, submitted). But substantially less attention has been given to the broader social context of coping beyond global indicators such as "social support" (*cf.* Silver *et al.*, submitted). Very little is known, for example, about the impact of responses from specific relationships (e.g., spouse, friend, sibling) on an individual's ability to adjust to traumatic events (see Brock *et al.*, 1996; Sarason *et al.*, 1997), and limited consideration has been given to dynamic interpersonal systems, such as the family (Norris *et al.*, 2002a, b).

When compared to other age groups, school-aged youth report the highest level of psychological impairment following trauma (Norris *et al.*, 2002b), and a growing body of literature explores coping with stressful life events among children and adolescents (e.g., see Garbarino *et al.*, 1991; Weisenberg *et al.*, 1993; Yule *et al.*, 2000). Yet despite this interest, few published studies have contrasted the adjustment processes of youth and their parents to the same trauma, and have examined how their responses mutually influence each other. As parental adjustment predicts children's adjustment beyond the effects of levels of exposure (Gleser *et al.*, 1981; McFarlane, 1987), and higher levels of parental support and warmth are associated with children's adjustment following exposure to violence (Gorman-Smith & Tolan, 1998; Kliewer *et al.*, 1998; Kliewer *et al.*, 2001), it is important to understand how dynamic family processes shape each family member's response.

Community traumas affect not only parents and adolescents individually, but also their relationships, which complicates the provision of support (Hawkins *et al.*, 2005). We expect long-term negative consequences of the traumatic experience to be exacerbated when parental distress is high and open discussion of the trauma is constrained (Kliewer *et al.*, 1998; Silver *et al.*, submitted).

After their exhaustive review of research on coping with disasters, Norris *et al.* (2002a, p. 249) concluded: "We need carefully conceived and theory-driven studies of basic process that are longitudinal in design.... We need more research that addresses the needs of diverse populations. We need more complex studies of family systems and community-level processes."

Our prospective longitudinal study is one of the first attempts to recruit and systematically follow a national sample of individuals shortly after a major traumatic event, and the only one to continue to do so for several years after September 11th. We address many of the aforementioned methodological limitations of prior research (see Norris *et al.*, 2002a, b). First, we have obtained access to data on physical and mental health collected *before* the terrorist attacks. Second, we collected data on stress and coping responses shortly after them (e.g., 9–14 days post-attacks). Third, our study is longitudinal (follow-up data have been collected at multiple intervals over several years post-attacks). Fourth, as our study is designed to track the influence of prior life events on adjustment to the attacks, we have assessed the pre-September 11th occurrence of a variety of personally experienced stressful life events during childhood and/or adulthood (e.g., witnessing someone being injured or killed, sexual assault). Because we anticipate that the prior experience of community trauma may also influence response to the events of September 11th (see Turner & Lloyd, 1995), we over-sampled from three US communities that previously experienced trauma, including large-scale interpersonal violence (i.e., the Columbine High School Shooting in Littleton, CO), terrorism (i.e., the bombing of the Murrah Federal Building in Oklahoma City, OK), and a natural disaster (i.e., Hurricane Andrew in Miami, FL). As immediate exposure to the events of September 11th may exacerbate responses to this atrocity (Yehuda, 2002), we over-sampled from New York City (NYC). Thus, we can compare responses to the terrorist attacks among three groups (NYC, previously traumatized communities, and the rest of the country), and can compare responses to subsequent traumas and highly stressful life events more generally between individuals and communities (e.g., NYC, Miami, Littleton/Denver, Oklahoma City) that have or have not had previous trauma. Through repeated assessments of stressful events that occur both individually and at a community level over the course of our study, comparisons of response before and after a variety of life events are possible. Fifth, our sample size provides us with sufficient power to examine processes within and across low-frequency groups and variables, and our study will broaden significantly the participation of underrepresented groups. Sixth, by studying a representative sample of Americans, we will also be able to examine how the traumatic event interacts with an individual's cognitive and social resources to predict long-term adjustment. Finally, because we have included a longitudinal sub-study of adolescents and their parents, we can explore the adjustment process within families over time.

Overview of methods

In collaboration with Knowledge Networks, Inc. (KN), a survey research organization that maintains a nationally representative web-enabled research panel of potential respondents, we have administered a web-based survey at several points in time since September 11th to a national sample of US residents. Respondents have completed several items exploring their specific 9/11-related experiences, including the severity of their exposure to and loss from the attacks, the hours per day they watched TV coverage of the attacks and their aftermath, and other behavioral responses surrounding the events of September 11th (e.g., volunteer efforts, church attendance). We have also examined the role of prior exposure to traumatic events, and the role of psychological and social processes that may affect psychological outcomes after the September 11th attacks. Specifically, participants have completed a trauma history questionnaire, measures of cognitive response following the attacks (e.g., searching for meaning, temporal disintegration, counterfactual thinking), emotional response (e.g., frequency and intensity of positive and negative emotions), and overall functioning (e.g., social, work-related limitations). To understand the role of social relationships in response to the attacks, the quality of social relationships available in the aftermath of this trauma have also been assessed (e.g., interpersonal conflict, support, and frequency of ventilation with several different social contacts). Prior research documents the importance of these variables in studies on coping with highly stressful or traumatic experiences (see Silver & Wortman, 1980; Terr, 1983; Steinglass et al., 1988; Baum, 1990; McCann & Pearlman, 1990; Herman, 1992; McIntosh et al., 1993; van der Kolk, 1996; Holman & Silver, 1998). Consistent with recent work on coping with trauma, we have also included an assessment of core beliefs about self, others, and the world using the World Assumptions Scale (Janoff-Bulman, 1989). In addition, a pre-9/11 mental and physical health history had been assessed on our sample via a survey completed by most KN Panel Members *prior to* the attacks (between September 2000 and September 2001). Respondents reported whether they had ever suffered from an anxiety disorder (obsessive compulsive disorder, generalized anxiety disorder) or depression, and whether they received such a diagnosis from a medical doctor. Respondents also indicated whether a medical doctor had ever diagnosed them with any disorders from a list of 28 physical ailments (e.g., asthma, diabetes, hypertension) (see Silver et al., 2002).

Since September 11, our study has examined the impact of the attacks on individuals' current psychological and emotional state, life satisfaction, world views, and perceptions of future risk. Below, we briefly discuss the levels and types of reactions to the attacks over time, and note how several selected individual (e.g., prior life stress) and social variables (e.g., adolescent social interactions with parent) are linked to various outcomes.

Data collection following 9/11/2001

KN administered an initial survey between September 20 and October 4, 2001, to identify early coping strategies employed and acute stress symptoms experienced by a national probability sample of individuals in the immediate aftermath of the events of September 11th. The survey consisted of the brief COPE (Carver, 1997), a measure of coping strategies, and a modified version of the Stanford Acute Stress Reaction Questionnaire (SASRQ; Cardena *et al.*, 2000), a measure used to assess acute stress disorder (ASD). In total, a sample of 3134 KN Panel Members completed the initial survey, including 2729 adults (78% participation rate) and 405 adolescents between ages 13 and 17 (41% participation rate; see Table 4.1 for a full summary of *N*'s and participation rates). Over 75% of respondents completed this survey within the first few days (9–14 days post-attacks); the remainder completed it the following week.

KN also administered a web-based self-administered survey designed by our research team between November 10 and December 3, 2001 (Wave 2). Budgetary constraints and lack of full panel availability precluded a follow-up of all Wave 1 participants. The sampling strategy employed in Wave 2 included a randomly drawn sample of KN adult panelists (ages 18 and over) who completed the Wave 1 measures, and a random sample of KN adult panelists drawn from each of four targeted communities: Littleton, CO and the surrounding Denver metropolitan community; Miami, FL;

Table 4.1. *N*'s and per-wave completion rates for each wave of data collection

	W1 September 2001		W2 November 2001		W3 March 2002		W4 September 2002		W5 March 2003		W6 September 2003		W7 September 2004	
	N	%	*N*	%	*N*	%	*N*	%	*N*	%	*N*	%	*N*	%
National sample	2729	78	933	87	846	91	2033	75	1666	78	1571	74	1950	79
Previously traumatized communities			449	78	355	87	333	76						
Adolescents	405	41			110	65	146	76						
Parents					151	86	166	86						

Oklahoma City, OK; and New York, NY. The Wave 2 sample included 1382 adults (overall participation rate was 84%). Individuals who did not respond to the survey were not significantly different from respondents in terms of income, education, gender, marital status, or ethnicity. Non-respondents were, however, significantly younger ($M = 40$ years) than respondents ($M = 48$ years; $t\,(1371) = -8.33$; $p < 0.001$). The survey assessed posttraumatic stress symptoms with the IES-R (Weiss & Marmar, 1997), global distress with the Hopkins Symptom Checklist (Derogatis et al., 1974), life satisfaction with the Satisfaction with Life Scale (Diener et al., 1985), and positive affect (Diener et al., 1995) (see Table 4.2 for a general timetable of assessments). Table 4.3 (modified from Silver et al., 2002) presents the demographic breakdown of participants from Waves 1 and 2 – both weighted and unweighted – and provides a comparison with September 2001 Current Population Survey (CPS) benchmarks from the US Census Bureau (2001).

A follow-up survey (Wave 3) was conducted between March 16, 2002 and April 11, 2002, using measures similar to Wave 2 (e.g., the BSI-18; Derogatis, 2001). All adult panelists who completed Waves 1 and 2, and who remained part of the KN sample

Table 4.2. Timetable of assessed variable categories for each wave of data collection

	Pre-9/11/2001	W1 September 2001	W2 November 2001	W3 March 2002	W4 September 2002	W5 March 2003	W6 September 2003	W7 September 2004
Physical health (disorders, ailments, utilization)	X			X	X	X	X	X
Mental health (e.g., depression, PTS symptoms, distress, positive affect, life satisfaction)	X	X	X	X	X	X	X	X
Coping strategies		X						
9/11 Exposure/loss			X		X			
Stressful life events (age, duration, type)			X	X	X	X	X	X
Social support/conflict			X	X	X	X	X	X
Anniversary exposure/response					X		X	X

Table 4.3. Demographic composition of the initial sample and comparisons with 2001 US Census Data (CPS, US Bureau of the Census, September 2001)

	Wave 1: 9–14 days			Wave 2: 2 months			US Census
	N	Unweighted %	Weighted %	N	Unweighted %	Weighted %	Weighted %
Gender							
Male	1322	48.4	47.8	676	48.8	48.2	48.0
Female	1407	51.6	52.2	706	51.2	51.8	52.0
Total	2729	100.0	100.0	1382	100.0	100.0	100.0
Age							
18–24	223	8.2	10.9	98	7.1	9.8	13.3
25–34	474	17.4	20.6	222	16.1	21.1	18.1
35–44	577	21.1	21.9	293	21.1	21.7	21.7
45–54	567	20.8	17.9	307	22.1	19.4	18.9
55–64	416	15.2	13.3	211	15.4	13.0	11.9
65+	472	17.3	15.3	251	18.2	15.0	16.1
Total	2729	100.0	99.9	1382	100.0	100.0	100.0
Race							
White	2138	83.2	80.0	1068	82.7	80.4	83.2
Black/African American	265	10.3	12.3	127	9.8	12.5	11.9
American Indian	38	1.5	1.7	32	2.5	2.4	0.9
Asian/Pacific Islander	42	1.6	1.9	23	1.8	1.6	4.0
Other	88	3.4	4.1	41	3.2	3.1	N/A
Total	2571	100.0	100.0	1291	100.0	100.0	100.0
Hispanic ethnicity							
Non-hispanic	2379	91.8	89.3	1200	89.4	86.6	89.2
Hispanic	213	8.2	10.6	142	10.6	13.4	10.8
Total	2592	100.0	99.9	1342	100.0	100.0	100.0
Education							
Less than HS	247	9.1	15.7	109	8.0	16.0	15.8
HS Diploma or equivalent	952	35.2	32.8	418	30.7	31.7	33.0
Some college	685	25.3	24.0	368	27.0	23.5	19.3
Associate Degree	119	4.4	3.5	72	5.3	4.3	7.8
Bachelor's Degree or beyond	703	26.0	24.0	395	29.1	24.5	24.1
Total	2706	100.0	100.0	1362	100.0	100.0	100.0

Table 4.3. (Continued)

	Wave 1: 9–14 days			Wave 2: 2 months			US Census
	N	Unweighted %	Weighted %	N	Unweighted %	Weighted %	Weighted %
Marital status							
Married	1691	62.9	61.3	772	57.5	57.6	57.1
Single	520	19.4	21.9	269	20.0	22.1	24.1
Separated, divorced, widowed	476	17.7	16.8	302	22.5	20.3	18.8
Total	2687	100.0	100.0	1343	100.0	100.0	100.0
Household income							
Under $10,000	133	4.9	5.6	73	5.4	6.5	7.4
$10,000 to $24,999	448	16.4	19.2	232	17.1	19.6	18.4
$25,000 to $49,999	1052	38.6	39.6	509	37.5	38.7	28.5
$50,000 to $74,999	612	22.5	20.8	308	22.6	21.0	20.0
$75,000 or more	480	17.6	14.8	237	17.4	14.2	25.7
Total	2725	100.0	100.0	1359	100.0	100.0	100.0
Region							
Northeast	558	20.4	19.7	285	20.6	19.4	19.1
Midwest	566	20.7	21.5	185	13.3	22.0	22.9
South	1016	37.2	36.4	593	43.0	36.1	35.6
West	589	21.6	22.4	319	23.1	22.5	22.4
Total	2729	100.0	100.0	1382	100.0	100.0	100.0

6 months after the attacks ($N = 1323$) were included in this data collection. Ninety percent of those fielded the survey completed it. Individuals who did not respond to the Wave 3 survey were not different from respondents in terms of gender, income, education, marital status, or ethnicity. Non-respondents to the Wave 3 survey were, however, significantly younger ($M = 45$ years) than respondents ($M = 49$ years; $t(930) = 2.33; p < 0.05$).

The Wave 1 sample also included 405 adolescents: 201 (49.6%) males and 204 (50.4%) females, ranging in age from 13 to 17 ($M = 15.35$ years). Seven months after the attacks (4/2/02–4/30/02), a sub-sample of these adolescents also participated in a parent–adolescent dyad study of coping within families. The Wave 3 adolescent sample included 54 (49%) males and 56 (51%) females ranging in age from 14 to

18 ($M = 15.89$). The adolescents who completed the survey did not differ significantly from non-participants in terms of gender, age, ethnicity, early coping strategies employed, or Wave 1 trauma symptoms. A randomly selected parent/guardian living in the same household with the adolescent was also recruited at the same time to complete a companion survey. Half the parents/guardians were male, and they ranged in age from 21 to 93 ($M = 44.56$ years). Twenty-two percent were college graduates, 39.5% had attended college, 32% had a high school diploma, and 6.5% had not completed high school. Household income ranged from less than $5,000 per year to over $125,000 per year with a median of $40,000–49,999. There were 104 matched dyads in which an adolescent and a parent/guardian from the same household participated.

The Wave 4 1-year anniversary data collection was fielded between September 20 and October 24, 2002. All Waves 1 and 2 adults ($N = 3170$) were eligible for this data collection. Although 17.5% ($N = 555$) of these individuals had left the KN panel by September 2002, we re-approached them for this follow-up data collection effort. These withdrawn panelists were given the opportunity to complete our survey online (via a password protected link) or via a paper and pencil version of our Wave 4 questionnaire. Over 32% of the withdrawn KN panelists were retrieved for this data collection (45% of whom completed the survey online). Overall, 75% of all eligible adults completed the 1-year anniversary data collection ($N = 2366$), which included measures similar to those included in earlier surveys. In addition, the PTSD Checklist (PCL; Weathers *et al.*, 1993) was used to assess posttraumatic stress symptoms 1 year after the attacks. Table 4.4 presents the demographic breakdown of the Wave 4 participants – both weighted and unweighted – and provides a comparison with 2002 Census data. At the 1-year anniversary data collection, we continued to maintain a sample that was nationally representative of the adult US population.

Another data collection took place 18-month post-attacks (Wave 5) that included similar measures to those in prior waves and was fielded between March 13 and April 9, 2003. All withdrawn and active panel members from Wave 4 ($N = 2138$) who had completed the Wave 1 survey and all NYC residents were eligible for this survey, and 78% ($N = 1666$) participated. This number included 55% of the withdrawn panelists (42% of whom completed the survey online). In response to the initiation of US hostilities against Iraq, an additional survey was fielded from March 27 (1 week after the first major US attacks) to April 6, 2003. Because the purpose of this data collection was to obtain rapid-response data on a timely national event, only active KN panelists were asked to complete this supplemental survey. It was fielded to 1801 panelists and 75% ($N = 1349$) participated. The war survey was shorter than the September 11th-related surveys, included a question to assess general war-related distress ("How distressed do you feel about the ongoing war in Iraq?" 1 = "Not at all"; 5 = "Extremely"), the SASRQ (Cardena *et al.*, 2000) for war-related acute stress symptoms, and a measure assessing the frequency with which respondents had seen 16 specific images of the war through their exposure to the media.

Table 4.4. Demographic composition of the 1-year sample and comparisons with 2002 US Census Data

	Wave 4 (12 months)			US Census[a]
	N	Unweighted %	Weighted %[b]	Weighted %[b]
Gender				
Male	993	48.8	48.2	48.0
Female	1040	51.2	51.8	52.0
Age				
18–24	96	4.7	9.0	13.3
25–34	274	13.5	21.9	17.8
35–44	414	20.4	21.2	21.1
45–54	452	22.2	18.3	19.0
55–64	359	17.7	13.5	12.7
65+	438	21.5	16.2	16.1
Marital status				
Married	1313	64.6	63.7	57.2
Single	315	15.5	19.5	24.1
Separated, divorced, widowed	405	19.9	16.8	18.7
Race				
White	1705	84.3	81.8	82.9
Black/African American	185	9.2	11.3	12.0
American Indian	43	2.1	2.6	1.0
Asian/Pacific Islander	48	2.4	2.0	4.1
Other	41	2.0	2.3	N/A
Hispanic ethnicity				
Non-hispanic	1867	92.0	89.9	88.9
Hispanic	162	8.0	10.1	11.1
Education				
Less than HS	175	8.6	13.6	15.9
HS Diploma or equivalent	679	33.4	35.9	32.3
Some college	661	32.5	27.2	27.5
Bachelor's Degree or beyond	518	25.5	23.3	24.3
Household income				
Under $10,000	126	6.2	8.3	7.4
$10,000 to $24,999	351	17.3	19.5	18.4
$25,000 to $49,999	723	35.6	36.2	28.5
$50,000 to $74,999	441	21.7	20.2	20.0
$75,000 or more	392	19.3	15.8	25.7
Region				
Northeast	427	21.0	19.4	18.9
Midwest	410	20.2	25.5	22.8
South	769	37.8	34.1	35.7
West	427	21.0	21.0	22.6

[a]*Data source*: CPS, US Bureau of the Census, December 2002.

[b]Weights adjust estimates for sampling design and post-stratification to Census characteristics. Some of the variables have missing data and the numbers do not add up to the total.

Finally, data collection efforts were also completed approximately 2 years (Wave 6) and 3 years (Wave 7) post-September 11th. We successfully maintained a substantial portion of the eligible adult sample at each wave (74% participation rate at Wave 6 and 79% participation rate at Wave 7).

Overview of analytic strategy

The following statistical analyses were conducted with STATA version 7.0, a program designed to handle weighted analyses of complex longitudinal survey data and provide the necessary adjustments of standard errors for these analyses. Data were weighted to adjust for differences in the probabilities of selection and non-response both within and between households. In addition, the post-stratification weights are calculated by deriving weighted sample distributions along various combinations of age, gender, race/ethnicity, region, metropolitan status, and education. Similar distributions are calculated using the most recent US Census Bureau's CPS data and the KN panel data. Cell-by-cell adjustments over the various univariate and bivariate distributions are calculated to make the weighted sample cells match those of the US Census and the KN panel. This process is repeated iteratively until there is convergence between the weighted sample and benchmark distributions from the 2001 CPS and the US Census Bureau.

Weighted rates of acute stress symptoms were examined using SASRQ symptom reports. Using the *Diagnostic and Statistical Manual of Mental Disorders, Fourth Edition (DSM-IV)* criteria B, C, D, and E for ASD (i.e., three or more dissociative symptoms, one or more re-experiencing/intrusive symptom, one or more avoidance symptom, *and* one or more arousal/anxiety symptom) (American Psychiatric Association, 1994), individuals who met these cut-offs were classified as having "high" levels of acute stress symptoms. Because we did not assess all *DSM-IV* criteria (e.g., feelings of fear, horror or helplessness; duration of symptoms), respondents were not assumed to have ASD. After Wave 1, a dichotomous index of high vs. low posttraumatic stress symptoms was calculated from the measure of posttraumatic stress symptomatology employed at the particular wave (the IES-R or PCL). Symptoms were considered positive if respondents reported having been at least "moderately" distressed by them in the prior week (2 on a 0–4-point scale) (Mollica *et al.*, 2001). Rates of high levels of posttraumatic symptoms were determined using *DSM-IV* criteria B, C, and D for PTSD: one or more re-experiencing symptom, three or more avoidance symptoms, *and* two or more arousal symptoms (American Psychiatric Association, 1994). Because we did not assess all *DSM-IV* criteria (e.g., degree of functional impairment, duration of symptoms), and because most respondents did not meet the basic requirement for direct exposure, they were not assumed to have PTSD.

Analyses were designed to address (1) levels of acute or posttraumatic stress symptoms and distress over the years following the attacks, and (2) how pre-September 11th physical and mental health status, lifetime and recent stressors, and September 11th-related experiences were associated with patterns of posttraumatic stress symptoms and psychological distress over the 18 months following the attacks. Generalized estimating equation (GEE) population-averaged models were used to identify predictors of (a) posttraumatic stress and (b) global distress symptoms over the 18 months following the attacks. Two time-varying, longitudinal outcome variables were created for these analyses using the standardized, continuous mean scores for posttraumatic stress and global distress, both measured at four time points (2, 6, 12, and 18 months post-9/11/2001). The time-varying posttraumatic stress symptom score was used as the outcome in the first set of analyses, and then was employed as a time-varying covariate in the analyses of global distress. This approach allowed us to examine predictors of global distress scores independent of the predictor-posttraumatic stress symptom relationship. In each analysis, significant predictors from five groups of variables (demographics, pre-9/11 health, lifetime and recent exposure to stressful events, 9/11-related exposure and loss, 9/11-related acute stress symptoms) were tested for inclusion in the final models. Non-significant variables ($p > 0.05$) were removed from final analyses to provide the most parsimonious model. All analyses were weighted and estimated adjusting for time. Tables present standardized Betas as the relative effect size for each variable. When appropriate, missing values were imputed within waves using the EM method to maintain the size and integrity of the sample (Little & Rubin, 1987). KN used the mean income score for each respondent's census block to impute missing cases for income.

Immediate response data

At Wave 1, respondents reported using several different strategies to cope with the attacks. The three most commonly reported were acceptance ($M = 3.31$, SD $= 0.72$), self-distraction ($M = 2.80$, SD $= 0.86$), and religion ($M = 2.60$, SD $= 1.11$). High levels of acute stress symptoms were present in 11.7% ($N = 368$) of the Wave 1 sample (Silver *et al.*, 2002).

Presence of posttraumatic stress symptoms

High levels of posttraumatic stress symptoms were reported by 17.0% of the Wave 2 respondents, by 5.8% of the Wave 3 respondents, by 5.2% of the Wave 4 respondents, by 3.3% of the Wave 5 respondents, by 4.4% of the Wave 6 respondents, and by 4.5% of the Wave 7 respondents. Additionally, at the 1-year anniversary of the September 11th attacks, 43.2% of respondents reported that the anniversary reactivated feelings that they experienced immediately post-September 11th at least "somewhat."

Predictors of posttraumatic stress symptoms

Table 4.5 presents results from the analysis of posttraumatic stress symptoms. The findings suggest that several variables were important in explaining the presence of these symptoms over time. After adjusting for the strong relationship between acute stress symptoms and posttraumatic stress symptoms, individuals reporting direct exposure to the attacks reported higher levels of posttraumatic stress symptomatology over the 18 months after the attacks. Pre-9/11 mental health and childhood trauma were also associated with higher levels of posttraumatic stress symptoms. Importantly, the number of recent traumatic life events experienced *following* the September 11th attacks were associated with higher levels of 9/11-related posttraumatic stress symptoms, even after adjusting for significant demographics (e.g., education, gender, income), pre-9/11 mental health and trauma, and acute stress symptoms. As shown in Table 4.5, both education and income served as protective factors – individuals with higher levels of education and income reported fewer posttraumatic stress symptoms over time.

Predictors of global distress

Table 4.6 presents results from the analysis of global distress symptoms after adjusting for the time-varying longitudinal posttraumatic stress symptom score. Not surprisingly, pre-9/11 mental health was the strongest predictor of global distress after adjusting for posttraumatic stress symptoms. Importantly, however, the next most powerful predictor of global distress was the number of recent traumatic life events – the more events a person reported experiencing during the period following the attacks, the higher their levels of global distress over time. Consistent with the research linking physical illness, depression, and anxiety, the number of pre-9/11 physician diagnosed physical ailments was associated with higher levels of global distress over time as well. Both age and income served as protective factors – older and wealthier individuals reported fewer global distress symptoms over time.

Rates of stressful life events

Over the course of our study we have collected lifetime exposure to stressful life events (other than the September 11th attacks) on our sample. Occurrence, timing and duration of stressful life events was assessed using a checklist of events derived from the Diagnostic Interview Schedule section on PTSD (Robins *et al.*, 1981) and supplemented with items derived from the open-ended coding of lifetime traumas

Table 4.5. Longitudinal GEE model of posttraumatic stress symptoms over 18 months following 9/11 attacks ($N = 1923$)*

	Model 1		
	β	z	p
Demographics			
Gender	0.09	4.20	0.000
Education			
High School	−0.10	−2.11	0.035
Some college	−0.13	−2.74	0.006
College Degree	−0.15	−3.62	0.000
Income	−0.06	−2.17	0.030
Self-reported pre-9/11 health			
Physician diagnosed mental disorder	0.11	3.47	0.001
Life events			
Total number of childhood stressful events	0.08	1.97	0.049
Total number of adulthood stressful events	0.06	1.84	0.066
Total number of recent stressful events	0.07	2.26	0.024
9/11-related exposure			
Direct exposure	0.14	4.59	0.000
Watching live TV	0.05	2.54	0.011
9/11 related responses			
Initial acute stress/functioning	0.24	7.73	0.000
Statistical value			
Model Wald χ^2	187.00		
p-value	<0.0001		

*$N = 1923$ cases, 4811 observations. The following groups of variables were tested for inclusion in the model: (1) demographics (i.e., gender, age, marital status, ethnicity, education, and income); (2) pre-9/11 mental and physical health status (i.e., MD diagnosed mental disorders/physical ailments); (3) total number of childhood stressful life events, total number of adult stressful life events, and total number of recent stressful life events (from the year *following* 9/11, September 2001 to September 2002); (4) 9/11-related experience (i.e., exposure to and distance from 9/11 attacks); and (5) immediate post-9/11 acute stress/functioning symptoms following the 9/11 attacks. Variables not listed in the table were not significant ($p > 0.05$) and were removed from the final model. Gender was coded 0: male; 1: female; individuals who did not complete high school comprise the reference group for the education comparisons; individuals who were not directly exposed through witnessing 9/11 events live or by watching live TV comprise the reference group for exposure to 9/11 attacks; β is the standardized regression coefficient, "z" is the significance test for "β".

Table 4.6. Longitudinal GEE model of psychological distress over 18 months following 9/11 attacks (*N* = 1923)*

	Model 1		
	β	z	p
Demographics			
Age	−0.11	−4.67	0.000
Gender	0.01	0.65	0.517
Income	−0.07	−3.37	0.001
Self-reported pre-9/11 health			
Physician diagnosed mental disorder	0.16	5.02	0.000
Physician diagnosed physical ailments	0.10	3.83	0.000
Life events			
Total number of childhood stressful events	0.01	0.48	0.631
Total number of recent stressful events	0.11	3.71	0.000
9/11-posttraumatic stress symptoms			
Posttraumatic stress symptoms	0.50	18.46	0.000
9/11-related responses			
Initial acute stress/functioning	0.05	2.18	0.029
Statistical value			
Model Wald χ^2	655.68		
p-value	<0.0001		

*N = 1923 cases, 4811 observations. The following groups of variables were tested for inclusion in the model: (1) demographics (i.e., gender, age, marital status, ethnicity, education, and income); (2) pre-9/11 mental and physical health status (i.e., MD diagnosed mental disorders/physical ailments); (3) total number of childhood stressful life events, total number of adult stressful life events, and total number of recent stressful life events (from the year *following* 9/11, September 2001 to September 2002); (4) 9/11-related experience (i.e., exposure to and distance from 9/11 attacks); and (5) immediate post-9/11 acute stress/functioning symptoms following the 9/11 attacks. Variables not listed in the table were not significant ($p > 0.05$) and were removed from the final model. Gender was coded 0: male; 1: female; β is the standardized regression coefficient, "z" is the significance test for "β".

reported by a primary-care community sample (Holman *et al.*, 2000). The measure provides a wider range of events than is typically found in measures of traumatic events and has produced overall lifetime rates of specific traumas in this sample comparable to epidemiological surveys conducted in other representative community samples (Norris, 1992; Kessler *et al.*, 1995; Breslau *et al.*, 1998). Overall, 93.4% of the sample reported experiencing at least one stressful event during their lifetime (e.g., natural disaster, domestic violence, lost a loved one to homicide or suicide).

While 6.6% of respondents reported never having experienced a stressful life event, 27.8% reported experiencing 1–4 events, 57.1% reported 5 or more events, and 24.8% reported 10 or more events. Nearly 60% reported at least one childhood trauma (e.g., childhood abuse or neglect, interpersonal violence, a loss prior to age 18). Over 86% of the sample reported having experienced at least one highly stressful event during adulthood. Finally, 41.4% of the sample reported having experienced at least one highly stressful event during the year after September 11th.

Community comparisons on posttraumatic stress symptomatology

The Wave 2 proportions of respondents reporting high levels of posttraumatic stress symptomatology across the four over-sampled metropolitan areas were 29% for NYC, 30% for Miami, 15% for Oklahoma City, 9% for Littleton/Denver, and 17% for the national sample outside these communities. At Wave 3, the proportions for the four over-sampled metropolitan areas were 16% for NYC, 17% for Miami, 6% for Oklahoma City, 3% for Littleton/Denver, and 6% for the national sample. Longitudinal logistic regression modeling indicated that, after adjusting for demographic characteristics, prior mental health, September 11th-related experiences and distance from ground zero, individuals in the Littleton/Denver area were 49% less likely (odds ratio (OR) = 0.51, 95% confidence interval (CI) = 0.25–1.04), and individuals in both Miami (OR = 2.35, 95% CI = 1.40–3.96) and NYC (OR = 2.21, 95% CI = 1.11–4.44) were more than twice as likely, to report high levels of posttraumatic stress symptomatology than individuals in the national sample. Residents of Oklahoma City reported levels of posttraumatic stress symptomatology comparable to the national sample. These findings suggest wide variability in responses to the September 11th attacks across communities and raise questions about the role of prior community-based trauma in inoculating vs. sensitizing individuals to the impact of future stressful or traumatic events.

Parent–adolescent study findings

At Wave 1, adolescents reported experiencing on average 4.42 (SD = 4.34; on a 26-item scale) 9/11-related acute stress symptoms. Seven months post-attacks, adolescents' levels of symptomatology were low, with adolescents reporting an average of 2.51 (SD = 4.19; 22-item scale) positive 9/11-related posttraumatic stress symptoms (scores of 2 or higher). The coping strategies most frequently employed by adolescents included acceptance, self-distraction, active coping, and religious coping. However, adolescents' patterns of coping in the immediate aftermath of the attacks were not associated with subsequent distress or posttraumatic stress symptoms 7 months later. After adjusting for adolescents' perceived threat associated with the attacks and acute stress symptoms at Wave 1, higher levels of parental distress ($\beta = 0.25$, $p < 0.01$), parental coping advice to seek advice and help from others ($\beta = 0.32$, $p < 0.001$), adolescents' perceptions of parental unavailability to talk ($\beta = 0.25$, $p < 0.01$), and adolescents' reports that discussions with their parents about the attacks were not helpful ($\beta = 0.25$, $p < 0.01$) were associated with higher levels of posttraumatic stress symptoms 7 months after the attacks (Gil-Rivas *et al.*, submitted).

Acute stress response during the Iraq war

As assessed by the SASRQ and the duration of participants' acute stress symptoms, 7.0% of war survey respondents exhibited war-related acute stress symptoms. After adjusting for pre-September 11th mental and physical health, the odds of experiencing acute stress symptoms were significantly higher for women (OR = 2.37, 95% CI = 1.23–4.58), lower income individuals (OR = 0.91, 95% CI = 0.84–0.97), and those who experienced high levels of acute stress symptoms in response to the September 11th attacks (OR = 3.37, 95% CI = 1.56–7.30). Another important predictor of acute stress was individuals' trajectories of change in posttraumatic stress symptoms following September 11th, with those experiencing a slower decline or even an increase in symptoms having greater odds of war-related acute stress (OR = 5.65, 95% CI = 2.86–11.18).

Summary

A terrorist attack psychologically targets an entire population, not merely those in physical proximity to the attack. Most research on reactions to traumatic events, natural disasters, and mass murders has focused on the impact on those immediately affected. Largely unexplored are the psychological consequences to the individuals beyond the immediate community in which the event occurs. In the case of the September 11th attacks, the population of the USA was the terrorists' intended psychological target. In this chapter, we described the extent to which this attack affected adults across the US and identified variables that predicted who was most likely to suffer greater long-term psychological consequences. These data underscore the importance of looking beyond the obvious, immediate samples typically examined in disaster research, and the need to consider effects beyond those populations directly affected by tragedy.

Our results over the first 18 months after the attacks suggest the importance of prior mental health history, prior life traumas, as well as the significant role of subsequent stressors, in explaining distress and symptomatology over time. In addition, our findings from the Iraq war survey suggest that stress symptoms in response to one event – in this case, the Iraq war – may be strongly related to responses to a prior event – the September 11th attacks. Prior research has been largely unable to examine the association between individuals' stress responses to multiple events over time. This limitation has potentially thwarted understanding of the unique roles played by intra- and interindividual factors in responses to particular events. Prospective assessments of responses to multiple stressful events provide an excellent opportunity to examine these factors.

A second purpose of this chapter has been to describe how we conducted this research, and to emphasize that such research is not only possible, but also crucial in studying risk and resiliency factors for psychological distress in populations outside a directly impacted community. Launching a national study quickly after an event is rare and expensive – but we have demonstrated it can be done, and only by collecting such immediate national data and following the sample over time can the true impact of terrorism be understood.

Together, the findings from this program of research also raise a number of important, unanswered questions about patterns of coping with highly stressful events. Broadly, we found that outcomes are multiply determined, and that there are several factors beyond mere exposure to the event that predict outcomes. Our work suggests that, to understand fully how trauma affects human functioning, we need to consider the unique roles of individual differences (e.g., coping responses, previous experience with trauma), and social interactions (e.g., social constraints, conflict, social support) in mediating the relations between specific events and subsequent outcomes. These processes need to be documented over time and ideally in response to multiple events. In our ongoing data analyses, we are addressing these issues prospectively in the context of coping with a variety of personal and community-based events. Ultimately, it is our hope that information collected in this effort can illuminate the coping process more generally so as to advance future conceptual work in this area. We also hope it can further our understanding of the unique needs of traumatized individuals and provide information to help identify those at risk for subsequent difficulties. With these data in hand, educational and intervention efforts that are designed and implemented in response to terrorism can be better informed, more cost-effective, and more sensitive to community needs.

Acknowledgments

Project funding provided by National Science Foundation grants BCS-9910223, BCS-0211039, and BCS-0215937.

REFERENCES

American Psychiatric Association (1994). *Diagnostic and Statistical Manual of Mental Disorders, Fourth Edition*. Washington, DC: American Psychiatric Press.

Baum, A. (1990). Stress, intrusive imagery, and chronic stress. *Health Psychology*, **9**, 653–675.

Breslau, N., Kessler, R.C., Chilcoat, H.D., Schultz, L.R., Davis, G.C. & Andreski, P. (1998). Trauma and posttraumatic stress disorder in the community: the 1996 Detroit Area Survey of trauma. *Archives of General Psychiatry*, **55**, 626–632.

Brock, D.M., Sarason, I.G., Sarason, B.R. & Pierce, G.R. (1996). Simultaneous assessment of perceived global and relationship-specific support. *Journal of Social and Personal Relationships*, **13**, 143–152.

Cardena, E., Koopman, C., Classen, C., Waelde, L.C. & Spiegel, D. (2000). Psychometric proper-ties of the Stanford Acute Stress Reaction Questionnaire (SASRQ): a valid and reliable measure of acute stress. *Journal of Traumatic Stress*, **13**, 719–734.

Carnelley, K.B., Wortman, C.B. & Kessler, R.C. (1999). The impact of widowhood on depression: findings from a prospective national survey. *Psychological Medicine*, **29**, 1111–1123.

Carver, C.S. (1997). You want to measure coping but your protocol's too long: consider the brief COPE. *International Journal of Behavioral Medicine*, **4**, 92–100.

Chemtob, C.M., Tomas, S., Law, W. & Cremniter, D. (1997). Postdisaster psychosocial interven-tion: a field study of the impact of debriefing on psychological distress. *American Journal of Psychiatry*, **154**, 415–441.

Compas, B.E., Connor, J.K., Saltzman, H., Thomsen, A.H. & Wadsworth, M.E. (2001). Coping with stress during childhood and adolescence: problems, progress, and potential in theory and research. *Psychological Bulletin*, **127**, 87–127.

Davis, C.G., Lehman, D.R., Silver, R.C., Wortman, C.B. & Ellard, J.H. (1996). Self-blame follow-ing a traumatic event: the role of perceived avoidability. *Personality and Social Psychology Bulletin*, **22**, 57–67.

Derogatis, L.R. (2001). *BSI-18: Administration, Scoring, and Procedures Manual*. Minneapolis, MN: NCS Assessments.

Derogatis, L.R., Lipman, R.S., Rickels, K., Uhlenhut, E.H. & Covi, L. (1974). The Hopkins Symptom Checklist (HSCL): a self-report inventory. *Behavioural Science*, **19**, 1–15.

Diener, E., Emmons, R.A., Larsen, R.J. & Griffin, S. (1985). The Satisfaction with Life Scale. *Journal of Personality Assessment*, **49**, 71–75.

Diener, E., Smith, H. & Fujita, F. (1995). The personality structure of affect. *Journal of Personality and Social Psychology*, **69**, 130–141.

Downey, G., Silver, R.C. & Wortman, C.B. (1990). Reconsidering the attribution–adjustment relation following a major negative event: coping with the loss of a child. *Journal of Personality and Social Psychology*, **59**, 925–940.

Galea, S., Ahern, J., Resnick, H., *et al.* (2002). Psychological sequelae of the September 11 terror-ist attacks in New York City. *New England Journal of Medicine*, **346**, 982–987.

Garbarino, J., Kostelny, K. & Dubrow, N. (1991). What children can tell us about living in danger. *American Psychologist*, **36**, 376–383.

Gil-Rivas, V., Silver, R.C., Holman, E.A., McIntosh, D.N. & Poulin, M. (submitted for publica-tion). Parental response and adolescent adjustment to the September 11th attacks.

Gleser, G.C., Green, B.L. & Winget, C.N. (1981). *Prolonged Psychological Effects of Disaster: A Study of Buffalo Creek*. New York: Academic Press.

Gorman-Smith, D. & Tolan, P. (1998). The role of exposure to community violence and devel-opmental problems among inner-city youth. *Development and Psychopathology*, **10**, 101–116.

Harlow, S.D., Goldberg, E.L. & Comstock, G.W. (1991). A longitudinal study of the prevalence of depressive symptomatology in elderly widowed and married women. *Archives of General Psychiatry*, **48**, 1065–1068.

Hawkins, N.A., McIntosh, D.N., Silver, R.C. & Holman, E.A. (2005). Early responses to school violence: a qualitative analysis of students' and parents' immediate reactions to the shootings at Columbine High School. *Journal of Emotional Abuse*, **4**, 197–223.

Herman, J.L. (1992). *Trauma and Recovery*. Scranton, PA: Harper Collins.

Holman, E.A. & Silver, R.C. (1996). Is it the abuse or the aftermath: a stress and coping approach to understanding long-term responses to incest. *Journal of Social and Clinical Psychology*, **15**, 318–339.

Holman, E.A. & Silver, R.C. (1998). Getting "stuck" in the past: temporal orientation and coping with trauma. *Journal of Personality and Social Psychology*, **74**, 1146–1163.

Holman, E.A. & Zimbardo, P. (submitted for publication). The social language of time: trauma, time perspective, and social relationships.

Holman, E.A., Silver, R.C. & Waitzkin, H. (2000). Traumatic life events in primary care patients: a study in an ethnically diverse sample. *Archives of Family Medicine*, **9**, 802–811.

Janoff-Bulman, R. (1989). Assumptive worlds and the stress of traumatic events: applications of the schema construct. *Social Cognition*, **7**, 113–136.

Janoff-Bulman, R. (1992). *Shattered Assumptions: Towards a New Psychology of Trauma*. New York: Free Press.

Kaniasty, K. & Norris, F.H. (1995). Mobilization and deterioration of social support following natural disasters. *Current Directions in Psychological Science*, **4**, 94–98.

Kessler, R.C., Sonnega, A., Bromet, E. & Nelson, C.B. (1995). Posttraumatic stress disorder in the National Comorbidity Survey. *Archives of General Psychiatry*, **52**, 1048–1060.

King, D.W., King, L.A., Foy, D.W. & Keane, T.M. (1999). Posttraumatic stress disorder in a national sample of female and male Vietnam veterans: risk factors, war-zone stressors, and resilience-recovery variables. *Journal of Abnormal Psychology*, **108**, 164–170.

Kliewer, W., Lepore, S.J., Oskin, D. & Johnson, P.D. (1998). The role of social and cognitive processes in children's adjustment to community violence. *Journal of Consulting and Clinical Psychology*, **66**, 199–209.

Kliewer, W., Murrelle, L., Mejia, R., Torres de G, Y. & Angold, A. (2001). Exposure to violence against a family member and internalizing symptoms in Colombian adolescents: the protective effects of family support. *Journal of Consulting and Clinical Psychology*, **69**, 971–982.

Koopman, C., Classen, C. & Spiegel, D. (1997). Multiple stressors following a disaster and dissociative symptoms. In *Posttraumatic Stress Disorder: Acute and Long-Term Responses to Trauma and Disaster*, eds. C.S. Fullerton & R.J. Ursano. Washington, DC: American Psychiatric Press, Inc., pp. 21–35.

Lehman, D.R., Wortman, C.B. & Williams, A.F. (1987). Long-term effects of losing a spouse or child in a motor vehicle crash. *Journal of Personality and Social Psychology*, **52**, 218–231.

Lepore, S.J., Silver, R.C., Wortman, C.B. & Wayment, H.A. (1996). Social constraints, intrusive thoughts and depressive symptoms among bereaved mothers. *Journal of Personality and Social Psychology*, **70**, 271–282.

Little, R.J.A. & Rubin, D.B. (1987). *Statistical Analysis with Missing Data*. New York: Wiley.

Maes, M., Mylle, J., Delmeire, L. & Janca, A. (2001). Pre- and post-disaster negative life events in relation to the incidence and severity of post-traumatic stress disorder. *Psychiatry Research*, **105**(1–2), 1–12.

McCann, I.L. & Pearlman, L.A. (1990). *Psychological Trauma and the Adult Survivor: Theory, Therapy, and Transformation*. New York: Bruner/Mazel.

McFarlane, A.C. (1987). Posttraumatic phenomena in a longitudinal study of children following a natural disaster. *Journal of the American Academy of Child and Adolescent Psychiatry*, **26**, 764–769.

McFarlane, A.C. & Yehuda, R. (1996). Resilience, vulnerability and the course of posttraumatic reactions. In *Traumatic Stress: The Effects of Overwhelming Experience on Mind, Body, and Society*, eds. B.A. van der Kolk, A.C. McFarlane & L. Weisaeth. New York: Bruner/Mazel, pp. 155–181.

McIntosh, D.N., Silver, R.C. & Wortman, C.B. (1993). Religion's role in adjustment to a negative life event: coping with the loss of a child. *Journal of Personality and Social Psychology*, **65**, 812–821.

Mendes de Leon, C.F., Kasl, S.V. & Jacobs, S. (1994). A prospective study of widowhood and changes in symptoms of depression in a community sample of the elderly. *Psychological Medicine*, **24**, 613–624.

Mollica, R.F., Sarajlic, N., Chernoff, M., Lavelle, J., Vukovic, I.S. & Massagli, M.P. (2001). Longitudinal study of psychiatric symptoms, disability, mortality, and emigration among Bosnian refugees. *Journal of the American Medical Association*, **286**, 546–554.

Murphy, S.A. (1984). Stress levels and health status of victims of a natural disaster. *Research in Nursing and Health*, **7**, 205–215.

Murphy, S.A. (1985). Health and recovery status of victims one and three years following a natural disaster. In *Trauma and Its Wake (Vol. II): Traumatic Stress: Theory, Research, and Intervention*, ed. C.R. Figley. New York: Bruner/Mazel, pp. 133–155.

Norris, F.H. (1992). Epidemiology of trauma: frequency and impact of different potentially traumatic events on different demographic groups. *Journal of Consulting and Clinical Psychology*, **60**, 409–418.

Norris, F.H. & Kaniasty, K. (1996). Received and perceived social support in times of stress: a test of the social support deterioration deterrence model. *Journal of Personality and Social Psychology*, **71**, 498–511.

Norris, F.H., Perilla, J.L., Riad, J.K., Kaniasty, K. & Lavizzo, E.A. (1999). Stability and change in stress, resources, and psychological distress following natural disaster: findings from Hurricane Andrew. *Anxiety, Stress, and Coping*, **12**, 363–396.

Norris, F.H., Friedman, M.J. & Watson, P.J. (2002a). 60,000 disaster victims speak. Part II: Summary and implications of the disaster mental health research. *Psychiatry*, **65**, 240–260.

Norris, F.H., Friedman, M.J., Watson, P.J., Byrne, C.M., Diaz, E. & Kaniasty, K. (2002b). 60,000 disaster victims speak. Part 1: An empirical review of the empirical literature, 1981–2001. *Psychiatry*, **65**, 207–235.

North, C.S. & Pfefferbaum, B. (2002). Research on the mental health effects of terrorism. *Journal of the American Medical Association*, **288**, 633–636.

North, C.S., Smith, E.M. & Spitznagel, E.L. (1997). One-year follow-up of survivors of a mass shooting. *American Journal of Psychiatry*, **154**, 1696–1702.

North, C.S., Nixon, S.J., Shariat, S., Mallonee, S., McMillen, J.C., Spitznagel, E.L. & Smith, E.M. (1999). Psychiatric disorders among survivors of the Oklahoma City bombing. *Journal of the American Medical Association*, **282**, 755–762.

North, C.S., Spitznagel, E.L. & Smith, E. (2001). A prospective study of coping after exposure to a mass murder episode. *Annals of Clinical Psychiatry*, **23**, 81–87.

Pennebaker, J.W. (1989). Confession, inhibition, and disease. In *Advances in Experimental Social Psychology*, Vol. 22, ed. L. Berkowitz. San Diego, CA: Academic Press, pp. 211–244.

Pritchard, M.E. & McIntosh, D.N. (2003). What predicts adjustment among law students? A longitudinal panel study. *Journal of Social Psychology*, **143**, 727–745.

Reifman, A., McIntosh, D.N. & Ellsworth, P.C. (2000). Depression and affect among law students during law school: a longitudinal study. *Journal of Emotional Abuse*, **2**, 93–106.

Robins, L.N., Helzer, J.E., Croughan, J., Williams, J.B.W. & Spitzer, R.L. (1981). *NIMH Diagnostic Interview Schedule: Version III*. Rockville, MD: National Institute of Mental Health.

Sarason, B.R., Sarason, I.G. & Gurung, R.A.R. (1997). Close personal relationships and health outcomes: a key to the role of social support. In *Handbook of Personal Relationships: Theory, Research and Interventions* (2nd ed.), ed. S. Duck. New York: John Wiley & Sons, pp. 547–573.

Schlenger, W.E., Caddell, J.M., Ebert, L., Jordan, B.K., Rourke, K.M., Wilson, D., Thalji, L., Dennis, J.M., Fairbank, J.A. & Kulka, R.A. (2002). Psychological reactions to terrorist attacks: findings from the National Study of Americans' Reactions to September 11. *Journal of the American Medical Association*, **288**, 1235–1244.

Schuster, M.A., Stein, B.D., Jaycox, L.H., Collins, R.L., Marshall, G.N., Elliott, M.N., Zhou, A.J., Kanouse, D.E., Morrison, J.L. & Berry, S.H. (2001). A national survey of stress reactions after the September 11, 2001 terrorist attacks. *New England Journal of Medicine*, **345**, 1507–1512.

Shalev, A.Y., Peri, T., Canetti, L. & Schreiber, S. (1996). Predictors of PTSD in injured trauma survivors: a prospective study. *American Journal of Psychiatry*, **153**, 219–225.

Silver, R.C., Holman, E.A., McIntosh, D.N., Poulin, M. & Gil Rivas, V. (2002). Nationwide longitudinal study of psychological responses to September 11. *Journal of the American Medical Association*, **288**, 1235–1244.

Silver, R.C., Holman, E.A. & Gil-Rivas, V. (submitted for publication). Social responses to ventilation following traumatic life events.

Silver, R.L. & Wortman, C.B. (1980). Coping with undesirable life events. In *Human Helplessness: Theory and Applications*, eds. J. Garber & M.E.P. Seligman. New York: Academic Press, pp. 279–340.

Silver, R.L., Boon, C. & Stones, M. (1983). Searching for meaning in misfortune: making sense of incest. *Journal of Social Issues*, **39**(2), 81–102.

Steinglass, P., Weisstub, E. & De-Nour, A.K. (1988). Perceived personal networks as mediators of stress reactions. *American Journal of Psychiatry*, **145**, 1259–1264.

Tait, R. & Silver, R.C. (1989). Coming to terms with major negative life events. In *Unintended Thought*, eds. J.S. Uleman & J.A. Bargh. New York: Guilford, pp. 351–382.

Taylor, S.E., Klein, L.C., Lewis, B.P., Gruenewald, T.L., Gurung, R.A. & Updegraff, J.A. (2000). Biobehavioral responses to stress in females: tend-and-befriend, not fight or flight. *Psychological Review*, **107**, 411–429.

Terr, L.C. (1983). Time sense following psychic trauma: a clinical study of ten adults and twenty children. *American Journal of Orthopsychiatry*, **53**, 244–261.

Turner, R.J. & Lloyd, D.A. (1995). Lifetime traumas and mental health: the significance of cumulative adversity. *Journal of Health and Social Behavior*, **36**, 360–376.

US Census Bureau (2001). Current Population Survey. Available at http://www.census.gov. Accessed September 2001.

US Census Bureau (2002). Current Population Survey. Available at http://www.census.gov. Accessed December 2002.

van der Kolk, B.A. (1996). The complexity of adaptation to trauma: self-regulation, stimulus discrimination, and characterological development. In *Traumatic Stress: The Effects of Overwhelming Experience on Mind, Body, and Society*, eds. B.A. van der Kolk, A.C. McFarlane & L. Weisaeth. New York: Bruner/Mazel, pp. 182–213.

Weathers, F.W., Litz, B.T., Herman, D.S., Huska, J.A. & Keane, T.M. (1993). *The PTSD Checklist: Reliability, Validity, and Diagnostic Utility*. Paper presented at the *Meeting of the International Society for Traumatic Stress Studies*, San Antonio, TX, October 1993.

Weisenberg, M., Schwarzwald, S., Waysman, M., Solomon, Z. & Klingman, A. (1993). Coping of school-age children in the sealed room during scud missile bombardment and post-war stress reactions. *Journal of Consulting and Clinical Psychology*, **61**, 462–467.

Weiss, D.S. & Marmar, C.R. (1997). The Impact of Event Scale – Revised. In *Assessing Psychological Trauma and PTSD*, eds. J.P. Wilson & T.M. Keane. New York: Guilford, pp. 399–411.

Wortman, C.B. & Silver, R.C. (1989). The myths of coping with loss. *Journal of Consulting and Clinical Psychology*, **57**, 349–357.

Wortman, C.B. & Silver, R.C. (2001). The myths of coping with loss revisited. In *Handbook of Bereavement Research*, eds. M.S. Stroebe, R.O. Hansson, W. Stroebe & H. Schut. Washington, DC: American Psychological Association, pp. 405–429.

Yehuda, R. (2002). Post-traumatic stress disorder. *New England Journal of Medicine*, **346**, 108–114.

Yule, W., Bolton, D., O'Ryan, D. & Nurrish, J. (2000). The long-term psychological effects of a disaster experienced in adolescence. I: Incidence and course of PTSD. *Journal of Child Psychology and Psychiatry and Allied Disciplines*, **41**, 503–511.

5

An epidemiological response to disaster: the post-9/11 psychological needs assessment of New York City public school students

Christina W. Hoven, Donald J. Mandell, Cristiane S. Duarte, Ping Wu and Vincent Giordano

Introduction

American school texts, quoting Emerson's *Concord Hymn* (1837), tell us that the rifles fired at Lexington and Concord, Massachusetts, in 1775 were "the shot heard round the world." In a more literal sense, given the virtually instantaneous transmission of current news events, September 11, 2001 has become for adults and children worldwide just such a universally acknowledged point of reference. The attack on the World Trade Center (WTC) towers in the financial center of New York City on September 11th occurred in the morning rush hours of a bright sunny September day, at which time hundreds of thousands of persons near to or inside the WTC were either already at work, at school, or still on their way. Because September 11th was, and probably will remain, a defining moment in American history, it is important to understand how society's leading agencies responded to this event and how and why they took specific actions. From such analyses we can better prepare for future disasters, and, thus, be in a better position to meet the psychological needs of those most affected in such times. In this chapter, we outline the background, development and major findings of the New York City Board of Education's (NYC BOE) epidemiological study of the psychological effects of September 11 on a representative sample of 8236 4th–12th grade public school students.

Without question, it was immediately understood that the terrorist attacks on September 11th had the potential to have a great psychological impact on children. But before comprehensive, long-term interventions could be planned and implemented, the precise extent and manifestations of these mental health effects needed to be assessed. Moreover, the NYC child mental health infrastructure had not previously been tested in addressing children's needs in a crisis of such magnitude. The needs of different populations of children (e.g., age, gender, race/ethnicity, language, culture, etc.), the degree of both direct and indirect exposure experienced, and the level of resources available for addressing the potential mental health sequelae, were all unknown in the immediate aftermath of September 11th. Hence, a major goal of this chapter is to examine the events and processes by which the NYC BOE 9/11 study was fashioned, how it evolved, and how it was ultimately influential in garnering intervention sponsors and key financial contributors, as well as a brief overview of the study's findings which so influenced subsequent policy.

Background

Prior to September 11, 2001, disaster literature chiefly focused on mental health sequelae in adult populations, in the aftermath of such natural disasters as earthquakes, floods, fires, tornadoes, and hurricanes. A relatively small body of literature revealed that children were also at high risk for developing mental health problems following large-scale disasters (Garmezy & Rutter, 1983; Pynoos *et al.*, 1987a; Shannon *et al.*, 1994; Goenjian *et al.*, 2001). These important works informed and influenced our thinking and were helpful in the design and planning phase of the NYC BOE study. The following provides a brief overview of other studies that informed the NYC BOE investigation, as well as more recent findings that have helped to guide the interpretation of our findings.

Pre-9/11 studies of psychopathological sequelae in children in the aftermath of disasters were mostly limited to measuring post-traumatic stress disorder (PTSD) and occassionally depression (Pynoos *et al.*, 1987a; Shannon *et al.*, 1994; Sack *et al.*, 1999; Bolton *et al.*, 2000; Vizek-Vidovic *et al.*, 2000; Goenjian *et al.*, 2001; Rothe *et al.*, 2002). In the first systematic evaluation of PTSD symptoms in children following a disaster, conducted after a school shooting, 60.4% of exposed children presented symptoms consistent with PTSD (Pynoos *et al.*, 1987b). These studies revealed age differences in vulnerability to psychopathology, as well as differences in type and severity of reactions among boys and girls. For example, it was found that preteen girls were more likely than boys to be at risk for developing PTSD (Davis & Siegel, 2000; Qouta *et al.*, 2003).

In the USA before 9/11, the literature about children's reactions to acts of terrorism centered on the 1995 Oklahoma City and the 1993 WTC terror bombings. In the 1995 terrorist bombing of the Murrah Building in Oklahoma City, PTSD reactions were found in 44–49% of children who knew someone killed (Pfefferbaum *et al.*, 1999a). Among 22 children who were evaluated after the WTC bombing in 1993, PTSD reactions were found in 66% of those evaluated after 3 months, with these symptoms persisting in 55% of these children 9 months later (Koplewicz *et al.*, 2002). As each of these investigations was based on convenience samples, rather than on samples representative of the general population, the overall rates of psychopathology in the larger population could not be determined. Note also that the reported rates in these studies were for assessed reactions or symptoms, not for diagnosed or probable disorder.

Prior studies showed that being in geographic proximity to the site of a disaster is associated with risk for PTSD in children (Dyregrov *et al.*, 2000; Kitayama *et al.*, 2000; Udwin *et al.*, 2000; Goenjian *et al.*, 2001; Smith *et al.*, 2001; Brener *et al.*, 2002). It has been reported that following natural disasters, children who were present and physically injured developed PTSD (Hsu *et al.*, 2002). Proximity or physical presence, however, may not be the only requirements for developing a post-traumatic reaction; exposure can also be indirect. Factors associated with children who developed PTSD after the Oklahoma terrorist acts included media exposure (Pfefferbaum *et al.*, 2000) and knowing someone who was injured or killed (Pfefferbaum *et al.*, 1999b). PTSD reactions have been observed in children who lost a household family member (Hsu *et al.*, 2002) and also in children living with a parent who survived a disaster but who presented significant post-traumatic symptoms (Stoppelbein & Greening, 2000). Children's reactions following exposure to war were shown to be influenced by other factors, such as lack of resources at home or in the community, and presence of school stressors (Barath, 2002). These studies point to the possible development of PTSD as the result of indirect exposure. An interesting example of the impact of indirect exposure to trauma was that, after the April 1999 Columbine shooting spree, 9th–12th graders throughout the USA reported feeling unsafe (Brener *et al.*, 2002). Most of these children lived far from Colorado and Columbine High School and experienced no direct exposure to the shooting. Although there was extensive media coverage of Columbine, many children were affected without ever viewing the incident on TV, but simply by learning that the event had occurred. Spree shootings, like Columbine, seem to be particularly effective in creating a general sense of fear, irrespective of the number of individuals wounded or killed (Johnson, 2000). Along the same lines, the 2003 sniper shootings in Washington, DC and in Maryland were also effective in inducing widespread fear (von Drehle *et al.*, 2003).

The effect of media coverage of disasters has also recently been studied. It has been found that exposure to media accounts of terrorist attacks is often associated with the development of psychopathology in children (Pfefferbaum *et al.*, 2003). Saylor *et al.* (2003) surveyed children 1 month after the 9/11 attack, and found that children who viewed Internet reports showing images of death or injury, as well as children who feared that a loved one might have died, experienced a considerable number of PTSD symptoms.

The most recent literature reporting children's reactions to disaster consistently show that the development of PTSD is a complex occurrence, often comorbid with other disorders, and has a tendency to cluster in families. Kolaitis *et al.* (2003) report that 6 months after the 1999 earthquake in Athens, Greece, 78% of elementary school students attending schools in the epicenter of the tremor endorsed severe to mild PTSD symptoms. Moreover, the rate of depression among these children was one third higher compared to a matched group of Greek students from schools not affected by the earthquake. Thus, it is important to note that PTSD is but one of several types of childhood psychopathology that can manifest in reaction to a traumatic event (Hoven *et al.*, 2003).

Prior exposure to traumatic situations is among the factors that influence the development of psychopathology in children (Asarnow *et al.*, 1999; Udwin *et al.*, 2000). Also noteworthy is the finding by Kilic *et al.* (2003) that disasters often affect the mental health status of an entire family. In that study which examined the effects of parental psychopathology and family functioning on child psychopathology 6 months after an earthquake in Bolu, Turkey, it was found that severity of PTSD in children was mainly affected by the presence of PTSD and depression in the father, particularly when the father's symptoms included detachment and irritability.

Correlatively, there are factors that also enhance resilience and/or impede development of psychopathology. Lahad *et al.* (2000) point out the importance of both community involvement and individual coping mechanisms in preventing the formation of psychopathology. In their chapter, "Coping and Community Resources in Children Facing Disaster," Lahad *et al.* present a model tested on Israeli populations, which emphasizes the salutary effects of individual and community resources in fostering resiliency. Shalev *et al.* (2004) find that both the severity of the trauma and the accessibility of support systems may affect long-term outcome.

A number of recent studies also show that the type of coping mechanism employed by children and adolescents is strongly related to the subsequent development of psychopathology. For example, Bokszczanin and Kaniasty (2002) found that the coping strategy employed by children after severe flooding in Poland served as an intervening variable between exposure to the stressor and subsequent psychological well being. Langley (2003) also addresses the issue of coping and degree of exposure. She found that PTSD in children related to a wildfire disaster varied with coping efficacy and coping strategies.

An important issue is whether the experience of life-threatening events and subsequent development of PTSD results in persistent psychopathology or is generally characterized by a decrease in severity over time. The matter remains controversial. On the one hand, Morgan *et al.* (2003) studied the long-term effects of surviving the 1966 coalmine accident in Wales. The study revisited survivors, aged 4–11 years at the time of the disaster, 33 years after a coal tip cascaded down a mountain, hitting an elementary school and killing 136 of the occupants. Forty-six percent of the survivors had had PTSD at some point since the disaster, and 36 years later, 29% continued to meet diagnostic criteria for current PTSD. Yule *et al.* (2000) also corroborates the possibility of long-term persistence, finding that PTSD symptoms may be exhibited years after the occurrence of a traumatic situation.

On the other hand, a number of older studies demonstrate that symptoms may decrease over time. For example, children who survived the Buffalo Creek dam collapse in 1972 were found to have fewer psychiatric symptoms of anxiety, belligerence, and agitation when they were reevaluated 17 years post-disaster (Green *et al.*, 1994). Similarly, in a study of Cambodian refugee trauma, re-interviewed children were found to still have PTSD, but the symptoms appeared less severe (Sack *et al.*, 1993).

Although a few pre-9/11 post-disaster studies assessed disorders other than PTSD and depression, most were influenced by the assumption that these two disorders would be the only important forms of psychopathology to emerge after a disaster and thus other diagnoses have not been well studied. Following the events of September 11, 2001, the NYC BOE offered an opportunity to go beyond this assumption.

NYC BOE response to September 11, 2001

There were many heroes on 9/11, including many individuals associated with the NYC BOE. For example, Ada Dolch, Principal of the High School for Leadership and Public Service, located in the Ground Zero Area (GZA), led students out from school and across the Brooklyn Bridge at the very time she fearfully anticipated that her own sister, Wendy Dolch, had died. Scarlet Tavares, a student in attendance at that school on that day, went on to testify before the US Senate's Health, Education, Labor and Pensions Committee and Senators Hillary Rodham Clinton and Jon Corzine about her own and other's experiences on 9/11 and to recount the heroism of Ada Dolch, whose sister did indeed die in the attack (Rosner & Markowitz, 2003; Degnan *et al.*, 2004).

For the NYC BOE, the drama of the WTC attack, just days after the opening of the fall semester, was a challenge of unprecedented magnitude. With nearly 1.2 million students, the NYC public school system is the largest in the USA, and probably the most racially and ethnically diverse anywhere. Evacuating students from school buildings in close proximity to the WTC and leading them to safety was a daunting challenge. Furthermore, because 750,000 students reached school each day by means of public transportation (especially to Manhattan schools), students from each of the five boroughs were caught in the general travel nightmare that ensued. Fortunately, prior to September 11, 2001, each of the more than 1,100 NYC schools was required to have a plan in place to deal professionally and compassionately with its students to minimize the confusion expected from a calamitous event. Without a doubt, nothing of the magnitude of September 11th had been anticipated.

The NYC BOE, however, met the unanticipated challenges on that day with superb professionalism (Degnan *et al.*, 2004). Immediately, messages of information, instructions, and assurance emanated from the Chancellor's office, and soon after the planes struck the WTC towers superintendents and principals addressed teachers and staff, sending out guidelines provided by leading psychological and psychiatric associations on how and what to convey to students in the aftermath of disaster. Strict rules to insulate and protect students from excessive journalistic interference were also immediately put into place, as parents, teachers, and students seized the opportunity to collaboratively sort out educational alternatives, such as moving schools *en masse* or by working together to explore bringing individual students back to neighborhood schools.

As would be expected, the NYC BOE commissioned a number of 9/11-related reports. As the potential mental health effects of September 11th on the school children of NYC were of immediate and compelling interest to the NYC BOE, Dr. Michael Cohen of Applied Research and Consulting (ARC), LLC was, within days, commissioned to conduct a survey of the psychological effects of 9/11 on students attending school in the GZA. ARC had a long history of doing targeted contract work for the BOE and was a natural choice to conduct such a study. ARC prepared a questionnaire to be administered to approximately 3000 students attending schools located in the immediate vicinity of the WTC, probing mostly for attitudes and feelings of loss. The instrument was intended to provide information about the general effect of the 9/11 WTC attack. Although informative, that study, as planned, would not have yielded an overall assessment of the extent of probable psychiatric disorders, level of functional impairment or identified variations in types of exposures and vulnerabilities among students throughout the five boroughs of New York City. Perhaps, most importantly, the study design would not have yielded a representative sample and thus it would not have been possible to extrapolate from that study's findings to the status of non-survey participant students.

Partnership for recovery of New York City schools

Prior research on the range of the potential effects of trauma on children's mental health was limited, and NYC lacked an adequate child mental health strategy to respond to a crisis of this proportion. Therefore, the NYC BOE, in conjunction with the Children's Mental Health Alliance, a private, non-profit agency in New York City, immediately set up the Partnership for the Recovery of NYC schools, with Dr. Pamela Cantor, a child psychiatrist, at its helm. The purpose of the Partnership was to collectively explore all avenues to assist the NYC BOE in its effort to identify and meet the psychological needs of NYC's public school students. Participating in the Partnership, with the support of Chancellor Harold Levy, were the BOE's leaders, including Deputy Chancellor Dr. Judith Rizzo; Ms. Francine Goldstein, Chief Executive for School Programs and Student Services Director; Mr. Vincent Giordano, Executive Director for School Programs and Student Services; Dr. Lori Mei, Director, Student Information; and Ms. Linda Weirmkoff, Deputy Superintendent, Special Education. Other Partnership members included psychiatrists Dr. Robert Abramovitz, Jewish Board of Family Services; Dr. Harold Koplowitz, New York University Child Study Center; and Dr. Reese Abright, St. Vincent's Hospital and Medical Center, heads of the three largest child mental health services in the GZA. Each of these three psychiatrists had been actively involved in rendering assistance in the GZA starting on 9/11. In the weeks that followed, they had also facilitated support for parents, teachers, and children returning to evacuated schools and subsequently helped to create a new curriculum that would enhance the ability of mental health professionals in school settings to address the needs of affected children. A number of other individuals representing a range of expertise and resources were also invited to join the Partnership, including Dr. Steven Marans from the Yale Child Study Center, who would arrange for the training of school personnel in every district in each of the five boroughs. Those training sessions were designed to improve the ability of staff to recognize and deal with mental health problems (especially PTSD) *in situ*, and to learn how best to refer children in need.

A major purpose of the Partnership was not only to help guide the provision of immediate assistance for psychological stress, but also to facilitate understanding of the scope of mental health needs of students consequent to 9/11. Hence, later in September 2001, upon the recommendation of Dr. Cantor, the Partnership enlisted the assistance of Lawrence Aber, PhD and Christina Hoven, DrPH to provide scientific oversight of the study already commissioned by the BOE to be conducted by ARC. Dr. Aber assumed the role of primary consultant to Dr. Cantor, focusing on policy and fundraising for mental health services, while Dr. Hoven, a child psychiatric epidemiologist, assumed the role of principal investigator of what quickly became a new NYC BOE study. Both Drs. Hoven and Aber were enlisted from the Mailman School of Public Health, Columbia University. Dr. Hoven also represented New York State Psychiatric Institute (NYSPI), where she was already working on an Office of Mental Health appointed September 11th Task Force, headed by Dr. Ezra Susser, to determine a methodology to predict the effect of 9/11 on the residents of New York State. Although the initial charge to Dr. Hoven by the NYC BOE and the

Partnership was to develop and implement a study that would reveal the scope and breadth of mental health needs of NYC public school children in the GZA subsequent to 9/11, she quickly determined that a citywide assessment would be required to adequately understand the mental health sequelae in NYC's school population. The rationale for conducting a citywide assessment was presented to the BOE leadership, which agreed to void the existing ARC contract and to support a citywide epidemiological investigation. Consequently, ARC received a new contract through which it would be compensated additionally for the extra data collection required for this new, citywide Mental Health Needs Assessment.

To effectively design the Needs Assessment, advice from all members of the Partnership was sought. Additionally, scientists and staff from the Mailman School Public Health of Columbia University, the NYSPI and other institutions were consulted to help develop a multi-faceted instrument and to expedite the process of launching a study which would truly portray the mental health status of NYC school children 6 months after 9/11. At Columbia University and the NYSPI, Drs. Hector Bird, Patricia Cohen, Cristiane Duarte, Renee Goodwin, Donald Mandell, and Ping Wu were particularly important in helping to select, review, and/or design instrumentation, with Dr. Chris Lucas providing the diagnostic screening measure (Lucas *et al.*, 2001). Dr. Fan Bin was recruited to provide data management and Mr. George Musa to work with the Centers for Disease Control and Prevention (CDC) for geographic consultation, monitoring, and sampling compliance. Ms. Judith Wicks contributed to instrument development and provided training of ARC interviewers.

Dr. Martin Frankel of the City University of New York and Dr. Patricia Cohen of Columbia University and the NYSPI generously provided the initial consultation concerning possible sampling parameters. Dr. Hoven subsequently requested and received the support and collaboration of the US CDC, which assigned Drs. Victor Balaban and Bradford Woodruff to the project. Their contribution was critical in ultimately fashioning the study's sampling design. Advice and consultation on the survey instrument was also sought and was enthusiastically provided by many individuals, such as Drs. Steven Marans of the National Center for Children Exposed to Violence, Yale University; Betty Pfefferbaum of the University of Oklahoma College of Medicine; Elissa Brown of the New York University Child Study Center; Robert Pynoos, William Saltzman, and Alan Steinberg of the National Child Traumatic Stress Network, UCLA; Ezra Susser of the Departments of Epidemiology and Psychiatry, Columbia University and the NYSPI; Claude Chemtob of the National Center for Post-Traumatic Stress Disorder, Pacific Island Division, Honolulu; and others, too numerous to mention. Dr. Michael Cohen, Ms. Victoria Francis, Ms. Nellie Gregorian, and Mr. Chris Bumcrot of ARC (currently known as the Michael Cohen Group) had the critical responsibility for fielding the study in the schools. Throughout the planning and implementation phases they provided insight and advice, but most importantly, they provided the level of collaboration required to guarantee the study's scientific integrity. From all advisors and collaborators, there was a genuine sense of commitment, collegiality, and generosity that ultimately determined the success of the study. Except for tasks performed by ARC, all work was provided *pro bono*. The US Department of Education School Emergency Response to Violence (SERV) Project funded the data collection, through monies provided to the NYC BOE as a result of 9/11.

Background to the needs assessment

The first responsibility when considering the best design for the NYC BOE Study was to thoroughly review the literature and to speak with experts in the assessment of childhood psychopathology following a disaster. Having done this, it became apparent that most of the studies previously launched in the aftermath of natural and human-influenced disasters failed to reveal all that they might have, had they been planned and conducted from a broad epidemiological perspective. Such an approach was particularly relevant for the proposed investigation, as it was not being conducted for the purpose of case finding, the reason for most previous post-disaster assessments. Additionally, research into the effects of 9/11 on children in NYC posed an unprecedented opportunity to consider a number of possible disorders, as well as a range of contextual factors, such as loss, level of personal and family exposure, prior exposure to traumatic events, media exposure, family member's involvement with rescue efforts, parental occupation, coexisting medical conditions, coping practices, school location vs. home location, etc., which might be associated with the mental health effects of 9/11.

At the outset of the planning process, it was realized that merely surveying students in schools that were situated in close proximity to the WTC would (1) fail to capture a broad representation of all students potentially affected by the attack and (2) fail to assess the effects felt by students who were not themselves in the eye of the attack, but who nonetheless suffered from loss of family or friends, or endured the sting of discrimination or changed economic condition. The NYC public school system is responsible for nearly 1.2 million students enrolled in both typical comprehensive schools and a host of schools with special curricula to which students may travel from any of the five boroughs of New York City. Therefore, to sample exclusively from GZA would be myopic.

The challenge, then, was to sample not only those children attending schools in the GZA or in other high impact areas presumed to be heavily affected by 9/11, but also to survey a probability sample of all NYC public school children. Our interest was to determine the level of psychopathology among NYC public school children

6 months after 9/11, so as to produce an accurate estimate of the kind and quantity of required ameliorative services: including where such services were needed and by whom. Our population of interest, therefore, was not only the students who themselves witnessed the attack in the GZA, but all students, including those whose family members may have been among the hundreds of thousands of workers who commuted to the GZA daily, who worked as a first responder, who were evacuated from the WTC towers, who themselves became absorbed in media coverage of the event, or who simply were present in NYC on September 11, 2001.

Study considerations

In addition to those students potentially at higher risk because of proximity to the attack or familial relationship to those immediately affected, the study team projected that particular areas and special populations would also potentially have a greater chance of being affected by the events of 9/11. For example, a disproportionate number of firemen resided in the Borough of Staten Island. Since loss of life was particularly high among firefighting personnel, Staten Island was an area to be over sampled. Another population at elevated risk was the residents of the area of Brooklyn along the East River facing the WTC, who could have had a direct view of the attack and of its aftermath. In addition, on November 12, 2001, there was the crash in Belle Harbor, Queens, of American Airlines flight No. 587 carrying passengers to the Dominican Republic. This crash was, at first, also thought to be related to terrorism and caused high levels of stress in both the section of Queens (Belle Harbor) where the crash occurred, as well as in the Washington Heights section of Manhattan, where many relatives of those killed in the crash resided or had immediate family.

Selecting the sample

It was determined that students below grade 4 would require a different assessment methodology, therefore the target group for this Needs Assessment were students enrolled in grades 4–12 (approximately 716,189 youth). Based on the previously described considerations, the sampling parameters were determined with assistance from the US CDC. Each of the 1,193 schools in the public school system with grade-eligible students was assigned to one of three sampling strata (see Figure 5.1). Stratum 1, GZA, consisted of the 15 grade-eligible schools located in the immediate vicinity of the WTC, including elementary, middle, and high schools. Stratum 2, High Risk Areas, included schools where students were considered to be at elevated risk due to family exposure, geography or other factors. This stratum consisted of

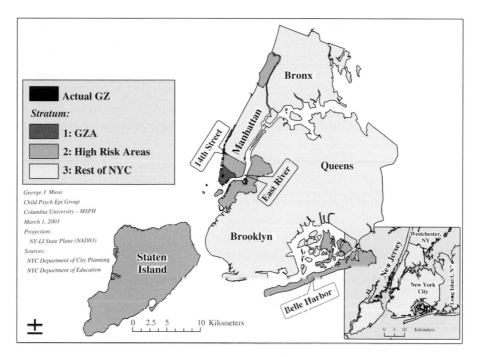

Figure 5.1   New York City Department of Education 9/11 Survey Strata. (*Modified from* Hoven *et al.*, 2005. Copyright © (2005), American Medical Association. All rights reserved.)

schools located in Manhattan above the GZA and below 14th Street; in Brooklyn in the area along the East River facing the WTC; Staten Island; Belle Harbor, Queens; and Washington Heights, Manhattan. The purpose of this stratum was to guarantee that these populations would be represented in sufficient numbers in the sample. Stratum 3 consisted of all other grade-eligible public schools located throughout NYC (excluding District 75 – special education). Mainstreamed special education students were eligible for selection. Details of the study sampling procedures are described elsewhere (Hoven *et al.*, 2002a; Hoven *et al.*, 2003; Hoven *et al.*, 2005).

The sampling plan was designed to allow for the study estimates, after being appropriately weighted, to truly represent the entire NYC school population of students in grades 4–12. The resulting representative sample consisted of 8,236 students in grades 4–12, drawn from 94 schools, selected randomly, proportional to school size, except in the GZA, where there was an effort to recruit all grade eligible schools. In Strata 2 and 3, three classrooms were randomly selected in each school, while the method was simple random selection of classrooms in in all grade-eligible GZA schools (Hoven *et al.*, 2002a; Hoven *et al.*, 2003; Hoven *et al.*, 2005).

The survey instrument

The primary goal of this study was to assess how many children in New York City public schools, as a result of the 9/11 attacks on the WTC, had a psychological reaction (probable psychiatric disorder) that included a negative impact on their daily functioning. Furthermore, we wished to determine how many children were exposed to the effects of the 9/11 attacks, either because they were physically exposed or because one of their family members had been exposed. We were also interested in identifying specific risk factors that could help school authorities and mental health workers recognize children with the highest need for mental health services. It was expected that the outcome of this research would reveal current mental health service need and utilization after the attack of 9/11, as well as the geographic distribution of these effects.

After careful review of the disaster literature and thoughtful consideration of which psychiatric disorders and associated factors should be assessed in the aftermath of this particular event, the NYC WTC BOE Needs Assessment Questionnaire was constructed (Hoven *et al.*, 2002b). In addition to assessing selected probable psychiatric disorders, this questionnaire was designed to elucidate a range of putative associated factors, such as demographics, health problems, discrimination, service need and utilization, school performance, coping practices, health status and conditions, support, home environment, safety issues, parental monitoring, and students' perspectives on the future. Information about different types of exposure to the 9/11 attack was also included, such as personal physical exposure, family exposure, and media use, as well as previous exposure to other traumatic situations.

Eight probable psychiatric disorders were identified as important to assess 6 months after the attack: PTSD, major depression, generalized anxiety, separation anxiety, panic disorder, agoraphobia, conduct disorder, and alcohol abuse/dependence. The assessment employed the Diagnostic Interview Schedule for Children (DISC) Diagnostic Predictive Scales (DPS; Lucas *et al.*, 2001), a screening measure derived from the National Institute of Mental Health (NIMH) DISC Version IV(DISC IV; Shaffer *et al.*, 2000), a structured diagnostic interview for children. The items in the DPS were derived by secondary analysis of a series of large data sets from studies containing DISC symptom, diagnostic, and impairment information. The screening performance of the DPS had been calculated in separate samples from those used for the screen's derivation and was also calculated separately for clinical and community, non-referred samples. DISC questions that were not originally part of the DPS major depression and conduct disorder scales were substituted for those addressing suicidal and criminal behavior, at the request of the BOE. The new items selected yielded the same overall psychometrics for each of these two disorders. For

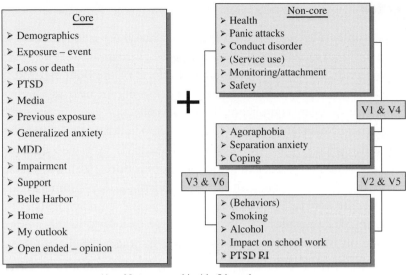

( ) = Not measured in 4th–5th grades

Figure 5.2   Survey measures: the WTC NYC student survey (Hoven *et al.*, 2002b).

the disorders assessed in this study, a test of the DPS in a community sample, showed acceptable psychometric properties. The DPS also includes a measure of children's impairment (seven global questions derived from the DISC), which is consistent with the Diagnostic and Statistical Manual for Mental Disorders-IV (DSM-IV) criteria (American Psychiatric Association, 1994) and is optimally included in epidemiological assessments of childhood psychiatric disorders, combined with symptoms, to define as a probable case (Bird *et al.*, 2000). As the DPS is a screening measure, psychiatric disorders identified in this Needs Assessment were to be considered "probable" disorders.

Because the NYC BOE allowed one class period (less than 1 hour) for the assessment, the full complement of desired questions could not be administered in the allotted time. Therefore, we decided upon a "planned-missing" design (see Figure 5.2) in which there was a core set of questions, and subgroups of non-core questions, only two-thirds of which would be combined with the core (Graham *et al.*, 1996; Schafer & Graham, 2002). This resulted in two of the three non-core sections (versions 1–3) plus the core section being randomly administered to students in grades 6–12. Similarly, with slightly modified (shorter) non-core sections, two of the three non-core sections (versions 4–6) plus the core were randomly administered in grades 4–5 (see Figure 5.2). This strategy allowed us to subsequently impute the missing information by applying the appropriate statistical techniques.

Data collection

Six months after September 11th, a time when most school officials were still trying to regain focus, it would have been easier for schools to refuse participation in this survey. Fortunately, the combined efforts of the BOE and ARC persisted in conveying the rationale that was key to obtaining the necessary individual school access and student compliance. In the data collection phase, it was the staff of ARC, especially Nellie Gregorian and Victoria Francis who coordinated the field work, and the leadership of Mr. Giordano of the NYC BOE who facilitated access to school superintendents and principals. These efforts permitted this study to proceed in a timely fashion, with excellent student participation rates.

All data were collected during a 6-week period from late January through early March 2002. In grades 6–12 the different versions (1–3) of the questionnaire were randomly distributed to students, whereas in grades 4–5 the random distribution of versions (4–6) was by classroom, as in these grades the questions were read aloud to students as they marked their responses. In grades 6–12, students read and marked their own questionnaires. In all instances, at least one monitor and the teacher were present during the survey administration to explain procedures and to answer questions.

Compliance

In general, school, parent, and student compliance with the Needs Assessment was excellent. However, school compliance in Stratum 1 was only 60%, resulting in an under representation of 4th–5th graders from that area. Perhaps, as might be expected, elementary school principals in the GZA who refused participation frequently noted that in their opinion it was better for the students to focus on schoolwork, not the events of September 11th. Strata 2 and 3 had 87% school compliance. The student response rate in Stratum 1 ($N = 2,044$) was 92.6% without absences (80.3% with absences); Stratum 2 ($N = 2,084$) was 88.1% without absences (76.7% with absences); Stratum 3 ($N = 4,138$) was 90.6% without absences (79.5% with absences). Absences during the Needs Assessment were consistent with non-survey absentee rates, so there is no reason to assume that students avoided school or that parents kept them home to avoid survey participation.

Approvals

Immediately following September 11th the NYC BOE's Institutional Review Board (IRB) decided to exercise extreme caution before allowing any school-based studies to occur. It was decided that this investigation would be the only assessment of students allowed to go forward, with any pending investigations or new requests delayed or refused.

This study was carried out in full compliance with all IRB requirements. Participation in the Needs Assessment was anonymous. Active, signed consent was obtained for students in grades 4–5 while parental notification, with an option to refuse, was employed for parents of students in grades 6–12. All students had the option to refuse participation at the time of the survey. Before the study was initiated, the NYC BOE IRB and the Columbia University and the NYSPI IRB approved the survey's methods and consent procedures. Also, the NYS Office of Mental Health, Disaster Research Review Committee for WTC-related Research reviewed and approved all aspects of the participation of Columbia University and the NYSPI investigators and staff.

Overview of initial findings

Prior to conducting in-depth analyses of these data, they were first compared to the entire BOE body student demographics for grades 4–12. Table 5.1 demonstrates how well the study's sample, drawn randomly from schools and classrooms as described earlier, matched the actual NYC public school student "population,"

Table 5.1. Socio-demographics: New York City public school students and survey sample, grades 4–12 (N = 8236)

	Sample size (unweighted)	Weighted percentage (SE)	NYC public schools grades 4–12[a]
Grade group			
4–5	1245	25.3 (9.6)	24.0
6–8	2924	33.7 (9.1)	34.4
9–12	4067	41.0 (10.0)	41.5
Gender (female)	4316	53.1 (2.8)	50.6
Race/ethnicity[b]			
African-Americans	1855	27.9 (5.3)	34.6
Latinos	2936	40.2 (4.4)	36.3
Whites	1489	13.4 (3.3)	15.8
Asians	1552	12.8 (3.2)	13.0
Mixed/others	404	5.7 (0.8)	0.3

[a]*Source*: www.nycenet.edu/Administration/Offices/Stats/Register/RegByEthnGndrJForm
[b]The NYC BOE used US Census 1990 race/ethnicity categories that does not include "mixed race." The "other" group reported by the BOE is Native American (0.3%). The study reported on here used US Census 2000 race/ethnicity categories and allows for mixed race. (*Modified from* Hoven *et al.*, 2005. Copyright © (2005), American Medical Association. All rights reserved.)

by grade group, gender, and race/ethnicity (with the exception of African-Americans), according to the NYC BOE statistics at the time of the Needs Assessment.

Our data corroborated the notion that children could be exposed to the WTC attack in several ways, besides being in a school in the GZA. The different types of exposure experienced by children in the GZA (Stratum 1) or in the rest of the city (Stratum 2 and 3) on September 11, 2001, are displayed in Table 5.2. As noted, although most children (81%) in the GZA were directly exposed to the attack, almost one quarter (24%) of the children in the rest of the city were similarly exposed. Considering family exposure, more family members of children going to

Table 5.2. Different types of exposures experienced by NYC public school children (grades 4–12) assessed 6 months after September 11, 2001 (*N* = 8,236)

Exposures	Total (%)	GZA (%)	Rest of the city (%)	*p*
Direct (two or more)	24.56	80.83	23.83	<0.0001
Personally witnessed the attack	7.56	55.94	6.93	<0.0001
Hurt in the attack	3.81	2.69	3.83	0.1695
In or near the cloud of dust and smoke	10.03	66.11	9.30	<0.0001
Evacuated to safety	31.71	88.07	30.97	<0.0001
Extremely worried about the safety of someone she/he love	47.91	37.31	48.03	0.0008
Family (any)	12.51	8.57	12.56	0.0006
Family member died	3.53	2.58	3.54	0.1184
Family member was hurt	3.89	2.24	3.91	0.0042
Family member escaped unhurt	15.81	11.20	15.87	0.0001
Television use (a lot)	63.35	60.66	63.38	0.3803
Belle Harbor plane crash	2.88	1.59	2.90	0.0582
Prior to 9/11 (ever, two or more)	30.60	22.11	30.71	0.0011
Badly hurt/killed in a violent/ accidental situation				
Self	14.28	9.91	14.34	0.0004
Close friend	25.74	20.88	25.80	0.0470
Family	24.99	17.90	25.08	0.0019
Seen anyone killed/seriously injured	35.35	26.45	35.46	0.0009
Lived in another country during a war	4.89	2.89	4.91	0.0080
Been in a big disaster	4.23	3.30	4.25	0.1315

Note: Weighted data; *p* values for Chi-square tests of GZA vs. rest of the city, adjusting for clustering in the sample design.

non-GZA schools were likely to be WTC evacuees. Approximately two-thirds of all the children watched "a lot" of TV about the attack. In addition, more children attending public schools outside the GZA were exposed to the Belle Harbor plane crash, or had had two or more exposures to traumatic events before September 11, 2001.

The primary purpose of this Needs Assessment was to determine if rates of any of the disorders assessed were elevated from expected rates. Table 5.3 shows the prevalence of probable psychiatric disorders in the NYC public school population in grades 4–12, 6 months after September 11, 2001. Unfortunately, a direct comparison with pre-9/11 rates of psychopathology among NYC children and adolescents was not possible, as these data had never been collected. In addition, national data that could provide comparative rates for the most important child psychiatric disorders in the USA did not exist. Fortunately, however, rates for at least some of

Table 5.3. Prevalence of probable mental disorder in grades 4–12, 6-months post-September 11th by exposure level, compared with USA pre-September 11th community rates (*N* = 8236)

Probable disorders[a]	NYC BOE		US community studies age in years (9–17)
	Estimated number of students	Total sample *N* = 8236 (%)	Pre-September 11, 2001 (%)
PTSD	75,916	10.6	3.3[e]
Major depression	58,011	8.1	2.1–5.9[b–e]
Generalized anxiety	73,767	10.3	3.4–5.5[d,e]
Separation anxiety	88,091	12.3	1.7–7.7[b–e]
Panic disorder	62,308	8.7	0.6–4.1[d,e]
Agoraphobia	105,996	14.8	1.3–4.5[b, e]
Any[f] anxiety/depressive	204,829	28.6	~
Conduct disorder	91,672	12.8	3.9–11.2[c–e]
Alcohol abuse/ dependence (6–12)	24,461	4.5	0.9–2.2[b,d,e]

Weighted data:

[a]Reported rates are with impairment, except for alcohol and conduct disorder.

[b]Bird *et al.* (1988); DSM III; 4–16 years; DISC 2 0; *N* = 777 (386).

[c]Cohen *et al.* (1993); DSM-III-R; 9–18 years; DISC 1 0; *N* = 776.

[d]Shaffer *et al.* (1996); DSM-III-R; 9–17 years; DISC 2 3; *N* = 356.

[e]Lucas *et al.* (2002), DPS validation report; DSM-IV; 9–17 years; DPS; *N* = 687; DISC IV; *N* = 191.

[f]Any is limited to PTSD, major depression, generalized anxiety, separation anxiety, panic, and agoraphobia.

(*Modified from* Hoven *et al.*, 2005. Copyright © (2005), American Medical Association. All rights reserved.)

Table 5.4. Prevalence of probable mental disorder by gender and grade group, New York City public school children 6 months after September 11th (*N* = 8236)

Probable disorders	Gender		Grade group		
	Girls (%)	Boys (%)	4–5 (%)	6–8 (%)	9–12 (%)
PTSD	13.3	7.4	20.1	9.1	5.9
Major depression	10.4	5.5	7.3	6.8	9.6
Generalized anxiety	12.8	7.5	10.9	9.2	10.8
Separation anxiety	16.0	8.2	20.2	12.1	7.6
Panic disorder	11.6	5.4	10.9	8.2	7.8
Agoraphobia	20.0	9.0	24.1	12.7	10.9
Any[a] anxious/depressive	34.7	21.8	34.1	27.8	26.0
Conduct disorder	10.6	15.3	9.6	12.4	15.1
Alcohol abuse/dependence (6–12)	4.3	4.8	–	1.8	6.8

Weighted data:

[a]Any is limited to PTSD, major depression, generalized anxiety, separation anxiety, panic, and agoraphobia. (*Modified from* Hoven *et al.*, 2005. Copyright © (2005), American Medical Association. All rights reserved.)

the major childhood psychiatric disorders were available from well-designed community studies, conducted using sound methodology, such as Cohen *et al.* (1993), Costello *et al.* (1998), Bird *et al.* (1991), Shaffer *et al.* (1996), and Offord *et al.* (1989, 1996). Note that rates for the disorders assessed in the NYC BOE study are all elevated over what might be expected based on these community studies assessing psychopathology in children of similar ages (9–17 years), prior to September 11, 2001. In fact, each probable disorder assessed in the NYC BOE Needs Assessment is approximately two to three times the expected rate.

The NYC BOE was particularly interested in learning about differences in the need for mental health service intervention among different student groups. According to Table 5.4 there were major differences in the prevalence of psychopathology by disorder, gender, and age groups. PTSD, generalized anxiety disorder, separation anxiety disorder, panic, and agoraphobia, as well as any anxious/depressive disorder, were higher for girls than boys, with the highest rates of probable disorder found in the youngest grade group.

Public health implications

The NYC BOE study demonstrates the need and feasibility of conducting epidemiological research in the aftermath of disasters. As in any carefully designed epidemiological investigation, consideration must be given to the context in which the study will be conducted. For example, this study took place in New York City, with approximately 750,000 children traveling to school through tunnels, over bridges and waterways each day on their way to school. Thus, it was only prudent to include agoraphobia as a disorder of interest. All disasters, however, present unique circumstances and contexts that must shape, not only the immediate interventions, but also the investigative response. Because of the NYC BOE Needs Assessment's inclusiveness and methodological rigor, it has been hailed as a landmark for the new light it has shed on the mental health consequences for children and adolescents in the aftermath of a large-scale disaster. However, until there are more epidemiological studies assessing the disorders included here, as well as other types of psychological impact, prejudging who will be affected with which mental health sequelae will most likely lead to limited, if not inappropriate responses (Costello *et al.*, 2004).

This study also highlights the need to rethink how mental health delivery systems can best reach out to children and adolescents following a disaster. The NYC BOE clearly demonstrates the importance of systematic screening for childhood psychopathology following a disaster. Because the greatest differences in expected levels of probable disorder in this study were found for the internalizing disorders, it is also prudent to consider these findings to be supportive of school-based screening, in general (Hoven *et al.*, 2002a). Specifically, this study also points out the need for improved, ongoing training of teachers and ancillary staff to recognize children with less obvious manifestations of post-disaster psychopathology. This study highlighted the need in NYC schools for strengthening teamwork in multi-component prevention programs for all children citywide. For example, in 2002, guided by the study's results, the BOE collaborated with The New York Academy of Medicine to start the *Moving From Crisis To Hope And Well-Being* Program, designed to train staff and teachers to implement school wide mental and emotional health promotion activities and to teach skills needed to cope, not just with this traumatic experience, but with a wide range of life situations. Developing mental health and mental illness curricula for students in all grades is paramount to engaging students themselves in recognizing when personal behavioral or emotional conditions warrant intervention. Because the general population has now become familiar with the fact that psychological disturbance is not uncommon following a disaster, using disaster-related training and preparation could serve as an opportunity to expand mental health education in general. Such curricula would also help to demystify mental illness and reduce the stigma associated with seeking help.

Another important lesson from this investigation should be an appreciation that proximity to a disaster is not the exclusive factor in determining which populations might be most affected. Failure to consider the larger context, both personal and geographic of those potentially affected by a disaster, inappropriately limits the scope of appropriate response and intervention. Similarly, the role of the media needs to be considered as an important form of exposure following any major disaster, regardless of where in the world the event occurs.

Limitations

It is most unfortunate that this study could only be anonymous and cross-sectional, rather than with full identification and longitudinal. Understandably, immediately after 9/11 there was great concern by the BOE that parents and children already adversely affected by the WTC attack itself should not be inundated with requests for interviews. That decision, which the NYC BOE itself later regretted, meant that we could neither return to the same study participants for follow-up, nor could we cross compare study responses with other NYC BOE data, such as academic performance. It is our hope that lessons learned in this important study, including its limitations, will inform future post-disaster investigations, so that we can better help children in need.

Acknowledgment

Without the NYC-BOE leadership, especially of Ms. Francine Goldstein, M.A., Chief Executive for School Programs and Student Services Director, as well as the superintendents, principals, teachers and, most of all, the students, this study could not have succeeded. We are most appreciative of their helping everyone to better understand the impact of 9/11. The authors also want to thank Ms. Anna Cheung and Ms. Judith Wicks for their assistance and constructive criticism during the preparation of this chapter.

REFERENCES

American Psychiatric Association (1994). *Diagnostic and Statistical Manual of Mental Disorders* (4th ed.). Washington, DC: American Psychiatric Association.

Asarnow, J., Glynn, S., Pynoos, R.S., Nahum, J., Guthrie, D., Cantwell, D.P. & Franklin, B. (1999). When the earth stops shaking: earthquake sequelae among children diagnosed for pre-earthquake psychopathology. *Journal of the American Academy of Child and Adolescent Psychiatry*, **38**, 1016–1023.

Barath, A. (2002). Children's well-being after the war in Kosovo: survey in 2000. *Croatian Medical Journal*, **43**, 199–208.

Bird, H.R., Canino, G., Rubio-Stipec, M., Gould, M.S., Riebra, J., Sesman, M., *et al.* (1988). Estimates of the prevalence of childhood maladjustment in a community survey in Puerto Rico. The use of combined measures. *Archives of General Psychiatry*, **45**, 1120–1126.

Bird, H.R., Gould, M.S., Rubio-Stipec, M., Staghezza, B.M. & Canino, G. (1991). Screening for childhood psychopathology in the community using the child behavior checklist. *Journal of the American Academy of Child and Adolescent Psychiatry*, **30**, 116–123.

Bird, H.R., Davies, M., Fisher, P., Narrow, W.E., Jensen, P.S., Hoven, C.W., Cohen, P. & Dulcan, M. (2000). How specific is specific impairment? *Journal of the American Academy of Child and Adolescent Psychiatry*, **39**, 1182–1189.

Bokszczanin, A. & Kaniasty, K. (2002). The impact of 1977 flood on children and adolescent symptoms of PTSD, depression, and loneliness. The role of coping strategies. *Studia Psychologiczne*, **40**, 21–39.

Bolton, D., O'Ryan, D., Udwin, O., Boyle, S. & Yule, W. (2000). The long-term psychological effects of a disaster experienced in adolescence. II: General psychopathology. *Journal of Child Psychology and Psychiatry, and Allied Disciplines*, **41**, 513–523.

Brener, N.D., Simon, T.R., Anderson, M., Barrios, L.C. & Small, M.L. (2002). Effect of the incident at Columbine on students' violence- and suicide-related behaviors. *American Journal of Preventive Medicine*, **22**, 146–150.

Cohen, P., Cohen, J., Kasen, S., Velez, C.N., Hartmark, C., Johnson, J., Rojas, M., Brook, J. & Streuning, E.L. (1993). An epidemiological study of disorders in late childhood and adolescence. I: Age- and gender-specific prevalence. *Journal of Child Psychology and Psychiatry, and Allied Disciplines*, **34**, 851–867.

Costello, E.J., Messer, S.C., Bird, H.R., Cohen, P. & Reinherz, H.Z. (1998). The prevalence of serious emotional disturbance: a re-analysis of community studies. *Journal of Child and Family Studies*, **7**, 411–432.

Costello, E.J., Erkanli, A., Keeler, G. & Angold, A. (2004). Distant trauma: a prospective study of the effects of September 11th on young adults in North Carolina. *Applied Developmental Science*, **8**, 211–220.

Davis, L. & Siegel, L.J. (2000). Posttraumatic stress disorder in children and adolescents: a review and analysis. *Clinical Child and Family Psychology Review*, **3**, 135–154.

Degnan, A.N., Thomas, G., Markenson, D., Song, Y., Fuller, F. & Redlener, I. (2004). Uncommon sense, uncommon courage: How the New York City school system, its teachers, leadership, and students responded to the terror of September 11. Columbia University, Mailman School of Public Health, New York City, New York.

Dyregrov, A., Gupta, L., Gjestad, R. & Mukanoheli, E. (2000). Trauma exposure and psychological reactions to genocide among Rwandan children. *Journal of Traumatic Stress*, **13**, 3–21.

Garmezy, N. & Rutter, M. (1983). *Stress, Coping, and Development in Children*. New York: McGraw-Hill.

Goenjian, A.K., Molina, L., Steinberg, A.M., Fairbanks, L.A., Alvarez, M.L., Goenjian, H.A., *et al.* (2001). Posttraumatic stress and depressive reactions among Nicaraguan adolescents after Hurricane Mitch. *American Journal of Psychiatry*, **158**, 788–794.

Graham, J.W., Hofer, S.M. & MacKinnon, D.P. (1996). Maximizing the usefulness of data obtained with planned missing value patterns: an application of maximum likelihood procedures. *Multivariate Behavioral Research*, **31**, 197–218.

Green, B.L., Grace, M.C., Vary, M.G., Kramer, T.L., Gleser, G.C. & Leonard, A.C. (1994). Children of disaster in the second decade: a 17-year follow-up of Buffalo Creek survivors. *Journal of the American Academy of Child and Adolescent Psychiatry*, **33**, 71–79.

Hoven, C.W., Duarte, C.S., Lucas, C.P., Mandell, D.J., Cohen, M., Rosen, C., *et al.* (2002a). *Effects of the World Trade Center Attack on NYC Public School Students – Initial Report to the New York City Board of Education.* New York: Columbia University, Mailman School of Public Health, New York State Psychiatric Institute and Applied Research and Consulting, LLC.

Hoven, C.W., Duarte, C.S., Mandell, D., Musa, G., Wicks, J., Wu, P., *et al.* (2002b). *WTC-NYC Child and Adolescent Questionnaire.* New York: Columbia University, New York State Psychiatric Institute.

Hoven, C.W., Mandell, D.J. & Duarte, C.S. (2003). Mental health of New York City public school children after 9/11: an epidemiologic investigation. In *September 11: Trauma and Human Bonds*, eds. S.W. Coates, J.L. Rosenthal & D.S. Schechter. Hillsdale, NJ: The Analytic Press, pp. 51–74.

Hoven, C.W., Duarte, C.S., Lucas, C.P., Wu, P., Mandell, D.J., Goodwin, R.D., *et al.* (2005). Psychopathology among New York City public school children six months after September 11. *Archives of General Psychiatry*, **62**, 545–552.

Hsu, C.C., Chong, M.Y., Yang, P. & Yen, C.F. (2002). Posttraumatic stress disorder among adolescent earthquake victims in Taiwan. *Journal of the American Academy of Child and Adolescent Psychiatry*, **41**, 875–881.

Johnson, C. (2000). Fear rules high school's hallways; Columbine-like threat hovers in Alameda. *The San Francisco Chronicle*. Retrieved April 18, 2005, from http://www.sfgate.com/cgi-bin/article.cgi?file=/chronicle/archive/2000/04/18/MN37785.DTL

Kilic, E.Z., Ozguven, H.D. & Sayil, I. (2003). The psychological effects of parental mental health on children experiencing disaster: the experience of Bolu earthquake in Turkey. *Family Process*, **42**, 485–495.

Kitayama, S., Okada, Y., Takumi, T., Takada, S., Inagaki, Y. & Nakamura, H. (2000). Psychological and physical reactions on children after the Hanshin-Awaji earthquake disaster. *The Kobe Journal of Medical Sciences*, **46**, 189–200.

Kolaitis, G., Kotsopoulos, J., Tsiantis, J., Haritaki, S., Rigizou, F., Zacharaki, L., *et al.* (2003). Posttraumatic stress reactions among children following the Athens earthquake of September 1999. *European Child and Adolescent Psychiatry*, **12**, 273–280.

Koplewicz, H.S., Vogel, J.M., Solanto, M.V., Morrissey, R.F., Alonso, C.M., Abikoff, H., *et al.* (2002). Child and parent response to the 1993 World Trade Center bombing. *Journal of Traumatic Stress*, **15**, 77–85.

Lahad, S., Shacham, Y. & Niv, S. (2000). Coping and community resources in children facing disaster. In *International Handbook of Human Response to Trauma*, eds. A.Y. Shalev & R. Yehuda. Dordrecht, The Netherland: Kluwer Academic Publishers, pp. 389–395.

Langley, A.K. (2003). Coping efforts and efficacy, acculturation, and posttraumatic symptomatology in adolescents following wildfire: a latent variable path analysis. Virginia Polytechnic Institute, Virginia.

Lucas, C.P., Zhang, H., Fisher, P.W., Shaffer, D., Regier, D.A., Narrow, W.E., *et al.* (2001). The DISC predictive scales (DPS): efficiently screening for diagnoses. *Journal of the American Academy of Child and Adolescent Psychiatry*, **40**, 443–449.

Lucas, C.P., Hoven, C.W., Greenwald, S. & Matteo, A. (2002). The DISC Predictive Scales: Depressive Symptoms Following 9/11. Paper presented at the *15th International Association for*

Child and Adolescent Psyciatry and Allied Professionals (IACAPAP) International Congress. New Delhi, India. October 30, 2002.

Morgan, L., Scourfield, J., Williams, D., Jasper, A. & Lewis, G. (2003). The Aberfan disaster: 33-year follow-up of survivors. *British Journal of Psychiatry*, **182**, 532–536.

Offord, D.R., Boyle, M.H. & Racine, Y. (1989). Ontario Child Health Study: correlates of disorder. *Journal of the American Academy of Child and Adolescent Psychiatry*, **28**, 856–860.

Offord, D.R., Boyle, M.H., Racine, Y., Szatmari, P., Fleming, J.E., Sanford, M., *et al.* (1996). Integrating assessment data from multiple informants. *Journal of the American Academy of Child and Adolescent Psychiatry*, **35**, 1078–1085.

Pfefferbaum, B., Moore, V.L., McDonald, N.B., Maynard, B.T., Gurwitch, R.H. & Nixon, S.J. (1999a). The role of exposure in posttraumatic stress in youths following the 1995 bombing. *Journal – Oklahoma State Medical Association*, **92**, 164–167.

Pfefferbaum, B., Nixon, S.J., Tucker, P.M., Tivis, R.D., Moore, V.L., Gurwitch, R.H., *et al.* (1999b). Posttraumatic stress responses in bereaved children after the Oklahoma City bombing. *Journal of the American Academy of Child and Adolescent Psychiatry*, **38**, 1372–1379.

Pfefferbaum, B., Seale, T.W., McDonald, N.B., Brandt Jr., E.N., Rainwater, S.M., Maynard, B.T., Meierhoefer, B. & Miller, P.D. (2000). Posttraumatic stress two years after the Oklahoma City bombing in youths geographically distant from the explosion. *Psychiatry*, **63**, 358–370.

Pfefferbaum, B., Seale, T.W., Brandt Jr., E.N., Pfefferbaum, R.L., Doughty, D.E. & Rainwater, S.M. (2003). Media exposure in children one hundred miles from a terrorist bombing. *Annals of Clinical Psychiatry*, **15**, 1–8.

Pynoos, R.S., Frederick, C., Nader, K., Arroyo, W., Steinberg, A., Eth, S., *et al.* (1987a). Life threat and posttraumatic stress in school-age children. *Archives of General Psychiatry*, **44**, 1057–1063.

Pynoos, R.S., Nader, K., Frederick, C., Gonda, L. & Stuber, M. (1987b). Grief reactions in school age children following a snipe attack at school. *The Israel Journal of Psychiatry and Related Sciences*, **24**, 53–63.

Qouta, S., Punamaki, R.L. & El Sarraj, E. (2003). Prevalence and determinants of PTSD among Palestinian children exposed to military violence. *European Child and Adolescent Psychiatry*, **12**, 265–272.

Rosner, D. & Markowitz, G. (2003). *September 11 and the Shifting Priorities of Public and Population Health in New York*. Milbank Memorial Fund, New York City, New York.

Rothe, E.M., Lewis, J., Castillo-Matos, H., Martinez, O., Busquets, R. & Martinez, I. (2002). Posttraumatic stress disorder among Cuban children and adolescents after release from a refugee camp. *Psychiatric Services*, **53**, 970–976.

Sack, W.H., Clarke, G., Him, C., Dickason, D., Goff, B. & Lanham, K. (1993). A 6-year follow-up study of Cambodian refugee adolescents traumatized as children. *Journal of the American Academy of Child and Adolescent Psychiatry*, **32**, 431–437.

Sack, W.H., Him, C. & Dickason, D. (1999). Twelve-year follow-up study of Khmer youths who suffered massive war trauma as children. *Journal of the American Academy of Child and Adolescent Psychiatry*, **38**, 1173–1179.

Saylor, C.F., Cowart, B.L., Lipovsky, J.A., Jackson, C. & Finch Jr., A.J. (2003). Media exposure to September 11: elementary school students' experiences and posttraumatic symptoms. *American Behavioral Scientist*, **46**, 1622–1642.

Schafer, J.L. & Graham, J.W. (2002). Missing data: our view of the state of the art. *Psychological Methods*, **7**, 147–177.

Shaffer, D., Fisher, P., Dulcan, M.K., Davies, M., Piacentini, J., Schwab-Stone, M.E., *et al.* (1996). The NIMH Diagnostic Interview Schedule for Children Version 2.3 (DISC-2.3): description, acceptability, prevalence rates, and performance in the MECA study. Methods for the epidemiology of child and adolescent mental disorders study. *Journal of the American Academy of Child and Adolescent Psychiatry*, **35**, 865–877.

Shaffer, D., Fisher, P., Lucas, C.P., Dulcan, M.K. & Schwab-Stone, M.E. (2000). NIMH Diagnostic Interview Schedule for Children Version IV (NIMH DISC-IV): description, differences from previous versions, and reliability of some common diagnoses. *Journal of the American Academy of Child and Adolescent Psychiatry*, **39**, 28–38.

Shalev, A.Y., Tuval-Mashiach, R. & Hadar, H. (2004). Posttraumatic stress disorder as a result of mass trauma. *Journal of Clinical Psychiatry*, **65**(Suppl. 1), 4–10.

Shannon, M.P., Lonigan, C.J., Finch Jr., A.J. & Taylor, C.M. (1994). Children exposed to disaster. I: Epidemiology of posttraumatic symptoms and symptom profiles. *Journal of the American Academy of Child and Adolescent Psychiatry*, **33**, 80–93.

Smith, P., Perrin, S., Yule, W. & Rabe-Hesketh, S. (2001). War exposure and maternal reactions in the psychological adjustment of children from Bosnia-Hercegovina. *Journal of Child Psychology and Psychiatry, and Allied Disciplines*, **42**, 395–404.

Stoppelbein, L. & Greening, L. (2000). Posttraumatic stress symptoms in parentally bereaved children and adolescents. *Journal of the American Academy of Child and Adolescent Psychiatry*, **39**, 1112–1119.

Udwin, O., Boyle, S., Yule, W., Bolton, D. & O'Ryan, D. (2000). Risk factors for long-term psychological effects of a disaster experienced in adolescence: predictors of posttraumatic stress disorder. *Journal of Child Psychology and Psychiatry, and Allied Disciplines*, **41**, 969–979.

Vizek-Vidovic, V., Kuterovac-Jagodic, G. & Arambasic, L. (2000). Posttraumatic symptomatology in children exposed to war. *Scandinavian Journal of Psychology*, **41**, 297–306.

von Drehle, D., Johnson, D. & Schulte, B. (2003, October 3). One year later, the memory of fear lingers; snipers shattered a sense of safety. *The Washington Post*. Retrieved April 18, 2005 from http://www.washingtonpost.com/ac2/wp-dyn?pagename=article&node=&contentId=A37134-2003Oct2

Yule, W., Bolton, D., Udwin, O., Boyle, S., O'Ryan, D. & Nurrish, J. (2000). The long-term psychological effects of a disaster experienced in adolescence. I: The incidence and course of PTSD. *Journal of Child Psychology and Psychiatry, and Allied Disciplines*, **41**, 503–511.

6

Historical perspective and future directions in research on psychiatric consequences of terrorism and other disasters

Carol S. North, Betty Pfefferbaum and Barry Hong

Introduction

This chapter will review the history of research on disasters and terrorism leading up to the state of the field at the time of the September 11th terrorist attacks and the methodological challenges faced in responding to this unprecedented event. This chapter will also discuss translations of empirical data to clinical intervention and policy, and the ramifications of disaster studies for future research and disaster planning.

Historical perspective

Catastrophic events have plagued mankind since the beginning of history. Emotional effects of disasters were recorded 4000 years ago in Egyptian cuneiform records (Kramer, 1969) and later in the Iliad of Homer (Shay, 1991). The Biblical floods of the Book of Genesis are even older, dating to approximately 5600 BC (Ryan & Pitman, 1998). Although history has provided ample opportunity to study psychiatric consequences of disasters, this area is a relatively new field of scientific inquiry.

The first medical literature on psychiatric sequelae of disasters can be found in descriptions of Railroad Spine Syndrome by John Erichsen in 1867 in connection with locomotive accidents in England (Fischer-Homberger, 1970; Trimble, 1981). At the time, Railroad Spine Syndrome was thought to be caused by physical damage to the spinal cord (Erichsen, 1875). It was not long, however, before experts identified psychiatric origins to the syndrome, attributing its manifestations to extreme fear (Page, 1885) or hysterical neurosis (Putnam, 1883), possibly representing the first modern recognition of psychiatric origins in posttraumatic syndromes.

War has provided opportunities to observe mass psychological casualties in soldiers. In the American Civil War, war-related symptoms were attributed not to the spine, but to the heart, which was thought to become irritated by battlefield fear and excitement (Hawthorne, 1863). Names given to the syndrome include Irritable Heart Syndrome, Da Costa Syndrome (Da Costa, 2003) Soldier's Heart, and Effort Syndrome. In the 20th century, 80,000 soldiers were discharged from World War I (Culpin, 1930) because of a nervous condition known as "Shell Shock" (Myers, 1915) thought at the time to require psychiatric as well as neurological intervention (The Medical Department of the United States Army in the World War, 1929). In World War II, extensive psychological manifestations were observed among prisoners of war and concentration camp survivors (Whiles, 1945; Bradford & Bradford, 1947; Bensheim, 1960). Later, the Vietnam War became a springboard for formalizing and popularizing posttraumatic stress disorder (PTSD) as a diagnosis, and interest in the syndrome grew substantially in the decades to follow (Lamprecht & Sack, 2002).

Although the psychological basis of these syndromes in soldiers was recognized as far back as World War I (MacKenzie, 1920; Mathers, 1942; Kinzie & Goetz, 1996), notions of physical disturbance as the basis of posttraumatic states persisted into the 20th century. The nervous condition known as hysteria at the time was then considered to represent a state of neurological damage caused by exposure to highly traumatic events (Ellenberger, 1970). Freud, Janet, and others, however, recognized the importance of fantasy and imagination in hysterical disorders and the related dissociative syndromes (Janet, 1907; Freud, 1953; van der Kolk & van der Hart, 1989; Kinzie & Goetz, 1996). These psychological processes distinguish hysterical and dissociative processes from the mental health effects of severely traumatic events in other populations – an important distinction not sufficiently appreciated today.

Since early in the 20th century (Stierlin, 1911), civilian victims of community-wide disasters such as earthquakes and workers in industrial and occupational accidents have also been known to suffer psychological consequences of these events. The first systematic study of psychological effects of major disasters was the study of the 1943 Coconut Grove fire in Boston (Adler, 1943). Several classical systematic studies of disasters followed this legacy in the following two decades (Langdon & Parker, 1954; Block *et al.*, 1956; Friedman & Linn, 1957; Bennett, 1970), before the formulation of PTSD as a recognized psychiatric illness.

PTSD epidemiology and disasters

The signature diagnosis of disaster mental health is PTSD. Although studies have documented many core features of PTSD, at present, this psychiatric diagnosis lacks validation through demonstration of unique features, distinction from other disorders, evidence of heritability in family studies, and consistency over time in longitudinal studies (Robins, 1990).

PTSD may not represent a unified construct. Even its symptom profile appears to vary in different populations and settings. For example, while studies of combat veterans have identified prominent re-experiencing symptoms such as flashbacks, studies of witnesses of abusive violence have demonstrated prominent denial (True et al., 1993), former prisoners of war have described hyperarousal, and rape victims have shown avoidance profiles (Henigsberg et al., 2001). While dissociative syndromes are commonly observed in patients presenting to clinical settings, they are not part of the usual presentation in disaster settings (Yargic et al., 1998; Zanarini et al., 2000). PTSD further varies across different populations in the psychiatric comorbidity associated with it. Cluster B personality features, especially borderline traits, are prevalent in patients who develop PTSD after community accidents, physical and sexual assaults, and present to clinical settings (Herman & van der Kolk, 1987). Premorbid psychiatric features such as personality traits and chaotic family background linked to risk for accidents and victimization may provide sources of bias in sampling in such settings (Breslau et al., 1991). Traumatic events do not strike randomly in community settings, but disaster settings provide opportunities to study the effects of exposure to severe trauma minimizing selection bias.

The level of exposure to a disaster agent has differential effects on various segments of the population. The segment of the population with the highest exposure burden can be expected to experience the most prevalent and severe mental health consequences (Frederick, 1980; Gleser et al., 1981; Baum et al., 1983; Beigel & Berren, 1985; Rubonis & Bickman, 1991; North et al., 1999) this may be true even of those with no prior psychopathology. Indirectly exposed and remotely exposed groups will generally be the most mildly affected psychiatrically, and those less directly exposed individuals who succumb to postdisaster psychiatric disorders will have high rates of pre-existing psychiatric problems (Breslau & Davis, 1992). Therefore, it is important to examine different exposure groups separately to determine the mental health effects of a large disaster on a community.

Numerous studies have examined populations directly exposed to disasters. Prevalence of PTSD has varied considerably from study to study, from 2% in a study of a volcano eruption (Shore et al., 1986), 4% following torrential rain and mudslides (Canino et al., 1990), and up to 8% in association with combined flooding and dioxin contamination (Smith et al., 1986), ranging up to 44% after a dam break and flood (Green et al., 1990), and 54% after an airplane crash landing (Sloan, 1988). Even with direct exposure to the most highly catastrophic events, however, the majority of people do not manifest serious psychiatric consequences. Less than one-half of people in the direct path of the bomb blast of the Oklahoma City bombing developed a psychiatric disorder, and only one-third experienced PTSD in association with it (North et al., 1999). Although the usual focus of such studies is on PTSD and other psychiatric illness, the relatively low rates of diagnosable psychopathology in the majority of people following the Oklahoma City bombing provides evidence of human resilience in the face of unimaginable trauma.

Most disaster research has focused on the most highly exposed groups. Prior to the September 11th terrorist attacks, less directly disaster-exposed groups had received little systematic mental health research. The psychological effects on the larger, indirectly exposed community are an especially salient issue in major terrorist incidents. Terrorism aims to evoke fear and intimidate a wider population than just those directly targeted physically (Pfefferbaum *et al.*, 2002), producing especially far-reaching and profound effects. Psychological effects have been reported on indirectly exposed and remotely affected members of the populations affected by the Oklahoma City bombing (Smith *et al.*, 1999; Pfefferbaum *et al.*, 2000; Sprang, 2001). Most studies of communities affected by terrorism have described symptoms of PTSD or other syndromes such as posttraumatic or depressive reactions. Research results suggest that symptoms and emotional distress are highly prevalent in nondirectly affected members in the community affected by terrorism (Pfefferbaum *et al.*, 2003).

Studies of disasters and terrorism have applied a plethora of instruments, most of which measure symptom counts, scale scores, or various approximations to diagnostic criteria for psychiatric disorders, making it difficult to interpret the data and compare findings inconsistently collected from one study to another. Without appropriate comparison data, the degree to which the measured symptoms and emotional upset reflect an increase of distress levels and specific responses to the event is unclear. Despite methodological limitations, studies suggest that disasters may have the anticipated effects on people not only directly exposed to such events but they may also have far-reaching effects on surrounding populations with less direct exposure. Disaster researchers and intervention planners must keep in mind that differences they observe in populations affected by disasters may be due to inconsistencies in research methodology such as variation in selection by disaster exposure rather than differences in population responses to disaster.

Disaster research has consistently identified two characteristics of individuals that have emerged as robust predictors of PTSD: female gender (Moore & Friedsam, 1959; Kasl *et al.*, 1981; Lopez-Ibor Jr. *et al.*, 1985; Weisæth, 1985; Steinglass & Gerrity, 1990; Rubonis & Bickman, 1991) and pre-existing psychopathology (Bromet *et al.*, 1982; Weisæth, 1985; McFarlane, 1989; Ramsay, 1990; Smith *et al.*, 1990; Southwick *et al.*, 1993; North *et al.*, 1994; North *et al.*, 1999; Chen *et al.*, 2001; Maes *et al.*, 2001; Liao *et al.*, 2002). Negative life events after disasters also appear to predict PTSD (Epstein *et al.*, 1998; North *et al.*, 1999; Maes *et al.*, 2001), although not with the predictive strength of female gender and pre-existing psychopathology.

Disaster research methods and diagnosis-focused investigation

Critical aspects of disaster research methods include time frame, sampling, comparisons, assessment tools, and interpretation of data. Review of disaster research methodology will follow this outline.

Timing of data collection is a primary consideration for disaster research. Studies that enter the field rapidly may have to sacrifice integrity of methods for early data collection (North & Pfefferbaum, 2002). However, the value of rapid entry into the field is that early data can be obtained only during a brief time period after a disaster, and if the information is not obtained then it will be lost forever. Practical and ethical difficulties obstruct research efforts to obtain early data. Respect for the study population's special and difficult circumstances and sensitivity to issues of appropriate timing may dictate delay in starting research while survivors address needs to locate loved ones, bury the deceased, seek shelter and secure their property, deal with insurance issues, and recover their possessions. Entry into the field before one month has passed faces the additional problem that diagnostic criteria requiring a one-month duration of symptoms mean that PTSD cannot be diagnosed during this period. Observation of the course of postdisaster mental health over time is also needed to help understand findings in the acute phase. Long-term outcomes may be very different from findings in the early postdisaster period. On the other hand, entering the field too late may yield corrupted and distorted data from research subjects. To determine the most appropriate time for conducting disaster research, researchers must balance obligations to victims at a particularly vulnerable time with the costs and benefits to society and future disasters.

Sampling issues present early barriers and obstacles to disaster research. Population samples that are easily accessible in the short run may yield limited data that are not well suited for generalization to other groups. Because disaster victims are considered emotionally fragile and vulnerable by the surrounding communities, researchers and outsiders may be barred from contact to establish systematic sampling strategies necessary for the conduct of methodologically sound research (North & Smith, 1994; Smith, 1996; North et al., 2002a). Recently heightened concern among institutional review boards for protection of research participants and new regulations for protection of personal privacy further complicate the sampling procedures in disaster research. The more severe, wide-reaching, and politically charged the event, the more difficult the issues pertaining to sampling become. For these reasons, terrorism presents greater challenges than other disasters to research.

In disaster studies, sampling must involve considerations of separate subpopulations based on exposure status. Directly and indirectly exposed populations require separate consideration because the mental health effects will be expected to vary. Aggregate findings will describe no segment of the population, instead characterizing a nonexistent amorphous average. Rescue worker populations have additional issues that distinguish them from other populations. For example, firefighters are selected as well as self-selected for their line of work that anticipates exposure to trauma, they may have accumulating experience with fire and trauma emergencies on the job, and they have pre-existing issues with alcohol (Boxer & Wild, 1993; Wagner *et al.*, 1998; North *et al.*, 2002b).

The selection of comparison groups is fundamental to most scientific research, but in disaster settings selection of comparison groups is innately problematic (North & Smith, 1994; North & Pfefferbaum, 2002). The goal is to choose a comparison group that is like the exposure group in every way except for not having had the exposure. In disaster research, either the comparison group is likely to be so different from the exposure group in other ways besides disaster exposure that it will be impossible to discern disaster-related effects from predisaster dissimilarities, or it is so closely related to the exposure group that it is tainted by some exposure to the disaster.

Contrasting postdisaster with predisaster mental health status is a critical comparison that involves temporal relationships. Without predisaster comparison (even with the flaws inherent in retrospectively obtained predisaster data), one cannot know what part of the postdisaster picture is due to the disaster and how much of it was pre-existing.

Selecting measurement instruments and deciding on a unit of measure are difficult tasks in disaster mental health research. It is important to consider both psychiatric disorders and emotional distress of nondiagnostic proportions along with many other variables, but the choice of instruments depends on the intended goals and purposes of the assessment. Instruments addressing psychiatric diagnosis need to assess all the diagnostic criteria in estimating the presence of disorders. Simple symptom counts or scales for which arbitrary thresholds are established fail to provide adequate diagnostic information. Assessment is required of other diagnostic features of PTSD, including discrimination of new symptoms from pre-existing symptoms that cannot be considered products of the traumatic event, determination of more than one month's duration of symptoms, and establishment of functional or clinical severity of the symptoms. Some instruments ask respondents to decide the relevance of the symptoms to an event rather than determining the onset of symptoms after the event. Judgment of causal determination is not part of diagnostic criteria, which require only that the symptoms be new after the event, which is a much more reasonable expectation of research participants.

The formal diagnosis of PTSD requires either direct exposure to or witnessing a traumatic event that threatens life or limb of those in its path, or vicarious exposure through the experience of loved ones directly in the path of the traumatic agent. Therefore, assessment of PTSD in populations lacking direct exposure or direct eyewitness experience must be limited to the select members of the population with loved ones directly exposed to the event, as described in *Diagnostic and Statistical Manual of Mental Disorders, Fourth Edition* (*DSM-IV*): "learning about unexpected or violent death, serious harm, or threat of death or injury experienced by a family member or other close associate (Criterion 1A)" (American Psychiatric Association, 1994, p. 424).

Assessment of indirectly exposed or remotely affected populations therefore encounters a unique dilemma in fitting the concept of PTSD to the experience of the individuals involved. Without fulfilling the exposure criterion, these individuals cannot meet PTSD criteria. In practice, however, the criterion symptoms of PTSD have often been counted and reported independently of the Criterion 1A exposure requirement as disembodied symptoms outside the context of exposure to a sufficient traumatic agent. Consideration of posttraumatic symptoms without the requisite context of a traumatic event is paradoxical and problematic for interpretation.

Screening instruments typically rely on symptom counts or scales. Screening scales are much easier to administer than full diagnostic assessment and they have utility for identification of subgroups with substantially increased risk of disorder for the purpose of further evaluation for diagnosis. This is only one part of assessment, however. Individuals who screen positive are of uncertain status until they receive more definitive assessment to determine their diagnostic status. Instruments that count symptoms or generate scales can also be used to follow symptoms over time in individuals *already* diagnosed. Discussion of symptoms outside of a disease construct lacks meaning and defies validation. Assessment of psychiatric symptoms without consideration of full diagnostic criteria does not approach adequate diagnostic assessment and should not be presented in diagnostic terms such as PTSD or "probable" caseness. Measurements based only on simple symptom counts, scales, or symptom thresholds should not be applied in assessment or to estimate disorders without some clear form of validation to determine the amount of error involved in such approximations.

Disaster exposure status may help determine the most suitable type of assessment tool for clinical or research evaluation. The type of instrument needed will depend on the research goals and outcomes to be studied as well as on the exposure level of the sample. For example, for evaluation of large population samples with low levels of exposure, an instrument with high sensitivity and low specificity such as a screening measure would help identify the at-risk proportion of the population most likely to benefit from more intensive evaluation and management. Such screening may spare valuable resources that would be wasted on formal diagnostic assessment of large numbers of people without a disorder that is difficult to accomplish and is prohibitively exhaustive of resources for the study of large samples.

Additionally, attempts at full diagnosis may be limited by failure to address significant subclinical and nonpsychiatric issues. For small, high-risk groups such as highly exposed individuals, however, full structured diagnostic assessment may be justified to estimate the incidence rates of specific disorders such as PTSD in relation to the disaster.

Exposure status itself should not be considered a proxy for diagnosis, however. People in the highest exposure groups, for example, are not automatically PTSD "cases." Even the most precise measure of exposure cannot determine the level of psychopathology in individuals. Exposure level has utility for predicting psychopathology in groups or populations but can be misleading if applied to individuals as an indicator of diagnosis.

Similar issues complicate the collection, interpretation, and reporting of substance abuse data. Differentiation must be made between patterns of *use* of alcohol/other drugs from *diagnoses* of abuse/dependence. Data reflecting use of substances or changes in patterns of use of substances without indicating how the patterns of use fit into diagnostic criteria such as through negative effects on employment, family relations, social and recreational activities, and health and legal status provide little useful information for clinical or research purposes. If, for example, after a community-wide catastrophe, an individual spends more time socializing and consumes moderately more alcohol and cigarettes than previously for a circumscribed period such as a week or two, this is not necessarily evidence of a problem requiring clinical response or intervention.

Interpretation of data is a vital part of disaster research that requires careful consideration. Potential pitfalls include inappropriate assumptions of causation from association, failing to differentiate disorders from normative distress, confusing predisaster issues with disaster-related outcomes, and lack of validity in assumptions of psychological morbidity in the context of the disaster setting. For example, the clinical significance of phobic symptoms is questionable in unusual and extreme settings of disaster when extreme fear may be a normative and expected response. Interpretation of the validity of such data can have profound implications for policy and practice in postdisaster interventions. Assumption of pathology in the fear response might suggest need for large-scale major mental health interventions for the affected population. Alternatively, understanding of fear as a normal yet distressing experience following extreme trauma might point interventions toward reassurance and education of the population.

The Oklahoma City bombing study: an empirical template for research

The Washington University study of survivors directly exposed to the 1995 Oklahoma City bombing (North *et al.*, 1999) is regarded one of the most authoritative sources for anticipating psychiatric effects in the population following the September terrorist attacks (e.g., Norris, 2002), especially because of its methodology. This study used formal diagnostic criteria for psychiatric disorders applied through structured interviews to a systematic sample of highly exposed individuals. One-third of the sample (34%) developed PTSD. The next most prevalent diagnosis was major depression, in 23%. No new cases of alcohol or drug abuse were identified after the bombing. The majority (55%) did not develop a postdisaster psychiatric disorder, exhibiting resilience even after surviving this severely traumatic experience. The major predictors of PTSD were female gender and a pre-existing psychiatric disorder. Major depression was found to have an extremely high likelihood of persistence or recurrence after the disaster.

Despite psychiatric resilience in this highly exposed population, symptoms and distress were nearly ubiquitous, with 96% reporting one or more PTSD symptoms. Avoidance and numbing (PTSD Group C) symptoms were pivotal to the diagnosis. While approximately 80% met criteria for intrusive re-experience (PTSD Group B) and hyperarousal (PTSD Group D) symptom clusters, only 36% met avoidance and numbing criteria.

Avoidance and numbing (Group C) criteria virtually defined PTSD, with 94% of those reporting 3 or more Group C symptoms meeting full criteria for PTSD. Avoidance and numbing symptoms were associated with indicators of illness including interference of the symptoms with activities, predisaster psychopathology, diagnostic comorbidity, receiving treatment, medication use, and use of alcohol for coping. These other variables were not associated with intrusive recollection (Group B) or hyperarousal (Group D) criteria in the absence of Group C criteria.

Initial onset of PTSD was rapid, with 76% of PTSD cases beginning the first day, 94% the first week, and 98% the first month. The early onset and chronicity of PTSD, the dominance of avoidance and numbing in the development of PTSD after disaster, and the lack of new cases of substance abuse are all consistent with findings of other disaster studies (North *et al.*, 1994; North *et al.*, 1999; McMillen *et al.*, 2000). PTSD was chronic as defined by *DSM-IV* (lasting 3 months) in 100% of cases. A followup study almost one year later, at 17 months postbombing, found that few of the PTSD cases had remitted (North, 2001).

Translation of empirical data to policy and intervention

A number of consistent findings have emerged from the research literature that can be directly applied to intervention and policy. First, trauma mental health research conducted in other settings may not apply to disasters. Confounding effects of pre-existing risk factors for trauma with predictors of mental health effects of trauma may render the findings inapplicable in disasters due to more random effects by disasters in involved populations than by individual traumatic events in general communities, much of what is known about posttraumatic response to other events may not apply to disaster settings. Therefore, interventions and policy are best informed by disaster research.

One of the most important, and often overlooked, findings of disaster research is that people are resilient, even after the most severe of traumatic events. Most people do not develop a new postdisaster psychiatric disorder (e.g., the Oklahoma City bombing). Despite this resilience, however, emotional distress may be ubiquitous among people exposed to community catastrophes, as observed in very high rates of PTSD symptoms reported and general expression of emotional upset among Oklahoma City bombing survivors.

This leads to the crucial distinction between psychiatric illness and emotional distress that forms the basis for developing interventions and planning disaster mental health responses. A central task of disaster mental health research and intervention is the differentiation of psychiatric illness from "subdiagnostic distress." In clinical settings, this differentiation provides direction for triage and treatment decisions. It allows psychiatrically ill individuals to be triaged to appropriate treatment while attending to subdiagnostic distress without pathologizing that distress. On the other hand, recognition of postdisaster distress apart from psychiatric illness avoids stigmatizing disaster populations. This differentiation prevents blanket application of uniform diagnosis of everyone with psychiatric illness while recognizing the importance of subdiagnostic distress and the potential for benefit from interventions involving education and reassurance. The phrase, "One size does not fit all" applies to the distinction between psychiatric illness and subdiagnostic distress and the decisions incumbent upon it.

Identification of psychiatric illness becomes possible through application of previous disaster research findings. The Group C criteria may have potential as a screening instrument. In the Oklahoma City bombing study, most people with any psychiatric disorder or PTSD were identified by Group C criteria (endorsement of at least three avoidance/numbing symptoms in association with the event). Other studies such as the study of the Northridge, California earthquake have reported similar findings (McMillen *et al.*, 2000). Further research, especially prospective studies, will be needed to confirm the utility of the approach to recognition of PTSD in populations through screening for Group C criteria.

PTSD is an important starting point because it is the most prevalent postdisaster psychiatric disorder in most populations, and because it identifies most of the cases of psychiatric illness following disasters (North *et al.*, 1999). PTSD is more often than not comorbid with other psychiatric disorders in postdisaster settings. The lesson to be learned from this is that although PTSD is the place to start to identify most of the psychiatric cases, one should not stop once PTSD has been diagnosed, because it is likely that another psychiatric disorder is present that may be at least as important as the PTSD to treatment and outcome. The comorbid cases appear to be those with greatest severity and may require the most intense treatment interventions.

Previous disaster research has repeatedly demonstrated that PTSD begins rapidly after disaster, indicating the value of commencing mental health intervention efforts promptly after a disaster. Although people with PTSD often delay in seeking treatment, these cases should not be assumed to represent delayed onset. The overwhelming chronicity of PTSD identifies need for services to continue to provide mental health services long term as the need persists.

Critical comments on research methods of studies of the September 11th terrorist attacks

This section provides relevant comments about the research literature pertaining to the September 11th terrorist attacks. A comprehensive review of this work is beyond the scope of this chapter, however. The outline structure of this chapter's earlier discussion of research methods will be followed in exploring post-9/11 research issues.

The early post-9/11 studies entered the research field quickly to obtain acute phase data during a brief interval that presented major obstacles to the conduct of research. In this context, difficult decisions had to be made to allow the data to be gathered. Early postdisaster research requires efficient data collection to succeed, but efficiency may conflict with ideal methodology, compromising the quality of the data to be obtained. Limitations in the data that may reduce the utility of the data must be considered in the interpretation of the results. The difficulties imposed by the temporal concerns may affect sampling, comparison, measurement, and interpretation of the data.

Early pursuit of post-9/11 data presented especially complex considerations for sampling efforts. A specific aspect of the September 11th terrorist attacks was the gradation of exposure level among differently affected subgroups of the population. Levels of exposure have previously received little consideration in sampling of disaster-affected populations. Most studies of mental health effects of disasters and terrorism have focused on high-exposure subgroups. Deciding who was affected by the September 11th attacks posed difficulties for selecting research samples. The profound magnitude and intensity of the event prevented systematic research access to the most highly exposed survivor groups. To date, the potentially most vulnerable subset of the population, those who escaped the Twin Towers during the terrorist attacks on them, has not yet been systematically examined for mental health effects. When data become available on the rescue workers, the findings may be compared with studies of the rescue workers from the Oklahoma City bombing, with the recognition that their exposure also involved direct threat to life and limb and massive traumatic bereavement issues not experienced by the Oklahoma City firefighters.

Post-9/11 research studies started with selecting random samples of the Manhattan residential population and national household samples from other metropolitan areas (Schuster *et al.*, 2001; Galea *et al.*, 2002; Schlenger *et al.*, 2002; Silver *et al.*, 2002). These initial post-9/11 research samples thus constituted mixed indirectly and distantly affected groups, with a few highly exposed individuals sprinkled among the more indirectly exposed samples. Random sampling of these groups cannot substitute for consideration of exposure level in sampling designs because exposure status is an important predictor of psychopathology. Stratification of 9/11 data by exposure and correlation of variables of interest with exposure might help manage mixed-exposure samples if they contain sufficient numbers of participants within the subgroups.

Sampling issues in post-9/11 research in turn are critical to comparability of data sets, choice of study instruments, and interpretation of the data. Inconsistent exposure levels present problems for comparing mental health effects across events. For example, a randomly selected sample of residents of households across Manhattan had inherently different exposure level to the 9/11 terrorist attacks than a sample of surviving Murrah Building occupants had to the bomb blast in Oklahoma City.

The random-digit-dial samples of household residents in the surrounding communities of the World Trade Center attacks could reasonably be compared with indirectly exposed members of the Oklahoma City community, but not with the Murrah Building occupants surviving the Oklahoma City bombing. Another appropriate comparison would be between those who escaped the Twin Towers after the terrorist attacks and occupants of the Murrah Building in the Oklahoma City bomb blast. In interpreting data from indirectly exposed samples, it is important to acknowledge limitations in utility of the data and to refrain from generalizing to directly exposed groups or comparison to directly exposed samples. Conversely, comparison or extrapolation from studies of directly exposed groups such as Murrah Building occupants in the Oklahoma City bombing to apply to indirectly exposed populations such as the population of Manhattan post-9/11 would inflate the anticipated effects.

Difficulties in using available measurement instruments as described in the research methods section were encountered in the early post-9/11 studies. Instruments are usually validated in other populations and settings pursuing various research goals and types of outcomes. The validity of the data obtained from these instruments in the post-9/11 setting may be uncertain. Additionally, no systematic study of psychiatric disorders in post-9/11 populations has been conducted. Estimates of PTSD provided to date are limited by lack of addressing one or more of the diagnostic requirements of *DSM-IV*: satisfying the exposure criterion, one-month duration of symptoms, new onset of the symptoms after the event, and clinically or functionally significant impact of the symptoms. As a result, it becomes difficult to differentiate emotional distress from psychiatric illness and to determine the degree to which the psychopathology has resulted from the terrorist attacks and not other sources of stress. Collective results of post-9/11 studies suggest that symptoms and emotional distress are nearly ubiquitous in affected populations (Associated Press, 2001; Schuster *et al.*, 2001; Galea *et al.*, 2002; Herman *et al.*, 2002; Schlenger *et al.*, 2002; Silver *et al.*, 2002).

In interpreting the data, researchers in this field can do much to help the public and policy planners avoid confusing emotional distress with formal psychiatric illness. These research precautions are especially appropriate for public health intervention planners because the findings may alternatively suggest divergent interventions such as a public media information to educate people about normative emotional responses and emphasize resilience vs. need for a large outpouring of resources for professional psychiatric assistance for hundreds of thousands of psychiatric casualties. Causal assumptions should be avoided when available data reveal simple associations among variables. Consideration of causal directionalities opposite to those assumed is needed as well as consideration of other variables that may confound or explain the apparent associations.

Ramifications of post-9/11 studies for subsequent research, intervention, and policy

Experience in disaster research and findings from recent studies suggest several recommendations to the research field. One of the most fundamental principles is differentiation of psychiatric illness from distress, through assessment of the complete set of DSM criteria for PTSD and other psychiatric disorders (rather than relying on symptom counts, symptom frequency, severity scales, or estimates from thresholds of symptom counts or scales). Psychiatric diagnostic assessment is resource intensive. Other means of adequate diagnostic approximation are needed.

Timing of entry into the disaster field deserves serious consideration to resolving competing desires to collect data before the data vanish forever and needs to develop optimal methods yielding quality data before entering the field for data collection.

Population subsets need separate study by exposure type, not only because they differ in exposure, but because they may differ in important ways not related to a particular disaster.

Consistent methodology, especially structured assessment instruments, should be repeated from study to study so that disasters can be compared. Collection of data should also consider special interests of disaster-related inquiry, such as current or postdisaster symptom count, symptom count, and diagnostic assessment in the immediate predisaster period for baseline comparison, and change in status related to the disaster that may not be routinely assessed in structured diagnostic interviews.

The September 11th terrorist attacks represented the first modern disaster research setting in which researchers might get in one another's way, inundate the survivor groups, and duplicate one another's efforts in research studies. After the Oklahoma City bombing, the Governor of Oklahoma set up a gatekeeper function for the conduct of research studies to protect the survivor population from these potential problems and from unworthy research efforts (Nixon *et al.*, 1998; Quick, 1998; Tucker *et al.*, 1998). Such control was not possible after September 11th terrorist attacks, and researchers have found themselves bumping into one another as they seek large samples of the most highly exposed groups. Coordination of efforts by the major research funding agencies might suffice to prevent many of these potential difficulties in future research on major disasters and terrorist attacks.

Coordination of interventions encounters parallel issues of duplication of efforts and potential for specialization in meeting the very different needs of individuals and subpopulations. While some segments of the population may need treatment for major psychiatric disorders following the event, other segments of the population may benefit from reassurance and education about their emotional responses. The population also needs efforts to build emotional resilience. The next disaster or terrorist attack will truly test the population's resilience.

Summary and conclusions

This chapter has reviewed the history of research on disasters and terrorism and the current methodological difficulties faced by the field in mounting organized research to respond to the September 11th terrorist attacks. Appropriate interpretation of carefully established empirical data is a necessary foundation for leaders in the field to develop the most effective mental health interventions and policy following disasters. The field has overcome many obstacles inherent in the conduct of disaster research, making important advances in methodology in recent decades. Numerous challenges remain, however, in organizing, planning, designing, and carrying out research on the mental health effects of disasters and terrorism. The unfortunate likelihood of future events demands that the field constantly update and maintain readiness to meet the next challenge.

REFERENCES

Adler, A. (1943). Neuropsychiatric complications in victims of Boston's Coconut Grove disaster. *Journal of the American Psychiatric Association*, **123**, 1098–1101.

American Psychiatric Association (1994). *Diagnostic and Statistical Manual of Mental Disorders* (4th ed.). Washington, DC: American Psychiatric Association Press.

Associated Press (2001). Poll: Americans depressed, sleepless. Washington, DC: Associated Press. Available at http://www.msnbc.com/news/631188.asp. 9-19-2001.

Baum, A., Fleming, R. & Davidson, L.M. (1983). Natural disaster and technological catastrophe. *Environment and Behavior*, **15**, 333–354.

Beigel, A. & Berren, M. (1985). Human-induced disasters. *Psychiatric Annals*, **15**, 143–150.

Bennett, G. (1970). Bristol floods 1968: controlled survey of effects on health of local community disaster. *British Journal of Medicine*, **3**, 454–458.

Benshcim, H. (1960). Die K.Z. Neurose rassisch Verfolgter: Ein Beitrag zur Psychopathologie der Neurosen [The concentration camp neurosis of the racially persecuted: a contribution on the psychopathology of neuroses]. *Der Nervenarzt*, **31**, 462–469.

Block, D.A., Silber, E. & Perry, S.E. (1956). Some factors in the emotional reaction of children to disaster. *American Journal of Psychiatry*, **412**, 416–422.

Boxer, P.A. & Wild, D. (1993). Psychological distress and alcohol use among fire fighters. *Scandinavian Journal of Work and Environmental Health*, **19**, 121–125.

Bradford, J.M. & Bradford, E.J. (1947). Neurosis in escaped prisoners of war. *British Journal of Medical Psychology*, **20**, 422–435.

Breslau, N. & Davis, G.C. (1992). Posttraumatic stress disorder in an urban population of young adults: risk factors for chronicity. *American Journal of Psychiatry*, **149**, 671–675.

Breslau, N., Davis, G.C., Andreski, P. & Peterson, E. (1991). Traumatic events and posttraumatic stress disorder in an urban population of young adults. *Archives of General Psychiatry*, **48**, 216–222.

Bromet, E.J., Parkinson, D.K. & Schulberg, H.C. (1982). Mental health of residents near the Three Mile Island reactor: a comparative study of selected groups. *Journal of Preventive Psychiatry*, **1**, 225–276.

Canino, G., Bravo, M., Rubio-Stipec, M. & Woodbury, M. (1990). The impact of disaster on mental health: prospective and retrospective analyses. *International Journal of Mental Health*, **19**, 51–69.

Chen, C.C., Yeh, T.L., Yang, Y.K., Chen, S.J., Lee, I.H., Fu, L.S., Yeh, C.Y., Hsu, H.C., Tsai, W.L., Cheng, S.H., Chen, L.Y. & Si, Y.C. (2001). Psychiatric morbidity and post-traumatic symptoms among survivors in the early stage following the 1999 earthquake in Taiwan. *Psychiatric Research*, **105**, 13–22.

Culpin, M. (1930). The need for psychopathology. *Lancet*, **2**, 725–726.

Da Costa, J.M. (2003). On irritable heart: a clinical study of a form of functional cardiac disorder and its consequence. *American Journal of Medical Science*, **16**, 17–52.

Ellenberger, H.F. (1970). *The Discovery of the Unconscious*. New York: Basic Books.

Epstein, R., Fullerton, C. & Ursano, R. (1998). Posttraumatic stress disorder following an air disaster: a prospective study. *American Journal of Psychiatry*, **155**, 934–938.

Erichsen, J. (1875). *On Concussion of the Spine: Nervous Shock and Other Obscure Injuries of the Nervous System.* [Reprinted in New York: William Wood; 1886, pp. 36–37]. London: Longmans, Green.

Fischer-Homberger, E. (1970). Railway Spine and traumatische neurose: seele and rückenmark [Railway Spine and traumatic neurosis: soul and spine]. *Gesnerus*, **27**, 96–111.

Frederick, C.J. (1980). Effects of natural vs. human-induced violence upon victims. *Evaluation and Change*, Special Issue, 71–75.

Freud, S. (1953). My views on the part played by sexuality in the aetiology of the neuroses. In *Standard, Edition, VII* (Original Work Published 1906), ed. J. Strachey. London: Hogarth Press.

Friedman, P. & Linn, L. (1957). Some psychiatric notes on the Andrea Doria disaster. *American Journal of Psychiatry*, **114**, 426–432.

Galea, S., Ahern, J., Resnick, H., Kilpatrick, D., Bucuvalis, M., Gold, J. & Vlahov, D. (2002). Psychological sequelae of the September 11 terrorist attacks in New York City. *New England Journal of Medicine*, **346**, 982–987.

Gleser, G.C., Green, B.L. & Winget, C.N. (1981). *Prolonged Psychosocial Effects of Disaster: A Study of Buffalo Creek.* New York: Academic Press.

Green, B.L., Lindy, J.D., Grace, M.C., Gleser, G.C., Leonard, A.C., Korol, M. & Winget, C. (1990). Buffalo Creek survivors in the second decade: stability of stress symptoms. *American Journal of Orthopsychiatry*, **60**, 43–54.

Hawthorne, H. (1863). On heart disease in the army. *American Journal of Medical Science*, **48**, 89–92.

Henigsberg, N., Folnegovic-Smalc, V. & Moro, L. (2001). Stressor characteristics and post-traumatic stress disorder symptom dimensions in war victims. *Croatian Medical Journal*, **42**, 543–550.

Herman, D., Felton, C. & Susser, E. (2002). Mental health needs in New York state following the September 11th attacks. *Journal of Urban Health*, **79**, 322–331.

Herman, J. & van der Kolk, B.A. (1987). Traumatic antecedents of borderline personality disorder. In *Psychological Trauma*, ed. B.A. van der Kolk. Washington, DC: American Psychiatric Press.

Janet, P. (1907). *The Major Symptoms of Hysteria: 15 Lectures Given in the Medical School of Harvard University.* New York: Macmillan.

Kasl, S.V., Chisholm, R.E. & Eskenazi, B. (1981). The impact of the accident at Three Mile Island on the behavior and well-being of nuclear workers. *American Journal of Public Health*, **71**, 472–495.

Kinzie, J.D. & Goetz, R.R. (1996). A century of controversy surrounding posttraumatic stress-spectrum syndromes: the impact on DSM-III and DSM-IV. *Journal of Traumatic Stress*, **9**, 159–179.

Kramer, S.N. (1969). A Sumerian lamentation. In *Ancient Near Eastern Texts Relating to the Old Testament*, ed. J.B. Pritchard. Trenton, NJ: Princeton University Press, pp. 455–463.

Lamprecht, F. & Sack, M. (2002). Posttraumatic stress disorder revisited. *Psychosomatic Medicine*, **64**, 222–237.

Langdon, J.R. & Parker, A.H. (1954). Psychiatric aspects of the March 7, 1954 earthquake. *Alaska Medicine*, **6**, 33–35.

Liao, W.C., Lee, M.B., Lee, Y.J., Wang, T., Shih, F.Y. & Ma, M.H. (2002). Association of psychological distress with psychological factors in rescue workers within two months after a major earthquake. *Journal of the Formosan Medical Association*, **101**, 169–176.

Lopez-Ibor Jr., J.J., Canas, S.F. & Rodriguez-Gamazo, M. (1985). Psychological aspects of the toxic oil syndrome catastrophe. *British Journal of Psychiatry*, **147**, 352–365.

MacKenzie, J. (1920). The soldier's heart and war neurosis: a study in symptomatology. *British Medical Journal*, Part II, 530–534.

Maes, M., Mylle, J., Delmeire, L. & Janca, A. (2001). Pre- and post-disaster negative life events in relation to the incidence and severity of post-traumatic stress disorder. *Psychiatry Research*, **105**, 1–12.

Mathers, A.T. (1942). The psychoneuroses in wartime. *Canadian Medical Association Journal*, **47**, 103–111.

McFarlane, A.C. (1989). The aetiology of post-traumatic morbidity: predisposing, precipitating and perpetuating factors. *British Journal of Psychiatry*, **154**, 221–228.

McMillen, J.C., North, C.S. & Smith, E.M. (2000). What parts of PTSD are normal: intrusion, avoidance, or arousal? Data from the Northridge, California earthquake. *Journal of Traumatic Stress*, **13**, 57–75.

Moore, H.E. & Friedsam, H.J. (1959). Reported emotional stress following a disaster. *Social Forces*, **38**, 135–138.

Myers, C.S. (1915). A contribution to the study of shell shock. *Lancet*, **i**, 316–320.

Nixon, S.J., Vincent, R., Krug, R.S. & Pfefferbaum, B. (1998). Structure and organization of research efforts following the bombing of the Murrah Building. *Journal of Personal and Interpersonal Loss*, **3**, 99–115.

Norris, F.H. (2002). Psychosocial consequences of disasters. *PTSD Research Quarterly*, **13**, 1–7.

North, C.S. (2001). The course of post-traumatic stress disorder after the Oklahoma City bombing. *Military Medicine*, **166**, 51–52.

North, C.S. & Smith, E.M. (1994). Quick response disaster study: sampling methods and practical issues in the field. In *Stressful Life Events II*, ed. T.W. Miller. New York: International Universities Press, pp. 295–320.

North, C.S. & Pfefferbaum, B. (2002). Research on the mental health effects of terrorism. *Journal of the American Medical Association*, **288**, 633–636.

North, C.S., Smith, E.M. & Spitznagel, E.L. (1994). Posttraumatic stress disorder in survivors of a mass shooting. *American Journal of Psychiatry*, **151**, 82–88.

North, C.S., Nixon, S.J., Shariat, S., Mallonee, S., McMillen, J.C., Spitznagel, E.L. & Smith, E.M. (1999). Psychiatric disorders among survivors of the Oklahoma City bombing. *Journal of the American Medical Association*, **282**, 755–762.

North, C.S., Pfefferbaum, B. & Tucker, P. (2002a). Ethical and methodological issues in academic mental health research in populations affected by disasters: the Oklahoma City experience relevant to September 11, 2001. *CNS Spectrums*, **7**, 580–584.

North, C.S., Tivis, L., McMillen, J.C., Pfefferbaum, B., Spitznagel, E.L., Cox, J., Nixon, S., Bunch, K.P. & Smith, E.M. (2002b). Psychiatric disorders in rescue workers after the Oklahoma City bombing. *American Journal of Psychiatry*, **159**, 857–859.

Page, H.W. (1885). *Injuries of the Spine and Spinal Cord Without Apparent Mechanical Lesions and Nervous Shock in Their Surgical and Medical Legal Aspects.* London: J.A. Churchill.

Pfefferbaum, B., Seale, T.W., McDonald, N.B., Brandt, E.N., Rainwater, S.M., Maynard, B.T., Meierhoefer, B. & Miller, P.D. (2000). Posttraumatic stress two years after the Oklahoma City bombing in youths geographically distant from the explosion. *Psychiatry*, **63**, 358–370.

Pfefferbaum, B., Pfefferbaum, R.L., North, C.S. & Neas, B.R. (2002). Does television viewing satisfy criteria for exposure in posttraumatic stress disorder? *Psychiatry*, **65**, 306–309.

Pfefferbaum, B., Seale, T.W., Brandt, E.N., Pfefferbaum, R.L., Doughty, D.E. & Rainwater, S.M. (2003). Media exposure in children one hundred miles from a terrorist bombing. *Annals of Clinical Psychiatry*, **15**, 1–8.

Putnam, J.J. (1883). Recent investigation into the so-called concussion of the spine. *Medical and Surgical Journal*, **109**, 217–220.

Quick, G. (1998). A paradigm for multidisciplinary disaster research: the Oklahoma City experience. *The Journal of Emergency Medicine*, **16**, 621–630.

Ramsay, R. (1990). Post-traumatic stress disorder: a new clinical entity? *Journal of Psychosomatic Research*, **34**, 355–365.

Robins, L.N. (1990). Steps toward evaluating post-traumatic stress reaction as a psychiatric disorder. *Journal of Applied Social Psychology*, **20**, 1674–1677.

Rubonis, A.V. & Bickman, L. (1991). Psychological impairment in the wake of disaster: the disaster-psychopathology relationship. *Psychological Bulletin*, **109**, 384–399.

Ryan, W. & Pitman, W. (1998). *Noah's Flood*. New York: Simon & Schuster.

Schlenger, W.E., Caddell, J.M., Ebert, L., Jordan, B.K., Rourke, K.M., Wilson, D., Thalji, L., Dennis, J.M., Fairbank, J.A. & Kulka, R.A. (2002). Psychological reactions to terrorist attacks: findings from the National Study of Americans' Reactions to September 11. *Journal of the American Medical Association*, **288**, 581–588.

Schuster, M.A., Stein, B.D., Jaycox, L., Collins, R.L., Marshall, G.N., Elliott, M.N., Zhou, A.J., Kanouse, D.E., Morrison, J.L. & Berry, S.H. (2001). A national survey of stress reactions after the September 11, 2001, terrorist attacks. *New England Journal of Medicine*, **345**, 1507–1512.

Shay, J. (1991). Learning about combat stress through Homer's Iliad. *Journal of Traumatic Stress*, **4**, 561–579.

Shore, J.H., Tatum, E.L. & Vollmer, W.M. (1986). The Mount St. Helens stress response syndrome. In *Disaster Stress Studies: New Methods and Findings*, ed. J.H. Shore. Washington, DC: American Psychiatric Press, pp. 77–97.

Silver, R.C., Holman, E.A., McIntosh, D.N., Poulin, M. & Gil-Rivas, V. (2002). Nationwide longitudinal study of psychological responses to September 11. *Journal of the American Medical Association*, **288**, 1235–1244.

Sloan, P. (1988). Posttraumatic stress in survivors of an airplane crash-landing: a clinical and exploratory research intervention. *Journal of Traumatic Stress*, **1**, 211–229.

Smith, D.W., Christiansen, E.H., Vincent, R. & Hann, N.E. (1999). Population effects of the bombing of Oklahoma City. *Journal of the Oklahoma State Medical Association*, **92**, 193–198.

Smith, E.M. (1996). Coping with the challenges of field research. In *Trauma Research Methodology*, ed. E.B. Carlson. Lutherville, MD: Sidran, pp. 126–152.

Smith, E.M., Robins, L.N., Przybeck, T.R., Goldring, E. & Solomon, S.D. (1986). Psychosocial consequences of a disaster. In *Disaster Stress Studies: New Methods and Findings*, ed. J.H. Shore. Washington, DC: American Psychiatric Association, pp. 49–76.

Smith, E.M., North, C.S., McCool, R.E. & Shea, J.M. (1990). Acute postdisaster psychiatric disorders: identification of persons at risk. *American Journal of Psychiatry*, **147**, 202–206.

Southwick, S.M., Yehuda, R. & Giller, E.L. (1993). Personality disorders in treatment-seeking combat veterans with posttraumatic stress disorder. *American Journal of Psychiatry*, **150**, 1020–1023.

Sprang, G. (2001). Vicarious stress: patterns of disturbance and use of mental health services by those indirectly affected by the Oklahoma City bombing. *Psychological Reports*, **89**, 331–338.

Steinglass, P. & Gerrity, E. (1990). Natural disasters and posttraumatic stress disorder: short-term vs. long-term recovery in two disaster-affected communities. *Journal of Applied Social Psychology*, **20**, 1746–1765.

Stierlin, E. (1911). Nervöse und psychische Störungen nach Katastrophen [Nervous and psychological disturbances following catastrophes]. *Deutsche Medizinische Wochenschrift*, **37**, 2028–2035.

The Medical Department of the United States Army in the World War (1929). *Neuropsychiatry.* Washington, DC: Office of the Surgeon General, US Army, 1966.

Trimble, M.R. (1981). *Post-traumatic Neurosis from Railway Spine to Whiplash.* Chichester: Wiley and Sons.

True, W.R., Rice, J., Eisen, S.A., Heath, A.C., Goldberg, J., Lyons, M.J. & Nowak, J. (1993). A twin study of genetic and environmental contributions to liability for posttraumatic stress symptoms. *Archives of General Psychiatry*, **50**, 257–260.

Tucker, P., Pfefferbaum, B., Vincent, R., Boehler, S.D. & Nixon, W.J. (1998). Oklahoma City: disaster challenges mental health and medical administrators. *The Journal of Behavioral Health Services and Research*, **25**, 93–99.

van der Kolk, B. & van der Hart, O. (1989). Pierre Janet and the breakdown of adaptation in psychological trauma. *American Journal of Psychiatry*, **146**, 1530–1540.

Wagner, D., Heinrichs, M. & Ehlert, U. (1998). Prevalence of symptoms of posttraumatic stress disorder in German professional firefighters. *American Journal of Psychiatry*, **155**, 1727–1732.

Weisæth, L. (1985). Post-traumatic stress disorder after an industrial disaster. In *Psychiatry – The State of the Art*, eds. P. Pichot, P. Berner, R. Wolf & K. Thau. New York: Plenum Press, pp. 299–307.

Whiles, H. (1945). A study of neurosis among repatriated prisoners of war. *British Medical Journal*, **2**, 697–698.

Yargic, L.I., Sar, V., Tutkun, H. & Alyanak, B. (1998). Comparison of dissociative identity disorder with other diagnostic groups using a structured interview in Turkey. *Comprehensive Psychiatry*, **39**, 345–351.

Zanarini, M.C., Ruser, T., Frankenburg, F.R. & Hennen, J. (2000). The dissociative experiences of borderline patients. *Comprehensive Psychiatry*, **41**, 223–227.

7

Capturing the impact of large-scale events through epidemiological research

Johan M. Havenaar and Evelyn J. Bromet

Introduction

Since the United States Civil War in the 19th century and World War I in the early 20th century, it has been recognized that some of the casualties of war are caused by the psychological impact of these experiences rather than just by their physical impact. Similarly, since the seminal descriptions of survivors of the Coconut Grove fire disaster in 1942 (Adler, 1943), many studies of natural and human-made disasters, including toxic exposures, have described their physical and psychological consequences (Havenaar et al., 2002). By their very nature, the recent terrorist attacks are specifically intended to induce fear (terror) in the population in addition to physical casualties and damage. Hence it is useful to consider the lessons learned from research on the diverse catastrophic experiences over the past 50 years.

The advent of structured interviews and clinical criteria in psychiatric research during the 1970s spurred a large number of epidemiological studies that have quantified the impact of disasters on mental health and well-being (Bromet & Dew, 1995; Galea et al., 2005; Van den Berg et al., 2005). The first study to use structured diagnostic interviews focused on the impact of the 1979 accident at the Three Mile Island nuclear power plant rates on major depression and generalized anxiety disorder (Bromet & Schulberg, 1986). Since then, the Diagnostic and Statistical Manual of Mental Disorders (DSM) classification system officially operationalized post-traumatic stress disorder (PTSD), and the ICD-10 introduced a similar category. Subsequently, much of the research on the psychological impact of disasters has tended to focus more or less exclusively on PTSD, even though it is increasingly recognized that the range of potential negative outcomes is far broader and includes affective, anxiety, and substance use disorders and non-specific medical symptoms. Thus, while the research over the past decades has produced a wealth of information documenting the prevalence of mental health problems in the aftermath of disasters, and identifying the major risk factors and protective factors determining outcome, the recent work has generally focused only on PTSD.

The terrorist attacks on New York and Washington, D.C. on September 11, 2001, have once again given rise to a wave of post-disaster studies. There are both empirical and public health reasons for conducting further descriptive epidemiological studies in the wake of these disasters (Morris, 1964; Fielder *et al.*, 2002). From a research perspective, the reasons include:

(a) ascertaining high-risk groups among children, adults, and the elderly;
(b) identifying risk and protective factors as well as potential unique aetiologic or pathogenic mechanisms;
(c) completing the clinical picture beyond people who present for treatment;
(d) identifying new syndromes.

Public health reasons include:

(e) estimating the prevalence of psychopathological reactions in the community for needs assessment purposes;
(f) gathering information that can be used for preparing and tailoring response programs;
(g) evaluating the effectiveness of interventions;
(h) monitoring the long-term health problems, particularly in cases involving exposures with uncertain future effects;
(i) addressing public concerns about the health effects of the event;
(j) responding to possible legal challenges.

In a recently published review of the disaster literature, we expressed the concern that contemporary disaster research has reached a point where further descriptive studies may be expected to yield little added value to what is already known (Bromet & Havenaar, 2002). We pointed out that recent studies tend to reconfirm findings that are well established. In part, this occurs because the majority of contemporary studies administer a core battery of interview schedules and questionnaires that contain pre-formatted questions and pre-determined answer categories. Thus, we suggested that except for the need for further studies about psycho-physiological mechanisms associated with adverse outcomes, especially in cases where the disaster involves exposure to toxic substances with potential negative effects on the central nervous system, the main reasons for doing further disaster studies are likely to be in the public health domain. Conceivably, a merger of quantitative and qualitative methods might yield some significant novel findings about disaster's impact. Along these lines, funding agencies, such as the National Institute of Mental Health (2002), are in fact more interested in studies designed to develop and evaluate post-disaster mental health interventions than in further descriptive epidemiologic post-disaster research.

Challenges in designing disaster studies

Disasters by their very nature are unanticipated. As such, a number of challenges arise in designing studies of their mental health sequelae.

Assembling a research team

The first such challenge is to identify collaborators and organize a research team. Relationships within any research team must be built on mutual trust and respect. In disaster studies, the team is likely to be assembled quickly and at the same time to find itself having to operate under extremely difficult circumstances and with major time constraints. Also, it is not unusual for some members of the research team or their relatives to be directly affected by the event. It is equally important to establish trust between the team and the affected population, as well as between the research team and people involved in relief work in the field. While this may seem obvious, these challenges are not easily achieved when both the research team and the affected population share the shock and devastation of the event. Thus, the research team needs to take stock of their own emotional responses and privacy needs as they consider how to deal with the same issues among potential study participants.

Timing

The design of an investigation will depend largely on the aims of the study and the conditions under which the study will take place. Most mental health studies will take place after the disaster occurs, and after the physical toll is known. Many recent studies have involved cross-sectional surveys, including telephone surveys. These studies try to show differences in rates of symptoms across time, but only longitudinal (follow-up) studies are capable of describing the course and outcome of post-disaster psychological effects, risk and protective factors, and benefits of intervention programs. The timing of the research, as well as of the follow-ups, will be determined by the specific research questions being addressed, as well as by the feasibility and availability of resources available for conducting the study.

So far, we have focused on post-disaster research. It is also important to consider the challenges involved in studying "potential" disasters, such as future bio-terrorist attacks in which the need for an entirely different type of study may arise. In this scenario, researchers may be confronted with an essentially unique situation, that is, to design an investigation of whether certain observed health problems are the result of an as yet unknown attack (Fielder *et al.*, 2002). This was the case in the initial days after the first cases of anthrax were diagnosed in Florida in the fall of 2001 and the source of the infection was unknown. This type of *cluster analysis* will not be further discussed here, but readers interested in this issue are referred to Fielder *et al.* (2002).

Exposure identification

The next step is to identify the relevant physical and psychosocial exposures. This issue is critically important because it will determine which end-points are to be assessed, that is, only psychological or psychiatric sequelae or also global and/or specific physical health outcomes. In the realm of mental health outcomes, it is important to consider a range of potential clinical and sub-clinical domains, including depression, anxiety, substance use and abuse, somatic symptoms, and PTSD. Recent research has demonstrated that medically unexplained physical symptoms (MUPS) are an under-researched outcome of disasters (Bromet & Havenaar, 2002; Van den Berg *et al.*, 2005). They may occur especially after disasters involving toxic exposure or in cultural settings where somatic complaints are the normative means for expressing distress. For each of the outcomes to be studied, the relevant competing risk factors, and the potential confounding variables, must be carefully measured as well. Often this means that the interviews or questionnaires will be lengthy, and this too poses a special challenge for disaster studies.

One of the important challenges in disaster research, which gives rise to continuous debates at all stages of the research, from design and instrument selection to data analysis and interpretation, is to bridge the gap between the psychological and psychiatric approaches. Psychologists tend to approach research from a dimensional and dynamic point of view, whereas psychiatric epidemiologists tend to focus on categorical disease end-points. To some extent, this will influence the sample size needed to achieve a specific result. More than that, these different approaches may give rise to incorrect use of terms, such as "PTSD" which is meant to be a clinical category but is often used to describe individuals with high scores on scales evaluating the intrusion, avoidance, and hyperarousal symptoms encompassed by the DSM-IV definition of PTSD.

Sample selection

Once the aim of the study has been set, and the study design decided upon, the next step is to define the affected population. This represents one of the most difficult tasks in disasters studies. The chaotic situation that occurs immediately after a disaster often makes it impossible to determine who exactly was affected and who was not. Immediately after the crash of the El Al Boeing 747 into a housing block in Amsterdam in 1992, killing 29 residents and 4 crewmembers, the authorities estimated that between 1000 and 1500 persons had directly experienced the crash. This included rescue workers who arrived during the early hours after the event. Six years later, after the endless rumours regarding the possible presence of toxic agents in the cargo was finally proven to be false, more than 6000 people came for a medical check-up because they feared that their health might have been compromized because of the event (Yzermans & Gersons, 2002). Because of the chaos and the need to maximize the number of people available at the disaster site, even tightly run organizations such as police and fire departments may be unable to produce accurate lists of officers who participated in relief work. Because of the difficulties in defining the sampling frame for a disaster study, many studies turn to convenience samples, such as litigants, web survey responders, telephone responders, insurance claimants, or clinic attenders. Prevalence estimates based on such samples are likely to be unreliable. For example, studies of help-seeking refugees from Cambodia residing in the United States produced prevalence rates of disasterrelated disorders ranging from 22% to 92% (Abueg & Chun, 1996).

Once the target sample is defined, it is often extremely difficult to identify an unaffected control group (or groups) who are similar in all respects except for exposure to the disaster. Usually control groups are selected from nearby towns. One obvious problem is that people in nearby towns may in fact be exposed via extensive media coverage, by working in or near the disaster area, or by having friends or family members living or working in the exposure site. For example, in a study of the effects of major floods in southern France, Verger and colleagues found that many control subjects from the unaffected villages nearby had family members or business interests in the flooded villages (Verger *et al.*, 2000). In disasters involving toxic exposures, the comparison sites should be screened for other contaminants that could lead to the same end-points. For example, one of the first western epidemiological studies of the health effects of the 1986 Chernobyl accident, the International Chernobyl Project (IAEA, 1991), evaluated the health status of five age groups living in rural contaminated communities with that of controls from "non-exposed" villages and found no significant differences in physical health (hematological, thyroid, and general health measures). After the report was disseminated in Ukraine, the authorities claimed that the control villages were polluted by dangerous levels of pesticides.

Challenges in instrument selection

Diagnosis vs. symptom checklists

Once the research questions, study design and relevant outcome domains have been determined, the next step is to select the specific measures. A large number of standardized diagnostic and symptom inventories are available, and certain measures, such as Diagnostic Interview Schedule (DIS), the General Health Questionnaire (GHQ), and the Impact of Events Scale (IES), have been administered in many disaster studies. Even though most of these instruments have been shown to have acceptable reliability and validity, it is important to realize that when different instruments are used to measure the same condition, or even when single instruments are used with different cut-off scores or diagnostic criteria, wide variation in prevalence rates may ensue. More specifically, in the recent National Comorbidity Survey-Replication, a sub-sample of those initially interviewed with the Composite International Diagnostic Interview (CIDI) were subsequently re-interviewed by clinicians over the telephone with an abbreviated 12-month version of the Structured Clinical Interview for DSM-IV (SCID) (Kessler *et al.*, 2003). Although 7.6% of the sample met DSM-IV criteria for major depressive disorder on the CIDI, 5.2% met the same criteria on the SCID, with a chance corrected agreement that was at best moderate (*kappa* = 0.6, 95% CI 0.2–0.6). It is therefore important to keep in mind that the variability in the prevalence rates achieved across different studies is in part attributable to the specific instruments included in the research.

Having made the choice between dimensional or categorical (diagnostic) measures, or the choice to use both, the next issue to decide upon is whether to use self-report or interview methods. Self-report questionnaires are convenient and relatively inexpensive to use. They tend to have good sensitivity but less favourable specificity. Interviews are more costly, and especially in the case of structured interviews, have reasonable specificity. The cut-points themselves may be culturally specific. For example, in the USA, when asked to rate your health, the majority of people in the general population answer excellent or very good; few people say moderate, fair, or poor. In Ukraine, the normative response is moderate, and the next most popular response is fair. Few people would evaluate their health as very good. In our Chernobyl research (Adams *et al.*, 2002), it was necessary to extend the low end of the scale by adding a "very poor" category in order to capture the full range of responses in a meaningful way.

To date, most disaster studies have been conducted in the West. Whether our measures are equally reliable and valid across race and ethnic groups is a topic that has rarely been studied. Thus, September 11 affected a diverse set of cultural and ethnic groups. Our lack of knowledge about the cross-cultural validity of western measures and the absence of culturally sensitive measures for most of these affected populations has limited what could be learned from this body of disaster research. Similarly because the majority of disasters occur in underdeveloped areas of the world, selecting appropriate instruments is a major challenge. Unfortunately, few disaster studies include an examination of cultural variations in idioms of distress or the cross-cultural validity of the instruments and assessment methods that are used (Van Ommeren, 2003). The best way to handle the issue is to include investigators on the research team who are part of the community that was affected by the disaster although even then, the arduous task of establishing cross-cultural reliability and validity may be beyond the grasp of the typical disaster study that is done under both time and budgetary constraints.

A further measurement issue is the assessment of the level of personal involvement and incurred stress as a consequence of the disaster. Usually in disaster studies, proximity to the disaster site is used as a proxy for exposure to stress emanating from the event. In addition, other information is collected to assess the level of personal involvement, such as whether the subject was injured, lost relatives or property, had to be evacuated, or witnessed dead or injured persons. When the exposure information is subjective (Did you feel threatened by the event?), recall bias may be a special problem because the response will be influenced by current affectivity. However, even when the exposure information is presumed to be objective, recall bias is an issue, especially over time. Southwick *et al.* (1997) interviewed veterans from the first Gulf War about their traumatic experiences 1 month and again 2 years after their return home. Eighty-eight per cent changed their response to at least one item of the questionnaire that asked about their experiences in the field.

Challenges in executing disaster studies

Access to remote areas

Not only it is difficult to define the affected population, in many cases it may also be difficult to reach the area. Many disasters in developing countries occur in remote areas, but even areas that are accessible under normal conditions might be difficult to reach because of disrupted transportation systems or restrictions imposed by the authorities regarding entry. Conducting telephone surveys may be a way to circumvent these problems, providing telephones are widely available and are functional. When the Chernobyl accident occurred in 1986, many people in Kiev had party lines, and thus there was no guarantee that privacy could be achieved. Conditions at the disaster site may also make it difficult to adequately monitor the fieldwork. Another problem is that affected populations or parts of them may have been evacuated or scattered.

Response rates

Even if eligible subjects can be reached, response rates may be low because people have other priorities and have no time to participate in a mental health study. The post-disaster period is often characterized by great turmoil, food and housing shortages, economic hardships, and battles for benefits. These can all lead to relatively low response rates and potentially biased samples. This is certainly not always the case, and response rates of more than 80% have been achieved (e.g., Adams *et al.*, 2002). In general, however, response rates from disaster follow-up studies have been disappointing. For example, in a 33-year follow-up after a mudslide in Aberfan, South-Wales, which killed 116 children, it was possible to trace 115 of the 145 survivors in the original cohort, but only 41 agreed to participate (28% of the total). Achieving a good response rate in the control group is sometimes more difficult because the motivation for participation is not as obvious. In the Aberfan study, only 19% of controls participated in the follow-up (Morgan *et al.*, 2003).

Informed consent

In settings where the population is not literate, or distrust in authorities is the norm, including a western-style informed consent procedure may be challenging. However, in our experience studying the effects of Chernobyl, while our colleagues in Ukraine, Belarus, and Russia expressed outrage at the concept, virtually everyone whom we studied was happy to hear about confidentiality and related issues and did not hesitate to sign the consent form.

A related concern that has been raised is whether trauma victims are able to give valid informed consent, especially immediately after the event. DuMont and Stermac (1996) found that 10–39 months later, 14 out of 15 survivors of sexual assault who had signed consent forms to participate in a trauma study could not remember having given consent. However, they also reported that they had no problem with being approached by the research team and were willing to participate. To date, there is no evidence to suggest that participation has negative effects on participants, even in the immediate aftermath of traumatic experiences, although more research needs to be conducted on this issue.

In a similar vein, several authors have suggested that trauma survivors may be too fragile to endure the painful memories and the stress evoked by participation in PTSD research (Templeton, 1993; DuMont & Stermac, 1996; Drauker, 1999). These concerns have largely been based on anecdotal evidence. The few empirical studies to investigate this issue found no negative effects of interviews among victims of interpersonal violence (Walker *et al.*, 1997; Newman *et al.*, 1999; Griffin *et al.*, 2003). In fact, in most studies participants tended to view participation as a positive experience, while only a minority reported that the emotions aroused during the interview were stronger than they expected. In the Bromet follow up 3 years after the Three Mile Island accident (Dew *et al.*, 1987), one control mother said that the questions previously asked about her marriage were extremely upsetting and she thus refused to participate again; however, no other respondent refusing the follow-up interview indicated that her decision was based on the content of the previous assessment.

Challenges in the analytic phase

Power

Many disaster studies are by their very nature designed and implemented on short notice. Usually no power analysis has been done beforehand. Power problems are particularly likely to be problematic in studies focused on clinical diagnoses with relatively low prevalence, such as somatization disorder. Thus, the two published prospective studies of subjects who had by chance participated in a mental health survey and subsequently experienced a disaster had relatively small numbers of subjects (Robins *et al.*, 1986; Smith *et al.*, 1986; Canino *et al.*, 1990; Escobar *et al.*, 1992). While these studies are very valuable from a methodological point of view, their relatively low N's have made it practically impossible to establish whether the disasters had an effect on clinically diagnosable disorders although symptom severity for these disorders increased significantly.

Multiple comparisons

An issue arising in any study involving extensive testing, and therefore also in disaster studies, is the multiple comparisons problem. This is further compounded by the fact that the measures themselves are highly intercorrelated (e.g., depression, anxiety, PTSD, and somatic complaints). To date, very few disaster studies have controlled for multiple comparisons, and it is important that future studies consider this issue when establishing cut-points for statistical significance.

False positive and misleading inferences

The widely used IES (Horowitz, 1990) and other PTSD scales contain measures of intrusion and avoidance symptoms. It is important to realize that with recurrent images of disasters shown on TV, high scores for intrusion may represent false positive answers, and instead may be tapping repeated exposure to images on the news networks. In a recently completed study of the mental health effects of an accident near Lviv, in western Ukraine, in which a jet fighter plane crashed into a crowd of families who had gathered to watch an air show, we found a modest but statistically significant correlation between the presence of intrusive symptoms on the IES and watching the event over and over again on TV (Bromet *et al.*, 2005). If the symptom inventories were not comprehensive in scope, false negatives can occur. Thus, for example, if acting out behaviours or substance abuse problems are not assessed, and anxiety and affective symptoms are evaluated, women will appear to have suffered more in relation to an event than men when in fact, the overall impact on psychological and substance morbidity may be similar.

Reporting mental health effects

In the situation of disasters, where the stress is collective, a public health perspective should be maintained when describing the psychological impact on a stricken community. For example, if the results show an increased rate of panic attacks in exposed vs. controls, it is important to clearly communicate that this does not imply that "the population was in a panic". Indeed, as Glass and Schoch-Spana (2002) commented, the findings generally suggest that panic is the exception, not the norm. As responsible citizens, it is our obligation as researchers to present a balanced picture of the impact of the event under study. Rarely do we include "positive" outcomes, rarely do we examine the functional consequences of psychological symptoms, and rarely are we mindful of the limitations of our measures. Thus in our opinion, it is important for investigators not to over-emphasize or over-dramatize the findings. Durodie and Wessely (2002) take this point one step further by suggesting that the strong emphasis placed on the negative impact of terrorist events by media and authorities – who mostly obtain their information from researchers and clinicians – may even be exploited by terrorist groups to their advantage (Durodie & Wessely, 2002; Gearson, 2002). Following these authors' line of reasoning, negative findings from disaster studies may send an unintended message to the public that massive psychopathology is likely to ensue.

As noted above, disaster studies usually do little justice to describing the overall resilience of the population, or the positive effects a disaster can have in strengthening community ties or sense of patriotism. In the worst-case scenario, studies emphasizing negative outcomes may instead strengthen victim identity among the survivors and/or suggest symptoms to future study subjects. In short, disaster research is a form of intervention, and like any intervention, it may have positive as well as negative effects which should be taken into consideration.

Discussion

In recent years many studies have been published about the health effects of disasters. The point has been reached where one might get the impression that every disaster either is or should be followed by a mental health study. As we indicated earlier, it is unlikely that studies that continue in the tradition of using the same standardized interviews with predetermined response categories will come up with new, clinically relevant information. Perhaps one of the main reasons that these studies are still being done is that they are a way for society at large, and mental health specialists in particular, to show their concern for the affected community. The study confirms for the victims that the outside world cares about them and may be a way to communicate the outcry of the affected population to the outside world.

From a scientific point of view, it is important that future studies be designed to investigate the effects of large-scale mental health interventions. After the terrorist attacks of September 11, numerous support services were set up in the New York area, although reportedly socially underprivileged neighbourhoods received far less mental health support than more affluent parts of the city. As researchers, we are in a position to recognize disparities in the provision of mental health care after disasters and other catastrophic events. Indeed, since most disaster studies are epidemiologic in nature, and epidemiology is the scientific arm of preventive medicine, it behaves us as disaster researchers to address this issue.

We also believe that it is timely to reconsider the need for rapid interventions in the intermediate aftermath of a disaster (Sensky, 2003). A number of studies have reported that "crisis support", that is, providing people who will listen and give practical and emotional support, has positive effects on well-being (e.g., Dalgleish *et al.*, 1996). Undoubtedly people from the affected population will appreciate the attention and support offered, whether this is provided by mental health professionals, clergy, or lay people. It remains to be seen, however, whether providing such support by mental health professionals makes sense from a public health point of view. There have been relatively few studies which have systematically investigated the effectiveness of mental health interventions, such as psychological debriefing, in a randomized controlled fashion. The studies that have been done were unable to consistently show a positive effect of this type of intervention (Wessely & Bisson, 2001). Two trauma studies, in fact, reported a negative effect of individual and group emotional debriefing (Carlier *et al.*, 2000). It remains to be investigated whether these results also hold true in disaster situations.

Even less is known about the effects of information provided by authorities about what occurs in the immediate aftermath of an event. In the Amsterdam airplane crash disaster described above, it was believe that failure of the authorities to credibly falsify rumours about the presence of toxic substances aboard the freighter was one of the crucial factors which fuelled uncertainty and fear in the public. Similar allegations have been made about the way the British government handled the bovine spongiform encephalitis crisis (Furedi & Taylor-Goodby, 2002). More research is needed about the most effective strategies for risk communication in the wake of disaster.

Despite our lengthy discussion of caveats and potential drawbacks of conducting disaster research, it is our experience that meeting the special challenges that disaster research poses is well worth the effort. Victims of disasters do need to talk, and researchers who listen (not just prejudge all the questions and possible responses) may contribute valuable insights about coping with horrific stress. From a scientific point of view because disasters are independent events, often occurring indiscriminately to subjects regardless of their personal histories or personalities, they offer epidemiology the rare opportunity to study the effects of a "natural" experiment. Most importantly, the results of carefully designed and interpreted studies can be used for planning public heath interventions in the future.

REFERENCES

Abueg, F.R. & Chun, K.M. (1996). Traumatization stress among Asians and Asian Americans. In *Ethnocultural Aspects of Posttraumatic Stress Disorder: Issues, Research and Clinical Applications*, eds. M.J. Marsella, M.J. Friedman, E.T. Gerrity & R.M. Scurfield. Washington, DC: American Psychological Association, pp. 285–299.

Adams, R.E., Bromet, E.J., Panina, N. & Golovakha, E. (2002). Stress and well-being in mothers of young children 11 years after the Chornobyl nuclear power plant accident. *Psychological Medicine*, **32**, 143–156.

Adler, A. (1943). Neuropsychiatric complications in victims of Boston's Coconut Grove disaster. *Journal of the American Medical Association*, **123**, 1098–1101.

Bromet, E.J. & Dew, M.A. (1995). Review of psychiatric epidemiologic research on disasters. *Epidemiological Reviews*, **17**, 113–119.

Bromet, E.J. & Schulberg, H.C. (1986). The TMI disaster: a search for high-risk groups. In *Disaster Stress Studies: New Methods and Findings*, ed. J.H. Shore. Washington, DC: American Psychiatric Press, pp. 2–19.

Bromet, E.J. & Havenaar, J.M. (2002). Mental health consequences of disasters. In *Psychiatry in Society*, eds. N. Sartorius, W. Gabael, J.J. Lopez-Ibor & M. Maj. Chichester, U.K: John Wiley & Sons, pp. 241–261.

Bromet, E.M., Havenaar, J.M., Gluzman, S.F. & Tintle, N.L. (2005). Psychological aftermath of the Lviv air show disaster: a prospective controlled study. *Acta Psychiatrica Scandinavica*, **112**, 194–200.

Canino, G., Bravo, M., Rubio-Stipec, M. & Woodbury, M. (1990). The impact of disaster on mental health: prospective and retrospective analyses. *International Journal of Mental Health*, **19**, 51–69.

Carlier, I.V., Voerman, A.E. & Gersons, B.P. (2000). The influence of occupational debriefing on post-traumatic stress symptomatology in traumatized police officers. *British Journal of Medical Psychology*, **73**, 87–98.

Dalgleish, T., Joseph, S., Thrasher, S., Tranah, T. & Yule, W. (1996). Crisis support following the Herald of Free-Enterprise disaster: a longitudinal perspective. *Journal of Traumatic Stress*, **9**, 833–845.

Dew, M.A., Bromet, E.J. & Schulberg, H.C. (1987). A comparative analysis of two community stressors' long-term mental health effects. *American Journal of Community Psychology*, **15**, 167–184.

Drauker, C.B. (1999). The emotional impact of sexual violence research in participants. *Archives of Psychiatric Nursing*, **13**, 161–169.

DuMont, J. & Stermac, L. (1996). Research with women who have been sexually assaulted: examining informed consent. *Canadian Journal of Human Sexuality*, **5**, 185–191.

Durodie, B. & Wessely, S. (2002). Resilience or panic: the public and terrorist attack. *The Lancet*, **360**, 1901–1902.

Escobar, J.I., Canino, G., Rubio-Stipec, M. & Bravo, M. (1992). Somatic symptoms after a natural disaster: a prospective study. *American Journal of Psychiatry*, **149**, 965–967.

Fielder, H.M.P., Palmer, S.R. & Coleman, G. (2002). Methodological issues in the investigation of chemical accidents. In *Toxic Turmoil: Psychological and Societal Consequences of Ecological Disasters*. New York: Plenum, pp. 185–197.

Furedi, F. & Taylor-Goodby, P. (2002). *The Assessment of Asymmetric Threat.* Canterbury: University of Kent.

Galea, S., Nandi, A. & Vlahov, D. (2005). The epidemiology of post-traumatic stress disorder after disasters. *Epidemiologic Reviews*, **27**, 78–91.

Gearson, J. (2002). The nature of modern terrorism. In *Political Quarterly*, ed. L. Freedman. Oxford: Blackwell, pp. 7–24.

Glass, T.A. & Schoch-Spana, M. (2002). Bioterrorism and the people: how to vaccinate a city against panic. *Clinical Infectious Disease*, **34**, 217–223.

Griffin, M.G., Resick, P.A., Waldrop, A.E. & Mechanic, M.B. (2003). *Journal of Traumatic Stress*, **16**, 221–227.

Havenaar, J.M., Cwikel, J.G. & Bromet, E.J. (2002). *Toxic Turmoil: Psychological and Societal Consequences of Ecological Disasters.* New York: Plenum.

Horowitz, M. (1990). Post-traumatic stress disorders: psychosocial aspects of the diagnosis. *International Journal of Mental Health*, **19**, 21–36.

IAEA (International Atomic Energy Association). (1991). *The International Chernobyl Project: An Assessment of Radiological Consequences and Evaluation of Protective Measures.* Vienna: IAEA.

Kessler, R.C., Berglund, P., Demler, O., Jin, R., Koretz, D., Merikangas, K.R., Rush, J., Walters, E.E. & Wang, P.S. (2003). The epidemiology of major depressive disorder. Results from the National Comorbidity Survey-Replication (NCS-R). *Journal of the American Medical Association*, **289**, 3095–3105.

Morgan, L., Scourfield, J., Williams, D., Jasper, A. & Lewis, G. (2003). The Aberfan disaster: 33-year follow-up of survivors. *British Journal of Psychiatry*, **182**, 532–536.

Morris, J.N. (1964). *Uses of Epidemiology* (2nd ed.). London: Livingstone.

National Institute of Mental Health (2002). *Rapid Assessment Post-impact of Disaster.* www.nimh.nih.gov.

Newman, E., Walker, E.A. & Gefland, A. (1999). Assessing the ethical costs and benefits of trauma focussed research. *General Hospital Psychiatry*, **21**, 187–196.

Robins, L.N., Fischbach, R.L., Smith, E.M., Cottler, L.B., Solomon, S.D. & Goldring, E. (1986). Impact of disaster on previously assessed mental health. In *Disaster Stress Studies: New Methods and Findings*, ed. J.H. Shore. Washington, DC: American Psychiatric Press, pp. 21–48.

Sensky, T. (2003). The utility of systematic reviews: the case of psychological debriefing after trauma. *Psychotherapy and Psychosomatics*, **72**, 171–175.

Smith, E.M., Robins, L.N., Pryzbeck, T.R., Goldring, E. & Solomon, S.D. (1986). Psychosocial consequences of a disaster. In *Disaster Stress Studies: New Methods and Findings*, ed. J.H. Shore. Washington, DC: American Psychiatric Press, pp. 49–76.

Southwick, S.M., Morgan III, A., Nicolaou, A.L. & Charney, D.S. (1997). Consistency of memory for combat-related traumatic events in veterans of Operation Desert Storm. *American Journal of Psychiatry*, **154**, 173–177.

Templeton, D.M. (1993). Sexual assault: effects of the research process on all the participants. *Canadian Family Physician*, **39**, 248–258.

Van den Berg, B., Grievink, L., Yzermans, J. & Lebret, E. (2005). Medically unexplained physical symptoms in the aftermath of disasters. *Epidemiologic Reviews*, **27**, 92–106.

Van Ommeren, M. (2003). Validity issues in transcultural epidemiology. *British Journal of Psychiatry*, **182**, 376–378.

Verger, P., Hunault, C., Rotily, M. & Baruffol, E. (2000). Risk factors for post traumatic stress symptoms five years after the 1992 flood in the Vaucluse (France). *Revue Epidemiologie Sante Publique*, **48**(Suppl. 2), 2S44–2S53.

Wessely, S. & Bisson, J. (2001). *Brief Psychological Interventions "Debriefing" for Trauma-Related Symptoms and Prevention of Post Traumatic Stress Disorder*. Oxford: The Cochrane Library.

Walker, E.A., Newman, E., Koss, M. & Bernstein, D. (1997). Does the study of victimization revictimize the victims? *Psychiatry and Primary Care*, **19**, 403–410.

Yzermans, J. & Gersons, B.P.R. (2002). The chaotic aftermath of an airplane crash in Amsterdam: a second disaster. In *Toxic Turmoil: Psychological and Societal Consequences of Ecological Disasters*, eds. J.M. Havenaar, J.G. Cwikel & E.J. Bromet. New York: Plenum, pp. 85–99.

8

Mental health research in the aftermath of disasters: using the right methods to ask the right questions

Sandro Galea

Introduction

Several research teams have documented the consequences of the September 11, 2001, terrorist attacks in New York City and throughout the country. The chapters in this part bring together reports from three of these research teams and summarize some of the key findings from each of their studies. Two commentaries offer perspectives on the challenges that this research faces and what these challenges suggest for post-disaster research in general. There are several key methodologic points that emerge from these preceding chapters. In this discussion I will synthesize the key methodologic issues that emerge both from the empiric papers and from the accompanying commentaries. Some of my comments are congruent with those already articulated in the preceding six chapters. I restate those comments here to reflect their importance and to present them as a part of a broader reflection on this area of research.

Overall, we can fruitfully consider the key methodologic issues at hand along two principal lines, namely issues pertaining to nature of the sample and issues that pertain to assessment methods used in the research.

Population sampling

Choosing the right sample to ask the right questions

We can consider that there are three principal types of samples that have, appropriately, been the focus of most post-disaster research. These are: samples of persons who were directly affected by a disaster (frequently referred to as "victims" in the literature), samples of rescue works (including police, fire-fighters and others), and general population samples. As noted by North *et al.* (this volume) in their commentary, studies that are implemented in each of these samples are not comparable and indeed neither should they be. We can readily imagine that persons in each of these three samples may be affected by a particular disaster in different ways. For example, the relation between intensity of traumatic event exposure and risk of post-traumatic stress disorder (PTSD) is well established (Brewin *et al.*, 2000; Galea *et al.*, 2005). It is to be expected that samples of those directly affected by a disaster will have higher prevalence of psychopathology than either of the other two samples. Similarly, the event exposures of general population samples are likely to be immensely heterogenous, ranging from direct personal exposure (i.e., some persons in the general population will have been direct victims) to no exposure whatsoever, and as such, the overall prevalence of psychopathology in general population samples would be expected to be far lower than that in victim groups.

These different types of samples present researchers with an opportunity to ask different questions in the aftermath of disasters. Samples of disaster victims allow inquiry about individual-level mechanisms that explain the associations between risk factors and risk of psychopathology. For example, recent work using such samples has explored both the role of social support in shaping post-disaster resilience (Tucker *et al.*, 2000) and the physiologic precursors of PTSD (Goenjian *et al.*, 2003).

Samples of rescue workers are marked by heterogeneity in exposures that is typically greater than that in victim samples. Rescue workers may include, for example, both fire-fighters who were directly involved in the extraction of persons from a disaster site and construction workers who were involved in cleanup operations. In many disaster instances, the September 11, 2001, terrorist attacks among them, rescue workers are exposed to disaster sites for a prolonged period after the disaster. Therefore, these samples are particularly suited to questions that pertain to the relations between nature of exposure and subsequent psychopathologic outcomes. In addition, rescue workers may be exposed to occupational hazards ranging from fine particulate matter that may result in respiratory disease to direct physical injury from unsafe work sites. Occupational and environmental health researchers then have a unique opportunity to better inform our understanding of the aftermath of disasters, and how the consequences of these events can be minimized both in magnitude and in duration.

Finally, general population samples introduce opportunities to consider the population burden of disaster consequences, to understand the determinants of population rates of disease, and to understand disasters (and their consequences) within multivariate and multilevel frameworks that can facilitate our understanding of the factors *beyond* the individual that influence post-disaster outcomes. Direct victim samples do little to elucidate the overall burden of mental health problems. This may be a particular concern in large disasters such as the September 11, 2001, terrorist attacks where, in the months following the event, state and federal officials needed population estimates of disease burden in order to implement adequate mental health relief resources. Population-based samples can assess both those who were directly affected as well as those who were less directly affected by the disaster, hence providing such estimates. Importantly, research using population-based samples needs to ensure that there is a well-conceived rationale as to why a particular general population sample may be affected by a disaster. As noted in some of the preceding chapters, there may be conceptual reasons why PTSD, which nosologically requires linkage to exposure, may not be plausibly present in distant populations (e.g., general US samples) after a disaster in New York City but may well be plausible in areas closer to the disaster site.

Epidemiologically, the determinants of population rates of disease may be different than the determinants of individual risk (Rose, 1992). Factors that have only small effects on individual risk of pathology may, by virtue of their ubiquity, be sentinel determinants of population rates. Population-based samples are then essential to identify such factors. For example, although controversial, there have been some provocative findings published recently which suggest that television exposure may be linked to a greater risk of psychopathology among direct victims of a disaster (Ahern et al., 2004). This observation was facilitated by the heterogeneity of a population-based sample; samples that studied only victims would not have been likely to isolate television viewing as a risk factor. The ubiquity of modern television exposure to disasters unfolding in real time suggests that television viewing may be a critical determinant of population rates of psychopathology after future disasters.

Although there has been a longstanding appreciation in the scientific literature that factors which influence post-disaster outcomes include community-level factors there is very little empiric research about factors at levels beyond the individual that may affect population prevalence of post-disaster pathology (Norris et al., 2002; Galea et al., 2005). The social context undoubtedly modifies the individual experience of disasters and elucidating the role of social context in these circumstances is emerging as one of the most promising areas of disaster research. In addition, community-level factors such as social cohesion have no individual analog and must be studied at the group level often necessitating a representative, large, population-based sample to test specific hypotheses.

In sum, there is much room for growth in disaster research, particularly in moving beyond the victim-based samples that have been the traditional focus of most of this research, to innovative use of other samples asking questions that extend what we understand in the area.

The relevance of different sampling strategies

A smaller, but important, consideration about choosing samples to inform disaster research relates to the methods that are used to collect these samples and the implications these methods have for inference from this data. Perhaps an easy example of this concern arises in the use of random representative samples and the so-called "convenience" samples. Although randomly selected representative population-based samples may provide us with an opportunity to generalize to populations at large, in contrast, convenience samples embed biases about reasons for participation that make it difficult to draw inference from such samples to other populations.

More subtle differences in sample selection may also make generalization from studies employing different sampling strategies challenging. For example, although both the studies conducted by Galea *et al.* and Silver *et al.* discussed in chapters in this part of the book, recruited population representative samples, the former used random-digit-dialing techniques for sample selection while the latter employed an existing Internet-based cohort that was originally recruited through random-digit-dialing techniques (Galea *et al.*, this volume; Silver *et al.*, this volume). Many factors, including computer literacy, personal need for ongoing incentives, and amount of free time, may influence ongoing participation in an Internet-based cohort. The epidemiologic experience with these methods is limited and it is difficult to fully know how to account for the potential factors that influence ongoing participant involvement in this cohort, and as a result, to draw firm conclusions about the comparability of these two samples, even though both may mirror their target population socio-demographically. This issue may be a particular challenge when considering sampling strategies employed across countries. For example, in a series of studies that have assessed the consequences of the Chernobyl nuclear meltdown in the Ukraine, Bromet *et al.* (2000) recruited samples that represented the populations of interest in the Ukraine. However, the incentives to participate in such a study within a rigidly regimented centrally controlled system are undoubtedly different than the incentives that motivate volunteers in the USA to participate in disaster research. The challenges in obtaining representative samples, and the specific implications of the decisions made by the investigators to obtain such samples need to be understood and carefully considered when interpreting results of post-disaster research. An upcoming volume that concerns itself with methodologic issues in post-disaster research addresses these issues in substantially more detail (Norris *et al.*, 2006).

Comparing data across studies

Inherent in this discussion is the fact that data obtained from different sampling frames is frequently not directly comparable and as such cross-study inference can only be made with judicious attention to the nature of the sampling frame and its components. In some ways this observation is self-evident. For example, it is clearly unwise to use data from samples of children, such as those presented by Hoven *et al.* in this volume, to extrapolate to potential findings in adults, or vice versa (Hoven *et al.*, this volume). Other cross-sample comparisons may be more tempting to make and may well lead to erroneous conclusions. This may be particularly relevant when considering general population samples given these samples' heterogeneity. For example, reviews of the empiric epidemiologic literature have long suggested that the psychological consequences of human-made disasters may be more pronounced than the consequences of natural disasters (Norris *et al.*, 2002). However, as has been previously noted (Galea *et al.*, 2005), the persons who have typically been enrolled in studies of human-made disasters (e.g., explosions) tend to be more directly affected by the events than studies of natural disasters (e.g., tornadoes), where the samples typically include persons in the general community whose exposure is more heterogeneous. It is likely that the reason for lower estimates of psychopathology in the latter samples is simply that these samples include more persons whose exposure was less marked than those in the former samples.

Limitations of cross-sample comparisons have somewhat limited the field. In some ways all disasters are unique and as such observations drawn from one disaster study and one particular sample may require replication in several subsequent disasters before we can draw generalizations confidently. It is worth noting though, that it is often possible to compare specific subsamples within larger studies. For example, in the series of studies after the September 11, 2001, terrorist attacks conducted by Galea *et al.* (and discussed in part in an earlier chapter in this volume), the prevalence of PTSD among the subset of persons in the general population sample who actually were in the World Trade Center complex during the attacks was 34% (Galea *et al.*, 2003), virtually identical to the prevalence of PTSD documented among victims of the Oklahoma City bombing (most of whom were in the Murrah Federal building during the bombing) studied by North *et al.* (1999). Such comparisons can increase our confidence in replicability of these epidemiologic findings and can be immensely helpful to public health planners.

Comparing data within studies

A parallel issue to the above, and one that has been the subject of some debate in research related to this issue, is the issue of within-sample comparison. As Havenaar and Bromet suggest in their chapter in this part (Havenaar & Bromet, this volume), identifying control communities that are exactly comparable to those affected by disasters is next to impossible. This becomes even more apparent when we consider the potential contributions of community-level factors to population rates of disease. The search for control communities that are comparable to affected communities both on individual socio-demographic parameters and on key contextual characteristics is almost certainly futile. General population samples then present a particularly important opportunity for within-study comparison of persons who were differently exposed to a disaster but all of whom may plausibly have been at risk for psychopathology after the event. For example, in the series of studies conducted by Galea *et al.* after September 11, 2001, a sampling frame that included New York City and the New York metropolitan area allowed the investigators to compare persons who were geographically closer or further from the disaster focus (as discussed in a chapter in this book). This sample also allowed for comparison between those who were highly exposed (e.g., close to the World Trade Center) and those who were at most only indirectly affected by the event. This then permits comparison to other studies that have sampled only persons who were direct victims of the event (as noted earlier in comparison to North *et al.*, chapter) and also allows for intra-study comparisons between exposure groups, testing hypotheses both about risk factors for individual psychopathology and population-level determinants of disease rates.

Assessment methods

Rigorous adherence to DSM-IV nosology

There is little question that the field of mental health epidemiology has been immeasurably advanced by the establishment of the *Diagnostic and Statistical Manual of Mental Disorders* (DSM), and in particular since the DSM-III which was published in 1980. The DSM provides diagnostic algorithms and, as a result, allows for comparability of diagnosis across clinicians. North *et al.* in their chapter, discuss the implications of the DSM nosology for PTSD (North *et al.*, this volume). I concur with North *et al.* that the DSM should provide the basis for assessment of psychopathology in disaster research. However, it is also worth noting that diagnosable disorders and diagnostic criteria within psychiatry have not been subjected to extensive validation. Several authors (e.g., see Rounsaville *et al.*, 2002) have addressed the uncertainties of validating psychiatric diagnoses as established in the DSM. In particular, the DSM assumes that "psychiatric disorders are discrete biomedical entities with clear phenotypic boundaries" (p. 8) (Rounsaville *et al.*, 2002; Pfefferbaum *et al.*, in press). The DSM itself acknowledges this issue and notes that diagnostic criteria are "meant to serve as guidelines to be informed by clinical judgment." (American Psychiatric Association, 2000, p. xxii). Epidemiologic studies attempt to obtain data from participants in a systematic and invariant manner. As a result, numerous structured instruments have been developed that allow researchers to systematically collect psychiatric data from participants in a reproducible fashion. However, clearly, none of these instruments allow for clinical judgment and *none* of them can make diagnoses. Probably the most broadly accepted full structured interviews today are the CIDI, Composite International Diagnostic Interview and the clinician-administered PTSD scale (CAPS) (a discussion of the properties of the CIDI is provided in the Havenaar and Bromet chapter in this volume). However, these instruments are too lengthy for use in most general population surveys, where the researcher must balance issues of volunteer burden and costs, and obtain valid information as efficiently as possible. As a result, general population studies usually rely on brief instruments that have been validated, typically in studies that have compared their discriminatory ability to clinician diagnosis. Beyond such validation, the choice of instrument used then must depend on the particular study exigencies, the questions that are being asked, and the methods that are being used. It is in turn the responsibility of the researchers to make sure their decisions and instruments are presented clearly and of the consumers of the research to evaluate the validity of these findings accordingly.

There are two final points worth making in this regard. First, while I concur wholeheartedly with North *et al.* discussion (in this volume) about the need for semantic caution in presenting findings about psychopathology, I would suggest that since no diagnosis can be established absent clinical assessment, the essence of careful research interpretation lies not in nomenclature used for mental heath status detected (i.e., whether the appropriate term is "probable PTSD" or not), but rather in judicious interpretation of the findings of studies with careful attention paid to what the measures used in a particular studies were and how they were implemented. Second, regardless of our potential concern for the nosologic implications of findings from general survey research in the general population, the fact remains that several studies have shown that a substantial proportion of persons in the general population reported psychopathologic symptoms after the September 11, 2001, terrorist attacks, and that a proportion of those persons reported that these symptoms reduced their functioning (Galea & Resnick, 2005). It seems to this author self-evident that we must then consider the implications of this observation, both for the purposes of public mental health planning, and as an occasion for critical reflection on our current DSM-IV nosology and its potential limitations.

Choice of screening instrument

A corollary, but important point to this thinking is that the choice of assessment instrument, dictated, as I note above, primarily by what the key questions of interest are and what the best methods might be to address these methods. Use of different instruments across studies inevitably further complicates cross-study comparison. The use of different assessments instruments is critical because structural differences between assessment methodologies may lead to meaningfully different population-based prevalence estimates and small differences in diagnostic prevalence can produce significant underestimates or overestimates of the post-disaster needs of a community. To illustrate, in the 1–2 months following the September 11 terrorist attacks, Schlenger *et al.* (2002), using the PTSD Check List (PCL) as an assessment instrument, estimated that 11.2% of New York City area residents met criteria for probable PTSD. This estimate was 50% higher than of the 7.5% prevalence of PTSD estimated by Galea *et al.* (2002) in a sample of Manhattan residents using the National Women's Study (NWS) as an assessment instrument. Applying each of these prevalences to the population of over 8 million New York City residents, one would estimate that approximately 900,000 (Schlenger *et al.*, 2002) vs. 600,000 (Galea *et al.*, .2002) persons met criteria for probable PTSD, a difference of 300,000 people. Clearly, a discrepancy of 3.7% points can have significant implications for public mental health planning and resource allocations. Subsequent analyses have shown that the NWS instrument is more specific than the PCL and it is likely that these differences between these two population representative studies are primarily a function of the assessment instrument used (Ruggiero *et al.*, in press). It is then important that studies conducted after disasters explicitly state the psychometric properties of the assessment measures used to enable consumers of the research to adequately assess how to evaluate results from individual studies and how to compare results across studies.

Conclusion

As discussed throughout this section, and indeed in the whole book, post-disaster research presents particular challenges that must be addressed in order for this work to adequately document and understand the consequences of these events. While some of these challenges are endemic to all work carried out after disasters and mass traumas, others are particular to specific events. Clearly, researchers interested in the aftermath of disasters need to consider these issues, develop and implement study designs that best address them, and derive the best-possible inference from their studies. Equally as important, however, is the careful interpretation of post-disaster research. Unfortunately, both consumers of research and researchers themselves often fail to consider the methodologic and conceptual nuances that are guiding a particular study. Results from studies conducted in New York City are frequently conflated with studies conducted across the USA. Clearly, persons in each of these sampling frames may be at risk for different consequences of the September 11 terrorist attacks for different reasons. Scrupulous attention to decisions and assumptions embedded in particular study designs would go a long way to judicious inference drawn from post-disaster research. Conversely, researchers have a responsibility to present their work clearly, in such a way that consumers of the research can understand both its limitations and the extent to which inference can be drawn from their work. As the field expands, and as particular attention to methodologic rigor in these areas becomes paramount, the contribution of the field will undoubtedly grow and we will come closer to the goal of minimizing human suffering after mass traumas and terrorism.

REFERENCES

Ahern, J., Galea, S., Resnick, H. & Vlahov, D. (2004). Television images and probable PTSD after September 11: the role of background characteristics, event exposures and peri-event panic. *Journal of Nervous and Mental Disease*, **192**(3), 217–226.

American Psychiatric Association (1994). *Diagnostic and Statistical Manual of Mental Disorders* (4th ed.). Washington, DC: American Psychiatric Association.

American Psychiatric Association (2000). *Diagnostic and Statistical Manual of Mental Disorders*, (4th ed. Revised). Washington, DC: American Psychiatric Association.

Brewin, C.R., Andrews, B. & Valentine, J.D. (2000). Meta-analysis of risk factors for post-traumatic stress disorder in trauma-exposed adults. *Journal of Consulting and Clinical Psychology*, **68**, 746–766.

Bromet, E.J., Goldgaber, D., Carlson, G., Panina, N., Golovakha, E., Gluzman, S.F., Gilbert, T., Gluzman, D., Lyubsky, S. & Schwartz, J.E. (2000). Children's well-being 11 years after the Chornobyl catastrophe. *Archives of General Psychiatry*, **57**, 563–571.

Galea, S., Ahern, J., Resnick, H., Kilpatrick, D., Bucuvalas, M., Gold, J. & Vlahov, D. (2002). Psychological sequelae of the September 11 terrorist attacks in New York City. *New England Journal of Medicine*, **346**, 982–987.

Galea, S., Vlahov, D., Resnick, H., Ahern, J., Susser, E., Gold, J., Bucuvalas, M. & Kilpatrick, D. (2003). Trends in probable posttraumatic stress disorder in New York City after the September 11 terrorist attacks. *American Journal of Epidemiology*, **158**(6), 514–524.

Galea, S. & Resnick, H. (2005). Post-traumatic stress disorder in the general population after mass terrorist incidents: considerations about the nature of exposure. *CNS Spectrums*, **10**(2), 107–115.

Galea, S., Nandi, A. & Vlahov, D. (2005). The epidemiology of post-traumatic stress disorder after disasters. *Epidemiologic Reviews*, **27**, 78–91.

Galea, S., Ahern, J., Resnick, H. & Vlahov, D. (this volume). Post-traumatic stress symptoms in the general population after a disaster: implications for public health. In *9/11: Mental Health in the Wake of a Terrorist Attacks*, eds. Y. Neria, R. Gross & R. Marshall. Cambridge, UK: Cambridge University Press.

Goenjian, A.K., Pynoos, R.S., Steinberg, A.M., Endres, D., Abraham, K., Geffner, M.E. & Fairbanks, L.A. (2003). Hypothalamic–pituitary–adrenal activity among Armenian adolescents with PTSD symptoms. *Journal of Traumatic Stress*, **16**(4), 319–323.

Havenaar, J.M. & Bromet, E.J. (this volume). Capturing the impact of large scale events through epidemiological research. In *9/11: Mental Health in the Wake of a Terrorist Attacks*, eds. Y. Neria, R. Gross & R. Marshall. Cambridge, UK: Cambridge University Press.

Hoven, C.W., Mandell, D.J., Duarte, C.S., Wu, P. & Giordano, V. (this volume). An epidemiological response to disaster: the New York City Board of Education's post 9/11 needs assessment. In *9/11: Mental Health in the Wake of a Terrorist Attacks*, eds. Y. Neria, R. Gross & R. Marshall. Cambridge, UK: Cambridge University Press.

Norris, F.H., Friedman, M.J., Watson, P.J., Byrne, C.M., Diaz, E. & Kaniasty, K. (2002). 60,000 disaster victims speak. Part I: an empirical review of the empirical literature, 1981–2001. *Psychiatry*, **65**, 207–239.

Norris, F., Galea, S., Friedman, M., Watson, P. (2006). *Research Methods for Studying Mental Health after Disasters and Terrorism* (forthcoming from Guilford Press).

North, C.S., Nixon, S.J., Shariat, S., Mallonee, S., McMillen, J.C., Spitznagel, E.L. & Smith, E.M. (1999). Psychiatric disorders among survivors of the Oklahoma City bombing. *Journal of the American Medical Association*, **282**, 755–762.

North, C.S., Pfefferbaum, B. & Hong, B. (in press). Historical perspective and future directions in research on psychiatric consequences of terrorism and other disasters. In *9/11: Mental Health in The Wake of a Terrorist Attacks*, eds. Y. Neria, R. Gross & R. Marshall. Cambridge, UK: Cambridge University Press.

Pfefferbaum, B., Stuber, J., Fairbrother, G. & Galea, S. (in press). Panic reactions to the September 11 attacks in adolescents. *Journal of Traumatic Stress*.

Rose, G. (1992). *The Strategy of Preventive Medicine*. New York: Oxford University Press.

Rounsaville, B.J., Alarcon, R.D., Andrews, G., Jackson, J.S., Kendell, R.E. & Kendler, K. (2002). Basic nomenclature issues for DSM-V. In *A Research Agenda for DSM-V*, eds. D.J. Kupfer, M.B. First & D.A. Regier. Washington DC: American Psychiatric Association, pp. 1–29.

Ruggiero, K., Rheingold, A.A., Resnick, H., Kilpatrick, D.G. & Galea, S. (in Press). Comparison between two widely-used PTSD screening instruments: implications for public mental health planning, *Journal of Traumatic Stress*.

Schlenger, W.E., Caddell, J.M., Ebert, L., Jordan, B.K., Rourke, K.M., Wilson, D., Thalji, L., Dennis, J.M., Fairbank, J.A. & Kulka, R.A. (2002). Psychological reactions to terrorist attacks: findings from the National Study of Americans' reactions to September 11. *Journal of the American Medical Association*, **288**, 581–588.

Silver, R.C., Holman, E.A., McIntosh, D.N., Poulin, M., Gil-Rivas, V. & Pizarro, J. (in press). Coping with a national trauma: a nationwide longitudinal study of responses to the terrorist attacks of September 11th. In *9/11: Mental Health in The Wake of a Terrorist Attacks*, eds. Y. Neria, R. Gross & R. Marshall. Cambridge, UK: Cambridge University Press.

Tucker, P., Pfefferbaum, B. & Nixon, S.J. (2000). Predictors of post-traumatic stress symptoms in Oklahoma City: exposure, social support, peri-traumatic responses. *Journal of Behavioral Health Services and Research*, **27**, 406–415.

Part III

Reducing the burden: community response and community recovery

9

Community and ecological approaches to understanding and alleviating postdisaster distress

Fran H. Norris

How do we even begin to understand the aftermath of events as malicious, catastrophic, and far-reaching as the terrorist attacks of September 11, 2001? How can mental health professionals even begin to meet needs that are at once so intense and pervasive? The sections in this chapter illustrate that neither question can be answered without a shift in our thinking that places the community at the crux of the matter. Community is one of those concepts that semantically has meaning for most people but is difficult to define precisely. Not always, but typically, a community is an entity that has geographic boundaries and shared fate. Communities are composed of built, natural, social, and economic environments that influence one another in complex ways. In introducing this section, I will draw upon past research to illustrate the importance of thinking ecologically and systemically with regard to understanding and alleviating the consequences of large-scale disasters.

Understanding the effects of disasters

Event and population dynamics

Understanding the nature and effects of disasters is inherently challenging because it requires attention to event dynamics, population dynamics, community dynamics, social dynamics, and ethno-cultural dynamics. The causes of disasters are many, including *natural forces*, such as floods, hurricanes, and earthquakes, *failures of technology*, such as nuclear, industrial, and transportation accidents, and *mass violence*, such as shooting sprees and peacetime terrorist attacks. Regardless of their cause, disasters damage local infrastructures and strain the ability of local systems to meet the population's basic needs. For the survivors, disasters may engender an array of stressors, including threat to one's own life and physical integrity, exposure to the dead and dying, bereavement, profound loss, social and community disruption, and ongoing hardship. As a result of both the high prevalence and high stressfulness of disasters, the question of whether they impact mental health has been of interest for decades, and a substantial literature has developed that identifies and explains these effects.

Norris and colleagues attempted to provide a synthesis of this vast literature (Norris *et al.*, 2002). Their review was restricted to quantitative studies published in English between 1981 and 2001, selected from various databases using the search term, *disaster(s)*. That analysis encompassed 160 distinct samples of disaster victims composed of over 60,000 individuals who experienced 102 different events. The range of consequences experienced by these disaster survivors was broad, including various *psychological problems*, such as depression, anxiety, and most notably post-traumatic stress disorder (PTSD), *physical health problems*, such as sleep disruption, somatic complaints, and impaired immune function, *chronic problems in living*, such as troubled interpersonal relationships and financial stress, and *resource loss*, such as declines in perceived control and perceived social support.

Of course, not all events are equally serious from a public health perspective. To reflect the collective consequences of disasters in the review, the results for each sample were classified on a four-point ordinal scale of severity of effects or impairment. A few samples (11%) showed only *minimal* or highly transient effects or impairment. The majority of the samples (51%) showed *moderate* effects or impairment, indicative of prolonged stress but little psychopathology. In these samples, depending upon the study's design, there were significant differences between exposed participants and some comparison group, changes between predisaster and postdisaster mental health measures, or significant correlations between exposure measures and mental health measures. The remaining samples showed *severe* (21%) or *very severe* (18%) impairment, indicative of a high (25–49%) or very high (50%+) prevalence of clinically significant distress (determined on the basis of percentages scoring above established cut-points on standardized scales) or criterion-level psychological disorder (determined on the basis on diagnostic instruments).

In a regression analysis, three factors – sample type, disaster location, and disaster type – together explained a good percentage of the variance (32%) in samples' severity of impairment. Relative to adult survivors, samples were more likely to be impaired if they were composed of youth and less likely to be impaired if they were composed of rescue and recovery workers. Relative to the USA, samples were more likely to be impaired if they were from either developing or other developed countries, but the effect of location in a developing country was particularly large. It might be noted that disasters in developing countries were often associated with high losses of life. Relative to natural and technological disasters, samples were more likely to be impaired if they had experienced mass violence.

Each of the 102 *events* in the database was classified by aggregating ratings from all samples experiencing that event. For example, 13 samples experienced

Hurricane Andrew; their severity ratings ranged from 2 to 4 and averaged 2.8. A relatively more subjective analysis of events similarly classified as of *low* (aggregate severity ratings of 1.5 or less), *moderate* (1.6–2.4), or *high* (2.5+) impact suggested that the effects of disasters were greatest when at least two of the following event-level factors were present:

(a) The disaster caused extreme and widespread damage to property.
(b) The disaster engendered serious and ongoing financial problems for the community.
(c) The disaster was caused by human intent.
(d) The impact was associated with a high prevalence of trauma in the form of injuries, threat to life, and loss of life.

The relevance of this prediction to the events of September 11, 2001, was immediately obvious.

The overall impact of disasters is not as dire as these results suggest because most individuals and communities do recover over time. In Norris' and colleagues' review, findings from 34 samples were most relevant for discerning the course of postdisaster symptomatology because they were true panels, meaning that the same individuals were assessed with the same measures at each wave, and effects were observed at some point over the course of the study (Norris *et al.*, 2002b). Symptoms declined, at least predominantly, in 27 panels (79%) and, in general, the first year was the time of peak symptoms or effects. However, the course of recovery was often not uniform. The downward trends were predominantly or simply linear in only 3 of the 13 samples that showed a general improvement over three or more postdisaster assessments. Sometimes, symptoms declined at first, then stabilized; or stabilized for a while, then began a new downward trend; or showed a quadratic or cyclical pattern. Factors that influence fluctuations in population- and event-level effects are not yet well understood, and much more longitudinal research on these dynamics is required.

Community dynamics

The challenge in disaster work is that these events bring harm, pain, and loss to large numbers of people simultaneously. For the most part, our research strategies have not acknowledged this, and we study survivors as if they each experienced separate stressful or traumatic life events. This approach misses the essence of what it means to be a victim of disaster. From an ecological perspective, an important question is this: When predicting individuals' psychological responses and recovery, do only their own losses matter or are they influenced by the severity of losses and degree of recovery experienced by the community-at-large? This may be the question that I personally was asked most often in the aftermath of 9/11, as "indirect" effects appeared to loom particularly large – and were later documented (Schuster *et al.*, 2001; Galea *et al.*, 2002; Silver *et al.*, 2002).

The issue of extra-individual exposure is concerned with the relative contributions of two aspects of disaster exposure: *personal loss* and *community destruction*. Certainly, past research has focused on personal loss, which is the extent to which a given individual has experienced trauma or loss. Most definitions of disaster, however, recognize the broader context in which these losses occur. For example, it is generally assumed that as the proportion of victims to non-victims within a community increases, the mental health consequences of the disaster increase (Green, 1982). As this proportion increases, it becomes more difficult for people to avoid being exposed to physical destruction and even death following the more severe catastrophes. Erikson (1976) proposed that the trauma experienced by survivors of the dam collapse in Buffalo Creek, West Virginia had two facets, *individual trauma*, the personal psychic impact of the disaster, and *collective trauma*, the impairment of the prevailing sense of community. Bolin (1985) observed that there are two broad categories of victims: *Primary victims* are those who directly experience physical, material, or personal losses. *Secondary victims* are those who live in the affected area but sustain no personal injuries or damages. From this conceptualization, it can be inferred that a disaster is more than an individual-level event but is also a community-level event with potential psychological consequences even for those persons who experience no direct losses.

Occasionally, severity of exposure has been assessed at the neighborhood or community level. Measures such as the respondent's proximity to the "epicenter" may be derived geographically but typically are used to group participants who had similar individual experiences and are not intended to reflect extra-individual experience. Three approaches to ecological assessment have been demonstrated in the literature: (1) participants have been asked to describe conditions in their neighborhoods or communities (Hanson *et al.*, 1995; Kaniasty, 2003); (2) data have been aggregated "up" from the individual to the neighborhood or community level (Perilla *et al.*, 2002); and (3) archival data have been collected that reflect collective loss independent of personal loss (Norris *et al.*, 1994). In general, such measures tend to have modest effects, yet they often do explain variance in outcomes over and above those of individual-level measures. For example, in their study of 10 flooded counties, Norris *et al.* (1994) showed that personal loss and community destruction interacted; victims who fared most poorly were those who experienced both high personal loss and high community destruction. More broadly, the psychosocial consequences of the disaster were not limited to primary victims, but extended to the community-at-large. Pfefferbaum *et al.* (2000) and Smith *et al.* (1999) similarly showed that the effects of the bombing in Oklahoma City reached far beyond the direct victims and their families.

It is important to not overstate these findings because severity of exposure is among the most consistent predictors of postdisaster distress in the literature overall (Norris *et al.*, 2002a). Persistent disaster-specific psychopathology appears to be rare in the absence of severe, personal trauma or loss. However, less serious consequences are not uncommon among secondary victims. Norris *et al.* (1994) documented community-wide tendencies for residents to feel less positive about their surroundings, less enthusiastic, less energetic, and less able to enjoy life in the aftermath of the disaster. No one would suggest that such consequences constitute psychopathology, but they do indicate that disasters may impair the quality of life in the community for quite some time.

The differences between the effects of individual- and community-level exposure may be more qualitative than quantitative in character, which points to a need for additional conceptual progress if the goal is to describe the community's mental health. A strict focus on diagnostic criteria may cause us to erroneously or prematurely conclude that the community has recovered from the event. Moreover, crude archival data are quite limited in their utility for assessing community-level impact and recovery. Although the field of trauma research has provided an abundance of instruments for assessing exposure and outcomes at the individual level, we do not have validated tools for assessing the ecology of these individuals' experience. This shortcoming is a fundamental impediment to gaining a scientific understanding of community recovery and makes a meaningful evaluation of community recovery initiatives almost impossible to do. As Shinn (1996) noted, advances in assessment are often prerequisites to advances in theory and understanding. Progress in understanding the collective aspects of disaster exposure may rest on making advancements in ecological assessment and analytic strategies that allow us to explore the transactions of individual, family, and community recovery.

Quite relevant to this discussion of community dynamics is the notion of "community resilience" that is emerging as a key concept in the field of public health, especially with regard to terrorism. Because the intent of terrorism is to demoralize people, induce chaos, and disrupt society (Hall *et al.*, 2003), activities that promote a sense of unity, purpose, and collective well-being hold promise as effective countermeasures to this disruption (Reissman *et al.*, in press). The concept of resilience – literally meaning to "bounce back" – is not new, but its application to larger systems, such as families, occupational groups, and entire communities, is of relatively recent origin. Community resilience refers to the capacity of a collective to overcome shared trauma or adversity as manifest in social cohesion, mutual support, hope, and the presence of communal narratives that give the experience meaning and purpose (Fullilove & Saul, this volume). People who have attempted to build community resilience have observed that in times of massive trauma, community resilience is challenged because primary connections are disrupted and resources are strained (Landau & Saul, in press). A related concept is *communal mastery*, defined as the sense that individuals can overcome life challenges and obstacles *through and because of* their being interwoven in a close social network (Hobfoll *et al.*, 2002). There is clearly more to these notions than social support. Nonetheless, social connectedness is perhaps their most fundamental component (Kaniasty & Norris, 2004).

Social dynamics

A step forward toward an ecologically valid understanding of disasters is to recognize that the individuals we are studying are connected and dependent upon one another's coping strategies. For many years now, my colleague, Krys Kaniasty, and I have attempted to do this by studying postdisaster social support, social functioning, and other social processes. Social support is a powerful protective factor (Brewin *et al.*, 2000) but is complicated after disasters (Kaniasty & Norris, 1999). Initially, there is a strong *mobilization* of social support, but later, paradoxically, there is a *deterioration* of social support. Several studies indicate quite strongly that declines in social support and social participation underlie lingering postdisaster distress (e.g., Kaniasty & Norris, 1993; Norris & Kaniasty, 1996).

In the immediate aftermath of disasters, high levels of mutual helping materialize, and previous conflicts and divisions in the community appear to fade away. Survivors sometimes initially experience euphoria at having survived in the face of death and destruction. Temporarily, at least, they forget old quarrels, spontaneously share experiences, and are intensely uplifted by the recognition that others care. This phase during which the mobilization of support predominates has earned a variety of heartwarming labels, such as "altruistic community," "heroic phase," "honeymoon phase," and "postdisaster utopia" (see Kaniasty & Norris, 2004, for a more detailed discussion and review).

In the longer period that follows, the realities of loss and the formidable challenges of recovery must be faced. The heightened level of helping and cohesion seldom last. The attentive media and generous outsiders leave to another crisis. With the passage of time, camaraderie is replaced by grief, anger, and disillusionment (Somasundarum *et al.*, 2003). Because resource loss is difficult to prevent and more powerful than resource gain (see Hobfoll, this volume), the initial mobilization of social support may not be sufficient to conquer the creeping deterioration in social relationships routinely experienced by disaster-stricken communities.

Many things can lead to postdisaster declines in social support and social functioning. Because disasters affect entire indigenous networks, the need for support may simply exceed its availability, causing expectations of support to be violated (Kaniasty *et al.*, 1990; Harvey *et al.*, 1995). Relocation and job loss – and even death following the most severe events – remove important others from victims' supportive environments. Disaster victims often abandon routine social activities, leaving fewer opportunities for companionship and leisure (Bolin, 1993; Kaniasty, 2003).

Social networks become saturated with stories of and feelings about the event and may escape interacting. Whereas victims want and need to be listened to, they and others in their social environments may not necessarily wish to be the listeners. Physical fatigue, emotional irritability, and scarcity of resources increase the potential for interpersonal conflicts and social withdrawal. Different groups of victims may sometimes find themselves at odds. Thus, over time, mutual helping, and cohesion yield to conflict and disharmony. The mobilization of support yields to deterioration of support.

The family is a critical context for understanding the social dynamics of disaster recovery. Families are the primary source of postdisaster support (Kaniasty & Norris, 2000) and the cornerstone of community resilience (Landau & Saul, in press). Unfortunately, the quality of intimate and familial relationships may deteriorate after disasters because coping with stressors creates a shared "energy field" wherein reactions of people inadvertently rub off on each other. Past research has shown that, compared to other combat veterans and their wives, veterans with PTSD and their wives have less satisfaction with their relationships, less intimacy, less communication, more marital problems, and more family violence (e.g., Mikulincer et al., 1995; MacDonald et al., 1999). Such effects are sometimes referred to as *secondary traumatic stress*, a highly systemic construct. Relatively little disaster research speaks directly to this issue, but a few studies provide corroborating evidence (Gleser et al., 1981; McFarlane et al., 1987; Brooks & McKinlay, 1992; Norris & Uhl, 1993; Cohan & Cole, 2002).

The deterioration of support is, fortunately, not inevitable. Norris and Kaniasty (1996) proposed a model of *deterioration deterrence* in which the positive relation between severity of exposure and received support (mobilization) to a greater or lesser extent *offsets* or *counteracts* the negative relation between severity of exposure and perceived support (deterioration) because received support protects perceived support (protective assistance); see Figure 9.1. Using data collected 12 and 24 months following Hurricane Hugo and 6 and 28 months following Hurricane Andrew, we found strong evidence for the hypothesized model. Although disaster stress led to deterioration of perceived support, the *total* effects of disaster on perceived support were *less severe than they might have been* because the stress of disaster was positively associated with received support, and received support was positive associated with subsequent perceived support. Victims who receive very high levels of help following a disaster are thus protected against salient erosion in their perceptions of belonging and expectations of support. This finding indicates that the more we can do to help disaster victims mobilize – and sustain – social support, the better will be their long-term outcomes.

Tangible, informational, and emotional forms of social support are all needed by disaster victims, regardless of the disaster's cause. Tangible support may be the

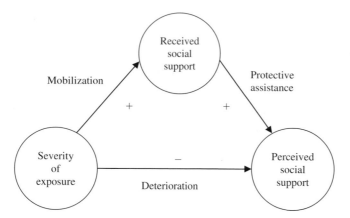

Figure 9.1   Simplified deterioration–deterrence model, showing that the positive impact of exposure on received support and the positive impact of received support on subsequent perceived support together may offset the negative impact of exposure on perceived support.

easiest form to provide. Indeed, both governmental and non-governmental agencies provide victims of disaster with essential shelter, food, money, and loans to hasten physical and fiscal recovery. The public's orientation to *do* something further augments the abundance of tangible support. However, informational support may be even more important than tangible support after human-caused disasters characterized by invisibility, confusion, and uncertainty. Information and messages promoted by authorities must be accurate and trustworthy. This point cannot be overemphasized. Otherwise, authorities will exacerbate processes (e.g., lack of consensus in appraisals, mistrust, misinformation, polarization, stress contagion) that contribute to support deterioration. Warning the public while simultaneously minimizing fear is extremely challenging. Altogether, for responding to terrorism and bioterrorism, risk communication and social marketing may emerge as the most critical strategies for interventions that target public – and social – health. Far more research is needed on how to apply these methods in the face of terrorist threats. Notwithstanding the essential role government agencies and other formal sources of support play in the aftermath of disasters, the greatest challenge lies in fostering naturally occurring social resources, which are most vital for disaster victims, especially with regard to the exchange of emotional support.

Ethno-cultural dynamics

The deterioration–deterrence model documents processes wherein helping activities counteract the forces of support deterioration. In one sense, it could be taken as a resilience model suggesting that communities can be trusted to provide ample support to their members in times of intense need. However, from an ecological perspective, it must also be recognized that various societal, cultural, and political dynamics interfere with the adequacy and equity of resource distribution. In fact, disaster-stricken communities are not always ruled in the most egalitarian way (Kaniasty & Norris, 1995). Ideally, the distribution or mobilization of support in a community follows the *rule of relative needs*, as represented in the figure by the path from severity of exposure to received support. Simply put, the most support goes to those who need it the most. More often, however, the distribution of support follows the *rule of relative advantage.* Factors such as ethnicity and economic status are key variables affecting distribution of social resources after disasters. Socially and economically disadvantaged groups are frequently too overburdened to provide ample help to other members in time of additional need. The abundant support that the public marshals in times of crisis should not obscure the fact that not all victims are fully participating in these emergent altruistic communities (Kaniasty & Norris, 1999). Sometimes, the neglect may be more imagined than real, as it is not uncommon for people from all walks of life to believe that other neighborhoods or groups received more – or more timely – formal assistance than they did. The distribution of helping resources is critical from a community perspective because many disaster studies have found that minority communities fare poorly in the aftermath of disasters or worse psychologically than do White communities (Bolton & Klenow, 1988; Green *et al.*, 1990; Palinkas *et al.*, 1993; Garrison *et al.*, 1995; Webster *et al.*, 1995; March *et al.*, 1997; Galea *et al.*, 2002; Perilla *et al.*, 2002; Chen *et al.*, 2003; Thiel de Bocanegra & Brickman, 2004).

Such findings also demonstrate the importance of cultural competence if the goal is to conduct community-centered or ecologically sound disaster research. Palinkas *et al.*'s (1993) study of the aftermath of the Exxon Valdez spill is a case in point. The investigation revealed significant differences between Native Alaskans and others in rates of postdisaster major depression, generalized anxiety, and PTSD that were not explained by exposure alone. The spill interrupted subsistence activities, and these disruptions had greater impact on natives because they feared losing long-held traditions that defined their culture and community. Perilla *et al.* (2002) similarly demonstrated that acculturation is a key variable for understanding ethnic differences in disaster-related distress. Also pertinent to this discussion are findings showing that culture shapes the effects of other important variables, such as gender and age, on postdisaster mental health outcomes (Norris *et al.*, 2001; Norris *et al.*, 2002c).

Alleviating the effects of disaster

What do these event, population, community, social, and ethno-cultural dynamics mean for planning mental health responses? Certainly, at minimum, they call for a public health approach that addresses the needs of the many, while simultaneously reaching out to individuals most at risk for long-term mental health problems. Chapters in this section address the critical importance of effective communication systems (LifeNet), public sector responses (Project Liberty), integration of medical and psychiatric care, and large-scale screening and treatment programs, and provide excellent illustrations of systemic approaches that reach out to entire communities.

The impact of trauma-related services rests not only on their clinical efficacy but also on the capacity of the system to deliver those services in an appropriate way, making research on the functioning of disaster mental health systems important from an ecological or public health perspective. Following major disasters, federal agencies, state offices of mental health, substance use prevention and treatment programs, victims' services, school systems, universities, and various community-based organizations may all be seeking to play a role in the recovery effort. Issues of coordination and cooperation are very real and are mentioned over and over again by professionals who have found themselves in the position of responding to major events in their communities (Hodgkinson & Stewart, 1998; Sitterle & Gurwich, 1998; Call & Pfefferbaum, 1999; Canterbury & Yule, 1999; Jacobs & Kulkarni, 1999; Bowenkamp, 2000). Gillespie and Murty (1994) noted that the failure of organizations to work together results in "cracks" in the postdisaster service delivery network, whereas an effective service delivery system provides a complete set of services and linkages in which such cracks do not appear. Norris and colleagues began their case studies of disaster mental health services with the assumption that providers who function within *coherent and supportive* systems will deliver services that are perceived to be credible, acceptable, accessible, and proactive, thereby maximizing the reach of the program to those in need (Norris *et al.*, 2005; Norris *et al.*, 2006).

Most of the programs described in this section aimed to provide relatively traditional dyadic counseling or psychiatric services, but they aimed to provide those services on an atypically large scale or in atypical places. I do imply criticism with this statement, as "clinical vs. community" debates are rather unproductive in the aftermath of disasters. I am periodically struck by how relevant Barbara Dohrenwend's (1978) model of psychosocial stress continues to be. Dohrenwend identified numerous potential points of intervention to reduce the impact of stressful events, ranging from political action to corrective therapy. One of the appealing features of her model was how seeming disparate activities took on, in Dohrenwend's words, "a satisfying coherence and directedness." The prevention/intervention activities were all directed at undermining the process whereby stress generates psychopathology, but *they tackled it at different points*. This is a crucial lesson for the overall ecology of postdisaster care. The professional clinician, paraprofessional outreach worker, and community activist are each essential to the effort, although they might not even be aware of their collaboration. The International Society of Traumatic Stress Studies (ISTSS) – UN Joint Initiative on Trauma (Green *et al.*, 2003) adopted a similarly integrative stance when it directed all committees (e.g., disasters, refugees) to conceptualize their recommendations on the basis of a pyramid that has the community at its base, the individual at its apex, and the family in between. Nonetheless, the scope of catastrophic disasters demands that we design community-level interventions for the population at large and conserve scarce clinical resources for those most in need (Norris *et al.*, 2002b). Thinking ecologically, one overlooks neither the community's functioning nor the individual's functioning but strives for a proper balance between the two.

In this volume, Fullilove and Saul provide the purest example of a community-based approach in their intriguing attempts to build community resilience in the aftermath of 9/11. Harvey (1996), Van den Eynde and Veno (1999), and Somasundarum *et al.* (2003) similarly advocated for postdisaster interventions that foster community competence and ownership of problems and solutions. Solomon (2003) summarized this viewpoint well: "Although professionals working in the mental health arena are seldom trained or prepared to work at a broader community level, the scale of these emergences may require abandoning dyadic interventions for those that can be implemented via community action using a public health approach." At present, empirical support for these principles of community intervention is meager, at best. Yet these initiatives can claim a basis in theory, as Hobfoll's contribution to this volume illustrates well. With regard to the conservation of resources, the primary goal of postdisaster interventions is to help people replace valued resources as quickly as possible. (Hobfoll & Lilly, 1993) Providing indigenous networks with the resources they need to help one another is (or should be) the primary objective of disaster mental health policy (Norris *et al.*, 1994; Somasundarum *et al.*, 2003).

From an ecological perspective, there is a critical need for further research that provides sound data about how to tailor responses to meet the needs of our increasingly diverse population. Norris and Alegria (2006) reviewed findings from research on psychiatric epidemiology, disaster effects, disparities in service use, and cross-cultural psychology to generate guidelines for culturally responsive postdisaster interventions. They concluded that ethnicity and culture influence mental health care at various points – on need for help; on availability and accessibility of help; on help-seeking comfort, and on the probability that help is provided appropriately. Norris and Alegria proposed that interventions for minority communities should give greater attention to socially engaged emotions and functioning. Notwithstanding the pain and stress they cause, disasters create opportunities to de-stigmatize mental health needs and build trust between providers and minority communities.

In closing, it is all too predictable but nonetheless necessary to say (again) that we must initiate more complex studies of community-level processes if we are to advance a scientific understanding of the psychosocial consequences of disaster. And, rising to an even greater challenge, we must find creative ways to test the effectiveness of postdisaster community interventions. Books, such as this one, that record the far-reaching consequences of terrorism – and give witness to the variety of ways in which professionals and activists respond to community needs – move us several, critical steps toward these goals.

Acknowledgment

Preparation of this chapter was supported by an Independent Scientist Award (K02 MH63909) to F.H.N. from National Institute of Mental Health.

REFERENCES

Bolin, R. (1985). Disaster characteristics and psychosocial impacts. In *Disasters and Mental Health: Selected Contemporary Perspectives*, ed. B. Sowder. Rockville, MD: National Institute of Mental Health, pp. 3–28.

Bolin, R. (1993). Natural and technological disasters: evidence of psychopathology. In *Environment and Psychopathology*, eds. A. Ghadirian & H. Lehmann. New York: Springer, pp. 121–140.

Bolton, R. & Klenow, D. (1988). Older people in disaster: a comparison of black and white victims. *International Journal of Aging and Human Development*, **26**, 29–43.

Bowenkamp, C. (2000). Coordination of mental health and community agencies in disaster. *International Journal of Emergency Mental Health*, **2**, 159–165.

Brewin, C., Andrews, B. & Valentine, J. (2000). Meta-analysis of risk factors for posttraumatic stress disorder in trauma-exposed adults. *Journal of Consulting and Clinical Psychology*, **68**, 748–766.

Brooks, N. & McKinlay, W. (1992). Mental health consequences of the Lockerbie disaster. *Journal of Traumatic Stress*, **5**, 527–543.

Call, J. & Pfefferbaum, B. (1999). Lessons from the first two years of Project Heartland, Oklahoma's mental health response to the 1995 bombing. *Psychiatric Services*, **50**, 953–955.

Canterbury, R. & Yule, W. (1999). Planning a psychosocial response to a disaster. In *Post-traumatic Stress Disorders: Concepts and Therapy*, ed. W. Yule. New York: Wiley & Sons, pp. 285–296.

Chen, H., Chung, H., Chen, T., Fang, L. & Chen, J.-P. (2003). The emotional distress in a community after the terrorist attack on the World Trade Center. *Community Mental Health Journal*, **39**, 157–165.

Cohan, C. & Cole, S. (2002). Life course transitions and natural disaster: marriage, birth, and divorce following Hurricane Hugo. *Journal of Family Psychology*, **16**, 14–25.

Dohrenwend, B.S. (1978). Social stress and community psychology. *American Journal of Community Psychology*, **6**, 1–14.

Erikson, K. (1976). Loss of communality at Buffalo Creek. *American Journal of Psychiatry*, **133**, 302–305.

Fullilove, M.T. & Saul, J. (this volume). Rebuilding communities post disasters in New York. In *9/11: Mental Health in the Wake of a Terrorist Attacks*, eds. Y. Neria, R. Gross & R. Marshall. Cambridge, UK: Cambridge University Press.

Galea, S., Ahern, J., Resnick, H., Kilpatrick, D., Bucuvalas, M., Gold, J. & Vlahov, D. (2002). Psychological sequelae of the September 11 terrorist attacks in New York City. *New England Journal of Medicine*, **346**, 982–987.

Garrison, C., Bryant, E., Addy, C., Spurrier, P., Freedy, J. & Kilpatrick, D. (1995). Post-traumatic stress disorder in adolescents after Hurricane Andrew. *Journal of the American Academy of Child and Adolescent Psychiatry*, **34**, 1193–1201.

Gillespie, D. & Murty, S. (1994). Cracks in a postdisaster service delivery network. *American Journal of Community Psychology*, **22**, 639–660.

Gleser, G., Green, B. & Winget, C. (1981). *Prolonged Psychosocial Effects of Disaster: A study of Buffalo Creek*. New York: Academic Press.

Green, B. (1982). Assessing levels of psychological impairment following disaster: consideration of actual and methodological dimensions. *Journal of Nervous and Mental Disease*, **170**, 544–552.

Green, B., Lindy, J., Grace, M., Gleser, G., Leonard, A., Korol, M. & Winget, C. (1990). Buffalo Creek survivors in the second decade. *American Journal of Orthopsychiatry*, **60**, 43–54.

Green, B., Friedman, M., De Jong, J., Solomon, S., Keane, T., Fairbank, J., Donelan, B. & Frey-Wouters, E. (2003). *Trauma in War and Peace: Prevention, Practice, and Policy*. New York: Kluwer Academic/Plenum Publishers.

Hall, M., Norwood, A., Ursano, R. & Fullerton, C. (2003). The psychological impacts of bioterrorism. *Biosecurity and Bioterrorism*, **1**, 139–144.

Hanson, R., Kilpatrick, D., Freedy, J. & Saunders, B. (1995). Los Angeles County after the 1992 civil disturbances: degree of exposure and impact on mental health. *Journal of Consulting and Clinical Psychology*, **63**, 987–996.

Harvey, J., Stein, S., Olsen, N., Roberts, R., Lutgendorf, S. & Ho, J. (1995). Narratives of loss and recovery from a natural disaster. *Journal of Social Behavior and Personality*, **10**, 313–330.

Harvey, M. (1996). An ecological view of psychological trauma and trauma recovery. *Journal of Traumatic Stress*, **9**, 3–23.

Hobfoll, S. (this volume). Guiding community intervention following terrorist attack. In *9/11: Mental Health in the Wake of a Terrorist Attacks*, eds. Y. Neria, R. Gross & R. Marshall. Cambridge, UK: Cambridge University Press.

Hobfoll, S. & Lilly, R. (1993). Resource conservation as a strategy for community psychology. *American Journal of Community Psychology*, **21**, 128–148.

Hobfoll, S., Jackson, A., Hobfoll, I., Pierce, C. & Young, S. (2002). The impact of communal-mastery versus self-mastery on emotional outcomes during stressful conditions: a prospective study of Native American women. *American Journal of Community Psychology*, **30**, 853–871.

Hodgkinson, P. & Stewart, M. (1998). *Coping with Catastrophe: A Handbook of Post-disaster Psychosocial Aftercare* (2nd ed.). London: Routledge.

Jacobs, G. & Kulkarni, N. (1999). Mental health responses to terrorism. *Psychiatric Annals*, **29**, 376–380.

Kaniasty, K. (2003). *Kleska zywiolowa czy katastrofa spoleczna? Psychospoleczne konsekwencje polskiej powodzi 1997 roku. (Natural Disaster or Social Catastrophe? Psychosocial Consequences of the 1997 Polish Flood)*. Gdansk, Poland: Gdanskie Wydawnictwo Psychologiczne.

Kaniasty, K. & Norris, F. (1993). A test of the support deterioration model in the context of natural disaster. *Journal of Personality and Social Psychology*, **64**, 395–408.

Kaniasty, K. & Norris, F. (1995). In search of altruistic community: patterns of social support mobilization following Hurricane Hugo. *American Journal of Community Psychology*, **23**, 447–477.

Kaniasty, K. & Norris, F. (1999). Individuals and communities sharing trauma: unpacking the experience of disaster. In *Psychosocial, Ecological, and Community Approaches to Understanding Disaster*, eds. R. Gist & B. Lubin. London: Bruner/Mazel, pp. 25–62.

Kaniasty, K. & Norris, F. (2000). Help-seeking comfort and the receipt of help: the roles of context and ethnicity. *American Journal of Community Psychology*, **28**, 545–582.

Kaniasty, K. & Norris, F. (2004). Social support in the aftermath of disasters, catastrophes, and acts of terrorism: altruistic, overwhelmed, uncertain, antagonistic, and patriotic communities. In *Bioterrorism: Psychological and Public Health Interventions*, eds. R. Ursano, A. Norwood & C. Fullerton. Cambridge, UK: Cambridge University Press.

Kaniasty, K., Norris, F. & Murrell, S. (1990). Perceived and received social support following natural disaster. *Journal of Applied Social Psychology*, **20**, 85–114.

Landau, J. & Saul, J. (2005). Facilitating family and community resilience in response to major disaster. In *Living Beyond Loss*, eds. F. Walsh & M. McGoldrick. New York: Norton, pp. 287–309.

MacDonald, C., Chamberlain, K., Long, N. & Flett, R. (1999). Posttraumatic stress disorder and interpersonal functioning in Vietnam War veterans: a mediational model. *Journal of Traumatic Stress*, **12**, 701–707.

March, J., Amaya-Jackson, L., Terry, R. & Costanzo, P. (1997). Posttraumatic symptomatology in children and adolescents after an industrial fire. *Journal of the American Academy of Child and Adolescent Psychiatry*, **36**, 1080–1088.

McFarlane, A.C., Policansky, S. & Irwin, C. (1987). A longitudinal study of the psychological morbidity in children due to a natural disaster. *Psychological Medicine*, **17**, 727–738.

Mikulincer, M., Florian, V. & Solomon, Z. (1995). Marital intimacy, family support, and secondary traumatization: a study of wives of veterans with combat stress. *Anxiety, Stress, and Coping*, **8**, 203–213.

Norris, F. & Alegria, M. (2006). Promoting disaster recovery in ethnic minority individuals and communities. In *Mental Health Intervention Following Disasters or Mass Violence*, eds. C. Ritchie, P. Watson & M. Friedman, New York: Guilford Press, 319–342.

Norris, F. & Kaniasty, K. (1996). Perceived and received social support in times of stress: a test of the social support deterioration deterrence model. *Journal of Personality and Social Psychology*, **71**, 499–511.

Norris, F. & Uhl, G. (1993). Chronic stress as a mediator of acute stress: the case of Hurricane Hugo. *Journal of Applied Social Psychology*, **23**, 1263–1284.

Norris, F., Phifer, J. & Kaniasty, K. (1994). Individual and community reactions to the Kentucky floods: findings from a longitudinal study of older adults. In *The Structure of Human Chaos: Individual and Community Responses to Trauma and Disaster*, eds. R. Ursano, B. McCaughey & C. Fullerton. Cambridge, UK: Cambridge University Press, pp. 378–400.

Norris, F., Perilla, J., Ibañez, G. & Murphy, A. (2001). Sex differences in symptoms of post-traumatic stress: does culture play a role? *Journal of Traumatic Stress*, **14**, 7–28.

Norris, F., Friedman, M. & Watson, P. (2002b). 60,000 disaster victims speak. Part 2: Summary and implications of the disaster mental health research. *Psychiatry*, **65**, 240–260.

Norris, F., Friedman, M., Watson, P., Byrne, C., Diaz, E. & Kaniasty, K. (2002a). 60,000 disaster victims speak. Part 1: An empirical review of the empirical literature, 1981–2001. *Psychiatry*, **65**, 207–239.

Norris, F., Kaniasty, K., Inman, G., Conrad, L. & Murphy, A. (2002c). Placing age differences in cultural context: a comparison of the effects of age on PTSD after disasters in the U.S., Mexico, and Poland. *Journal of Clinical Geropsychology* (special issue on trauma and older adults), **8**, 153–173.

Norris, F., Hamblen, J., Watson, P., Ruzek, J., Gibson, L., Pfefferbaum, B., Price, V., Stevens, S., Young, B. & Friedman, M. (2006). Understanding and creating systems of postdisaster care: a case study of New York's mental health system's response to the World Trade Center disaster. In *Mental Health Intervention Following Disasters or Mass Violence*, eds. C. Ritchie, P. Watson & M. Friedman. New York: Guilford Press, 343–364.

Norris, F., Watson, P., Hamblen, J. & Pfefferbaum, B. (2005). Provider perspectives on disaster mental health services in Oklahoma City. In *The Trauma of Terror: Sharing knowledge and Shared Care*, eds. Y. Danieli, D. Brom & J.B. Sills. Binghamton, NY: The Hawarth Press, 649–662.

Palinkas, L., Downs, M., Petterson, J. & Russell, J. (1993). Social, cultural, and psychological impacts of the Exxon Valdez oil spill. *Human Organization*, **52**, 1–13.

Perilla, J., Norris, F. & Lavizzo, E. (2002). Ethnicity, culture, and disaster response: Identifying and explaining ethnic differences in PTSD six months after Hurricane Andrew. *Journal of Social and Clinical Psychology*, **21**, 28–45.

Pfefferbaum, B., Seale, T., McDonald, N., Brandt, E., Rainwater, S., Maynard, B., *et al.* (2000). Posttraumatic stress two years after the Oklahoma City bombing in youths geographically distant from the explosion. *Psychiatry*, **63**, 358–370.

Reissman, D., Spencer, S., Tanielian, T. & Stein, B. (2005). Integrating behavioral aspects into community preparedness and response systems. In *The Trauma of Terror: Sharing Knowledge and Shared Care*, eds. Y. Danieli, D. Brom & J.B. Sills. Binghamton, NY: The Hawarth Press. pp. 707–720.

Schuster, M., Stein, B., Jaycox, L., Collins, R., Marshall, G., Elliott, M.N., Zhou, A.J., Kanouse, D.E., Morrison, J.L. & Berry, S.H. (2001). A national survey of stress reactions after the September 11, 2001, terrorist attacks. *New England Journal of Medicine*, **345**(20), 1507–1512.

Shinn, M. (1996). Ecological assessment: introduction to the special issue. *American Journal of Community Psychology*, **24**, 1–3.

Silver, R., Holman, E.A., McIntosh, D., Poulin, M. & Gil-Rivas, V. (2002). Nationwide longitudinal study of psychological responses to September 11. *Journal of the American Medical Association*, **288**, 1235–1244.

Sitterle, K. & Gurwich, R. (1998). The terrorist bombing in Oklahoma City. In *When a Community Weeps: Case Studies in Group Survivorship*, eds. E. Zinner & M. Williams. Philadelphia, PA: Brunner/Mazel, pp. 161–189.

Smith, D, Christiansen, E., Vincent, R. & Hann, N. (1999). Population effects of the bombing of Oklahoma City. *Journal of the Oklahoma State Medical Association*, **92**, 193–198.

Solomon, S. (2003). Introduction. In *Trauma in War and Peace: Prevention, Practice, and Policy*. New York: Kluwer Academic/Plenum Publishers, pp. 3–16.

Somasundarum, D., Norris, F., Asukai, N. & Murthy, R. (2003). *Trauma in War and Peace: Prevention, Practice, and Policy*. New York: Kluwer Academic/Plenum Publishers, pp. 291–318.

Thiel de Bocanegra, H. & Brickman, E. (2004). Mental health impact of the World Trade Center attacks on displaced Chinese workers. *Journal of Traumatic Stress*, **17**, 55–62.

Van den Eynde, J. & Veno, A. (1999). Coping with disastrous events: an empowerment model of community healing. In *Response to Disaster: Psychosocial, Community, and Ecological Approaches*, eds. R. Gist & B. Lubin. Philadelphia, PA: Bruner/Mazel.

Webster, R., McDonald, R., Lewin, T. & Carr, V. (1995). Effects of a natural disaster on immigrants and host population. *Journal of Nervous and Mental Disease*, **183**, 390–397.

10

What is collective recovery?

Mindy Thompson Fullilove and Lourdes Hernández-Cordero

George Engel, in his classic article on the biopsychosocial model of psychiatry, argued that a patient's full recovery might depend on interventions in systems outside of the individual's body, such as in the family system, the hospital system or other social systems within which the individual is nested (Engel, 1980). He pointed out that these systems were organized hierarchically, with larger systems acting to constrain smaller systems, as, for example, the family can constrain the actions of the individual. At each level of the hierarchy, we find systems that are self-integrated. At the same time, each system is interconnected with other higher and lower order systems. Following on Engel's seminal work, it has become clear that individual health is formed by interactions among systems. Analysis of these systems – and the formulation of intervention   depends on the examination of each system, or level of scale, on its own merits and with regard to other systems in the hierarchy.

Large-scale disasters, such as the attacks on the World Trade Center of September 11, 2001, demand this kind of multi-level analysis and intervention. Although the individual is the unit of most interest to biomedical practitioners, the injury that results from disaster is not limited to the system of the individual. Larger social groups, such as the family and the neighborhood, are also injured by disaster and implicated in recovery. In fact, the solution to the problems of the individual may lie at a level of scale at some remove from the single person.

To be more specific, when the Twin Towers collapsed, the neighborhood that was housed in those enormous buildings was disrupted.[1] All of the interactions and interconnections that went on within the many-storied Twin Towers were disassembled, as were the connections among the businesses within and without the

---

[1] When we say "neighborhood" with reference to the World Trade Center, people tend to think of the whole of Lower Manhattan. But neighborhoods in New York City are often much smaller than that, consisting of two or three blocks. In this discussion here, we are considering the Twin Towers as a neighborhood, specifically a central business district. Hence, we are examining the consequences of the destruction of an entire neighborhood.

Twin Towers. In sum, the social organization that was housed at the World Trade Center was sundered. The remaining elements were dispersed to the four corners of the region.

Similarly, the loss of the neighborhood of the Twin Towers had dramatic effects on other neighborhoods in the city and the region. Those located circumjacent to the disaster found themselves in a profound paralysis. The economy of Chinatown, for example, did not recover for many months. But neighborhoods at some remove were also affected. Some lost substantial numbers of people. Others were affected by job loss, particularly among low-income workers. Still others were caught up in budget cuts as the city scrambled to manage a $6 billion deficit.

Given that neighborhoods were affected, let us turn our attention to describing the kinds of injury that occur at that level of scale. Urban neighborhoods differ dramatically in their composition, but all are composed of structures used by homes and/or businesses that are located close to and interact with one another. As a result of these interactions, a neighborhood develops a fine pattern of daily interconnections among residents, workers and passersby.

One of the many kinds of relationships that develops is "familiarity among strangers," what the great urbanist Jane Jacobs dubbed a "sidewalk ballet." In her book, *The Death and Life of Great American Cities*, she wrote:

The stretch of Hudson Street where I live is each day the scene of an intricate sidewalk ballet. I make my own entrance into it a little after eight when I put out the garbage can, surely a prosaic occupation, but I enjoy my part, my little clang, as the droves of junior high school students walk by the center of the stage dropping candy wrappers. (How do they eat so much candy so early in the morning?)

While I sweep up the wrappers I watch the other rituals of morning: Mr. Halpert unlocking the laundry's handcart from its mooring to a cellar door, Joe Cornacchia's son-in-law stacking out the empty crates from the delicatessen, the barber bringing out his sidewalk folding chair, Mr. Goldstein arranging the coils of wire which proclaim the hardware store is open, the wife of the tenement's superintendent depositing her chunky three-year-old with a toy mandolin on the stoop, the vantage point from which he is learning the English his mother cannot speak… It is time for me to hurry to work too, and I exchange my ritual farewell with Mr. Lofaro, the short, thick-bodied, white-aproned fruit man who stands outside his doorway a little up the street, his arms folded, his feet planted, looking solid as earth itself. We nod; we each glance quickly up and down the street, then look back to each other and smile. We have done this many a morning for more than ten years, and we both know what it means: All is well. (Jacobs, 1993).

Some version of this sidewalk ballet took place in the corridors, elevators and plazas of the World Trade Center. A young woman, who had changed trains at the World Trade Center during her high school years, remembered stopping with friends to sit on the benches in the plaza to review the school day. This travel ritual was a key part of those years; in the aftermath of the disaster, transitions over bridges and in elevators became very difficult for her. There are a million stories of this sort, all stories of the Twin Towers' particular sidewalk ballet.

A sidewalk ballet is largely composed of what sociologists call "weak ties," the slight connections such as that between a coffee seller and his regular customers (Granovetter, 1972). Such a connection depends on place. Robert Browning's triumphant, "God's in His heaven, all's right with the world!" depends on God and the world being in their designated spots. While they are a very particular kind of social relationship, these weak ties are the social foundation of a neighborhood.

An important feature of an urban neighborhood is that neighbors are likely to differ from one another, and this is true even within the constraints of a highly segregated city. Neighbors eat different vegetables, celebrate different holidays and pray to different Gods. The injunction in the Judeo-Christian tradition – "Love thy *neighbor* as thyself" – is directed at helping urban people know what to do with people who are neither family nor tribe. In that formulation, propinquity becomes a new basis for courtesy. In a successful urban neighborhood, such as the one embedded in the World Trade Center, these courtesies were, indeed, observed. As Jane Jacobs makes clear, the relationships of propinquity and passage are highly satisfying. The familiar face provides an anchor in the naked city.

Finally, these relationships are enabling relationships. The expression "six degrees of separation" refers to the ability of the ordinary person to contact another person. When we ponder the chain that would link the average Joe to the President of USA, one link is a storekeeper. The link to the storekeeper is created by the sidewalk ballet. It is weak links that move the nation. Weak links, in turn, are created by patterns of movement in well defined places.

Within a neighborhood, a set of social relationships are created that are particular to that level of scale. They are neither the close ties of family nor the even weaker ties of nationalism. They are the ties that are formed by daily routine, and they depend on place. It goes without saying that the destruction of a place destroys the material basis for the place-based relationships. What will endure are the relationships of strong ties, that is the ties to work, family, church or school. But these are not the ties that link across groups, the ties that connect the local to the national. They are circumscribed ties, which belonging to a particular group. By definition, they are not shared with others. Strong ties are tribal ties, but it is weak ties that make cities function.

It is a matter of some urgency, therefore, to recreate weak ties in the aftermath of disaster. While it is beyond the scope of this present work to examine the effects of neighborhood destruction on each level of scale, we may surmise that there are unique losses, parallel in importance, though different in content, to weak ties. Suffice it to say that recreation of these essential linkages is at the heart of collective recovery.

Principles of collective recovery

As it is used here, "collective recovery" refers to the recovery of a community from injuries to its internal organization and its connections to other groups (Hernandez-Cordero, 2003). Because there are interactions among all levels of scale, recovery of the collective will have important implications for recovery of individuals. But it cannot be inferred that recovery of the collective will happen as a result of the recovery of many individuals. The following principles provide a basis for planning and carrying out collective recovery.

Principle 1: There is no "there," no "them"

Theories of complex systems have helped us understand that all things in the world are interrelated and small changes in initial conditions can lead to vast differences in the final outcomes. This leads to the idea that a butterfly flapping its wings in one part of the world can change the weather in another (Fullilove et al., 1997). Thus, the idea that a disaster happened to "other" people is incompatible with current ecological thinking. While it may be difficult to recognize the ways in which a disaster that happened somewhere else will affect "my" place, the working assumption should be that it will. The slogan of Project Liberty,[2] "We're all in this together," exemplified this ecological perspective.

Principle 2: The collective is not the tribe

The sundering of social ties at the neighborhood level of scale breaks inter-tribal relationships, and people fall back on their tribal connections in order to survive. The collective that has been injured is a supra-tribal entity. The repair of this system requires reconnections among groups and people who have lost the neighboring which was what they had in common.

Principle 3: The injury is not solely to the self

Though individuals experience enormous pain at the loss of a neighborhood, the injury of interest to collective recovery is the injury to the collective, that is the system of the neighborhood, itself. Oddly enough, this injury is obscured both by the obvious grief of many people and by the disappearance of neighborhood. It is hard to see the injury in something that has disappeared. Because people find new places, within which they continue their lives, the focus moves from the "then" place to the "now" place. In this strange configuration of lost place and present anguish, people

---

[2] Project Liberty was sponsored by the Federal Emergency Management Agency to provide mental health services to those affected by 9/11.

find it hard to grasp the collective injury. But, when the collective is repaired, people prosper again with a rapidity that we would not have thought possible.

Principle 4: The festival heals the collective

Just as individual therapy has identified a number of tried and true modalities, so too have practitioners of collective recovery begun to identify the modalities that lead to new ties among strangers. One of the most important is that of the "festival" (Memmi, 1991; Cantal-Dupart, 1994).[3] Though it may seem counterintuitive to have a party-like event in a time of tragedy, this turns out to be what is needed, and the need for this grows as time goes by. The festival is, first of all, at the right level of scale. Second, it is able to encompass soothing and inspiring interactions that enable people to re-envision the manner in which they will live together.

Putting collective recovery into action

Putting collective recovery into action is a challenging undertaking. Perhaps the greatest challenge is that a commitment to the recovery of the collective must take precedence over separatism, which is such a profound part of modern societies. The practice of "divide-and-conquer" has characterized Western colonial societies for hundreds of years, affecting both the colonizer and the colonized (Memmi, 1991). It is accepted as axiomatic that people have deep and important differences due to race, class, gender and religion. Asking that people act from solidarity across difference goes against centuries of acculturation in distrust. Furthermore, the philosophy of "divide and conquer" was implemented because it was advantageous to the ruling group. Ruling groups continue to benefit from division, and are suspicious of efforts to unite the populace.

This problem is reminiscent of the problem known as the "tragedy of the commons," that is the human tendency to act from self-interest to the detriment of group survival. The specific example is that of farmers who graze their cows on common land. If one farmer adds a cow to his herd, he will get richer. But the others, seeing his new wealth, will emulate his actions. In the end, the number of cows will exceed the carrying capacity of the land and lead to disaster for all (Hardin, 1968).

In this vein, if political leaders find separatism useful, they may not want to give it up for the sake of collective recovery. Yet, the failure of collective recovery will increase the impact of the disaster and its detrimental effects on society. Thus, leaders can choose a path that offers short-term power but long-term social disaster. There were numerous examples of New York City's leadership acting to impede

---

[3] We are indebted to Hirofumi Minami, an environmental psychologist from Hiroshima, Japan, for this formulation.

collective recovery, and these actions started almost immediately after the disaster. The very first was targeted at Union Square, which had become a gathering point for people seeking solace from their distress. Within days, the park was hung with posters from all over the country, expressing people's reactions to the events of 9/11. The Parks Department swept away the posters, thus undoing the sense that Union Square was the antidote to 9/11. Such actions ultimately inhibited collective recovery, a set of decisions that will affect the city and the region for many generations.

Implications for research and practice

Norris and colleagues, in an article reviewing mental health effects of disasters, concluded, "We need to identify and investigate novel approaches to community intervention, where the intervention itself has been designed to produce collective rather than individual improvements" (Norris *et al.*, 2002). We agree.

Moving out of treatment models that are focused on the individual, we will need to have clear models of the kinds of interrelationships that occur at different levels of scale, as well as ideas of interventions that recreate such connections once they have been disturbed or sundered. This is, at one and the same time, a work of description and invention.

While the public health community is placing increasing reliance on "evidence-based" models of intervention, we think that many kinds of evidence should be considered, and not simply the scientist's darling, the randomized, controlled, clinical trial. We can draw on history for solutions to these problems. We can draw on history for motivation not to neglect this crucial work. We can draw on the vast experience that resides among community organizations that have faced such crises and overcome them. The wealth of experience collected by gay community organizations during their decades-long fight against the AIDS epidemic holds many lessons for others concerned with carrying out collective recovery (Petrow *et al.*, 1990, p. 453). Similarly, the redevelopment of neighborhoods devastated by disinvestment can teach us a great deal about the struggle to reknit social networks sundered by disaster (Freedman, 1993).

Finally, collective recovery is a very exciting process. It offers the opportunity not only to repair injuries from new disasters, but also to fix problems inherited from centuries of intergroup exploitation due to colonialism and other forces. Collective recovery is the solution to the tragedy of the commons and offers us the possibility of a sustainable future, in which the human race pulls back from ecological catastrophe and learns to live in harmony with the natural world. This is a useful project for all of us.

REFERENCES

Cantal-Dupart, M. (1994). *Merci la Ville!* Bordeaux: Investigations Le Castor Astral.

Engel, G.L. (1980). The clinical application of the biopsychosocial model. *American Journal of Psychiatry*, **137**, 535–544.

Freedman, S.G. (1993). *Upon This Rock: The Miracles of a Black Church.* New York: HarperCollins.

Fullilove, R.E., Edgoose, J.C. & Fullilove, M.T. (1997). Chaos, criticality, and public health. *Journal of the National Medical Association*, **89**(5), 311–316.

Granovetter, M. (1972). The strength of weak ties. *American Journal of Sociology*, **78**, 1360–1380.

Hardin, G. (1968). The tragedy of the commons. *Science*, **162**, 1243–1248.

Hernandez-Cordero, L. (2003). Fostering collective recovery. In *Socio-Medical Sciences.* New York: Columbia University.

Jacobs, J. (1993). *The Death and Life of Great American Cities.* New York: Random House.

Memmi, A. (1991). *The Colonizer and the Colonized.* Boston: Beacon Press.

Norris, F.R., Friedman, M.J., Watson, P.J. (2002). 60,000 disaster victims speak. Part II. Summary and implications of the disaster mental health research. *Psychiatry*, **65**, 240–260.

Petrow, S., Franks, P. & Wolfred, T.R. (1990). *Ending the HIV Epidemic: Community Strategies in Disease Prevention and Health Promotion.* San Francisco: Network Publications.

11

Rebuilding communities post-disaster in New York

Mindy Thompson Fullilove and Jack Saul

What happened on September 11th?

Most clinicians and mental health professionals would say that what happened on September 11, 2001, was a terrorist attack that traumatized people at rates relative to their exposure to the event. Based on this assumption, the mental health system enumerated symptoms and mobilized resources for individual treatment. This was the driving logic of post-disaster response and it led to an investment of millions of dollars in a narrowly defined effort to treat the trauma suffered by individuals.

But we hope to argue here that, on 9/11, a keystone urban neighborhood was destroyed, an act that threatened the health and well-being of the New York metropolitan region, as well as the nation. Based on this assumption, an array of actions were required that would serve to re-knit the social, economic, and cultural linkages of the city, the region and the nation. This approach, though a minor part of the early disaster relief, is an essential component of long-term urban rehabilitation. We assert that the nature of long-term recovery will be influenced by the degree to which re-knitting interventions are ultimately instituted.

In this chapter, we will describe the rational for community-level interventions, and we will illustrate these ideas using examples from our work in Lower Manhattan and in the larger region.

What is a keystone?

Perhaps the central concept in the argument we are making is that of a "keystone," a concept that ecologists adopted from architects to describe the entity that gives stability to a complex system, similar to the manner in which a keystone gives stability to an arch. Urban ecologists have noted a keystone neighborhood will affect the well-being of the city and even the region within which the neighborhood is embedded (Fullilove, 1999–2000).

The World Trade Center certainly qualified as both a neighborhood – specifically a central business district – and a keystone. The World Trade Center was the worksite for 50,000 people, and a daily crossroads for an additional 100,000 people. Befitting a central business district, it was a transportation hub, connected by ferry, bus, subway, and train to an enormously large region, a fact we can see in the maps of the home communities of those who died on 9/11. In addition to its commercial role, the World Trade Center exerted enormous psychological influence as an icon of the city and the region. Countless trucks and pizzerias were decorated by murals featuring the World Trade Center towering over Lower Manhattan. An August 2001 cover of *The New Yorker* depicted people building sand castles modeled after the World Trade Center, complete with a stick to signify the signature antenna the North Tower. As a center of work, tourism, transportation, and as a symbol of the ego of the city, the World Trade Center functioned to meld the New York City (NYC) region into a social, economic, and cultural unit.

What happens when a keystone is eliminated?

Because of the keystone's central organizing function, the elimination of the keystone undermines the integrity of the larger system. At the level of ecosystems, the observation has been made that the disappearance of the key part of the food chain will affect all of the other plants and animals that are part of the linkage. In the case of neighborhoods, the destruction of a keystone neighborhood threatens the health and well-being of the larger urban system of which it is a part. There are two conclusions that follow from these observations. First, although the keystone is what is destroyed in these examples, the implications of its destruction reach far beyond the immediate area. Second, the ecosystem, as a whole, is faced with the task of reorganizing to stabilize itself in the absence of an essential member. Its ability to carry out these tasks in a timely manner will determine the manner in which the system proceeds into the future.

Pitirim Sorokin, chairman of the Department of Sociology at Harvard University in the 1940s, examined these issues extensively in his seminal book (Sorokin, 1942). Following the short- and long-term consequences of hundreds of disasters over several millennia, he observed that the actions of society were crucial to recovery. His remarks on famine are of particular relevance to considerations of the losses that accompanied the attacks on the Twin Towers. He concluded his assessment of the management of famine with the following words:

The practical lesson of history is this: the orderly ways of an integrated society are always more successful and less costly in dealing with famine than are the various disorderly modes resulting in huge mortality. If the starving society is wise, if its governing and well-to-do classes are unselfish, it will always seek a combination of the rational and less painful ways out of famine, never would it turn to revolutions, war, and other similar "medicine" which cure the sickness by killing the patient. Unfortunately, many a society does not possess this wisdom of temporary sacrifice. They turn to pseudo-measures and pay the terrible penalty for their foolishness and egotism, their lack of sociality and mutual help. (Sorokin, 1942)

In sum, the central need, in the aftermath of the destruction of a keystone neighborhood, is unselfishness and temporary sacrifice, that is, the expression of interdependence and mutual concern. Such actions are not only essential to rebuilding the society, but also are curative for the symptoms of trauma-related illnesses. Overcoming aloneness, feeling the support of the larger group, having a manifestation of the higher power that lies in collective action are the best antidotes to lingering feelings related to terror. Furthermore, the collective can use its energy to enact targeted solutions to trauma recovery, such as creating inclusive narratives of the traumatizing events. In many societies post-calamity, affected people have struggled to articulate to their would-be rescuers that recovery lay in group interactions, not in individual therapy.

How is interdependence to be expressed in a society of individualism and warring groups?

The USA, though known for episodes of sacrifice, has a dominant culture that is a mixture of individualism and tribalism. Though people are taught to stand on their own two feet, they are also conscripted into identification with tribal groups defined by complex mixtures of social class, occupation, ethnic origin, skin color, age, and religion, what the market researchers have affectionately labeled "target audiences." These subgroups are socially signified by "lifestyle choices," which range from favorite jeans to neighborhood of residence, as signaled by the all-important "zip + four"[1]. Because the subgroups live apart from each other and see themselves as different, the potential sympathy for the crisis of another's neighborhood is limited, as is the likelihood of the expression of mutuality after neighborhood disaster.

The uneven effects of the disaster added a new layer of difference to those already existing. In Figure 11.1, we present a pictorial representation of the region viewed from the perspective of the immediate damage created by trauma. In this view, the epicenter is the most heavily affected and the people there are most heavily traumatized. Other affected neighborhoods are those that lost substantial numbers of citizens, or were tightly connected by culture or economics to the World Trade Center.

---

[1] The "zip + four" refers to the seven digit zip code, plus four digits signifying an area within the zip code. It turns out that these areas tend to be homogeneous for many lifestyle measures, like supermarket, preferred automobile, etc. Market analysis has divided the US into approximately one hundred market categories, based on analysis of the buying patterns by zip + four areas.

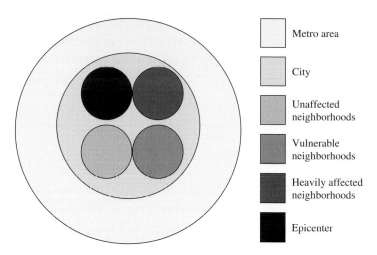

Metro area

City

Unaffected
neighborhoods

Vulnerable
neighborhoods

Heavily affected
neighborhoods

Epicenter

Figure 11.1 Nested systems and their relative injury

Vulnerable neighborhoods (those that were home to minorities or illegal immigrants) faced elevated risks from the economic fall-out of the disaster.

Despite these layers of distinction, shared concern for "my" city overcame tribalism to a remarkable extent. People felt a common pain and despair and turned to each for comfort. In this unique hiatus, black people smiled at police, rich people cared about poor people, and Jews were concerned about attacks on Arabs. In Lower Manhattan, people helped each other to find shelter, to search for loved ones, and to endure months of uncertainty and displacement. In other parts of the city, people made *impromptu* contact in parks, subways, and fire stations.

Thus, two tendencies could be discerned. One was a tendency to differentiate among groups, but the other was a remarkable tendency towards unity. This impulse towards togetherness created the possibility for healing not only from 9/11, but also from the pre-existing divisions. In this setting, the sense of common injury was the lever to use to overcome prior antagonisms and promote collective recovery.

What is the ecosystems approach to healing?

In the ecosystems approach, "treatment" should be directed at rebuilding the strength of social groups, including families, school communities, neighborhoods, and the city and region as a whole. The clinical approach can be distinguished from an ecosystems, or community, approach in a number of ways. The clinical approach focuses almost exclusively on the individual as the client, and particularly in a post-disaster context is easily stigmatizing, as people do not necessarily want to be identified as having a mental health problem. It usually offers a limited range of possibilities for healing. Clinical services are usually not oriented to the stated needs of clients, but to the services the clinicians are interested in providing. The clinical perspective emphasizes enhancing the expertise of the providers and little attention is paid to enhancing the competence of clients to recognize and find solutions to their own difficulties.

In the ecosystems, or community approach, the client is the social environment and the focus is on strengths, resources, and continuity. One of the most important assumptions behind this approach is that communities have the capacity to heal themselves and that the greatest resources for recovery are community members. The activities supported by such an approach are often those that community members are already engaged in and thus non-stigmatizing. In coming together around practical concerns, the connections between people may be enhanced, and as we have recognized both internationally and in New York, these become the sites for sharing information, expressing emotion, and providing mutual support.

In the following two sections, we will first examine efforts to use community mobilization to aid people at the epicenter and second examine efforts to develop methods for mobilizing organizations throughout the region to cope with the consequences of 9/11.

Lower Manhattan post-catastrophe: the Ground Zero Initiative

People living in Lower Manhattan bore the immediate brunt of exposure to the attack and its aftermath. As a psychologist with a long professional commitment to trauma recovery, Jack Saul found himself in a new role: that of "victim" rather than "helper." He realized that what he wanted and needed for his own healing was the mobilization of the local community. He thought that, among his friends and neighborhoods, there was the raw talent for doing what was required. He found it off-putting that people were arriving in droves from outside the neighborhood to "care for" the residents of the area.

The initial approach of the NYC Board of Education followed in the same vein, with a focus on screening children for post-traumatic stress disorder and offering therapeutic services to those who were identified as having difficulties. Not only had very little attention been paid to the impact of these events on teachers and parents, but neither group had been engaged in giving input into the evaluation process of the children. While the mental health of children became the focus of the school system's efforts, there were no places for parents to discuss their concerns as a group. Thus, Saul, like many other parents and teachers, found himself disenfranchised and unsupported. In response, they joined together to create family support committees that developed community forums for parents, teachers, and school staff from the downtown elementary schools.

Under the rubric of the "Ground Zero Initiative," Saul worked, first and foremost, with his children's school community. That school was quite close to Ground Zero. Teachers, students and administrators had experienced the immediate horror of running from the collapsing Towers, as well as the long-term stress of being displaced from their school building. The school of 600 children was offered a vacant school building as a temporary measure. In one weekend the parents came together and cleaned, painted and moved furniture into the vacant school, making it usable for the children to attend the following week. The sense of togetherness and of taking action in the context of practical activities were repeated numerous times during the year and were seen by many parents as some of the greatest contributors to returning to a sense of well-being. By doing for their children, the parents were able to reassert their own agency and thereby regain some sense of power and control.

Saul also worked with other parents, teachers, and residents in the Lower Manhattan area to develop community forums. Their goal was to expand the notion of healing from one primarily focused on individual stress reactions to a broader notion of community recovery. Parents of children from the schools in the vicinity of the World Trade Center, who were also mental health professionals, established drop in support programs where parents could get help with difficulties they were having with their children or in their families. These family support programs made connections across school communities to share ideas about how to address the emotional issues faced by children and parents as a consequence of the events that had taken place.

In January 2002, with the plan to return the children to their home schools, many parents were feeling distress about going back for the first time to the place where they had experienced the horror of 4 months earlier. Some families had already moved back into their homes near Ground Zero, while others were still displaced from their homes. Some people were more ready than others to have their children return to the school, and the differences among peoples' feelings about the safety of the environment and the visibility of the destruction were topics that caused tension in the community. To address these issues, a community forum was organized to give parents and teachers an opportunity to talk about the issues that were on their minds.

The family support group invited Dr. Claude Chemtob, a child psychologist and disaster specialist, to facilitate the meeting. As part of introducing a concept of community recovery, Dr. Chemtob presented a framework to orient participants about stages through which a community might pass following a disaster:
(1) An initial stage of shock and then coming together, sharing, and letting one's guard down, called the "united we stand" stage;
(2) As people start to get tired and irritable, stresses accumulate and tempers flare and people retreat into groups within which they feel safer, referred to as the "molasses and minefields" stage and it became apparent that there were things people could do to reduce tensions and better work together;

(3) A stage in which communities come together to create a positive vision of recovery.

Thus, Dr. Chemtob introduced the idea that recovery was not a passive process, but a consequence of the community actively coming together for a common purpose.

During the meeting the parents broke up into small groups to discuss their concerns and to consider how they might increase their skills as parents and teachers. This included a collective conversation about how parents and teachers could take care of themselves and support each other as well. A community needs assessment was conducted with the close to one hundred participants of the meeting. The community forum thus accomplished several goals: it deepened participants' understanding of the process of disaster recovery, it offered an opportunity to talk through concerns, and it collected data on community needs. The forum, at one and the same time, served for healing, problem solving, and needs assessment.

Through these activities, the Ground Zero Initiative demonstrated that disaster victims could heal themselves by engaging actively and collectively with the series of environmental challenges that had, literally, descended upon them. With each action, the group gained clarity and sanity, pulling out of the chaos of the disaster, a new basis for order. Empowerment, agency, engagement, initiative: these are some of the key words that describe the work of community recovery carried out by the Ground Zero Initiative.

Regional reconnections: NYC RECOVERS

The pain of 9/11 was felt throughout the metropolitan area, but people outside of the epicenter were urged to "get back to normal." This was specifically encoded in messages telling people to: (1) tell others to go to therapists if they had symptoms, (2) support the economy by shopping, taking an airplane and going to the theater, and (3) accept, without discussion, the decisions politicians were making about rebuilding Ground Zero. As these official instructions left vast numbers of people sitting on their pain, Mindy Fullilove thought that an alternative was essential. The major question she posed was, "How might we know what people are concerned about and how best to intervene?" The answer she acted on was that offered by urban theorist Louis Wirth, who noted that organizations are the key intermediaries between a city and its diverse and divided subpopulations (Wirth, 1964). In conjunction with Jennifer Stevens Madoff, Mindy Fullilove initiated NYC RECOVERS (NYCR), an alliance of organizations concerned with NYC's social and emotional recovery.

The central thesis of NYCR – and here we find a key resonance with Jack Saul's ideas – was that the wisdom of recovery lay in organizations. Organizations, which were integral to the myriad communities that comprised the regional ecosystem, had the ability to assess the needs of their constituents, and institute appropriate remedies. Furthermore, organizations had the capacity to form linkages with other organizations, thus recreating the social and organizational framework that had been damaged by 9/11.

NYCR Coordinating Team

The NYCR Coordinating Team consisted of a small group of staff and volunteers of the Community Research Group, a unit of the New York State Psychiatric Institute and the Mailman School of Public Health of Columbia University. Prior to 9/11, members of the Coordinating Team were engaged in a study of neighborhood obliteration due to urban renewal, a federal program of the 1950s and 1960s (Fullilove, 2004). The team's work had demonstrated that prominent among the long-term effects of urban renewal was a slow but inexorable dissolution of social bonds. In the cases under study, no efforts at social recovery had been made. Because the work on urban renewal was then unpublished, and thus unavailable to the general public or the disaster relief community, the team felt an obligation to share the need for social recovery with others who might implement this intervention.

Members of the alliance

NYCR sought to mobilize all organizations in the New York metropolitan area. Organizations of all kinds were of interest, from schools, churches, and other non-profit organizations to commercial and government enterprises. Organizations and individuals that joined in the effort were called "partners." Organizations and individuals who became associated with the effort, without formally joining, were called "friends." About 100 organizations established formal ties with NYCR. As many of these were themselves coalitions, with ties to other organizations, the effective range of NYCR's network was about 1000 organizations.

The bowl of NYCR

NYCR' Coordinating Team developed and offered to partners a "bowl," that is, a holding structure, or concept, which they might fill as they chose. The over-arching concept that guided the first year of work was that of "Year of Recovery," designed to counter two major ideas that emanated from city officials: (1) that the disaster had affected a small area of the city, and a small number of "heroes and victims," and (2) that the job of the "unaffected" was to "get back to normal" within days of the disaster. NYCR argued that all people in the metropolitan area had lost a neighborhood that was important to them and had a right to consider themselves injured. Furthermore, NYCR argued that such injuries did not heal quickly or that it was not even possible to get "back" to normal: rather, people needed to work together to envision and create the recovered city and region.

The Year of Recovery was devoted to tasks that are within the purview of groups in many cultures around the world, that is, mourning losses, learning what had caused the disaster, rebuilding social connections, and preventing the development of scapegoating and prejudice. The shorthand, "remember, respect, learn, and connect," was used to keep these core tasks at the forefront of the alliance's concern. The Coordinating Team initially proposed that these tasks might follow the seasons of the year, with winter devoted to conferences for learning and preventing prejudice, spring to rebuilding connections, and autumn to mourning, as the region encountered the first anniversary of the disaster. It became apparent as the year progressed that, contrary to initial assumptions, this was not a serial process. "Remember, respect, learn, and connect" were each observed in every NYCR gathering.

Filling the bowl

NYCR did not offer specific initiatives to partners. Rather, NYCR urged organizations to consider the idea, "We are all in pain. You know how to help your people. If we each pitch in, we'll all feel better." It was the partners' initiatives that gave content to the Year of Recovery, and this worked in two ways. In some cases, organizations began activities at the urging of members of the Coordinating Team. In other cases, the initiatives of organizations drew in the NYCR Coordinating Team and partners. Whatever the case, it was the organizations that created the events and gave them character and meaning. Through regular meetings, e-mail messages, and a large conference, the Coordinating Team worked to help organizations learn about and learn from the efforts of others, thus building a collective knowledge base of how organizations might promote recovery. A few examples will demonstrate the range of events that were held.

The Walk to Honor and Heal

Held on November 12, 2001, to honor the third month anniversary of 9/11, the Walk to Honor and Heal was led by a coalition of organizations active in the South Bronx. The Walk started at a local fire station that had been an important site of community struggle in the past. The Walk covered approximately 20 blocks through three commercial areas and ended in a labyrinth painted in a church parking lot at a major intersection. The Walk started shortly after Flight 587 crashed at Rockaway Beach in Queens, killing all on board. The crash created an atmosphere of fear and tension. As many of those who died had friends and relatives in the South Bronx, the crash took on deeper and more immediate importance in the days that followed. Despite the tension from the crash, the adults and children who walked together created a joyous and enthusiastic presence in the streets of the neighborhood. In a culminating moment, participants released white balloons in the blue November sky and watched them float off, past tenements into the stratosphere.

The Novena for Flight 587

Washington Heights, a neighborhood at the northern tip of Manhattan, lost many people in the crash of Flight 587. Alianza Dominicana, an early and important partner of NYCR, organized a Novena, which is a Dominican mourning ritual. In this instance, to honor the community's pain, 7 days of public Novenas were organized. Each day, the Novena started in a public park and was followed by a procession to a nearby church. NYC RECOVERS urged leaders of the nearby Columbia-Presbyterian Medical Center to join the Novena for the final day. Approximately 200 people from the Medical Center, including many of its major leaders, joined the procession.

The Luncheon of Champions

The American Express Open the Small Business Network was displaced from its Lower Manhattan offices, which made life difficult for staff already traumatized by the tragedy. Staff used dollars from a community relations fund to plan a special luncheon. They joined with another NYCR partner, the Washington Heights/ Inwood Coalition on Aging, to sponsor a "Luncheon of Champions," held at a Lower Manhattan restaurant that had just reopened after an extensive clean-up (and, as it turned out, did not accept American Express). The American Express hosts planned a delicious menu and a wonderful activity. Most of the guests were monolingual Spanish speakers and most of the hosts were monolingual English speakers. As one of the organizers commented, "It could have been a disaster." However, goodwill and sociability overcame the language barrier. The activity – decorating cakes with New York themes – created what the organizer called "a third language" of images and laughter.

Together we heal: community mobilization for trauma recovery

The most ambitious activity undertaken by the Coordinating Team was the organization of a conference on community resilience. The conference was sponsored by Project Liberty, and organized with support from the NYC Department of Mental Health and Mental Retardation, and the New York University International Trauma Studies Program (Jack Saul's program). It brought together 200 people from organizations of all kinds. The concept of community mobilization was presented and its application to planning for the anniversary of 9/11 was discussed. Out of the conference emerged the concept of "September Wellness," an effort to embed the anniversary in a larger period of healing mind, body, and spirit through wellness activities.

Learning from each other

A major finding of the work of NYCR was that organizations learned from each other. As communication and trust developed, people examined each other's ideas, and freely adopted and adapted those that seemed to suit. Walking labyrinths appealed to many people, hence Camino de Paz, the South Bronx labyrinth builders and one of the sponsors of the Walk to Honor and Heal, was invited to events around the city, such as the Riverside Church September Wellness Festival. Organizations might copy an activity for a first effort, but then return to report something they had created for a later event. Thus, a body of experience was created that helped to identify "best practices." In general, what emerged from the Year of Recovery was a distinct preference for recovery events organized according to a "festival model" – featuring activities, fellowship, and food – rather than a "heroic model" – featuring honors and ceremony.

The barrier-free city

The Coordinating Team was interested in engaging many kinds of organizations, hence outreach was made in a great number of directions. A surprise to the team, which was previously occupied with research in poor, minority communities, was that the city was nearly free of barriers in the immediate aftermath of 9/11. It was possible to meet with the very rich, as well as the very poor, and it was possible for them to meet together.

The major barriers to free exchange, in fact, were those erected by the officials of the City. As one example, it took months for NYCR to establish effective linkages with the Department of Health. While those linkages resulted in a very successful conference, other initiatives that partners and team members deemed equally important were stymied. In practice, the "heroes and victims" formulation narrowed attention and concern to a very small group of people. Many of those who found themselves outside of those narrow groups tended to accept the "unaffected" designation. This, in turn, appeared to disenfranchise those groups from the post-disaster political process, which included decisions around where the budget axe would fall.

Battle fatigue

One of the reasons partners developed the concept of "September Wellness: Healing Mind, Body, and Spirit," was the broad recognition of the onset of fatigue related to a long series of crises beginning with 9/11, but quickly expanding to include the fear of new attacks, the city budget deficit, the anthrax scare, the war on terrorism and the threat, followed by the reality, of war with Iraq. All of these problems were complicating lives already lived at the fast and demanding pace of NYC. Furthermore, some of the post-disaster sources of solace, like comfort food, and psychotropic drugs, had their own side effects that needed to be countered. September Wellness opened a door to self and community care, but also clearly revealed the need for long-term support for managing the new regional situation. Hence, a second year of recovery, called "Take Heart," was initiated.

Healer, Heal Thyself

The Coordinating Team of NYCR consistently implemented its own advice, working hard to help its parent organization, the Community Research Group, remember, respect, learn, and connect. Like other organizations, the Community Research Group felt the strain of piling new tasks related to launching NYCR onto a large body of other work. Using events to sustain and nourish the group, the Community Research Group was able to weather significant challenges it faced post-9/11, while continuing to produce scientific papers and community educational materials, and to compete successfully for new funding.

Conclusion

Community members have many advantages over outside providers. It has been said that they are five times more powerful to affect change. They have greater access to the local knowledge of existing resources and social networks and often are already engaged in positive social processes that build community solidarity and cohesion. These efforts have a greater possibility of success because they are driven by the community members' priorities and preferences. Because they live in the community and have greater investment in its development, their initiative and involvement is often crucial for the sustainability of such programs.

Thus, the role of the community-oriented provider is to offer structure and support that promotes positive connection and social process. The provider helps to build new connections between constituencies in the community and recognizes and enhances existing resources for recovery. This recognition can be one of the most humbling experiences for mental health professionals working in a post-disaster context. It is often very difficult for such professionals to shift their thinking from a mental health to a disaster context and accept that they do not have a monopoly on the processes of psychosocial recovery. In such a context, mental health professionals are one set of resources among many that exist in the community, and participate with different occupational groups in promoting the well-being of community members.

The community harbors a spectrum of opportunities for healing: community members with a diversity of skills and ages contribute in different ways to the resilience of the community. The elderly bring the memories of coping with previous tragedies, while children bring the capacity for play and spontaneity. People bring a diversity of strengths and skills based on occupation and talents – from the artistic to organizational management skills, from the sublime to the mundane – to enhance the process of recovery. Thus, healing can be seen as a creative process arising from the synergy of various community actors coming together to work toward a common purpose.

Community resilience approaches are systematically focused but at the same time address multiple levels and themes in the process of recovery. One of the shortcomings of many trauma programs is that they address trauma primarily at the level of the individual while ignoring the larger contexts – the family, work group, and other groups – in the community. The disruptions that take place to family systems, work organizations, and communal structures are given short shrift, even though the stresses related to the social trauma are often the most debilitating for individuals. In some cases, the system's response to traumatic events (i.e. fragmentation, conflict, stigmatization, and destabilization) may be even more painful and psychologically harmful than the primary traumatic event itself. This was frequently the case in the aftermath of the terrorist attacks in NYC, where fragmentation and conflict in the work setting and in schools and families themselves were described by many as having been more problematic than the events people experienced on 9/11. The disruption of such social systems was ignored in favor of individual approaches.

A community resilience approach following massive psychosocial trauma usually encompasses the following four themes (Landau, 2002; Madoff, 2002; Saul, 2002):

(1) *Building community and enhancing social connectedness*: It is a foundation for recovery. The foundation of community recovery is the reweaving of social connections that have been disrupted by traumatic events. Referred to as the matrix of healing, Judith Landau emphasizes the re-establishment of old community connections while facilitating new ones (Landau, 2002). This includes strengthening the system of social support, coalition building, and information and resource sharing.

(2) *Collectively telling the story of the community's experience and response*: An important part of the communal healing process is about having one's story validated and becoming a part of the collective story that emerges after a complex and horrible tragedy. This affirmation by the community at large is often described by those who survive major disasters as a crucial step in recovering their sense of well-being. As we have seen in NYC following 9/11, the emerging story after such events needs to respect and to encompass the stories experienced by many different people – those who have lost family and friends, who have lost their homes, who were far away from Ground Zero but still were deeply affected, those who were confused, and those who suffered discrimination and injustice as a result of the events. It can be problematic when the larger narrative is narrow, rigid or marginalizes some segments of the population. This has been the case in particular for the Arab speaking and Muslim communities where many members faced harassment, detention, and deportation. Often it is those people who do not have a voice in society that end up becoming the most victimized after a collective tragedy.

(3) *Re-establishing the rhythms and routines of life and engaging in collective healing rituals*: The spontaneous neighborhood vigils, anniversary rituals, and community events marking seasonal changes and holidays became important times for communities to reconnect with established temporal rhythms and to process the dissonant feelings associated with these events due to the loss and other experiences associated with the traumatic events of 9/11.

(4) *Arriving at a positive vision of the future with renewed hope*: Many of the collective responses to 9/11 were attempts to re-establish hope in the future. One of the most important questions faced by communities after a catastrophe is, "how do we move from haunting memories of the tragedy to a vision of the future that incorporates the new realities that we are facing?"

The efforts described here – the work of the Ground Zero Initiative and NYCR – were efforts carried out with minimal personnel and modest funding. The vast resources that were made available to pay for individual counseling of various kinds were not available for the community mobilization efforts we are describing. Nor were funds available to assess the effects of the work we are describing. Despite these limitations, we think that such community mobilization is the central focus for recovery of the city and the region in the years to come. In particular, the bright moment of togetherness that followed 9/11 was allowed to slip away by leaders who chose to use divisive interventions rather than promote mutuality and unselfishness. Thus, we can expect ripple effects that will endure for decades, if not centuries.

At the same time, we can say with confidence that it is possible to mobilize communities to work together in a highly effective manner, inventing creative and satisfying ways for healing trauma and envisioning the future of the city and the region.

REFERENCES

Fullilove, M.T. (1999–2000). Death and life in a great American city. *International Journal of Mental Health*, **28**, 20–29.

Fullilove, M.T. (2004). *Root Shock: How Tearing up City Neighborhoods Hurts America and What We Can Do About It*. New York: Ballantine Books/One World.

Landau, J. (2002). Terror and trauma: enhancing family and community resilience. *American Family Therapy Academy Annual Conference*, New York City, June 2002.

Madoff, J.S. (2002). Together we heal: community mobilization for trauma recovery. *Conference Summary*, NYC RECOVERS, April 16, 2002.

Saul, J. (2002). Promoting community recovery in downtown Manhattan. *American Family Therapy Academy Annual Conference*, New York City, June 2002.

Sorokin, P. (1942). *Man and Society in Calamity: The Effects of War, Revolution, Famine, Pestilence upon Human Mind, Behavior, Social Organization and Cultural Life*. New York: E.P. Dutton.

Wirth, L. (1964). Urbanism as a way of life. In *On Cities and Social Life: Selected Papers by Louis Wirth*, (2nd edn.). ed. A.J.J. Reiss. Chicago: The University of Chicago Press.

12

Journalism and the public during catastrophes

Elana Newman, Joanne Davis and Shawn M. Kennedy

When we think about the events of September 11, 2001, we visualize images of the World Trade Center Twin Towers falling down, the fractured Pentagon, and a large crater with wreckage in Shanksville, Pennsylvania. We envision firefighters, police, emergency rescue workers, smoke, rubble, and ashen-covered people. Sounds come back – confused and shocked voices explaining what is and is not known about these events, and the voice of a telephone operator describing a group of passengers overtaking a plane. For many of us our understanding, very memories, and images of these events are derived from a set of professional people first on the scene: journalists. These reporters, photographers, broadcasters, writers, and people behind the scenes accompanied emergency workers in order to bring the world the images and stories depicting 9/11 in real time.

Long before the events of 9/11 terrorism was a regular beat for journalists around the world (Bull & Newman, 2002). In recent US history, for example, American journalists covered the 1990 abortion clinic bombings, the 1993 World Trade Center bombing, and the 1995 bombing of the Murrah Federal Building in downtown Oklahoma City (Bull & Newman, 2002). While organizations such as the Dart Center for Journalism and Trauma (see www.dartcenter.org) have attended to the nature and effect of trauma-related reporting for several years, the 9/11 terrorist attacks significantly advanced the role of the media during traumatic times into the forefront of public and professional discourse. This chapter reviews the roles of American journalists during times of crisis, the emerging empirical and clinical literature on the relationship between media consumption and distress among the public, and the impact of covering trauma upon journalists themselves. The chapter concludes with recommendations for future scholarship and practice for the public and journalists.

Journalists' role

Journalists play a critical and multifaceted role in communities during times of destruction, war, and chaos (Newman, 2002b). First and foremost, journalists provide the public with information and analysis about traumatic events including community responses to these events. Often in the immediacy of a catastrophe, although not by design, the media become the primary means of crisis communication. This was readily apparent in the aftermath of September 11, 2001, when broadcast media conveyed information about safety, transportation routes, and volunteer needs. Tom Brockaw believed, "the most reassuring thing I could do was to get as much information to the audience as factually and as swiftly as I possibly could, and try to place it in perspective" (Gilbert *et al.*, 2002). Following the immediate crisis stage of a catastrophe, the role of journalists changes to that of "public watchdogs," investigating and providing truthful, verified information about public and private responses focusing on the tragedy while independently monitoring those in power (Kovach & Rosensteil, 2001). For example, journalists provided information about the health effects of the burning debris from the World Trade Center and the problems and successes of benefit disbursement to survivors and their families. Furthermore, journalists offer a forum for public dialogue, commentary and engagement about disaster-related experiences (Kovach & Rosensteil, 2001). Numerous columns, letters to the editors, editorial pieces, Internet-based dialogues and interactive broadcast programs that focused on the events of 9/11 promoted this public discourse. Finally, journalists provide the first draft of the history of particular calamities. The work of countless journalists who interviewed and documented the struggles and triumphs of survivors, family members, witnesses, rescue workers, experts, and politicians involved in 9/11 events will provide substantive material for future scholars. In all these roles, the American journalists' primary professional duty is to supply verified, comprehensive and proportional information about events in the service of assuring that citizens and communities have accurate information to make informed decisions and engage in democratic processes (Kovach & Rosensteil, 2001). Traditionally, journalism emphasizes this need to serve the public (Kovach & Rosensteil, 2001).

Covering terrorism is no easy task for even the most adroit professionals. Journalists and photojournalists may arrive at the scene before rescue personnel, both placing them in physical danger, and in ethical quandaries of whether to intervene or document the situation (Cote & Simpson, 2000). Once information is gathered, the journalist needs to accurately and objectively present pertinent information about these shocking events with a careful restraint as to not further the terrorists' goal of producing widespread panic (Bull & Newman, 2002). They need to depict horrific acts yet avoid sensationalism. A broad range of practical and emotional impediments can obstruct this process.

Firstly, as in the case of September 11th, information can be difficult to access when communication systems such as cellular phones, facsimiles, Internet, and telephone services are disrupted. Furthermore, the ability to provide information about the disaster to colleagues and the newsroom may be severely compromised. For example, the entire newsroom of the Wall Street Journal was moved to the New Jersey location when the World Trade Center area was evacuated. The emergency command center for New York City, which was based at the World Trade Center, had to be relocated, causing temporary disruption in communication of vital information. The need to be accurate and verify information that is pouring in every minute can also be quite taxing, especially since journalists recognize the potential harm to the public in disseminating falsehoods. Dan Rather wrote that on the morning of September 11th, he thought, "Clearly this is going to be a day in which every bit of information would have to be double- and triple checked...then again, when you get into this kind of coverage, you face a deadline every nanosecond. There were going to be mistakes. The most responsible thing you could do was to keep them to a minimum" (Gilbert *et al.*, 2002, p. 93).

Second, while journalists aim to be objective, the tragedies they cover may be personal ones, directly affecting their workplace, home, community, and loved ones (Gilbert *et al.*, 2002). Many experienced war correspondents who covered the events of 9/11 told the staff at the New York office of the Dart Center for Journalism and Trauma that covering "a hometown atrocity" challenged their emotional and professional ability to remain objective and detached. Business writers were confronted with the deaths of many of their longstanding sources. Even those reporters who are not personally involved as victims, but bear professional witness to horrific scenes of destruction, are emotionally affected by work that they do (Cote & Simpson, 2000). Given these realities, journalists who covered the events of 9/11 had to confront essential professional dilemmas in examining the degree to which journalists can be truly "objective." Further, many journalists had to confront their own ambivalence about documenting pain and tragedy instead of comforting and aiding victims. While it is not a stated mission of journalists to heal, some may conceptualize their reporting as assisting individuals. Elizabeth Cohen of CNN explained that telling stories about the families of those missing was "something she could do and something that helped the families in a way" (Sylvester & Huffman, 2002, p. 149). Although journalists feel the human tendency to provide comfort and aid, their professional commitment is to document and communicate the event if others are present who can assist those in harms way. It may be difficult to have the clarity that photographer, Peter Turnley (2001, p. 9) had during the midst of turmoil:

At the World Trade Center, there were other people who were much better prepared than I was to rescue the victims. I felt that what I could best do with my energy was pay tribute to the men and women who got out in those difficult conditions and made those gestures of help. The reason I would justify that cameramen and photographers and journalists be present in these situations is not because they are making money or because they're parasites. It's because fifty years from now, it's important that people contemplate the decency that so many people demonstrated in trying to do the right thing in a situation that was difficult. I don't know how that can be communicated without images, without words, without film.

Clearly, journalists face multiple challenges in obtaining and communicating verified information, appraising the overall impact of disasters, coping with their own responses to calamity, and ethically reporting on the events to serve the public at large.

Public response

Mass disasters and catastrophes are unique traumas in a number of ways and may have unique effects on the public. For example, 9/11 may have resulted in significantly greater distress than any previous disaster due, in large part, to the extent of vicarious exposure via the extensive media coverage. As Schuster and colleagues (2001) postulated, many Americans may have identified these events as personal attacks directed toward themselves, and not solely toward those who were injured or killed, a phenomenon which has been noted in other disasters (e.g., Dixon *et al.*, 1993). Many watched the shocking events unfold live on television and continued to access up-to-date information through the media, with a mean of 8.1 hours of viewing time for adults and 3.0 hours for children on September (Schuster *et al.*, 2001). In a survey of 988 New York City residents, 87% reported seeing the image of the airplane hitting the World Trade Center a mean of 7 times and a median of 36 times in the first week following the attacks (Ahern *et al.*, 2002). The image of the World Trade Center collapsing was seen a median of 29 times, whereas images of people jumping was viewed a median of 2 times. Furthermore, a poll conducted by the Pew Research Center (2001) of 1200 American adults from September 13 to 17, 2001, revealed that 63% of survey respondents reported that they "could not stop watching" news about the terrorist attacks. In fact, 81% reported keeping a television or radio tuned to the news for updates on the crisis and 46% reported that they read the newspaper more closely. The poll also revealed a variety of emotional responses to the coverage: 92% of the sample reported experiencing feelings of sadness, 77% reported feelings of fright, and 45% reported feeling "tired out" while watching such news.

These reactions are typical of many people during times of stress, and also typical of people learning about horrific events. Whether individual or collective stress, human beings have two basic and opposing coping tendencies: to avoid or to approach the stressful information (Roth & Cohen, 1986). Both coping strategies have potential advantages and disadvantages. Avoiding stressful material (e.g., not talking about the event, avoiding people, places, and situations that serve as reminders of the event) can help the person focus on tasks at hand and manage emotional reactions in the short term, but can prevent the person from incorporating this information to make important decisions and adequately cope with the trauma in the long term. Approaching such material (e.g., talking about it, experiencing it on emotional and intellectual levels) can be emotionally taxing in the short term, at times even overwhelming, but may permit the person to integrate the experience into their understanding, or change their understanding of the situation based on the information, thereby reducing long-term negative consequences (Roth & Cohen, 1986).

Although only a minority of direct trauma survivors experience long-lasting psychological distress severe enough to qualify them for a psychiatric disorder (e.g., Kessler *et al.*, 1995), this distress is typically related to difficulty with regulating approach and avoidance of the situation and its reminders. Post-traumatic stress disorder (PTSD), seen in about 9% of the general population (Breslau *et al.*, 1991), is a disorder comprised of distressing re-experiencing symptoms related to the trauma, avoidance and numbing to trauma-related cues, and general states of hyperarousal. Similarly, in acute grief states, grieving individuals are both overcome with memories of the deceased, sensitive to painful emotions when reminded of the deceased, and prone to avoidance of thinking about the deceased. In the aftermath of 9/11, individuals both directly and indirectly involved in the terrorist attack found themselves trying to balance the need to make sense of the experience and the need to avoid it. This balance was particularly difficult to achieve due to the overwhelming amount of media coverage.

The "public" that journalists serve is a heterogeneous group with a diverse set of interests, needs, and vulnerabilities with respect to approaching and avoiding stressful information. Research has only begun to delineate the important demographic, social, health-related, and historical variables that may discriminate differing responses and needs of individuals. To fully explore the public's response to terrorism-related news coverage, it is important, at minimum, to distinguish four groups: adult survivors, child survivors, adult non-survivors, and child non-survivors of traumatic events.

Adult survivors

Clearly, news reports contain the types of reminders or trauma-related cues (e.g., sounds, images) that may affect survivors and those grieving the loss of loved ones. Exposure to reminders of traumatic events can be distressing to survivors, and many may find it difficult to "calm down" after such exposure. During the Gulf War for example, many Vietnam Veterans experienced a reactivation of distressing war-related symptoms (Long *et al.*, 1994). Although research has primarily focused on survivors of the same event, clinical experience points to a generalized response to current trauma-related cues among individuals with a history of various types of trauma. For example, a rape survivor may be affected by cues from other traumas (e.g., war, terrorism). This may be related to several factors including a failure to integrate information regarding the previous trauma, a general feeling of hyperarousal, and/or a further example of the individual's view that the world is not a safe place.

Adult survivors of a disaster or catastrophe may find it difficult to avoid reminders of the event. Carrie Lemack, whose mother was killed in the collapse of the World Trade Center, described her response to the images in the news (Lemack, personal communication, July 24, 2002):

Each time they show her plane hit the World Trade Center, I have to hide, cover my eyes, or quickly change the channel. I cannot watch my mother die, and every time I watch television I sit ready, in a state of preparedness, in case a news broadcast, news journal, or other program decides to air the horror of her final moments.

In fact, Ms. Lemack launched an advocacy campaign with families of September 11th, urging broadcast media to issue a visual or verbal warning each time they were about to show planes crashing into buildings, people jumping from buildings or buildings collapsing (http://www.familiesofseptember11.org/news/news2.asp?s=6).

Trauma specialists tend to concur that viewing trauma-related media can adversely affect trauma survivors. McFarlane (1986) postulated that media exposure may increase the risk of developing or maintaining chronic PTSD among survivors. He postulated that media exposure may "reinforce the victim's feelings of vulnerability and fixate their images of death and destruction." Alternatively, feelings of guilt, blame, or shame may be reinforced by media depictions. A fact sheet prepared by the International Society of Traumatic Stress Studies (2002) suggests that "media reminders that occur without warning are particularly troublesome for survivors because they contribute to a sense of helplessness, emotional imbalance, and lack of control. In the face of these events, opportunities to anticipate and exercise choice and control with regard to exposure to potential triggers can aid survivors in regaining a sense of agency and control over their lives." Regardless of cause, there is some clinical consensus that survivors should monitor consumption of trauma-related media and prepare for such exposure with a plan for ways to reduce resultant distress (e.g., Hamblen, 2001; ISTSS, 2002).

Despite these opinions, there is only one published study of adult survivors that documents a relationship between trauma-related media exposure and trauma-related distress. Specifically, in a cross sectional random digit dial survey of 1008 adult residents of Manhattan surveyed between October 16 and November 15, 2001, frequency of viewing "people jumping from the towers of the World Trade Center" media images was correlated with trauma-related distress. Among those who directly experienced loss or witnessed the event in person, individuals who watched this broadcast image more frequently were more likely to report symptoms of PTSD (22.5%) and depression (21.3%) than those who did not (3.6% and 11.7%, respectively) (Ahern *et al.*, 2002).

Adult non-survivors

As stated above, nearly all Americans were vicariously exposed to 9/11 through media coverage. Many mental health professionals and others feared that this exposure would result in tremendous numbers of individuals reporting significant trauma-related distress. However, as reported in the study by Ahern *et al.* (2002), while there was a strong relationship between viewing traumatic images among New York City survivors, this was not the case for those not directly involved or affected by the attacks. In contrast, a poll of Americans conducted 3–5 days after the attacks, documented that extensive television viewing was associated with stress reactions (Schuster *et al.*, 2001). As Pfefferbaum *et al.* (2002) elucidate, indirect victim's reactions to early media coverage may have nothing to do with the media's representations of the event, but be a sign of the appropriate horror experienced when learning about an atrocity.

Mixed sample of survivors and non-survivors

Among the general public, which includes some survivors, it appears that viewing terrorism-related images and news is not necessarily associated with increased rates of PTSD or depression, but instead may be associated with temporary anxiety.

In a study of 237 Israeli adults, half the group was randomly selected to watch television clips of terrorism and the other half watched news clips not related to terrorism. While it was not noted what percent of the sample was directly exposed to terrorism-related events, individuals who watched the terrorism-related news clips reported more anxiety than those who watched the other types of news clips. Although the differences were statistically significant, the level of anxiety was not in the pathological range (Sloan, 2000). Similarly, in a nationally representative sample of 2773 adults (some who were directly affected by the terrorist attacks), clinically significant distress was associated with hours of terrorism-related television watched each day and the number of different types of graphic terrorism-related content viewed, although this distress was not greater than that seen in typical community samples. Furthermore, in a subset of 691 New York City dwellers surveyed 2 months post-9/11, number of hours of terrorism-related television coverage watched was significantly associated with higher PTSD symptom endorsement, but the type of graphic imagery viewed was not (Schlenger *et al.*, 2002). Among 85 individuals seeking mental health services for any reason in Oklahoma City after the bombing, numbers of hours viewing bomb-related television was not related with increased PTSD symptomatology (Tucker *et al.*, 2000).

Child survivors

More extensive research across disasters has examined the relationship between trauma-related television consumption and distress among child survivors. The results are mixed, suggesting that the relationship between viewing, distress, and psychopathology may not be linear. First, Oklahoman children related to deceased persons from the Murrah Federal Building bombing, had considerably more difficulty settling down after watching bomb-related television than those who did not experience a personal loss (Pfefferbaum *et al.*, 1999a, b; 2001). Furthermore, among Oklahoman children in grades 6–12 who lost a relative, those that watched more terrorism-related television reported more PTSD symptoms 7 weeks post-bombing than those who watched less terrorism-related television. Nevertheless, the prevalence of PTSD among these children was not related to the extent of bomb-related news consumption (Pfefferbaum *et al.*, 1999a, b). In contrast, PTSD severity was correlated with amount of television exposure to graphic images of mutilation among 51 Kuwaiti children and adolescents exposed to a military occupation (Nader *et al.*, 1993).

Child non-survivors

Research studies have found increased distress related to amount of viewing time of bomb-related news even among children who were not direct victims and did not experience a personal loss in the Oklahoma City bombing. (Pfefferbaum *et al.*, 1999a, b; 2001). Specifically, among Oklahoman children (grades 6–12), who did not lose a relative, those who watched more bomb-related television reported more PTSD symptoms 7 weeks post-bombing than those who watched less bombing-related television. Surprisingly, in a study of 2000 Oklahoman children, in grades 6–8, bomb-related television watching was associated with PTSD symptoms only among those who were not personally affected (e.g., lost a relative, witnessed it) by the Oklahoma City bombing. However, as Pfefferbaum *et al.* (2002) recently noted, terrorism-related news consumption accounted for a small part of the relationship to distress among those children not personally affected by the Oklahoma City bombing.

In a survey of adults 3–5 days after September 11th, 34% of parents had limited their children's access to viewing September 11th news coverage. It is interesting to note that children's concern about safety of self and others was not related to either parent's restriction of television viewing or number of hours that the child viewed terrorism-related television (Schuster *et al.*, 2001). In a study of children who watched the Challenger Space Shuttle explode on television, Terr *et al.* (1999) also documented traumatic symptoms 5–7 weeks later among children who had no personal connection to the event. Likewise, 45% of a sample of 137 parents living Wisconsin reported that their child was frightened by news coverage of the 1990 Desert Storm war on Iraq (Cantor *et al.*, 1993). These results suggest that shocking news of events not directly affecting children may be particularly difficult to assimilate, depending on the cognitive and emotional development of the child. For example, young children who viewed repeated images of airliners crashing into the Pentagon and the World Trade Center may not have recognized that these were repeated images of one event. Then again, perhaps children directly affected may receive explanations from family members that help them understand the tragedy, while those who are not directly affected receive no such guidance.

Critique and summary of literature

Although there are only a handful of studies that examine the relationship between news consumption and symptoms, these studies revealed different results for adults and children when comparing victims and non-victims. For adults, it appears that direct victims evidence an association between symptoms of PTSD and amount of disaster-related news coverage consumed, whereas indirect victims do not. It does appear, however, that news consumption is related to temporary increases in anxiety in the general public. Children, however, appear to be equally affected by news coverage, regardless of the extent of their involvement in the disaster. However, despite these correlations between distress and news consumption, the majority of individuals directly and indirectly affected did not report lasting symptoms (Michels, 2002).

Although a relationship between the amount of terrorism-related news consumed (especially broadcast images) and trauma-related distress clearly exists, the direction of causality is unknown. Specifically, it is unknown if watching terrorism-related television contributes to trauma-related symptoms, or if those with trauma-related symptoms choose to watch more televised depictions of terrorism. It is possible that exposure to constant terrorism coverage or unexpectedly repeated images of a loved one's demise may impede the natural recovery process, preventing adaptive dosing between approach and avoidance. Perhaps those who are in high states of arousal seek out news coverage to maintain that state of arousal. Alternatively, those affected may be searching for information to help them locate a loved one, better understand the event, pay tribute to their loved ones, or atone for guilt for surviving when others did not. Possibly another related mechanism that has not yet been identified might explain this relationship, such as personality traits, or amount of available social support. Finally, there is also a possibility of a reporting bias, memory bias, or attention bias such that those who endorse more trauma-related distress endorse more exposure to media-related images and vice versa.

Given these findings, it may be tempting, but erroneous, to pathologize individuals and blame the media for their difficulties. Learning about the death, injury, and devastation associated with terrorism is an upsetting experience. It is perfectly appropriate, and adaptive, to experience negative feelings in the face of such atrocities. Moreover, when journalists communicate such information, the news communication may not be the cause for this distress, just the messenger of this upsetting news. Since it is difficult to disentangle to what degree the news itself, rather than the communication of that news, contributes to distress, we need to be cautious not to blame the messenger. Trying to separate the content and the communication of these messages will be a challenging task for scientists to examine in future research.

Unfortunately, the empirical literature thus far has been mostly limited to visual broadcast materials; therefore the effects of newspaper, magazine, radio, and Internet news on the public is unknown. In addition, future studies need to be contextualized with respect to the timing of assessment in relation to the event to clarify if these are transient or long-lasting reactions. It would be important to evaluate if warnings about the risks of viewing such images would actually increase or decrease public anxiety to assist empirically based policy about this matter. Finally, it will be important to examine the positive effects, and not solely negative effects of terrorism-related news coverage to have a complete understanding of the public health implications. For instance, verbalizing the event for others, especially early on, may have a calming effect on the larger community. Although these research efforts may take substantial time and money, the potential gains are well worth the investment.

Journalists as witnesses

When journalists cover catastrophic events like those of 9/11, they bear witness to horrific deaths, destruction, and profound grief. No published research has examined the effects of the terrorist events of 9/11 specifically upon correspondents, although it is safe to assume that that journalists' responses would be similar to others groups (Schuster *et al.*, 2001; Schlenger *et al.*, 2002). Thus, a subgroup of those who directly witnessed or experienced loss will have long-term psychological difficulties, and a large number will have experienced temporary difficulties that abate over time or linger at levels that do not cause impairment. Thus far, journalists' testimonies suggest that these events affected individual correspondents at least temporarily (e.g., Bull & Erman, 2002; Gilbert *et al.*, 2002; Sylvester & Huffman, 2002), and that particular symptoms linger at sub-clinical levels, at least for a few journalists. For example, Jim Pensiero, Vice President, News Operations of *The Wall Street Journal*, told an American Society of Newspaper Editors panel on April 9, 2001, that after witnessing people jumping from the World Trade Center that, "you don't get rid of [those] pictures, they keep coming back."

In general, research about journalists' occupational risks is still in its infancy. Thus far, there are six published studies investigating journalists' long-lasting and deleterious responses to covering traumatic stories (Freinkel *et al.*, 1994;

Simpson & Boggs, 1999; McMahon, 2001; Feinstein, Owen & Blair, 2002; Newman *et al.*, 2003; Pyevich *et al.*, in 2002). Several studies document (Simpson & Boggs, 1999; Newman *et al.*, 2003; Pyevich *et al.*, 2003) that most journalists are exposed to events that mental health professionals would deem traumatic (e.g., involved death, destruction, and injury while evoking fear, horror and helplessness). Among reporters not covering war or conflict zones, vehicular accidents are rated as the most stressful news to cover (Simpson & Boggs, 1999; Newman *et al.*, 2003; Pyevich *et al.*, 2003). Short-term distress (Freinkel *et al.*, 1994), and long-term distress have been noted among journalists covering traumatic assignments (Simpson & Boggs, 1999; McMahon, 2001; Feinstein *et al.*, 2002; Newman *et al.*, 2003; Pyevich *et al.*, 2003). Elevated rates of trauma-related symptoms have been documented among journalists (Simpson & Boggs, 1999; Newman *et al.*, 2003; Pyevich *et al.* 2003), with war correspondents demonstrating the greatest estimated prevalence of PTSD (Feinstein *et al.*, 2002). War correspondents also reported significantly higher alcohol consumption than non-war journalists (Feinstein *et al.*, 2002). Risk factors for increased distress included higher amounts of professional and personal trauma exposure (Simpson & Boggs, 1999; Newman *et al.*, 2003; Pyevich *et al.*, in press) and decreased social support (Newman *et al.*, 2003).

A consistent strength of the studies reviewed is the use of standardized outcome measures of psychological difficulties, which is especially notable given the breadth of disciplines of the authors. Notwithstanding the groundbreaking content, these studies all suffer from the methodological shortcomings of most emerging literatures – small samples sizes, poor response rates, and potential selection biases. In addition, since all participants but a sub-sample of the war correspondents were assessed with self-report measures (Feinstein *et al.*, 2002), factors such as concentration problems, self-presentation issues, and other test-taking biases may affect the quality of data obtained. Moreover, these self-report instruments are screening devices rather than clinical diagnostic assessments, which yield less precise estimates of disorders. In addition, since all these studies are cross-sectional and retrospective, it is unknown if any of these journalists had difficulties prior to covering these difficult events. Nonetheless, these studies provide a beginning foundation of consistent information about journalists' needs in covering terrorism.

In sum, the emerging evidence indicates that most journalists are extraordinarily resilient in the face of covering trauma-related assignments. In fact, it is somewhat remarkable that in the face of high trauma exposure only a few journalists develop long-lasting disorders. However this does not negate the fact that PTSD is an important problem for some, especially those that repeatedly cover traumatic events or work in war zones. Strikingly, there is a discontinuity between the extant empirical research, which focuses upon significant clinical pathology among journalists and the testimonies of journalists who focus on long-lasting sub-clinical distress.

Understanding journalists' acute and chronic responses to covering traumatic stories is a vital area of continued study since vicarious traumatization has been demonstrated to affect the quality of care delivered (Pearlman & McCann, 1995; Stamm, 1997), but it is unknown if such responses affect journalists' work quality. It is unknown, for example, if journalists who are struggling with their own avoidance and numbing symptoms may be brusquer when interviewing survivors or fail to represent certain issues in their coverage. Further, there is currently no systematic evidence available illustrating whether or not trauma-related symptoms affect the journalists' quality of work, although this is likely since both testimony of journalists (Sylvester & Huffman, 2002) and studies of other groups (e.g., Stamm, 1997) document such difficulties.

There are many important areas for future research about risks and protective factors among journalists that are consistent with evidence about general risk factors for traumatic stress. For example, in the face of disaster, those who feel helpless and out of control typically are more vulnerable to intense distress than those who have a sense of self-efficacy (Norris *et al.*, 2001). Given journalists' testimonies about the pride and satisfaction experienced when providing excellent coverage of the September 11th attacks (Gilbert *et al.*, 2002; Sylvester & Huffman, 2002), it is likely that the journalistic role and endeavor itself may shield some journalists from harm who are exposed to horrific events. Similarly, both one study about photojournalists (Newman *et al.*, 2003) and the overall literature on disaster survivors (Norris *et al.*, 2001) suggests that good social support buffers the development of traumatic symptoms. This is an extremely important finding to pursue as it may guide inexpensive and effective prevention efforts.

Summary and future practice

Although distress is correlated with viewing media coverage of terrorism, especially among those vulnerable (e.g., children, direct victims), the causal relationship is unknown. It is unknown if those with greater distress or vulnerability seek out more news coverage or if coverage creates greater distress over and above than would be elicited by the particular tragedy itself. The key issue for future scholarship is to further examine if media coverage of catastrophes may promote or hinder long-lasting problems, and if so, what kind of problems, for whom, and under what circumstances. Moreover, caution is warranted when examining these issues, because distress, while unpleasant is not necessarily pathological – it may be a sign of health to feel appropriate negative emotions when learning about atrocities befalling others. As research examines the role of the news, it is vital to examine the role, training, and reactions of journalists and media organizations to understand how reactions of individuals and the organizational culture of newsrooms affect news production.

The next section will review implications for journalists, public health workers, and the public. As we explore evidence-based practice, gaps of knowledge, and issues, our commitment is to foster collaboration in areas of mutual concern, while respecting the different needs and goals of these three groups.

Implications for public health workers

Whether intentional or not, journalists are part of the immediate and the long-term public health response in the wake of trauma. Given this reality, public health officials need to consider the informational needs of journalists in crisis planning. Appointing a public spokesperson to coordinate regular opportunities to meet with print, radio, television, Internet, and cable media, representatives will help update the community, ultimately saving time and confusion.

In advance, it may be useful to provide opportunities to those journalists interested in learning more about health risk communication. Alternatively, it might be useful to ask journalists to participate in emergency response drills.

The issue of media policy and formal media liaisons is one that needs to be approached cautiously within each locality. Journalists are appropriately cautious that when establishing any formal media liaisons, they run the risk of becoming public relation agents, losing their important and valued autonomy and investigatory capacity. Therefore, journalists and news organizations may decline formal participation in an emergency response plan. Nonetheless, asking different media outlets to explain their needs at a planning meeting can help public health and disaster response professionals create a feasible emergency plan. Since needs vary by medium and focus, it is important to ask a wide range of journalists for input, since needs vary by medium and focus. Freelance journalists and photojournalists should be an integral part of this process as they represent two different and unique groups within the media. Although public health professionals cannot possibly meet the needs of all media organizations, much is to be gained, if major needs are anticipated and accordingly met.

Safety and security of sites, people, and evidence is essential after a crisis. Nevertheless, journalists should be allowed to access the site as soon as it is feasible. If journalists can provide information to the public about the crisis site, fewer non-essential personnel are likely to inundate the disaster scene and interfere with emergency responders. Similarly, it is important for the public to connect the event with real human victims. Journalists have the capacity to help citizens understand the full extent of the tragedy and set volunteer and civic action in motion through accurately and compassionately conveying the impact of the event upon real people. Therefore if the event involves families and survivors at the scene, it may be helpful to plan locations for journalists to converge that simultaneously promotes the privacy of survivors and access to journalists should the survivors want to talk to the media. The model of positioning families in a closed tent with a rope several yards away where journalists congregate has worked successfully at airline disaster sites (Robert Frank, personal communication October 2001).

After the acute phase of a disaster, continued fair and safe access to the site by multiple journalists is also a worthy consideration. Potential conflict can arise among journalists when only a select few are granted access to the site. Alternatives such as rotating a pool of journalists with press credentials at certain hours of the day may be a more viable solution that can meet multiple needs of journalists and the public.

As public health organizations prepare disaster response plans, the physical and psychological health of journalists may need to be considered. For example, many journalists were at the World Trade Center vicinity immediately after the attacks where they were possibly exposed to dangerous toxins, but they were not initially included in health assessments of high-risk groups.

As Putnam (2002) suggests, the scientific community must continue to examine the role of graphic disaster media coverage, with support from agencies such as the National Institute of Mental Health who should make this a funding priority.

Implications for journalists

In light of the emerging relationship between audience response and exposure to trauma-related images, journalism is faced with new professional issues to explore. Ethics codes, like those of the Society of Professional Journalists, emphasize the importance of minimizing harm by treating "sources, subjects and colleagues as human beings deserving of respect" (http://spj.org/ethics_code.asp). Interestingly, the focus of ethics codes has not been on minimizing harm to the sources and subjects, not the audience. Yet more journalists and news corporations are addressing issues related to potential harm to the audience, even though this has not formally entered the ethical code. For example, both immediately after, and in the days following 9/11, many news organizations voluntarily chose not to show images of people jumping from the World Trade Center or repeat images of the plane crash, in the service of the public's health. In the service of minimizing harm, the industry will need to assess to what degree attending to the psychological response of the audience serves the public and does not compromise their commitment to verified, accurate, and proportional information. Furthermore, if it indeed turns out that trauma survivors and their families access the news in greater numbers than non-trauma survivors, the industry needs to consider if they want to present the news with an awareness of the particular needs of this viewing audience.

Despite the key role that journalists play in times of uncertainty and chaos like the events of 9/11 journalists actually receive little preparatory training about covering violence, interviewing victims, and the field of traumatic stress studies. This is a critical omission because the taught skills needed to cover those in public office differ radically from untaught skills needed to cover disempowered individuals caught up in emotionally wrenching tragedies (Cote & Simpson, 2000). Similarly, without appropriate training, reporters may make well-intentioned mistakes regarding crisis needs that hinder rescue and relief efforts. For example, journalists should not convey needs mentioned casually by sources, but wait until public officials detail precise community needs and ways of providing for those needs. Cote & Simpson (2000) provide numerous examples regarding how well-intentioned journalists amplified, rather than reduced, public health problems in the wake of disaster by offering a call for unneeded assistance. Given the necessity for such trauma-related journalism education, several leading journalism schools have added trauma training into to the curriculum (Cote & Simpson, 2000) and a pilot study suggests that the doing so increased short-term knowledge about traumatic stress and trauma-related reporting (Mills *et al.*, 1999). Longitudinal examination of changes in behavior to determine whether such programs actually change conduct in the field is needed.

Although continuing education for professionals has lagged behind that of students, the events of 9/11 have created new opportunities for professional training, and increased interest in trainings that are regularly offered. For example, in the wake of 9/11, the Dart Center for Journalism opened a satellite office in New York City dedicated to supporting the trauma-related professional needs of journalists (Monseu & Newman, 2002; Newman, 2002a). In addition several news companies and professional associations are conducting trainings about reporting on violence. For the past 4 years, mid-career and senior journalists could earn a special fellowship to engage in intensive education about the science of traumatic stress and its implications for newsgathering (http://www.Dartcenter.org). Although changes are slow, more opportunities are evolving for journalists to consider trauma-related reporting.

Clearly to advance reporting of terrorism, the culture of the newsroom may need to be altered. The traditional newsroom culture is one where the stoic, objective, and a "need to get the job done" zeitgeist prevails. In this cultural mythology, expression of emotion is seen as an impediment to truth, so personal responses to work, subjects, and sources are ignored. This cultural norm may prevent journalists from acknowledging distress caused by job-related exposure to horrible events and fostering social support in response to job-related trauma exposure. Journalists, unlike fire, police, and emergency safety have no culture of receiving interventions after covering harrowing events. Increasingly, newsrooms and professional organizations are offering peer counseling, ombudspersons, and counselors for staff when covering major tragedies, although this is far from universal (Smyth & Hight, 2002), and there are invisible and visible barriers to accessing these services. For example, in the work conducted at the New York office of the Dart Center for Journalism and Trauma, several journalists reported that although debriefing was available in the days after September 11, 2001, they were not able to use it, since they were so busy working on the story (Monseu & Newman, 2002). Furthermore, some journalists perceive that their editor's actively discouraged staff from using offered crisis related services (Barbara Monseu, personal communication, November 10, 2002). As Chris Cramer has emphasized, it is important for management to help change the culture so that good journalists can seek emotional support as needed so they can continue to contribute to the profession (Cramer, 2002).

Similarly, the culture of objectivity may obstruct journalists' ability to tell the story of victims in ways that are simultaneously truthful, sensitive to victims, and capable of mobilizing efforts to help (Ochberg, 1996). While emotional restraint is indeed needed in journalism, emotions can offer vital information about how to interview sources, understand survivors' experiences, and avoid clichés about trauma. The struggle to balance humanity and professionalism in the service of objectivity is not unique to journalism. Training in research-based service professions, such as psychology, use models in which explicit training about handling one's feelings and how those emotions can be useful and harmful in clinical decision-making are addressed. It may be useful to examine the degree to which other professional models can be successfully integrated into the service of good journalism.

Implications for public

Although not definitive, the results of extant studies do suggest that it may be prudent for adults and children to limit exposure to trauma related images as much as possible. In particular those with a direct connection to the event may want to limit their exposure. Children, regardless of relationship to the event, should be encouraged to watch less terrorism-related news coverage. In addition, it makes sense to discuss with children their understanding of trauma-related events and try to make them feel as safe as possible.

The public, as consumers of journalism, also bear some responsibility for providing the news industry with feedback. Reader opinion and response can shape coverage as journalists become more aware of community and readership standards. Therefore registering both complaints and compliments of good coverage with news organizations can be an effective strategy. The public can also provide feedback by choosing which media outlets to financially support through subscriptions.

Final Remarks

It is clear that journalists fulfill an important role in the wake of disasters mediating public awareness and response to catastrophes. Accurate communication about the immediate and long-term catastrophe is a fundamental component of the public health response plan that should be respected and supported. Clearly, collaboration across professionals and non-professionals is needed to promote public health. As such, journalists have an ethical duty to examine their responsibilities to the public, their profession, and to see the ways in which they can become more effective in this role. Similarly, public health officials need to plan and support the role of journalists, both in practice and research. Finally, the public also needs to be informed consumers, who choose what news to watch under what context.

REFERENCES

Ahern, J., Galea, S., Resnick, H.S., Kilpatrick, D.G., Bucuvalas, M., Gold, J. & Vlahov, D. (2002). Television images and psychological symptoms after the September 11 terrorist attacks. *Psychiatry*, **65**, 289–300.

Breslau, N., Davis, G.C. & Andreski, P. (1991). Traumatic events and post-traumatic stress disorder in an urban population of young adults. *Archives of General Psychiatry*, **48**, 216–222.

Bull, C. & Newman, E. (2002). Covering Terrorism. http://www.dartcenter.org/special_features/terrorism.html

Bull, C. & Erman, S. (2002). *At Ground Zero: 25 Stories From Young Reporters Who Were There.* Emeryville, CA: Avalon Publishing Group, Inc.

Cantor, J., Mares, M.L. & Oliver, M.B. (1993). Parents' and children's emotional reactions to TV coverage of the gulf war. In *Desert Storm and the Mass Media*, ed. B.S. Greenberg & W. Gantz. Cresskill, NJ: Hampton Press, Inc, pp.325–340.

Cote, B. & Simpson, R. (2000). *Covering Violence: A Guide to Ethical Reporting About Victims and Trauma.* NY: Columbia University Press.

Cramer, C. (2002). We have a long way to go. In *Sharing the Front Lines and the Back Hills: International Protectors and Providers: Peacekeepers, Humanitarian Aid Workers and the Media in the Midst of Crisis*, ed. Y. Danieli. Amityville, NY: Baywood Publishing Company, Inc, pp. 275–280.

Dixon, P., Rehling, G. & Shiwach, R. (1993). Peripheral victims of the herald of free enterprise disaster. *British Journal of Medical Psychology*, **66**, 193–202.

Feinstein, A., Owen, J. & Blair, N. (2002). A hazardous profession: war, journalists, and psychopathology. *American Journal of Psychiatry*, **159**, 1570–1575.

Freinkel, A., Koopman, C. & Speigel, D. (1994). Dissociative symptoms in media eyewitnesses of an execution. *American Journal of Psychiatry*, **151**, 1335–1339.

Gilbert, A., Hirschkorn, P., Murphy, M., Walensky, R. & Stephens, M. (2002). *Covering catastrophe: broadcast journalists report September 11th.* Chicago: Bonus Books.

Hamblen, J. (2001). How the community may be affected by media coverage of the terrorist attack: a national center for PTSD fact sheet. http://www.ncptsd.org/facts/disasters/fs_media_disaster.html

International Society of Traumatic Stress Studies Fact Sheet. (2002). What does the news industry need to know about the science related to survivors, the public and news consumption? http://www.istss.org/terrorism/news_consumption.htm

Kessler, R.C., Sonnega, A., Bromet, E., Hughes, M. & Nelson, C.B. (1995). Posttraumatic stress disorder in the national comorbidity survey. *Archives of General Psychiatry*, **52**, 1048–1060.

Kovach, B. & Rosensteil, T. (2001). *The Elements of Journalism*. NY: Three Rivers Press.

Long, N., Chamberlain, K. & Vincent, C. (1994). Effects of the Gulf war on reactivation of adverse combat-related memories in Vietnam veterans. *Journal of Clinical Psychology*, **50**, 138–144.

McFarlane, A.C. (1986). Victims of trauma and the news media. *Medical Journal of Australia*, **145**, 664.

McMahon, C. (2001). Covering disaster: a pilot study into secondary trauma for print media journalists reporting on disaster. *Australian Journal of Emergency Management*, **16**, 52–55.

Michels, R. (2002). Commentary: exposure to traumatic images: symptoms or cause? *Psychiatry*, **64**, 304–305.

Mills, L.J., Simpson, R., Newman, E., Reynolds-Ablacas, P., Scherer, M., Maxson, J. & Boggs, J. (1999). Examining the effectiveness of a trauma training program for journalists, presentation in *F. Ochberg's Journalism and Trauma Symposium on 15th Annual Convention of the International Society for Traumatic Stress Studies*, Miami.

Monseu, B. & Newman, E. (2002). Understanding journalists' experience of September 11, 2001: the need for a research agenda. Dart Center for Journalism and Trauma (unpublished report).

Nader, K., Pynoos, R., Fairbanks, L., Al-Ajeel, M. & Al-Asfour, A. (1993). A preliminary study of PTSD and grief among the children of Kuwait following the Gulf crisis. *British Journal of Clinical Psychology*, **32**, 407–416.

Newman, E. (2002a). Psychologists at Ground Zero assess effects on journalists covering 9/11 attacks. *International Psychologist*, **13**, 4–5.

Newman, E. (2002b). The bridge between sorrow and knowledge. In *Sharing the Front Lines and the Back Hills: International Protectors and Providers: Peacekeepers, Humanitarian Aid Workers and the Media in the Midst of Crisis*, ed. Y. Danieli. Amityville, NY: Baywood Publishing Company, Inc, pp. 305–322.

Newman, E., Simpson, R. & Handschuh, D. (2003). Trauma exposure and post-traumatic stress disorder among photojournalists. *Visual Communication Quarterly*, **10** (1), 4–13.

Norris, F.H., Byrne, C.M., Diaz, E. & Kaniasty, K. (2001). Risk factors for adverse outcomes in natural and human-caused disasters: a review of the empirical literature. National Center for Posttraumatic Stress Disorder. http://www.ncptsd.org/facts/disasters/fs_riskfactors.html

Ochberg, F. (1996). A primer on covering victims. *Nieman Reports*, **50**, 21–26.

Pearlman, L.A. & McCann, L. (1995). Vicarious traumatization: an empirical study of the effects of trauma work on trauma therapists. *Professional Psychology: Research and Practice*, **26**, 558–565.

Pew (2001). American psyche reeling from terror attacks. Pew Research Center for the People & the Press. http://people-press.org/reports/print.php3?ReportID=3, September 19.

Pfefferbaum, B., Moore, V., McDonald, N., Maynard, B., Gurwitch, R. & Nixon, S. (1999a). The role of exposure in posttraumatic stress in youths following the 1995 bombing. *Journal of the State Medical Association*, **92**, 164–167.

Pfefferbaum, B., Nixon, S., Tucker, P., Tivis, R., Moore, V., Gurwitch, R., Pynoos, R. & Geis, H. (1999b). Posttraumatic stress response in bereaved children after the Oklahoma City bombing. *Journal of the American Academy of Child and Adolescent Psychiatry*, **38**, 1372–1379.

Pfefferbaum, B., Nixon, S., Tivis, R., Doughty, D., Pynoos, R., Gurwitch, R. & Foy, D. (2001). Television exposure in children after a terrorist incident. *Psychiatry*, **64**, 202–211.

Pfefferbaum, B., Pfefferbaum, R.L., North, C.S. & Neas, B.R. (2002). Commentary: Does television viewing satisfy criteria for exposure in posttraumatic stress disorder. *Psychiatry*, **64**, 306–309.

Putman, F.W. (2002). Commentary on "Television images and psychological symptoms after the september 11 terrorist attacks." Televised trauma and viewer PTSD: implications for prevention. *Psychiatry: Interpersonal and Biological Processes*, **65**, 310–312.

Pyevich, C., Newman, E. & Daleidan, R. (2003). The relationship among cognitive schemas, job-related traumatic exposure, and PTSD symptoms in journalists. *Journal of Traumatic Stress*, **16**, 325–328.

Roth, S. & Cohen, L.J. (1986). Approach, avoidance, and coping with stress. *American Psychologist*, **41**, 813–819.

Schlenger, W.E., Caddell, J.M., Ebert, L., Jordan, B.K., Rourke, K.M., Wilson, D., Thalji, L., Dennis, J.M., Fairbank, J.A. & Kulka, R.A. (2002). Psychological reactions to terrorist attacks: findings from the national study of Americans' reactions to September 11. *Journal of The American Medical Association*, **288**, 581–588.

Schuster, M., Bradley, D., Stein, M., Jaycox, L.H., Collins, R.L., Marshall, G.N., Elliott, M.N., Zhou, A.J., Kanouse, D.E., Morrison, J.L. & Berry, S.H. (2001) A national survey of stress reactions after the September 11, 2001, terrorist attacks. *New England Journal of Medicine*, **345**, 1507–1512.

Simpson, R. & Boggs, J. (1999). An exploratory study of traumatic stress among newspaper journalists. *Journalism and Communication Monographs*, **1**, 1–24.

Sloan, M. (2000). Response to media coverage of terrorism. *Journal of Conflict Resolution*, **44**, 508–522.

Smyth, F. & Hight, J. (2002). Tragedies & journalists: a guide for more effective coverage. Dart Center for Journalism and Trauma.

Stamm, B.H. (1997). Work-related secondary traumatic stress. *PTSD Research Quarterly*, **8**, 1–6.

Sylvester, J. & Huffman, S. (2002). *Women Journalists at Ground Zero: Covering Crisis*. NY: Rowman & Littlefield Publishers, Inc.

Terr, L.C., Bloch, D.A., Michel, B.A., Shi, H., Reinhardt, J.A., Metayer, S.A. (1999). Children's symptoms in the wake of challenger: a field study of distant-traumatic effects and an outline of related conditions. *American Journal of Psychiatry*, **156**, 1536–1544.

Tucker, P., Pfefferbaum, B., Nixon, S. & Dickson, W. (2000). Predictors of post-traumatic stress symptoms in Oklahoma City: exposure, social support, peri-traumatic response. *Journal of Behavioral Health Services and Research*, **27**, 406–416.

Turnley, P. (2001). September 11th, 2001: telling stories visually. *Nieman Reports*, **55**, 6–9.

13

Effective leadership in extreme crisis

Richard E. Boyatzis, Diana Bilimoria, Lindsey Godwin,
Margaret M. Hopkins and Tony Lingham

As he ran, the tears on his cheeks were not from crying. He was too scared to cry. They were from the acrid smoke and ash. There were bodies lying on the street – some were getting help, some were beyond help. People were yelling, "Run, run." He thought this is what it must have been like in London during the blitz. But he kept running toward the center of trouble. It was his job.

Having traded days off with a friend, David Simms decided to start sunny September 11, 2001, jogging in a park near his home on Long Island. A neighbor stopped him and said, "Aren't you with the New York Fire Department?" to which David nodded. "A plane just hit one of the World Trade Center buildings." David is a Lieutenant in New York City's Fire Department, Ladder Company 20. So he did what he thought was needed. He drove downtown to his station and found firemen standing around confused. He told them to get their equipment and move out. All of their vehicles were gone so he commandeered a truck to get them as close to Ground Zero as possible. When the truck could no longer get through, they ran.

What he didn't know at the time he was running down the street toward the World Trade Center with his men was that 14 of his comrades were already dead, including the man who had taken his place that day. The next 30 hours were as horrible as can be imagined, but the most challenging aspects of the event were yet to hit David. The nightmares, ever present guilt, flashbacks of shock and deep sorrow plagued him for weeks.

Talking to others helped. Focusing on his wife and daughter helped. After all, his brother and father, also New York firefighters were safe, but so many were not. He found himself confronting life's larger questions: What did this mean? How can anyone make sense of such bizarre events? Reflection on these questions and talking with others helped. He spent a lot of time talking with his men and the media. He estimated that he had conducted over 140 media interviews during the 5 weeks following 9/11.

David Simms was a leader on 9/11 and in the months immediately following. He mobilized the remaining firefighters of Ladder Company 20 into action so that they could do their job and help others. He helped them also deal with the grief, anguish, and confusion resulting from the horrible events of that day and the haunting replays that kept reoccurring day after day.

Effective leadership is a relationship. It is a resonant relationship (Goleman *et al.*, 2002). A resonant relationship is one in which the leader is in tune with the people around him or her. David Simms did not have to consciously consider what needed to be done as he entered the Fire House on 9/11. Similarly, he did not have to consult psychological texts to know that talking about the events was a healing process for his men, as well as for himself. He was in tune with the firefighters of Ladder Company 20. His actions and comportment both reflected and addressed the feelings of others around him.

Research on leadership shows that effective leaders create an overall positive emotional tone with those around them and are in touch with these others (Goleman *et al.*, 2002). A person's emotional intelligence enables them to be in such relationships and, as a leader, to initiate them.

Since human cognition is most often associated with emotions, emotional intelligence can be defined as "the intelligent use of one's emotions" (Le Doux, 1996; Damasio, 1999; Goleman *et al.*, 2002). Specifically, emotional intelligence is a cluster of abilities, or competencies. Two clusters of the competencies describe a person's Self-Awareness (e.g., emotional self-awareness, self-confidence) and Self-Management (e.g., emotional self-control, transparency, optimism, adaptability). They determine the degree to which he or she can engender a positive emotional state within him- or herself, and then using the contagion of emotions to spread it to others. The other two clusters of competencies describe a person's Social Awareness (e.g., empathy, system awareness) and Relationship Management (e.g., inspirational leadership, conflict management, building bonds, teamwork and collaboration). Clusters of competencies allow individuals to get and stay in touch with others around them and to be sensitive to the thoughts and feelings of others (Goleman *et al.*, 2002). These competencies have been shown to predict outstanding performance of leaders, managers, and executives (Boyatzis, 1982; Kotter, 1982, 1988; Spencer & Spencer, 1993; Goleman, 1998).

Describing reality and giving hope: Ken Chenault[1]

Visiting the Salt Lake City office, Ken Chenault, Chairman and CEO of American Express was on the phone with a colleague in the New York headquarters on the morning of September 11, 2001. Suddenly, the phone call is interrupted. A plane

---

[1] The descriptions of the behavior, statements, and leadership effectiveness of the people described in this chapter are primarily derived from press and media accounts at the time, with the exception of Ken Chenault for whom additional personal interviews were conducted. The following analysis should not be construed to be an assessment of each person's leadership in general, but rather how they acted and the consequences at this highly unusual, but critical moment in time surrounding the events of September 11, 2001.

just crashed into one of the Twin Towers, which is across the street from their head-quarters. Chenault asked to be transferred to security. He told them to evacuate the more than 4000 employees immediately. Unable to get back to headquarters for 2 days, he managed the company via hourly conference calls (Byrne & Timmons, 2001; McGeehan, 2001).

While assuming leadership of the company only months before September 11, 2001, Chenault had already begun to receive accolades from critics about his attrib-utes as a good leader (Byrne & Timmons, 2001; Future Banker, 2001; McGeehan, 2001). "In a time of crisis you can't manage by manual; you have to manage by values and beliefs," contended Chenault (Chaffin & Larsen, 2001).

In the chaotic days that followed the collapse of the Twin Towers, American Express acted quickly. They waived millions of dollars in delinquent fees, increased credit limits to people in need, and helped over half a million cardholders get home. American Express often went above and beyond what would typically be expected from corporate America, they chartered airplanes and buses to get people home across the country (Bloom, 2001).

Just days after his company had been evacuated from their headquarters and forced into cramped, temporary spaces in New Jersey, he stated in an interview on September 14, 2001, "We've been around for 150 years. This is clearly an incredible tragedy, but I said to the organization, we will survive and we will prosper, because of the character and strength and courage of our people" (Francis & Viles, 2001). Chenault was able to acknowledge the tragedy, while still instilling a positive vision of the future.

Despite his inability to be in New York on 9/11, his employees recalled that "he was there, and he was in the middle of it" (Byrne & Timmons, 2001). Once back home, Chenault wasted no time, rolling-up his sleeves and getting involved with his company and his city. Maintaining a presence with his people, Chenault set up an office for himself in each of the six locations the company was dispersed to, spending a couple of days in each one, getting to know his employees personally by making "the rounds" (Ingram, 2002).

On September 20, 2001, Chenault organized a "town hall" meeting of 5000 American Express employees at New York's Paramount Theater. While others had doubts about the timing and location of this meeting, fearing that people were not ready to reassemble in Manhattan, Chenault simply stated, "The employees needed to hear from me about how I felt about them and the state of the company. It was a way to begin the healing process" (McGeehan, 2001).

During this meeting, Chenault expressed his own emotions, as well as those of his grief-stricken employees. He admitted his feelings of despair, sadness, and anger; embracing upset employees, saying, "I represent the best company and best people in the world. You are my strength and I love you" (Byrne & Timmons, 2001). At this meeting, Chenault also promised to donate $1 million of the company's profits (despite the fact that profits would decrease after the crisis) to the families of American Express victims, showing his faith in the company financially, as well as his desire to support the company emotionally.

Both his actions in convening a meeting in downtown New York when others would not and his honest and heartfelt words evoked a sense of hope in a time of uncertainty. In addition to being in touch with the emotions of his employees, he also recognized that they would have needs above and beyond his ability to help. Therefore, he had the company providing a series of counseling services to the employees to make sure that their emotional and psychological needs were met (MacCallum, 2002).

Chenault's resonant leadership did not cease once the ashes and dust had settled. He continued to inspire and promote a sense of hope not only within American Express, but within New York and the nation as well. On October 3, 2001, Chenault was at President Bush's side as millions of TV viewers watched. Chenault again declared that, "We will not succumb to this evil … We believe in the American promise, and we will do everything to build on that promise" (Federal News Service, 2001).

In May 2002, he announced that American Express would move back into its headquarters across the street from Ground Zero. His company led businesses moving back. "If we can get people down here, I think the confidence increases about the rebuilding of downtown New York … that's why we are sponsoring events like the Tribecca Film Festival and River to River" (MacCallum, 2002).

Creating and managing an overall positive emotional tone in the environment require being in an authentically positive state oneself. To inspire others, the leader must be in this hopeful state to communicate it and spread it, consciously and unconsciously, and verbally and non-verbally (Goleman *et al.*, 2002). In times of crisis, the leader has to convey enormously difficult information acknowledging the traumatic emotional realities of the day, while simultaneously reassuring others that things are moving in a positive direction – engendering hope, not fear; control, not chaos; resilience and the sense of overcoming great odds, not confusion, anxiety or paralysis; unity, not fragmentation; and compassion, not hatred.

A crisis precipitates a condition of threat, fear, and stress. An extreme crisis provokes extreme stress. This often results in many of the same psychological and physiological symptoms of chronic stress. People often turn to others for assurance or interpretation of their feelings (Schachter, 1959; Taylor *et al.*, 2002). Without others to ameliorate or interpret this condition, continued stress would lead to various forms of clinical anxiety and inhibition of action.

The physical presence of a positive and calm leader during a crisis is particularly reassuring; by emotional contagion it creates an immediate positive and calming effect on others. Similarly, demonstrating courage in the face of imminent danger, threat, or stress sets a high example and inspires others to also serve with courage.

Effective leaders thus shift the mood and overall emotional tone in stressful events. They do it by shifting their own reaction and then it spreads to others, both intentionally and unintentionally. An effective leader is inspirational in this regard. He or she is on the same wavelength with others around them. Their emotions are the medium for their message. Since emotions are contagious, their emotional tone spreads to others (Hatfield *et al.*, 1994). They do not have to "align" people to their vision or strategy. They are in tune with the people around them.

Stories of great leadership emerge when people face extreme crises. It can be as clear as Winston Churchill reassuring a frightened nation and their allies while bombs were falling in England during the early years of World War II. When people did not know that there was to be an end of the bombing or worse that it might end with an invasion, they listened to their radios and passed along any information they could collect. Times of crisis raise the level of uncertainty to uncomfortable or intolerable degrees. Certain leaders can respond to the feelings of others with the intensity needed. Charismatic leaders often emerge in such times to help create meaning (Bass & Stogdill, 1990).

Dissing your colleagues: Dr. Bernandine Healy

Dr. Bernadine Healy, President and CEO of the American Red Cross, tried to help the nation deal with the terrible tragedy. Soon after 9/11, criticism began about Dr. Healy's actions. "The same steely qualities that Healy displayed during the September 11th attacks have left ruffled feelings in the aftermath" (Farhi, 2001). It was claimed that Dr. Healy had a "go it alone" style that led her to be overly aggressive, redundant and premature in her gung-ho fundraising efforts (Farhi, 2001).

Dr. Healy's response to these criticisms did not help to ease anxiety both within the Red Cross and in public. She did not show as much empathy for co-workers or fellow blood bank colleagues as they wished for or needed, but rather saw the "public spiritedness" of the crisis aftermath as an opportunity on which to capitalize, stating, "In the best of times, we have a 3-day supply of blood in this country. I kept thinking, 'You ding-dongs. You had an opportunity to drive the inventory to 10 or 14 days.' What really gets my Irish up is that everyone in America was saying, 'What can I do to help?' And the response they were getting was, 'Come back later'" (Farhi, 2001). Such words were not inspirational to employees or colleagues, who themselves were experiencing the after-effects of the national trauma.

Dr. Healy's critics claimed that she has been so aggressive in appealing for blood that was not needed that some blood had actually expired (Seelye & Henriques, 2001). Others criticized her flip-flopping on whether the Red Cross should join a non-profit, central database keeping track of how much victims' families would be receiving from donations raised after the attacks (Seelye & Henriques, 2001).

Those around her were seeking to calm these criticisms. However, her comments were often not calming, but rather focused on the pressures she personally faced in her job: "It is not exciting to be in this job. It's intense. In a quiet moment, you get a deep fulfillment, but it's linked with just a sense of heavy responsibility. It's that obligation that keeps you from ever being too pleased or satisfied ..." (Farhi, 2001).

This was a trying time for everyone, including Dr. Healy. A leader's personal reactions often may cloud their perception or sensitivity to others' needs. Coupled with her task-focused management style, sentiments about her were injured beyond repair when she ordered a separate special fund to be set up for terrorism-related relief efforts. This led to confusion and bad will toward the Red Cross (and philanthropy associated with other 9/11 relief efforts) from donors who did not agree with how Dr. Healy earmarked their money. Where donors believed they were giving money directly to victims, she designated funds to be used for projects like terrorist prevention, increasing the Red Cross's telecommunications, and a variety of other services (Koppel, 2001; Seelye & Henriques, 2001). Ultimately, Dr. Healy was asked to resign in October, 2001 (Koppel, 2001; Zahn, 2001).

Leadership is a power-oriented role (McClelland & Boyatzis, 1982). The leader is called upon to inspire and "influence" others. This can be stressful even on a calm day. But during a crisis, the power-stress of the role is added to the compounding stress of the events. In a major tragedy, the stress increases geometrically.

There are few antidotes to stress syndrome. One is the experience of compassion. When a person empathizes and cares for another person, it ameliorates the arousal effects of the stress syndrome (Goleman, 2003). Normally, this would help a leader rebalance their internal sensations and feelings. But in time of a major tragedy, a leader is faced with hundreds, or in the case of 9/11, thousands of grieving people needing compassion. This can be overwhelming to the leader and push him or her back into a stress syndrome.

In addition to alleviating stress, compassion and empathy is a second aspect of resonance. In a crisis, a resonant leader is attuned to the emotional needs of others. Crises are characterized by heightened limbic and emotional arousal, and the feelings are typically negative – horror, shock, terror, fear, disbelief, sadness, withdrawal, anger, hatred, powerlessness, and vulnerability. Reaction times are truncated. The contagion and reaction to the leader's expressed emotions are heightened because people are emotionally fragile: "responses to such events and preparations for future ones have critical consequences for the health and well-being for both their employees and their organizations" (American Psychological Association, 2003). Even when a leader thinks he or she is "putting up a good face," they are usually telegraphing their negative effect through facial micro-muscles (Ekman, 2003).

Effective leadership in a time of crisis thus requires being in touch with the thoughts, feelings, and reactions of others affected by the crisis. Beyond this sensitivity, a leader should communicate understanding of and empathy with the feelings of the victims and their families, as well as the feelings of crisis survivors. In large-scale disasters, leaders have to immediately address the feelings of emergency and rescue workers, as well as the overall mood of the general public. Drawing on Social Awareness and Relationship Management competencies, effective leaders in a crisis build a large trust radius, conveying a compelling dual message of concern and taking action that comes across as both authentic and reliable to others.

It is through such leadership that the people in the organization or community can begin to deal with the crisis and heal. Resiliency of the human spirit and people's ability to return to typical life functioning appears to be related to their ability to recover from the trauma. Initial research suggests that the speed with which a person can move thoughts from neural circuits emanating through the right prefrontal cortex to the left may be a signal of their progress in healing the wounds of a stress (Davidson *et al.*, 2000; Goleman, 2003). The resonant leader, by inspiring hope, helps people to refocus their thoughts and feelings in this way.

Primal leadership

In the wake of the 9/11 crisis, organizational leaders themselves began to view their positions and responsibility differently. For example, in 2000, a survey of 194 CEOs revealed that 42% said it was "very important" for them to be a spokesperson in a crisis, with 10% indicating that it was "not necessarily important". However, in a 2001 post-9/11 world, 50% of the CEOs surveyed stated that it was "absolutely vital" for them to be the spokesperson in a crisis, with 46% saying it was "very important" and none replied that it was "not necessarily important" (Bloom, 2001).

An entire consulting industry seems to be arising to help leaders deal with crisis management. Web sites, company promotions, and books are offering "how to" advice. Some of these books are scholarly reviews of how people have handled other crises, such as the nuclear accident at Three Mile Island (Fink, 2000), the chemical disaster in Bhopal, India, the arsenic-laced Tylenol, NASA's Challenger and Columbia disasters, and the oil spill from the Exxon Valdez (Mitroff & Anagros, 2000). But amazingly, no empirical studies seem to have been completed to test ideas and help us understand which advice seems most critical. On some topics, all of these case studies agree. Leaders must be visible, authentic, speak to the feelings as well as thoughts of those around them, speak to as many of their organization's stake-holders as possible, focus on shared values, and emphasize the mission or purpose of the organization.

But the complexity of major or extreme crises, in which thousands are involved directly and millions indirectly, is still a puzzle. Hindsight makes it easier to see what worked and what did not, but when the event is unfolding, a leader is still a person. He or she must deal with their own fear and frustration while trying to convey a spirit of hope and help others cope or deal with events.

Given the critical role of awareness and management of emotions in leadership, Goleman, Boyatzis & McKee (2002) propose a framework of *primal* leadership that encompasses the resonant (i.e., effective) leadership profile. These authors draw attention to the primordial nature of effective leadership: leadership that is emotionally compelling. The leader serves as the group's emotional guide by positively engaging self and others, and by being attuned to the emotional needs of others.

However, not all leadership is resonant. Dr. Bernadine Healy's actions created distance and discord among her staff at the Red Cross, their donors, and the public. Others took dissonance to greater extremes, even if they did not intend it.

Blamestorming: Rev. Jerry Falwell

Rev. Jerry Falwell, a Baptist minister appearing on the religious program "700 Club" 2 days following the 9/11 terror attacks, pointed the finger at "those who have tried to secularize America" (Niebuhr, 2001, p. A18). He said, "The abortionists have got to bear some burden for this because God will not be mocked. And when we destroy 40 million little innocent babies, we make God mad. I really believe that the pagans, and the abortionists, and the feminists, and the gays and the lesbians who are actively trying to make that an alternative lifestyle, the A. C. L. U., People for the American Way, all of them who have tried to secularize America, I point the finger in their face and say 'You helped this happen'" (Goodstein, 2001, p. A15).

Rev. Falwell expressed his own anger and beliefs in an emotionally charged way that likely matched the needs of some enraged followers seeking to explain the horror they felt. However, by channeling his message in a harsh and negative criticism of people and groups that had nothing to do with the events of 9/11, Rev. Falwell created an overall negative emotional tone, arousing hatred among his followers and ridicule among those he attacked. Instead of helping to move beyond hatred to healing, Rev. Falwell's comments tapped into the undercurrents of fear and powerlessness experienced in the wake of 9/11, and further stoked the fires of fear and escalated the stress that was already at an unbearably high level.

In a subsequent interview following the televised program, Rev. Falwell stated that he was simply making a theological statement. Later, he issued an apology over the controversy.

From resonant to dissonant leadership and maybe back again: Howard Lutnick

On September 11, 2001, Howard Lutnick, CEO of Cantor Fitzgerald was late to work after dropping off his 5-year-old son for his first day of kindergarten. As he was leaving the school, he got a call informing him that a plane had crashed into the World Trade Center. He got there as fast as he could. Seeing that the damage was worse than he had imagined, he walked around Ground Zero like a zombie after the second tower collapsed – lost and caked with dust – only to find out later that all his employees who were working that day had perished in the flames (including his brother Gary). Two days later, in an interview with ABC-TV's Connie Chung, Lutnick mentioned that his life had changed and that he needed to direct his energies to the families who have suffered such loss. He said, "there's 700 families. 700 of my families. I can't say it … 700 of my families, 700 … what do I do? This is too many. It's too many, too many" (Howard Lutnick, 2001a). Although deeply affected by the overall attack, Lutnick still managed to focus on the need to help the 700 families.

Lutnick did not sink into depression. He truncated his personal emotional distress and managed to act swiftly by reopening Cantor Fitzgerald for business, even among such anguish and loss ("Tough bond trader," 2001). To provide emotional support, Lutnick immediately made available his home telephone number to the affected families and employees, encouraging people to call. Lutnick opened a family services center at the Pierre Hotel in New York City, where on the first day he made an emotional appearance in a black suit, sharing hugs and weeping openly. He also told his employees the reality that all rumors of rescued Cantor employees were untrue. He went further to create the Cantor Fitzgerald Foundation to aid the families of anybody who had died in the disaster, no matter where they worked. Lutnick himself donated 1 million dollars to this foundation.

Paul Ofman, the Red Cross chairman of emergency services for Greater New York mentioned that in such a situation "a firm's leadership has to be very visible and communicate a great deal. Management has to be a palpable presence throughout the organization; they have to be empathic, thoughtful, and sincere. Howard Lutnick was an example of such leadership" (Colaruuso, 2001). Yet, such exemplary leadership took a turn only a few days later.

On September 15, 2001, Lutnick mentioned that he was not going to pay the salaries of the missing employees. When asked why he cut the salaries after vowing to look after the employee's families, he said that it was the most difficult decision he had to make. "It was not," he said, "a business or personal decision – it was an everything decision" (Raphael, 2001).

Lutnick's decision to cut the pay of the missing employees caused strong reactions. In a news broadcast, NBC News asked several of the employees and families of the deceased employees if they still felt that Lutnick was going to take care of them. An employee answered that he has not seen it in the deeds; he has heard the words but not seen the deeds. Another woman said that she hopes and prays that Mr. Lutnick is a man of his word, because if he is not, they're left with nothing. Another woman mentioned that she did not need another false hope (Howard

Lutnick, 2001b). Some family members who lost their loved ones in the tragedy mentioned that they were disgusted as they were not given the time to grieve; and that Lutnick never treated anyone kindly in the firm and was not liked by the company. Others mentioned that he was trying to gain sympathy by sobbing on national TV (Raphael, 2001). In response to the reactions people had, Lutnick said, "Anyone who has anything to say, I hope they never have to walk in my shoes … but they shouldn't say anything until they close their eyes and try" (Knox, 2001).

It seemed strange that a caring man is remembered mainly for stopping the pay-checks of his dead employees (Johnston, 2002). Lutnick had shifted to become a dissonant leader. To his credit, Lutnick tried to turn this around. Beginning in October 2001, he began paying for the first 10 years of promised health insurance (Bay, 2001). Six months later, Lutnick made his first distribution of a percentage of profits to the affected families (about $6000 each) (Schoolman, 2002). A year later, Cantor's profit contributions to its families totaled just under $25 million; still providing a decade of health insurance coverage to the affected families; and also providing a relief fund to hand out cash grants to cover many other financial needs (Henriques, 2002). His efforts since that week have appeared extraordinary and compassionate. But whether out of his own confusion or an impulse to preserve what financial security he could for the company, damage had been done and lingering doubts or shadows about his leadership during that time remain in some people's minds.

From dissonant to resonant leadership: Rudy Giuliani

These days it seems hard to believe that the former Mayor of New York, Rudolph W. Giuliani, was the subject of countless negative headlines during his years in office prior to 9/11. He was accused of fueling racial tensions in the city for his reactions to allegations of police brutality. His private life became daily tabloid fodder in the latter years of his mayoralty (CNN.com, 2001). Reflecting upon his early years in office, he said "People didn't elect me to be a conciliator … They wanted someone who was going to change this place. How do you expect me to change it if I don't fight with somebody? You don't change ingrained human behavior without confrontation, turmoil, anger" (Pooley, 2001, p. 4). In New York's darkest days, Giuliani became a resonant leader.

Mayor Giuliani rushed to the scene of the World Trade Center disaster and arrived just after the second plane struck. He immediately set up a command center with his top safety officials and nearly got trapped in that building from the destruction and debris. Covered with smoke and ash from the South Tower's collapse, he kept his composure. He led officials north in a blizzard of debris to set up another operation center in a nearby firehouse (Perez-Pena, 2001).

Mayor Giuliani reflected later that "I was so proud of the people I saw on the street. No chaos, but they were frightened and confused, and it seemed to me that they needed to hear from my heart where I thought we were going. I was trying to think, where can I go for some comparison to this, some lessons on how to handle it? So I started thinking about Churchill, started thinking that we're going to have to rebuild the spirit of the city, and what better example than Churchill and the people of London during the Blitz in 1940, who had to keep up their spirit during this sustained bombing? It was a comforting thought" (Pooley, 2001, p. 1).

Throughout the day and night of September 11, 2001 "Giuliani took to the airwaves to calm and reassure his people, made a few hundred rapid-fire decisions about the security and rescue operations, toured hospitals to comfort the families of the missing and made four more visits to the apocalyptic attack scene" (Pooley, 2001, p. 1).

At a late afternoon press conference with Governor Pataki on 9/11, the Mayor warned that feelings of anger and hatred are responsible for today's actions and urged that all rise above it, as one people, to recover from this tragedy. Later that same evening, he said "It's going to be a very difficult time. I don't think we yet know the pain we're going to feel. But the thing we have to focus on now is getting the city through this and surviving and being stronger for it. New York is still here." (Ripley, 2001, p. 5). "Tomorrow New York is going to be here," he said. "And we're going to rebuild, and we're going to be stronger than we were before" (Pooley, 2001, p. 2). He referred to the strong role of hope that a leader provides to his people: "Look, in a crisis you have to be optimistic." When I said the spirit of the city would be stronger, I didn't know that. I just hoped it. There are parts of you that say, "Maybe we're not going to get through this." He pauses, "You don't listen to them" (Pooley, 2001, pp. 2–3)

Mayor Giuliani consistently urged the public to draw on their compassion and humanity in the face of utmost grief and shock, calling them to a higher standard of service and courage: "Again, we ask all New Yorkers to cooperate and to try to help each other. There are going to be a lot of people today who need help and need assistance, either because of the fact that they know people that were lost in the terrible tragedy or because they are frightened of what may happen. If you could comfort them, help them and assist them, that might be a way in which all New Yorkers could lend a hand… I think for the people in New York, the best way to deal with this tragedy right now, is not only to deal with all their own grief, which we all feel and have, but to show that we're not going to be in any way affected by this, that we're not going to be cowed by this, that we're not afraid. We are going to go about our business and lead normal lives and not let those cowards affect us in any way" (NYC.gov, 2001).

Effectively balancing an awareness of his and others' emotions with the management of both his and others' emotions is the embodiment of an emotionally intelligent leader (Goleman *et al.*, 2002). Mayor Giuliani showed confidence, optimism, and humor along with empathy and self-control in the hours and days following the terrorist attacks. He demonstrated an acute awareness of what New Yorkers (and indeed Americans and people throughout the world in general) were thinking and feeling, and responded to those emotions in ways that acknowledged them, soothed them, and moved them. At the same time, the mayor was dealing with his own personal loss of many friends and colleagues. He spoke of these multiple realities honestly and forthrightly. His leadership was steadfast and inspirational. "He inhabited the role of wartime leader with a fine mixture of brisk compassion and gritty command presence" (Alter, 2001, p. 1).

Acting at once as chief operating officer of the city – personally monitoring, for instance, how many pounds of debris have been removed by the hour to securing low-interest loans to rebuild the city – to city psychologist, trying to assure a grief-stricken and terrified population that they are safe and that he knows they are hurting, the mayor had almost unilaterally managed to create the sense that the city and by its proxy, the nation, are scratching their way back to normalcy (Steinhauer, 2001a, p. A2). He was a whirlwind of activity, never once forgetting that the dominant emotion he and others were feeling was grief and how quickly that can turn to anger. He, through his actions and words, turned the grief into compassionate action.

"The mayor has also demonstrated a very soft and human side that seems to act as a balm on the frayed and mournful souls of the city. Here is the mayor imploring the city to dig deep and move on live television. Next, he is walking the sister of a fallen firefighter down the aisle in the brother's stead" (Steinhauer, 2001b, p. B9) "Since the catastrophe, he has exerted the leadership which he's always had. What was different was that he was sensitive and warm and compassionate and showed nuances with respect to emotion that he never showed before," said Ed Koch, a former New York Mayor and Giuliani rival (CNN.com., 2001).

Leaders with the best results use multiple leadership styles and understand the appropriate roles to play in any given situation (Goleman, 2000). One test of an effective leader is his ability to demonstrate contrary behaviors. Mature leaders develop more "balanced repertoires" (Denison *et al.*, 1995; Hooijberg, 1996), or a wide array of functions, that allow them to respond to complex demands. In addition to having a portfolio of behaviors, outstanding leaders are able to differentiate the most effective roles to play depending upon the situation.

Particularly in times of crisis, where extreme emotions are aroused, leaders may channel these emotions or further amplify them. With Rev. Falwell we saw someone who turned the grief and shock into immediate anger. With Dr. Healy, we sensed her not being connected with the people working for her organization, the Red Cross, as well as the public. Howard Lutnick seemed to be connected and then broke the connection with one decision, and seems to have rebuilt it after a great deal of work following that week. Like Ken Chenault, Mayor Giuliani established the connection, turned the grief and shock into action and compassion, and then mobilized a city and the millions of people watching the events on television. Instead of inflaming the negative emotions of anger, retribution, and stereotyping associated with it, Giuliani and Chenault created a positive emotional tone in the midst of a disaster.

Great leaders are made not born

As elusive as effective leadership can be, especially in moments of crisis, we offer a message of hope. Adults can develop emotional intelligence competencies (i.e., the habits or behavior patterns described in these competencies). Moreover, they can develop them in ways that are sustainable.[2] Longitudinal studies at the Weatherhead School of Management have shown that a person who sustains improvement in their emotional intelligence goes through a process described as Intentional Change Theory (it was called Self-Directed Learning from 1967 through to 2002), shown in Figure 13.1 (Boyatzis *et al.*, 1995; Goleman *et al.*, 2002).[3] Because of the discontinuous nature of sustained change, the process is experienced as five discoveries. The first discovery is one's Ideal Self, that is what he/she wants out of life and work – what his/her dreams and aspirations are (i.e., Personal Vision). Following development of the ideal, each participant works toward the second discovery, awareness of his or her Real Self, their strengths and weaknesses (i.e., Personal Balance Sheet). With the help of coaches, each person converts their Personal Vision and Balance Sheet into a Learning Plan for their development as a leader – this is the third discovery in the process. The fourth discovery is the actual experimentation and practice with the new behavior. The fifth discovery in the process is actually a continuous discovery throughout the entire process – the development of trusting relationships that help and encourage the person at each step in the process.

Concluding thought

Emotionally intelligent, or resonant leaders, can have an immensely positive influence on those around them. While acknowledging the horror that people have gone

---

[2] The Consortium for Research on Emotional Intelligence in Organizations searched the scientific literature for examples of programs that helped people developed such behavior (see their web site www.eiconsortium.org). They found 15 programs, of which five were still functioning at the time of publication of their findings (Cherniss & Goleman, 2001).

[3] One of the programs cited has 14 longitudinal studies of 25–35-year-old managers, 2 longitudinal studies of 38–42-year-old executives, and 4 longitudinal studies of 45–65-year executives as part of the Weatherhead School of Management's programs. These programs have shown that not only can adults develop emotional intelligence competencies, as measured through behavioral coding of audiotape work samples from critical incidents and videotapes of group simulations, but also have shown that these changes were sustainable up to 7 years after taking the course (Boyatzis *et al.*, 2002; Boyatzis *et al.*, 1995). These same programs have been extended to develop leaders through emotional intelligence in specific organizations (Boyatzis & Van Oosten, 2003).

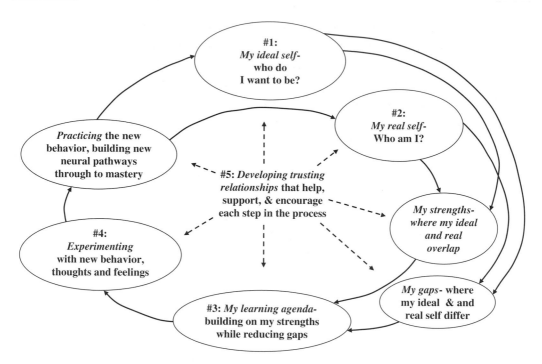

Figure 13.1   Boyatzis' Intentional Change Theory.

through, resonant leaders try to psychologically move people from fear to hope. This helps people spiritually, emotionally, and physically by setting into motion internal processes that strengthen their immune system.

To accomplish this feat, resonant leaders are physically present in times of crisis and are able to inspire and arouse a sense of compassion and humanity in their followers. Our profiles of Rudy Giuliani and Ken Chenault as resonant leaders during the 9/11 crisis echo the American Psychological Association's (2003) position that, "the most effective leaders are visible, convey a sense of hope and optimism while being realistic, and are calming, all the time communicating both what is known and what is not known. Successful leaders also involve their employees in developing disaster and recovery plans and profoundly affect outcomes when they ensure that organizational supports are in place and that they themselves are accessible, supportive, and empathic". Using the analogy of the immune system, resonant leaders in crisis situations not only help eradicate the harmful germs of negativity and disconnection, but have the ability to transform these germs into vaccines that build human resilience in the present moment and may help people in future crises.

Just as resonant leaders are positive and in touch with the emotions of those around them, there are also less effective or even ineffective leaders, who engage in negative emotional messages and/or are out of touch with the emotional climate around them. In times of crisis these leaders may act unintentionally or deliberately, but they invariably belittle the trauma that individuals have experienced or ineffectively pay attention to the emotional needs of their followers. Some dissonant leaders are paralyzed by their own panic or anger, or even worse, they exacerbate the anxiety and fear that ensue post crisis, becoming a contagion of negative emotions. At the extreme, these toxic leaders turn into demagogues, who reflect, channel, and amplify the negative feelings of the public into destructive ends. The people around them suffer the negative health effects of the trauma that are made worse by the continued arousal of destructive emotions.

September 11, 2001, served as an unexpected and traumatic public stage on which these different types of leadership played out. It is a source of hope that effective leaders emerge, when needed, to help us endure life's traumas and remember our humanity not our frailty.

REFERENCES

Alter, J. (2001). Lifesaver hero: Rudolph Giuliani. *Newsweek* (September 24), p. 1.

American Psychological Association. Task Force on Workplace Violence. (2003). "Responses to Workplace Violence Post 9/11: What Can Organizations Do? http://www.apa.org/pubinfo/post911workplace.html

Bass, B.M. & Stogdill, R.M. (1990). *Handbook on Leadership: Theory, Research, and Managerial Implications* (3rd ed.). NewYork: Free Press.

Buy, W. (2001). Encore presentation: Howard Lutnick delivers on his promises. CNN, CNN Pinnacle 16:30, transcript No. 083100CN.V39. (August 31).

Bloom, J. (2001). CEOs: leadership through communication. *PR Week* (November 26), Section: CEO Survey 2001, p. 20.

Boyatzis, R.E. (1982). *The Competent Manager: A Model for Effective Performance*. New York: John Wiley & Sons.

Boyatzis, R.E., Cowen, S.S. & Kolb, D.A. (1995). *Innovations in Professional Education: Steps on a Journey from Teaching to Learning*. San Francisco: Jossey-Bass.

Boyatzis, R.E., McKee, A. & Goleman, D. (2002). Reawakening the passion for work. *Harvard Business Review*, **80**(4), 86–94.

Boyatzis, R.E. & Oosten, E.V. (2003). "Developing leaders with emotional intelligence and the emotionally intelligent organization." In *International Executive Development Programmes* (7th ed.). ed. Roderick Millar. London: Kogan Page Publishers.

Boyatzis, R.E., Stubbs, E.C. & Taylor, S.N. (2002). Learning cognitive and emotional intelligence competencies through graduate management education. *Academy of Management Journal on Learning and Education*, **1**(2), 150–162.

Byrne, J. & Timmons, H. (2001). Tough Times for a New CEO. *Business Week* (October 29), Section: Cover Story, p. 64.

Chaffin, J. & Larsen, P.T. (2001). Rebuilding the house of cards: interview with Kenneth Chenault, *American Express* (October 17, Wednesday late edition), Section: Insider Track, p. 17. Retrieved from Lexis Nexis database.

Cherniss, C. & Goleman, D. (2001). *The Emotionally Intelligent Workplace.* San Francisco: Jossey-Bass. CNN.com. (2001). Rudolph Giuliani Profile: New York Mayor Winds Up on Top. Retrieved 4/17/03 from CNN.com.

Colaruuso, D. (2001). The struggle to rebuild: uncharted territory in every direction. *Investment Dealers Digest* (September 24), Securities Data Publishing.

Damasio, A. (1999). *The Feeling of What Happens: Body and Emotion in the Making of Consciousness.* New York: Harvest Books.

Davidson, R.J. (2003). Personal communication (April 23).

Davidson, R.J., Jackson, D.C. & Kalin, N.H. (2000). Emotion, plasticity, context, and regulation: perspectives from affective neuroscience. *Psychological Bulletin*, **126**(6), 890–909.

Denison, D.R., Hooijberg, R. & Quinn, R.E. (1995). Paradox and performance: toward a theory of behavioral complexity in managerial leadership. *Organization Science*, **6**, 524–540.

Ekman, P. (2003). *Gripped by Emotion*, ed. Henry Holt, New York: Times Books.

Farhi, P. (2001). In the face of disaster, Red Cross President Bernadine Healy activated her troops – and riled her critics. *The Washington Post* (October 4), Thursday Final edition. Section: Style, p. C01.

Federal News Service. (2001). Remarks by President George W. Bush; Kenneth Chenault, CEO, *American Express* (October 3), and Betsy Holden, CEO, Kraft Foods Following Meeting with U.S. Business Leaders. Section: White House Briefing.

Fink, S. (2000). *Crisis management: Planning for the Inevitable.* New York: iUniverse.com.

Francis, B. & Viles, P. (2001). American Express Chairman & CEO. *The NEW Show* 5 pm EST.

Future Banker. (2001). No. 1 Ken Chenault, CEO, *American Express* (May); Overhauled the executive suite, then he went to work. Section: Twenty-five most influential personalities in financial services, p.20.

Goleman, D. (1998). *Working with Emotional Intelligence.* New York: Bantam Books.

Goleman, D. (2000). Leadership that gets results. *Harvard Business Review*, March–April, 78–90.

Goleman, D. (2003). *Destructive Emotions: How Can We Overcome Them? A Scientific Dialogue with the Dalai Lama.* New York: Bantam Books.

Goleman, D., Boyatzis, R.E. & McKee, A. (2002). *Primal Leadership: Realizing the Power of Emotional Intelligence.* Boston: Harvard Business School Press.

Goodstein, L. (2001). Falwell's finger-pointing inappropriate, Bush says. *The New York Times* (September 15), p. A15.

Hatfield, E., Cacioppo, J.T. & Rapson, R.L. (1994). *Emotional Contagion.* New York: Cambridge University Press.

Henriques, D.B. (2002). Threats and responses: the bond trader; from devastation to determination. *The New York Times* (September 10), Tuesday, late final edition. p. 1; column 2.

Hooijberg, R. (1996). A multidirectional approach toward leadership: an extension of the concept of behavioral complexity. *Human Relations*, **49**, 917–946.

Howard Lutnick, CEO of Cantor Fitzgerald, defends the promises he made to the 733 employee's families that were lost in the World Trade Center terrorist attack, to take care of them. (2001a). *NBC Today* (October 10) (7:00 AM ET), NBC news transcripts.

Howard Lutnick, chairman and CEO of Cantor Fitzgerald, discusses the 700-plus employees he lost on the 101st floor. (2001b). *NBC Today* (September 14) (7:00 AM ET), NBC news transcripts.

Ingram, Leah. (2002). "Thinking Outside the Blue Box." *Continental* (June), p. 31–33. In the shadow of death, a life changes. (2001). *Toronto Star* (September 14), Friday Ontario edition. p. E09.

Johnston, J. (2002). We used to make money for the kicks … now it's because it matters; broker boss on why a quarter of his profits go to 9/11 families. *The Mirror* (May 15), (Ist ed.). pp. 8–9.

Knox, N. (2001). Cantor battles back from tragedy. *USA Today* (November 12), Money. http://www.usatoday.com/money/covers/2001-11-12-bcovmon.htm

Koppel, T. (2001). Did she quit or was she pushed, and why as America fights back: Dr. Bernadine Healy of the American Red Cross resigns. *ABC News: Nightline* (October 26), Friday 11:35 pm.

Kotter, J.P. (1982). *The General Managers*. NewYork: Free Press.

Kotter, J.P. (1988). *The Leadership Factor*. New York: Free Press.

LeDoux, J. (1996). *The Emotional Brain: The Mysterious Underpinnings of Emotional Life*. New York: Touchstone Books.

MacCallum, M. (2002). *American Express* – CHMN. & CEO. Interview. (May 13; Monday). CNBC/Dow Jones Business Video.

McClelland, D.C. & Boyatzis, R.E. (1982). Leadership motive pattern and long term success in management. *Journal of Applied Psychology*, **67**(9), 737–743.

McGeehan, Patrick. Sailing Into a Sea of Troubles; No Grace Period for New Chief of American Express. (2001). *The New York Times* (October 5), Section C; Page 1; Column 3; Business/Financial Desk.

Mitroff, I.I. & Anagnos, G. (2000). *Managing Crises Before They Happen. What Every Executive and Manager Needs to Know about Crisis*. New York: AMACOM.

Niebuhr, G. (2001). U.S. 'secular groups set tone for terror attacks, Falwell says. *The New York Times* (September 14), p. A18.

NYC.gov. (2001). Remarks by Rudolph Giuliani following the attack at the WTC. Retrieved 4/17/03 from NYC.gov (September 12).

Perez-Pena, R. (2001). Trying to command an emergency when the emergency command center is gone. *The New York Times* (September 12).

Pooley, E. (2001). Mayor of the world. *Time*. Person of the Year Issue.

Raphael, R. (2001). Keeping His Word: CEO of hard-hit company to compensate victim's families. http://abcnews.go.com/sections/2020/2020/2020_011010_lutnick.html (October 10).

Ripley, A. (2001). We're Under Attack. *Time*. Person of the Year Issue.

Schachter, S. (1959). *The Psychology of Affiliation*. San Francisco: Stanford University Press.

Schoolman, J. (2002). Cantor looking to get workers back to city. *Daily News* (February 14), p.71.

Seelye, K. & Henriques, D. (2001). A Nation Challenged: The Charity; Red Cross President Quits, Saying that the Board Left Her No Other Choice. *The New York Times* (October 27), Section B, p. 9, Column 1: National Desk; Saturday, Late edition. Retrieved from Lexis Nexis database.

Spencer Jr., L.M. & Spencer, S.M. (1993). *Competence at Work: Models for Superior Performance.* New York: John Wiley & Sons.

Steinhauer, J. (2001a). Giuliani Takes Charge, and City Sees Him as the Essential Man. *The New York Times* (September 14), p. A2.

Steinhauer, J. (2001b). Comforting and Cajoling to a Chant of "4 More Years". *The New York Times* (September 18), p. B9.

Taylor, S.E., Klein, L.C., Lewis, B.P., Gruenewald, T.L., Gurung, R.A.R. & Updegraff, J.A. (2002). Biobehavioral responses to stress in females: tend or befriend, not fight or flight. *Psychological Review*, **107**(3), 411–429.

Tough Bond Trader Shows Tender Side. (September 15, 2001). *Desert News* (Salt Lake City, Utah), p. A02.

Zahn, P. (2001). Bernadine Healy to Resign as Red Cross Head. *CNN Breaking News* (October 26), Friday 9:29. Retrieved from Lexis Nexis database.

14

Guiding community intervention following terrorist attack

Stevan E. Hobfoll

Clearly many nations have faced terrorism's modern form for decades. Israel has faced terrorist attack against civilian targets since before its inception as a state. India is attacked daily by Muslim separatists from Cashmere, Spain has faced *Euskadi ta Askatasuna* (*ETA*) for decades, and Russia and China have faced terrorist attack from separatist movements that have brought violence and death to their major cities.

What is different about September 11th is that terrorists attacked the most powerful nation on earth using its own technology of aircraft and structural physics in a way that in minutes ended the lives of thousands in New York and nearly 200 lives at the Pentagon. The attack was the first on American soil since the all but forgotten attack by Japan on the Aleutian Islands during World War II, and even that attack and Pearl Harbor were not on the continental USA. Moreover, and easily forgotten, because no one knew what might occur in the wake of the aircraft genocidal attacks, the secondary threat was the belief that "anything was possible" in the hours, days, and weeks following the attack. Television news talked of possible, or even probable, secondary attack that could take the form of more airplanes, suicide bombers, chemical or biological weapons, or even an atomic attack. The US security establishment was clearly caught unprepared. Fully 5 hours after the attack (1:44 p.m. EST), the first warship and aircraft carriers were ordered dispatched from the US Naval Station in Norfolk, Virginia (US Department of State, 2002). These facts are critical if we are to understand the public response to the attack. Specifically, as terrible as the loss of life was and as great as was the physical devastation, the public feared much more and the follow-up anthrax attacks were easily linked in people's minds to a proliferation of the terrorist attack in a way that could kill millions. It is not hyperbole to say that many believed that the thousands killed in the World Trade Center and the Pentagon was only the beginning.

Need for a threat-loss-response model

The unexpected nature and magnitude of the attacks of September 11th raises a critical point for a mental health response to terror. Specifically, any response or plan for the future that is merely the adoption of "lessons learned" from prior instances is likely to be obsolete before it enters the field because of the potential for unique variations of attacks. Yet, this is indeed the model being formulated by the few policymakers who are even bothering to contemplate what to do in case of future attacks. So, web sites have proliferated from the two APAs (American Psychological Association and American Psychiatric Association) about care for victims of terror, but these are essentially amalgams of clinical wisdom and provide few if any guidelines for communities and for policy *per se*. Despite the fact the homeland security depends on the response of citizens of the homeland, I know of no plans or allocations for this aspect of homeland security.

Paradoxically, traumatic stress treatment has been one of the most theoretically articulated and carefully researched areas of clinical intervention (Foa & Meadows, 1997; Foa *et al.*, 2000). However, the extrapolation of these efforts to populations who have been exposed to terrorist attack who have developed clinical levels of disorder or, perhaps more importantly on the community level, to victims who are subclinical, but under high levels of distress, has not been followed, despite prior publications that carefully consider these issues (deJong, 1995; Hobfoll & de Vries, 1995; Weisæth, 1995). Clinical psychology and psychiatry have weak, almost nonexistent, public mental health wings, and community psychology has all but abandoned interest in clinical-community intervention. This leaves community response policy an orphan at a time when it is the most pressing area of mental health concern. Still, the clinical model is probably the major approach that has been adopted for addressing community level responding to terrorist attack.

COR theory and its application to community trauma

I have argued elsewhere that stress-appraisal theory (Lazarus & Folkman, 1984) provides an excellent model on the clinical level, but a partial model for more major stressors and where large numbers of people are involved (Hobfoll, 1988, 1989, 1998). There are a number of reasons that I have lodged this criticism against this valuable and popular theory. First, if we need to wait for appraisals, then we need to wait for the event to occur. Second, appraisals mix personal evaluations of threat, circumstances, and resources, so that these important factors cannot be disentangled. Third, appraisals tell us critical information about the individual, but little about the group or classes of people. Finally, appraisal theory has, in practice, relocated the focus of stress research from structural elements of the stressor and resources to cognitions. This is consistent with clinical intervention that motivates people to reframe events, but at odds with the viewpoint that it is change in the actual structural elements that cause or perpetuate the stress. The clinician works with rape victims' feelings, not with making streets safer. The cognitive revolution in psychology has moved us away from social policy and community change, and placed the problem as one of individuals' cognitions.

COR theory (Hobfoll, 1988, 1989, 1998, 2002) offers an alternative to stress-appraisal theory which may help guide community intervention following major traumatic events such as terrorist attack. The basic tenet of COR theory is that individuals strive to obtain, retain, protect, and foster those things that they value.

These valued entities are termed resources, and one way of dividing them is into object (e.g., car, home, clothing), condition (e.g., employment, marriage), personal characteristic (e.g., self-esteem, optimism, job skills), and energy (e.g., credit, knowledge, stamina) resources. Resources are not individually determined, but are both transcultural and products of any given culture. Our research uncovered 74 basic resources (see Table 14.1) that represent a comprehensive, but certainly not exhaustive, set (Hobfoll, 1998). It follows that psychological stress will occur in one of three instances and that these are all represented when we refer to the community impact of terrorism.

Table 14.1. COR resources and evaluation

Resources	Extent of actual loss[a]	Extent of threat of loss[b]
1. Personal transportation (car, truck, etc.)		
2. Feeling that I am successful		
3. Time for adequate sleep		
4. Good marriage		
5. Adequate clothing		
6. Feeling valuable to others		
7. Family stability		
8. Free time		
9. More clothing than I need		
10. Sense of pride in myself		
11. Intimacy with one or more family members		
12. Time for work		
13. Feelings that I am accomplishing my goals		
14. Good relationship with my children		
15. Time with loved ones		
16. Necessary tools for work		
17. Hope		
18. Children's health		
19. Stamina		
20. Necessary home appliances		
21. Feeling that my future success depends on me		

(cont.)

Table 14.1. (cont.)

Resources	Extent of actual loss[a]	Extent of threat of loss[b]
22. Positively challenging routine		
23. Personal health		
24. Housing that suits my needs		
25. Sense of optimism		
26. Status/seniority at work		
27. Adequate food		
28. Larger home than I need		
29. Sense of humor		
30. Stable employment		
31. Intimacy with spouse or partner		
32. Adequate home furnishings		
33. Feeling that I have control over my life		
34. Role as a leader		
35. Ability to communicate		
36. Providing children's essentials		
37. Feeling that my life is peaceful		
38. Acknowledgment of my accomplishments		
39. Ability to organize tasks		
40. Extras for children		
41. Sense of commitment		
42. Intimacy with at least one friend		
43. Money for extras		
44. Self-discipline		
45. Understanding from my employer/boss		
46. Savings or emergency money		
47. Motivation to get things done		
48. Spouse/partner's health		
49. Support from co-workers		
50. Adequate income		
51. Feeling that I know who I am		
52. Advancement in education or job training		
53. Adequate financial credit		
54. Feeling independent		
55. Companionship		
56. Financial assets (stocks, property, etc.)		
57. Knowing where I am going with my life		
58. Affection from others		
59. Financial stability		
60. Feeling that my life has meaning/purpose		
61. Positive feelings about myself		

Resources	Extent of actual loss[a]	Extent of threat of loss[b]
62. People I can learn from		
63. Money for transportation		
64. Help with tasks at work		
65. Medical insurance		
66. Involvement with church, synagogue, etc.		
67. Retirement security (financial)		
68. Help with tasks at home		
69. Loyalty of friends		
70. Money for advancement or self-improvement (education, starting a business, etc.)		
71. Help with child care		
72. Involvement in organizations with others who have similar interests		
73. Financial help if needed		
74. Health of family/close friends		

My resources: 0: not at all/not applicable; 1: to a small degree; 2: to a moderate degree; 3: to a considerable degree; 4: to a great degree.
[a] To what extent have I experienced *actual loss* during the past 6 months/since "name of event"? (Asked again on separate page for resource gain).
[b] To what extent have I experienced *threat of loss* during the past 6 months/since "name of event"?

Stress will occur:
(1) when individuals' resources are threatened with loss,
(2) when individuals' resources are actually lost,
(3) where individuals fail to gain sufficient resources following significant resource investment.

This means that when threat of terror or terror occurs, a basic motivation of individuals is disturbed. This follows because terror is meant to threaten both the physical reality of those it kills or maims, but more so the underlying belief that people can conduct their lives in a way that allows them to obtain, retain, foster, and protect their resources. Terror attempts to challenge people's belief that they can preserve these lifelong resource caravans that they have so carefully created and that their government is obliged to protect. Nor is this only a perception. Terrorism in Israel in the Al-Aqsa Intifada has crippled Israel's economy and September 11th has cost Americans billions of dollars in disruption of business and the costs of added security.

A number of principles and corollaries follow from COR theory. They are presented in Table 14.2. The empirical support and more complete justification of these principles are detailed elsewhere (Hobfoll, 1991, 1998, 2001, 2002). These principles and corollaries form a roadmap by which to predict and respond to threat of resource loss that is an inevitable part of terrorist threat and attack and outline a strategy for initiation of the gain cycles that can be initiated to respond to such attack.

Principle 1 of COR theory (see Table 14.2) emphasizes the primacy of resource loss. *It states that resource loss is disproportionally more salient than resource gain* (Hobfoll & Lilly, 1993; Wells *et al.*, 1999). This means that in the face of terrorist attack that the other gains that people are making in their lives become less salient for them and the treat to resource loss or actual loss that accompanies attack is magnified, often well beyond the purely rational nature of the threat. Hence September 11th quickly took on the attributes of a doomsday scenario. Although many news media discussions and politicians emphasized that America was strong and we would overcome this attack as we had Pearl Harbor, the very reference to an attack that destroyed the US Pacific Fleet and entered the US into a major world war is illustrative of the degree to which loss is exaggerated. In part due to media

Table 14.2. Principles and corollaries of COR theory

Principles

1. The primacy of resource loss
   The first principle of COR theory is that resource loss is disproportionally more salient than resource gain.

2. Resource investment
   The second principle of COR theory is that people must invest resources in order to protect against resource loss, recover from losses, and gain resources.

3. Increased salience of gain in the face of loss
   Gain increases in salience in the context of loss, because the loss makes the gain more critical.

Corollaries

1. Those with greater resources are less vulnerable to resource loss and more capable of orchestrating resource gain. Conversely, those with fewer resources are more vulnerable to resource loss and less capable of resource gain.

2. Loss cycles: Those who lack resources are not only more vulnerable to resource loss, but that initial loss begets future loss. At each iteration of the cycle they have fewer resources to use to mount a defense against ongoing resource challenges that occur. Further, because resource loss is more potent than resource gain, loss cycles will be more impactful and more accelerated (i.e., occur at greater speed) than gain cycles.

3. Those who possess resources are more capable of gain, and initial resource gain begets further gain. However, because resource loss is more potent than resource gain, gain cycles will be less impactful and have less acceleration than loss cycles.

4. Those who lack resources are likely to adopt a defensive posture to conserve their resources.

sensationalizing, and in part due to the true nature of the tragedy, fears of loss to the self and loved ones, and even to one's way of love for omnipresent following the events of September 11th.

Extrapolating this principle to the community level, we can see that not only is resource loss more salient than gain for the community, the weight of loss is multiplied by the collective experience. This has been shown in what Riley and Eckenrode (1986) termed the process of *stress contagion* and what Hobfoll and London (1986) termed the *pressure cooker* effect. Stress contagion occurs on the individual level, whereby the stress experience is shared by those who occupy a common social space. The pressure cooker effect further indicates that when stress contagion occurs that the sharing of the stress experience increases its power because it comes to define reality – stress is everywhere one turns.

It is also notable that Norris (2001) in establishing a template for research that was promoted by National Institute of Mental Health (NIMH) adapted the COR theory loss of resources scale as a critical element that all research projects concerning September 11th should include. This scale addressed personal loss, social loss, economic loss, and psychological loss (e.g., diminished hope). The long tail of this loss sequence is also illustrated by the accumulating number of crisis calls over time, even a year after September 11th as noted by Katz *et al.* and Draper *et al.* in this volume.

The primacy of loss is also noted in the study of the impact of September 11th in New York City by Galea *et al.* (2002). They found that degree of loss, proximity to the World Trade Center, and ethnic minority status (which is related to lack of available resources) were key risk factors for development of post-traumatic stress disorder (PTSD). These findings, and the very study approach, are consistent with COR theory and quite different than the approach that would be taken by appraisal or clinical theories which would instead rely on individual difference variables. This said, individual difference variables are also important, but many of the key individual differences are central personal (e.g., optimism and self-efficacy), social (e.g., social support, marital ties), or condition (e.g., insurance, having stable employment) resources.

The second principle of COR theory (see Table 14.2) states that *people must invest resources in order to protect against resource loss, recover from losses, and gain resources* (Hobfoll, 2002). So, people may invest self-esteem to offset a threat to self-esteem or can invest social support to offset loss of self esteem. Translating the concept of resource investment to a community level presents special problems and opportunities, however. First, the opportunities should be considered. Specifically, people can rely on collective resources when a terrorist attack occurs. The resources of state, church, organizations, the workplace, and neighborhood are typically available to victims of terrorist attack because it is considered an attack on the collective.

These are all critical to aid lagging resources of individuals who can be easily over-whelmed by terrorist attacks, and especially of large scale attack such as September 11. Second, people in more everyday circumstances may fail to respond to threat because they can forestall change and because the threat of even some major stres-sors (e.g., divorce, work layoffs) can be vague. Terrorist attack offers a clear threat with a clear need to respond.

Turning to the obstacles to resource investment, the principal obstacle to respond-ing with resource investment to terrorist attack is that individual and collective coping responses are seldom articulated or practiced for individuals and commu-nities for events of such magnitude or scale. For New York City, September 11th represented an entirely new scenario that was outside New Yorkers' or New York City institutions' coping repertoires. This was not just because of the scale of attack. Even an attack of one-tenth the magnitude would have been outside the repertoires people and institutions had for coping. Even in Israel there is no stan-dard, disseminated, practiced, let alone institutionalized response repertoire to ter-rorist attack in terms of people's or institutions' coping responses.

Because individuals' families', organizations', and institutions' coping responses are outstripped when terrorist attack occurs, there is an added feeling of chaos, threat, and doom. "Not only have we been targeted for attack, we don't know what to do and neither do those institutions whom we depend upon." Initial responding is often altruistic (Kaniasty & Norris, 1995), but that does not make it organized or effective. Still, and importantly, Principle 2 of COR theory tells us that individuals and groups will mobilize resources to respond to offset the impact of resource loss. That is, they will move into an action, mobilization phase if at all possible, whether or not they know their direction or are clear on either means or goals. When this is a directed effort, as in the several community programs discussed in this volume by Fullilove and Saul, it is most effective. Fullilove and Saul (this volume) illustrate how experts should form a partnership with the healthy natural tendencies of the community and can redirect the unhealthy sequelae and pathways that people might otherwise adopt.

To suggest that resource gain is also critical when COR theory emphasizes the primacy of resource loss over resource gain appears paradoxical. It is clarified by Principle 3, which is stated outright as a principle of COR theory for the first time here (previously it was nested in the primacy of loss). Recent work on traumatic stress due to threat of life from AIDS (Billings *et al.*, 2000) and in the case of long-term gains when major life stressors are considered (Holahan *et al.*, 1999) indicate the importance of resource gain in the context of loss. Specifically, *Principle 3 states that resource gain becomes more salient for people when they face significant losses and when they can sustain gains over long periods (e.g., obtain a better marriage, improve their education, increase their internalized sense of self-efficacy)* (Wells *et al.*, 1999).

When terrorism or other traumatic community events occur, the world can quickly become painted black and this blackness and doom seems to reach out to the long horizon. A common perceptual bias invades the population in which it is easy to feel that "all is lost," "our dreams are crushed," "the terrorists are so powerful; we'll never be able to stop them." For this reason, even small gains in the wake of major resource loss are critical. Individuals are biased to overweight loss compared to gain (Tversky & Kahneman, 1974; Ito *et al.*, 1998). However, this in part also increases their search for instances of gain and increases the value they place on gain when loss is omnipresent.

The increased salience of resource gain in the face of loss suggests the need for interventionists to encourage messages of resource gain by public officials in public statements. These should not be exaggerated because, if found false, they undermine the potency of future such communication. Similarly, families and organizations can be aided in paths that they can take to initiate family and organizational gain cycles, and a similar process can be encouraged in individual counseling. This is very different than what cognitive therapy calls "reframing." Instead, gain initiatives should be real, involve personal and social action, and as much as possible have consequences that are clear to those involved.

DeJong (2002) argues persuasively that interventionists should not stop at working for small, local wins. Rather, groups should work on making major gains such as organizing to work for tolerance of others, working on the fight against the causes that breed terrorism in some cases (e.g., Israelis working together for peace with Palestinians; Irish Catholics and Protestants working on equal housing and employment opportunities). This is critical because terrorism also makes people feel small and inconsequential on the plane that the attack involves. Citizens naturally feel that these are political problems that are out of their control and to some extent this is true, but it is a hurdle that can and should be crossed. This is clearly illustrated in the chapter by Fullilove and Saul (this volume) who emphasize how working with the community, sharing expertise, and reminding people of their efficacy to solve local problems are critical gain steps. This can be compared with the clinical model which places therapists as knowing experts and citizens as hapless victims as clinical models are consistently focused on addressing psychopathology, as opposed to building resilience (Rappaport, 1981).

Protecting the most vulnerable

In addition to COR theory's primary principles, COR stipulates a number of related corollaries that follow from these principles.

Corollary 1 of COR theory states that *those with greater resources are less vulnerable to resource loss and more capable of orchestrating resource gain. Conversely, those with fewer resources are more vulnerable to resource loss and less capable of resource gain.* This means that intervention following terrorist attack must act quickly to protect vulnerable populations. Those who already lack resources, such as those who are poor, have a history of psychological disorder, are more dependent on social institutions (e.g., the elderly, those on welfare, the physically handicapped), ethnic minority, and immigrant populations are particularly susceptible to resource loss following major traumatic events such as terrorism. Events quickly can escalate for them into rapid resource loss cycles as indicated in Corollary 2 which states that *those who lack resources are not only more vulnerable to resource loss, but that initial loss begets future loss.* At each iteration of the cycle they have fewer resources to use to mount a defense against ongoing resource challenges that occur. *Further, because resource loss is more potent than resource gain, loss cycles will be of more impact and more accelerated (i.e., occur at greater speed) than gain cycles.*

Loss cycles are especially powerful and accelerate rapidly because people's loss of resources is stressful and because people employ their resource reservoirs to forestall the negative impact of resource loss. On a community level people can call on insurance, government institutions, and their workplace to aid them when terrorist attack occurs. However, the more disenfranchised and disempowered they are, the less capable they are of mobilizing such resources. Those with few resources are most likely to have their few resources quickly overwhelmed. Then, in the wave of secondary losses and threat to loss that occur following such major events as terrorist attack, they have few reserves to mount an emotional, material, or social defense of further resource loss. Thus, it is not surprising that Galea *et al.* (2002) found that following the attack of September 11th that those in Manhattan who had greatest risk of PTSD were of Hispanic ethnicity, had low social support, lost a family member or friend in the attack, and lost a job due to the attack. Moreover, as indication of the net effect of drained resources, those who had two or more prior major life stressors were also more vulnerable to PTSD. These findings clearly indicate how resource loss and possessing limited psychological resistance resources combine to increase psychological risk, striking the most vulnerable populations.

COR theory also indicates in Corollary 3 that *those who possess resources are more capable of gain, and initial resource gain begets further gain.* However, because resource loss is more potent than resource gain, gain cycles will be of less impact and have less acceleration than loss cycles. This translates to a process whereby gain cycles tend to be difficult to catalyze, perpetuate, or accelerate in speed. Gain cycles tend to be slow moving. Following terrorist attack, even more resilient individuals must invest much of their resource armamentarium just to sustain themselves and their loved ones and prevent further loss. Much of their resources and resource energy must be invested in limiting the slide of loss cycles. This is where intervention can be so critical, however. Interventionists have the professional training and experience to understand the difficulty of initiating and sustaining resource gain. They can therefore use their own resources to make wise investments in critical community, family, and individual processes as illustrated so well by Fullilove and Saul in this volume.

The fourth and final corollary of COR theory states that *those who lack resources are likely to adopt a defensive posture to conserve their resources.* This is a critical postulate of COR theory for events such as September 11th or disasters that seriously and perilously invade people's resources. To understand the nature of this corollary we must consider that people are not necessarily altruistic, and indeed may become quite selfish following an attack. The fear of further loss of resources, once loss occurs, may instead motivate extreme measures which can be short-sighted and negative. This helps explain the emotional call for action to attack the attackers following September 11th. This can be seen in the calls to bomb "them" that emerged as soon as al-Qaeda and Afghanistan's Taliban regime was a recognized source of the attack. Even more sinister, the tendency to form a defensive posture can result in attacks against local Muslims or anyone else that appears like "them." The defensive posture accentuates in-group–out-group differences as a knee jerk defensive reaction. In this way people's defensive posture results in their wanting an enemy who they can do something about directly in order to insure their own future safety.

Following major threat or loss, people "hole up" and "dig in" both metaphorically and actually. It can become difficult to get them to take the risks involved in investing resources for recovery. Long after the attack people may avoid flying, going to tall public buildings, and visiting abroad. Despite the lack of serious follow-up attacks and the greater likelihood of other health concerns being in actuality of greater threat, we see security remain a major political agenda item in the polls long after a more realistic viewpoint would otherwise inform people of their risk. It is for this reason that a major part of military training is aimed at training troops to continue following orders after their own responsive system would have them withdraw physically and psychologically. In the case of civilian non-combatants this is of course more problematic as they are neither trained nor feel that they have "signed up" for the duty.

Principles of intervention in the community

COR theory can be used to devise several intervention principles for major community threats such as terrorist attack (Hobfoll *et al.*, 1995). For the sake of brevity, these are simply listed here and I refer readers back to the original source for details:

(1) Act to halt loss cycles.
(2) Initiate gain strategies.
(3) Act early and with sufficient magnitude. Minor or late intervention will have little impact.

(4) Expect secondary loss chains; these will accumulate and gain negative momentum.

(5) Resource losses are intertwined. Pay attention to the web of resource's connections.

(6) Expect odd, defensive strategies.

(7) Don't ignore those who are initially coping well.

(8) Loss cycles have long tails. Intervention must continue downstream of the original "event."

(9) Pay attention to political processes. They are not always munificent and often represent the gain/loss advantages of entrenched in-groups.

Conclusion

The events of September 11th highlight the need to revitalize community psychiatry and community psychology which have both atrophied and ignored training in disaster preparedness. New thought must now be given to the response to terrorism and this must be translated to public health policy and inform pre- and post-terrorism.

COR theory provides one theoretical outlook for organizing the promotion of resilience and combating the many losses and negative psychological sequelae that come in terrorism's wake (Hobfoll, Canetti-Nisim & Johnson). We must also revitalize the work on dogmatism and authoritarianism of Rokeach (1960) and others, as we have allowed such study to lie fallow, sanguine that we successfully confronted Naziism, communism, and McArthyism. There are many more "isms" whose supporters will use to perpetrate their view on the world through violence, denial of human rights, and political process that psychology and psychiatry can do much to combat.

REFERENCES

Billings, D.W., Folkman, S., Acree, M. & Moskowitz, J.T. (2000). Coping and physical health during care-giving: the roles of positive and negative affect. *Journal of Personality and Social Psychology*, **79**, 139–142.

deJong, J.T.V.M. (1995). Prevention of the consequences of man-made or natural disaster at the (inter)national, the community, the family, and the individual level. In *Extreme Stress and Communities: Impact and Intervention*, eds. S.E. Hobfoll & M.W. de Vries. Dordrecht, The Netherlands: Kluwer, pp. 207–227.

deJong, J.T.V.M. (2002). Public mental health, traumatic stress, and human rights violations in low-income countries. In *Trauma, War, and Violence: Public Mental Health in Socio-cultural Context*, ed. J.T.V.M. deJong. New York: Plenum, pp. 1–91.

Foa, E.B. & Meadows, E.A. (1997). Psychosocial treatment for posttraumatic stress disorder: a critical review. *Annual Review of Psychology*, **48**, 449–480.

Foa, E.B., Keane, T.M., Friedman, M.J., Bisson, J.I., McFarlane, A., Rose, S., Rothbaum, B.O., Meadows, E.A., Resick, P., Foy, D.W., Davidson, J.R.T., Mellman, T.A., Southwick, S.M., Cohen, J.A., Berliner, L., March, J.S., Chemtob, C.M., Tolin, D.F., van der Kolk, B.A., Pitman, R.K., Glynn, S.M., Schnurr, P.P., Jankowski, M.K., Wattenberg, M.S., Weiss, D.S., Marmar, C.R., Gusman, F.D., Kudler, H.S., Blank, A.S., Krupnick, J.L., Courtois, C.A., Bloom, S.L., Penk, W., Flannery, R.B., Cardena, E., Maldonado, J., Van der Hart, O., Spiegel, D., Riggs, D.S. & Johnson, D.R. (2000). Guidelines for treatment of PTSD – introduction (reprinted from effective treatments for PTSD). *Journal of Traumatic Stress*, **13**, 539–588.

Fullilove, M. & Saul, J. (2005). Rebuilding communities post-disaster. In *9/11: Mental Health in the Wake of a Terrorist Attacks*, eds. Y. Neria, R. Gross & R. Marshall. Cambridge, UK: Cambridge University Press.

Galea, S., Ahern, J., Resnick, H., Kilpatrick, D., Bucuvalas, M., Gold, J. & Vlahov, D. (2002). Psychological sequelae of the September 11 terrorist attacks in New York City. *New England Journal of Medicine*, **346**, 982–987.

Hobfoll, S.E. (1988). *The Ecology of Stress*. New York: Hemisphere Publishing Corporation.

Hobfoll, S.E. (1989). Conservation of resources: a new attempt at conceptualizing stress. *American Psychologist*, **44**, 513–524.

Hobfoll, S.E. (1991). Traumatic stress: a theory based on rapid loss of resources. *Anxiety Research: An International Journal*, **4**, 187–197.

Hobfoll, S.E. (1998). *Stress, Culture, and Community. The Psychology and Philosophy of Stress*. New York, NY: Plenum.

Hobfoll, S.E. (2001). The influence of culture, community, and the nested-self in the stress process: advancing conservation of resources theory. Lead article. *Applied Psychology*, **50**, 337–370.

Hobfoll, S.E. (2002). Social and psychological resources and adaptation. *Review of General Psychology*, **6**, 307–324.

Hobfoll, S.E. & de Vries, M.W. (1995). *Extreme Stress and Communities: Impact and Intervention*. Dordrecht, The Netherlands: Kluwer Academic.

Hobfoll, S.E. & Lilly, R.S. (1993). Resource conservation as a strategy for community psychology. *Journal of Community Psychology*, **21**, 128–148.

Hobfoll, S.E. & London, P. (1986). The relationship of self-concept and social support to emotional distress among women during war. *Journal of Social and Clinical Psychology*, **4**, 189–203.

Hobfoll, S.E., Briggs, S. & Wells, J. (1995). Community stress and resources: actions and reactions. In *Extreme Stress and Communities: Impact and Intervention*, eds. S.E. Hobfoll & M.W. de Vries. Dordrecht, The Netherlands: Kluwer Academic, pp. 137–158.

Hobfoll, S.E., Canetti-Nisim, D. & Johnson, R.J. (in Press). Exposure to terrorism, Stress-related health symptoms and defensive coping among Jews and Arabs in Israel. *Journal of Consulting and Clinical Psychology*.

Holahan, C.J., Moos, R.H., Holahan, C.K. & Cronkite, R.C. (1999). Resource loss, resource gain, and depressive symptoms: a 10-year model. *Journal of Personality and Social Psychology*, **77**, 620–629.

Ito, T.A., Larsen, J.T., Smith, N.K. & Cacioppo, J.T. (1998). Negative information weighs more heavily on the brain: the negativity bias in evaluative categorizations. *Journal of Personality and Social Relationships*, **75**, 887–900.

Kaniasty, K. & Norris, F. (1995). In search of altruistic community: patterns of social support mobilization following Hurricane Hugo. *American Journal of Community Psychology*, **23**, 447–477.

Katz, C.L., Smith, R., Herbert, R. & Levin, S. (2005). The World Trade Center worker/volunteer mental health screening program. In *9/11: Mental Health in the Wake of a Terrorist Attacks*, eds. Y. Neria, R. Gross & R. Marshall. Cambridge, UK: Cambridge University Press.

Lazarus, R.S. & Folkman, S. (1984). *Stress Appraisal and Coping*. New York: Springer Publishing Company.

Norris, F. (2001). Measuring exposure to the events of September 11, 2001: pretest results and stress/loss norms obtained from a minimally exposed by diverse sample of college students. Available at http://obssr.nih.gov/activities/911/attack

Rappaport, J. (1981). In praise of paradox: a social policy of empowerment over prevention. *American Journal of Community Psychology*, **9**, 1–25.

Riley, D. & Eckenrode, J. (1986). Social ties: subgroup differences in costs and benefits *Journal of Personality and Social Psychology*, **51**, 770–778.

Rokeach, M. in collaboration with Richard Bonier and others (1960). *The Open and Closed Mind; Investigations into the Nature of Belief Systems and Personality Systems.* New York, NY: Basic Books.

Tversky, A. & Kahneman, D. (1974). Judgement under uncertainty: heuristics and biases. *Science*, **185**, 1124–1131.

Weisæth, L. (1995). Preventive psychosocial intervention after disaster. In *Extreme Stress and Communities: Impact and Intervention*, eds. S.E. Hobfoll & M.W. de Vries. Dordrecht, The Netherlands: Kluwer, pp. 401–419.

Wells, J.D., Hobfoll, S.E. & Lavin, J. (1999). When it rains it pours: the greater impact of resource loss compared to gain on psychological distress. *Personality and Social Psychology Bulletin*, **25**, 1172–1182.

Part IV

Outreach and intervention in the wake of terrorist attacks

15

Science for the community after 9/11

Randall D. Marshall

"… men [and women] of science are becoming conscious of the responsibility towards society conferred by their knowledge, and are feeling it a duty to take a larger part in the direction of public affairs than they have hitherto done."

– Bertrand Russell, *The Scientific Outlook*, 1931 (p. 233)

Public health models after large-scale disaster always consider the problem of "surge capacity" – that is, how effectively will a community be able to absorb a sudden increase in a particular need for medical intervention. Before the 9/11 disaster, models of such an event – the complete collapse of two of the world's tallest skyscrapers along with the destruction of surrounding buildings would literally have focused on surge capacity for medical treatment, for basic needs (food, clothing, shelter for persons displaced from contaminated dwellings) and social services after dwellings. The totally unexpected public health problem, was the need to address surge capacity for mental health problems and disorders. These chapters document only a few of the programs developed in response.

All epidemiological studies of the mental health consequences of the 9/11 attacks found significant rates of new-onset 9/11 related posttraumatic stress disorder (PTSD) in those directly and indirectly exposed in New York, and, surprisingly, also in persons across the US. Several groups have replicated this finding independently over time (Neria *et al.*, this volume; Galea *et al.*, this volume; Hoven *et al.*, this volume; Cohen-Silver *et al.*, this volume). Because the population base is so large, small percentages translate into large absolute numbers (e.g., a rate of 0.9% in the New York area = 142,000 persons).

The term epidemic is defined as a disease "produced by some special causes not generally present" (*Oxford English Dictionary*, 2002); and, in common usage, "wide-spread." The 9/11 attacks created an epidemic of mental disorder, by both usages of the term (see Part II of this volume). Consider the public health response that might result after detection of 5000 new cases of West Nile virus (0.06% of the New York City population). Would sensible people be arguing over whether it should be called an epidemic? That there is such a debate, in both the popular media and the scientific literature, reflects the stigma associated with mental disorders and PTSD in particular, the nascent state of our public health models, and the politicization of the tragedy, and both are unfortunately shadow players on the larger national and mental health stages.

The chapters in this section document a spectrum of largely institutional responses to the early findings that hundreds of thousands of people were extremely distressed after 9/11, and might benefit from community-based, social-support in its place focused services, and that a smaller proportion of persons (still many tens of thousands) would benefit from specialized treatment for serious mental disorders such as PTSD, depression, and complicated grief. In most cases, these programs illustrate productive partnerships between academia and other institutions (hospitals, service providers, philanthropy, government) – a striking and effective 9/11 phenomenon in itself (see Rosenthal introduction, this volume; Marshall, this volume). Taken together, they represent a massive outpouring of services efforts directed at improving mental health outcomes in a community struggling with an economic depression, living in constant fear of additional attacks, and interspersed with tens of thousands of persons whose natural capacity for resilience had been overwhelmed by their 9/11 experience, and the multiple stressors faced in the months afterwards.

In many ways, 9/11 brought into sharp relief several major deficiencies in the US mental health care system, and in the state of our science. Little is known about actual practices in the community in treating all serious mental disorders including PTSD – and for that matter, little is known about medical outcomes in the community, in general. Everything we do know suggests that PTSD remains underdiagnosed in its place in the community (96–100% of cases) and is therefore almost certainly inadequately treated. In an urban outpatient psychiatric clinic, Davidson and Smith found that 22% ($n = 12/54$) were diagnosed with PTSD and another 9% had subthreshold symptoms; none had been diagnosed by the clinic (Davidson & Smith, 1990). A similar study found that 40% (72/181) of outpatients in an urban psychiatric clinic met structured interview diagnostic criteria for PTSD (but only three had been diagnosed in the clinic (Switzer et al., 1999). Finally, Al-Saffar et al. (2002, 2003) studied a Swedish psychiatric outpatient clinic and found the prevalence of PTSD to be 46% ($n = 53$) based on a self-report questionnaire; none had been diagnosed.

In other words, the attacks on 9/11 evoked an urgency about the lack of high quality, evidenced-based care in the community that ideally should have been there already. It is hoped that the different types of treatment interventions and programs described in this section have created permanent highly competent service delivery systems and programs. Eventually, evidence-based practices for PTSD should become core competency requirements in mental health and medical training programs so that sufficient expertise is embedded in the community. Until that time, however, we believe that *ad hoc* training and treatment programs will be needed whenever there is a sudden surge in serious mental disorder due to disasters and mass violence events. Moreover, *ad hoc* programs will always be needed to address surge capacity problems in a community after a large-scale disaster or terrorist attack.

Thus, after 9/11, treatment efforts were needed because (1) PTSD was not being adequately treated prior to 9/11 and (2) both informed estimates, and then epidemiological research pointed to a sudden and dramatic surge in need for treatment that would overwhelm community capacity to provide evidence-based services. So 9/11, in essence compounded a services shortage that was already in existence.

Two models of intervention

This section reflects the dual emphasis of post-9/11-programs. First, public health programs emphasized psychodirectional programs focusing on resilience in the general population, promoted healthy coping strategies that included the use of social support (see Felton *et al.*, this volume; Brewin *et al.*, 2000) and made use of an outreach model with embedded community members (with or without mental health training) wherever possible. Although this perspective generated much sound and fury in the super-specialized New York community initially, with much skepticism expressed about the capabilities of untrained laypersons, the scientific basis for this approach is reasonable (in that it overcomes a major source of stigma) and has a long tradition in disaster services. Simultaneously, treatment programs were attempting to expand capacity to treat the subgroup of persons who would suffer with serious mental disorders (e.g., PTSD).

Because these two approaches can seem diametrically opposed on the surface ("you can get better on your own with the help of friends and family" vs. "you should seek professional help"), they have been confounded in the treatment community, in the media, and even among experts in the field. It is our view that, after large-scale disaster and if there are preliminary data suggesting that community capacity to treat serious mental disorder will be exceeded, programs that aim to address both public health problems should be launched simultaneously. *Most importantly, research methodology should be embedded within such programs from the beginning so that some measure of quality assessment will be possible. Only this will allow the field of postdisaster intervention services to be advanced based on real-world outcomes.*

An effort to ensure that purported objectives are actually being met within a clinical program does not constitute "R"esearch in the traditional sense the

"R" word. In reality, most services programs prior to 9/11 did not routinely assess diagnosis and treatment progress, and after 9/11 the focus was on getting services to the community. Visionary leaders in government, like Sharon Carpinello and Chip Felton (New York State Office of Mental Health) and Lloyd Sederer (Division of Mental Hygiene, New York City) found ways to integrate evidence-based principles into systems, and to encourage clinicians to make use of simple assessment methodologies that allow a measure of quality control, and thus provide a rational basis for improving services.

Still, it is a trenchant critique of the services model in the US to note that *not one of these efforts can document that effective community services were in fact provided on a meaningful scale.*

This is of course a very easy criticism to launch, and an extremely difficult problem to address in the postdisaster environment, in the US (in which there is no centralized health care system), and in a multiethnic community (Marshall & Suh, 2003). Services researchers have documented, and are attempting to understand, the multiple barriers to moving effective treatments into the community, and to getting these treatments to the people who need them, and to assessing the outcome of these treatments once they have been successfully disseminated. To study all of these problems in the postdisaster environment, with no prior planning, we freely admit was too lofty a goal. We hope that these chapters, in documenting the process of outreach, implementation, and dissemination programs, can contribute to the services literature and advance this field, so that no other community will have to start from scratch in mounting such large-scale efforts.

REFERENCES

Al-Saffar, S., Borga, P. & Hallstrom T. (2002). Long-term consequences of unrecognised PTSD in general outpatient psychiatry. *Social Psychiatry and Psychiatric Epidemiology*, **37**, 580–585.

Al-Saffar, S., Borga, P., Edman, G. & Hallstrom, T. (2003). The aetiology of posttraumatic stress disorder in four ethnic groups in outpatient psychiatry. *Social Psychiatry and Psychiatric Epidemiology*, **38**, 456–462.

Brewin, C.R., Andrews, B. & Valentine, J.D. (2000). Meta-analysis of risk factors for posttraumatic stress disorder in trauma-exposed adults. *Journal of Consulting and Clinical Psychology*, **68**, 748–766.

Cohen-Silver, R., Holman, E.A., McIntosh, D.N., Poulin, M., Gil-Rivas, V. & Pizarro, J. (this volume). Coping with a national trauma: a nationwide longitudinal study of responses to the terrorist attacks of September 11th. In *9/11: Mental Health in the Wake of Terrorist Attacks*, eds. Y. Neria, R. Gross & R. Marshall. Cambridge, UK: Cambridge University Press.

Davidson, J. & Smith, R. (1990). Traumatic experiences in psychiatric outpatients. *Journal of Traumatic Stress*, **31**, 459–475.

Felton, C.J., Donahue, S., Lanzara, C.B., Pease, E.A. & Marshall, R.D. (this volume). Project liberty: responding to mental health needs after the World Trade Center's terrorist attacks. In *9/11: Mental Health in the Wake of Terrorist Attacks*, eds. Y. Neria, R. Gross & R. Marshall. Cambridge, UK: Cambridge University Press.

Galea, S., Ahren, J., Resnick, H. & Vlahov, D. (this volume). Posttraumatic stress symptoms in the general population after a disaster: implications for public health. In *9/11: Mental Health in the Wake of Terrorist Attacks*, eds. Y. Neria, R. Gross & R. Marshall. Cambridge, UK: Cambridge University Press.

Hoven, C.W., Mandell, D.J., Duarte, C.S., Wu, P. & Giordano, V. (this volume). An epidemiological response to disasters: the NYC board of education's post 9/11 needs assessment. In *9/11: Mental Health in the Wake of Terrorist Attacks*, eds. Y. Neria, R. Gross & R. Marshall. Cambridge, UK: Cambridge University Press.

Marshall, R.D. (this volume). The New York consortium for effective trauma treatment. In *9/11: Mental Health in the Wake of a Terrorist Attacks*, eds. Y. Neria, R. Gross & R. Marshall. Cambridge, UK: Cambridge University Press.

Marshall, R.D. & Suh, E.J. (2003). Contextualizing trauma: using evidence-based treatments in a multicultural community after 9/11. *Psychiatric Quarterly*, **74**(4), 401–420.

Neria, Y., Gross, R., Olfson, M., Gameroff, M., Das, A., Shea, S. & Weissman, M. (2005). PTSD in low-income, predominantly Hispanic, primary care patients in NYC one year after 9/11 attacks. In *9/11: Mental Health in the Wake of Terrorist Attacks*, eds. Y. Neria, R. Gross & R. Marshall. Cambridge, UK: Cambridge University Press.

Rosenthal, J. (this volume). The New York Times Company Foundation. In *9/11: Mental Health in the Wake of Terrorist Attacks*, eds. Y. Neria, R. Gross & R. Marshall. Cambridge, UK: Cambridge University Press.

Russell, B. (1931). *The Scientific Outlook*. New York, NY: W.W. Norton & Company.

Switzer, G.E., Dew, M.A., Thompson, K., Goycoolea, J.M., Derricott, T. & Mullins, S.D. (1999). Posttraumatic stress disorder and service utilization among urban mental health center clients. *Journal of Traumatic Stress*, **12**, 25–39.

New York area

16

PTSD in urban primary care patients following 9/11

Yuval Neria, Raz Gross, Mark Olfson, Marc J. Gameroff, Amar Das, Adriana Feder, Rafael Lantigua, Steven Shea and Myrna M. Weissman

Introduction

Mass violence disasters, especially terrorist events in urban areas, are hypothesized to have greater impact on mental health than either natural or technological disasters due to their intentional nature (Norris *et al.*, 2002). The density of the urban environment, its ethnic diversity, and expected support deterioration, might exacerbate the disaster effects (Norris, 2002). Studies focused on the exposure to terrorist events in recent years: the 2001 World Trade Center (WTC) disaster (Schuster *et al.*, 2001; Galea *et al.*, 2002; Schlenger *et al.*, 2002; Silver *et al.*, 2002; Vlahov *et al.*, 2002), and the 2000–2002 terrorist attacks in Israel (Bleich *et al.*, 2003), have documented significant psychological problems, in the short term, in both directly and indirectly exposed individuals.

A recent review concluded that the health effects of disasters are wide and adversely affect several aspects of health including generalized distress, psychiatric disorders, physical illness, and interpersonal problems (Norris *et al.*, 2002). Mass violence was found to have greater psychosocial impact than natural or technological disasters, due to its intentional character (Norris *et al.*, 2002). For example, 6 months following the Oklahoma bombing (North *et al.*, 1999) adults injured in that event had markedly elevated rates of post-disaster mental health disorders (45%), including post-traumatic stress disorder (PTSD, 34%).

Political terrorism, and especially suicide terrorism, has emerged as a highly detrimental international problem. As a well planned and executed violent event, suicide terrorism is deliberately intended to cause massive destruction and gruesome death; induce fear and helplessness; diminish safety and stability; weaken crucial social bonds; and disrupt the economic, political, and social order (Kaniasty & Norris, 2004; Neria *et al.*, 2005). For example, Bleich *et al.* (2003) have studied the effect of an ongoing exposure to suicide and other terrorism acts in Israel, and found significant signs of general distress together with a deterioration in a sense of safety.

The 9/11 attacks were aimed directly at two prominent symbols of the Western World, and shocked American society and the world community. The huge loss of human lives; unprecedented destruction; and the broad, live, continuous media coverage may have contributed to the impact of these events on the mental health of the general population. The impact may have been especially acute for specific populations including the bereaved, evacuees, rescue personnel, and clean-up workers, and those with fewer resources (North *et al.*, 2002).

As expected, all September 11 studies to-date have demonstrated elevated prevalence of 9/11-related stress symptoms. The first national survey (Schuster *et al.*, 2001), conducted 3–5 days after the attacks, used a sample of 560 adults (73% response rate) obtained by random digit dialing. The results indicated extensive PTSD symptoms across the nation. Specifically, 44% of the adults reported at least one of the five PTSD screening symptoms, and 90% reported at least some stress symptoms. Proximity to the epicenter of exposure was related to the severity of the emotional reaction.

A random-digit telephone survey of New Yorkers below 110th Street in Manhattan conducted 4–8 weeks after the attacks, reported that 7.5% of adults met provisional criteria for PTSD (Galea *et al.*, 2002). In addition, 9.7% of the sample reported symptoms of current depression while 3.7% met criteria for both disorders. Of special relevance to the proposed study, PTSD was significantly more common among Hispanics than non-Hispanics and among persons who had two or more stressors preceding 9/11. In addition, 10% of the respondents reported an increase in frequency of visits to a mental health professional in the month following 9/11, compared to the month before, and 3.4% reported new use of psychotropic medications during this time period (Galea *et al.*, 2002). Importantly to the proposed study, although the prevalence of PTSD symptoms was consistently higher among persons who were more directly affected by the attacks, a substantial number of persons who were not directly affected by the attacks also met criteria for probable PTSD.

A national, web-based community survey (Schlenger *et al.*, 2002) conducted 1–2 months after 9/11 attacks on a larger sample ($N = 2733$, 73% response rate) found the prevalence of current PTSD to be higher in the New York City (NYC) metropolitan area (11.2%) than in Washington, DC (4.0%). Being in NYC on the day of the attacks was associated with a 2.9 fold increase in the likelihood of PTSD.

A time-related decline in the rate of PTSD has also been observed in a longitudinal, nationwide study (Silver *et al.*, 2002). According to this web-based survey, 2 months after the attacks 17% of the population outside NYC experienced acute or post-traumatic stress symptoms; 6 months after the attacks prevalence had declined to 5.8%. Overall, the findings suggested persistent stress symptoms, across the nation and in persons who were, mostly, only indirectly exposed to the attacks.

No study to date has investigated the effects of WTC disaster in primary care patients. A greater understanding of the risk and protective factors for the development of PTSD in an exposed low-income immigrant primary care population will facilitate planning for targeted primary care-based interventions.

The aim of the study described in this chapter was to study a systematic sample of low-income, mostly Hispanic patients attending an urban general medicine clinic in NYC. The specific aims of this study were to: (1) estimate the current prevalence of patients who receive a positive screen results for current 9/11-related PTSD; (2) compare demographic, 9/11 trauma exposure, clinical, treatment, and service use characteristics of patients who screen positive for current PTSD with those who do not; and (3) report on comorbidity, impairment, and health functioning of screen positive patients.

Trauma and PTSD in primary care

As compared with the general population, poor, and ethnic populations are at increased risk for a range of mental disorders, including PTSD (Brewin *et al.*, 2000; Ortega & Rosenheck, 2000). Low-income minority populations also tend to disproportionably rely on primary care services for the provision of mental health care (Olfson & Pincus, 1996), and they are less likely to seek (Howard *et al.*, 1996) and to receive treatment from mental health specialists (Gallo *et al.*, 1995; Leaf *et al.*, 1998).

In recent years, it has become increasingly evident that individuals with trauma related mental health problems are likely to be seen in primary care (Fifer *et al.*, 1994; Dickinson *et al.*, 1998; Samson *et al.*, 1999; Stein *et al.*, 2000; Bruce *et al.*, 2001; Mcquaide *et al.*, 2001; Taubman-Ben-Ari *et al.*, 2001; Yang *et al.*, 2003). In one primary care study, PTSD was the most common anxiety disorder: 17% of the study group met criteria for PTSD (Fifer *et al.*, 1994). In a second study, 38.6% of primary care patients referred for mental health services met criteria for PTSD (Samson *et al.*, 1999). In a study of affluent primary care outpatients, Stein and colleagues found that 11.8% of the sample met criteria for PTSD (Stein *et al.*, 2000). Primary care studies in Israel ($n = 2975$) (Taubman-Ben-Ari *et al.*, 2001) and Taiwan ($n = 663$) (Yang *et al.*, 2003) have found PTSD in 9% and 11% of the cases, respectively.

Although considerable research has shown that a large percentage of people who go to their primary care doctor have a mental health diagnosis including PTSD, the psychosocial impact of mass violence events in urban area, such as 9/11 attacks, has not been studied in the primary care setting to date. To the best of our knowledge this is the first study to propose the examination of the psychological sequelae to mass violence in the primary care setting.

Ethnicity, acculturation, and PTSD

Ethnicity may be significantly related to the experience of large-scale trauma and its aftermath. For example, as compared to Whites, African Americans were found to be exposed to fewer traumatic events, but were more likely to develop PTSD (Green, 1990; Norris, 1992). Since Hispanics are now the largest minority in the USA, exploring the relationships between ethno-cultural factors and mental health is increasingly important (Ortega *et al.*, 2000). Recent literature suggests that Hispanics are more likely to be exposed to life stressors and adversities (Ruef *et al.*, 2000), and to suffer from psychiatric distress following the exposure than Whites (Penk *et al.*, 1981; Kulka *et al.*, 1990; Ortega & Rosenhack, 2000; Ruef *et al.*, 2000; Pole *et al.*, 2001; Perilla *et al.*, 2002).

Socio-economic status (SES) may also mediate the relationships between the exposure and PTSD symptoms and thus worthwhile to study. In the disaster literature, lower SES indicators (e.g., education, income, literacy, occupational status) were found to be related to adverse effects (e.g., Bolin & Klenow, 1988; Hanson *et al.*, 1995; Epstein *et al.*, 1998; Armenian *et al.*, 2000; Caldera *et al.*, 2001; Norris *et al.*, 2002).

African Americans and Hispanics are known to face elevated levels of stress (e.g., racism), but appear to have lower rates of PTSD than Hispanics (Kulka *et al.*, 1990; Galea *et al.*, 2002; Perilla *et al.*, 2002). It has been suggested that the increased rates of PTSD among Hispanics compared to their White and African American counterparts, may represent an over-expression of symptoms rather than a true increase in disorder prevalence (Ortega *et al.*, 2000).

A greater vulnerability to PTSD among Hispanics may be related to their higher level of fatalism and acculturative stress: their discomfort in dealing with members from other ethnic groups. If true, this might affect seeking social support and professional help in times of stress (Norris *et al.*, 2002). It has also been suggested that Blacks may feel more empowered to cope with adversities (Ruef *et al.*, 2000), and discrimination due to the Civil Rights and the "Black Power" movements.

Health utilization, trauma, and PTSD

The study of trauma, PTSD, and health utilization has been similarly focused on war veterans (Kulka *et al.*, 1990; Litz *et al.*, 1992; Marshall *et al.*, 1998; Deykin *et al.*, 2001). There is a dearth of relevant information concerning low-income ethnic minority patients. Post-9/11 research conducted by Galea *et al.* (2002) found that 10% of the respondents in their study of the general community in NYC, have increased the frequency of their visits to mental health professionals after September 11, and 3.4% have reported the use of new psychiatric medications in the month after September 11.

Another study (Rosenheck & Fontana, 2003) examined use of mental health services by veterans with PTSD after 9/11 attacks. They found no significant increase in the use of Veterans Administration (VA) services or change in the pattern of services for the treatment of PTSD or other mental disorders or in visits to psychiatric and non psychiatric clinics in NYC. An important limitation of this study, not present in our proposal, is use of registry database, and thus lack of information on symptoms, distress, and impairment. Another limitation of that study is lack of data on use of emergency and informal services. In our study data on emergency room (ER) visits will become available through cross-linkage to the hospital's computerized database; data on informal services will be obtained by means of structured questions.

Structural barriers, such as low rates of insurance and lack of providers have been suggested to impede access to care for low-income individuals and Hispanics (Norquist & Wells, 1991; Miranda *et al.*, 1996), and studies have emphasized the key role of cultural factors in modulating predisposing, enabling, and need-related barriers to care (Kleinman, 1980). Hispanics show significantly lower utilization than those with greater connection to mainstream US society, even after controlling for differences in socio-demographic and economic status, physical and mental health status, and type of insurance (Vega *et al.*, 1999).

Study design, recruitment, and sample characteristics

The study was conducted at the Associates in Internal Medicine (AIM) clinic of New York Presbyterian Hospital (Columbia Presbyterian Medical Center), New York. The AIM clinic is the faculty and resident group practice of the Division of General Medicine at College of Physicians and Surgeons of Columbia University. Each year AIM serves approximately 18,000 patients from the surrounding northern Manhattan community.

The initial study design for this survey took place before the 9/11 attacks, and did not include an assessment of trauma exposure and PTSD. Following the attacks we added questions assessing exposure to the WTC attacks and a PTSD instrument. All data forms were translated from English to Spanish and back by a bilingual team of mental health professionals. Institutional review boards of both Columbia University and The New York State Psychiatric Institute approved the survey methods and procedures, and a signed informed consent was obtained from all participants at the beginning of the interview.

Subject recruitment started on April 1, 2002, and was completed on January 16, 2003. Patients seeking primary care who presented to the AIM clinic waiting room, were invited to participate in the study. Eligible patients were between 18 and 70 years of age, had made at least one prior visit to the practice, could speak and understand

Spanish or English, and were waiting for scheduled face-to-face contact with their primary care physician. Patients were excluded from the study if their current general health status prohibited completion of the survey form.

A systematic sample of consecutive adult patients seeking primary care who presented to the waiting rooms of the AIM practice was invited to participate over the time period of 7–16 months after the 9/11 attacks. Eligible patients were between 18 and 70 years of age, had made at least one prior visit to the practice, could speak and understand Spanish or English, were waiting for scheduled appointment with a primary care physician, and were able to complete the survey. Of the 1118 patients who met eligibility criteria, 992 (88.7%) consented to participate, and of these, 930 (93.8%) provided detailed data with regard to their location on 9/11 and PTSD symptoms, and therefore comprise the analytic sample. All assessment forms were translated from English to Spanish and back-translated by a bilingual team of mental health professionals. The Spanish forms were reviewed and approved by the Hispanic Research and Recruitment Center at Columbia Presbyterian Medical Center. The Institutional Review Boards of the Columbia Presbyterian Medical Center and the New York State Psychiatric Institute approved the study protocol, and all participants gave informed written consent. Subject recruitment started on April 1, 2002, and was completed on January 16, 2003.

Study survey

All participants completed a history form to assess socio-demographic characteristics and family psychiatric history. Type of exposure to the 9/11 disaster was determined by questions inquiring whether the patient was in Lower Manhattan (below 14th Street); directly witnessed the WTC attacks; had a loved one or somebody close to them at the WTC during the attacks; knew somebody who was killed in the WTC attacks; was involved in the recovery efforts; and knew somebody who was involved in the recovery efforts. Exposure to trauma prior to 9/11/2001 was determined based on (1) a positive report of at least one trauma exposure from a modified version of the Life Events Scale (Kessler *et al.*, 1995) ("happened to me" or "witnessed it"); and (2) age of patient at which the "earliest exposure occurred" was at least 2 years earlier than the subject's current age, to verify that the exposure occurred prior to 9/11. An item following the Life Events Check List format was added to assess exposure to the plane Crash of Flight 587 to the Dominican Republic that crashed in Rockaway, New York, on November 12, 2001, killing all 265 passengers ("having a loved one or somebody close to you on the plane").

The PTSD Check List – Civilian Version (PCL-C) (Weathers *et al.*, 1993) was used to screen for probable current 9/11-related PTSD. The PCL-C consists of 17 items corresponding to each Diagnostic and Statistical Manual of Mental Disorders,

Fourth Edition (DSM-IV) PTSD symptom rated from 1 (not at all) to 5 (extremely) to the extent to which the symptom bothered the patient in the last month with regard to the WTC attacks. This instrument has been widely used as a PTSD screen and has been shown to have good internal consistency, high correlations with other measures of PTSD (Weathers et al., 1994; Blanchard et al., 1996; Andrykownsky et al., 1998; Forbes et al., 2001) and high diagnostic efficiency (Manne et al., 1998). Following a previous 9/11 survey (Schlenger et al., 2002), a cut-off score of 50 was used to determine a diagnosis of probable PTSD.

The survey forms included the Primary Care Evaluation of Mental Disorders (PRIME-MD) Patient Health Questionnaire (PHQ) (Spitzer et al., 1994) to assess current symptoms of DSM-IV Major Depression (MD), Panic Disorder (PD), Generalized Anxiety Disorder (GAD), and past-year probable alcohol abuse/dependence. A probable drug abuse/dependence section patterned after the PRIME-MD PHQ alcohol use disorder assessment was also given. Suicidal ideation was positive for subjects who reported on the PHQ that they had been bothered by "thoughts that you would be better off dead or thoughts of hurting yourself in some way" for at least several days in the last 2 weeks. There is good agreement between PHQ diagnoses and those of independent mental health professionals (for the diagnosis of any one or more PHQ disorder, kappa = 0.65; overall accuracy, 85%; sensitivity, 75%; and specificity, 90%) (Spitzer et al., 1999).

Physical and mental health functioning were measured with the Physical and Mental Component Summary scores of the Medical Outcome Study 12-Item Short Form Health Survey (SF-12) (Ware et al., 1996). Impairment was evaluated with the 10 point self-rated social life and family life/home responsibilities subscales of the Sheehan Disability Scale (0 = none, 1–3 = mild, 4–6 = moderate, 7–9 = marked, and 10 = extreme) (Leon et al., 1995). Significant impairment for each subscale was defined by a rating of 7 or greater. Because only 152 (20.0%) of the patients were gainfully employed, the work subscale of the Sheehan Disability Scale was not used in the following analyses. An assessment was conducted for the number of days in the past month that patients had missed work (paid or unpaid) or school. Work loss (yes or no) was based on missing seven or more days in these activities. Self-report information was collected on mental health diagnoses of first-degree family member(s) including "bipolar disorder", "manic depression", "depression", "anxiety/bad nerves", and/or "alcohol/drug use problems", or previous diagnosis of these same disorders given to the patient by a health professional. In addition, self-report information was collected on mental health treatment and hospitalization history. The latter section included information on past month use of psychotropic medication.

In order to examine whether patients with 9/11-related PTSD had increased utilization of services during the first year post-9/11, a cross-linkage to the Columbia

University Medical Center's computerized database enabled the analysis of data concerning (1) visits (number and dates) to the primary care clinic and to the ER (both general and psychiatric); and (2) information on hospitalizations (including admission and discharge dates) during this time frame.

Analytic strategy

Subjects with a PCL-C score of 50 or above were classified as having current PTSD. The rates of MD, PD, GAD and alcohol use were based on diagnostic algorithms for the PRIME-MD PHQ (Spitzer *et al.*, 1994; 1999). A similar algorithm was developed for drug use disorder.

Prevalence of current PTSD was stratified by age, gender, race/ethnicity, immigrant status, marital status (defined as married or cohabiting vs. not), educational attainment, annual household income, employment status, and family psychiatric history. Age was categorized into four groups: 18–44 years, 45–54 years, 55–64 years, and 65–70 years. Race/ethnicity was based on self-designated national origin and race. Patients were categorized as Hispanic if they identified their nation of origin as Spain or a Latin American country or if they chose to complete the study forms in Spanish. In addition, patients of Hispanic origin were divided into three groups (1) Dominicans, (2) Puerto Ricans, and (3) others. Non-Hispanic patients were divided into two groups: (1) Blacks and (2) Whites or others.

We restricted our analysis of post-9/11 health care utilization to patients who had received services at New York-Presbyterian Hospital at least 1 year prior to 9/11. Because of the small number of subjects with one or more ER visits or hospital admissions during the time frame examined, use of each of these services was coded as a binary outcome (1 = any, 0 = none).

Chi-square analysis was used to compare patients with and without PTSD on background variables that included demographic characteristics, presence of family psychiatric history, and presence of any pre-9/11 trauma. Fisher's exact test was used when any cell had an expected count less than 5. Binary logistic regression was used to assess the effect of three types of trauma exposure on the likelihood of PTSD (1 = present, 0 = absent): proximity to the WTC on 9/11 (3 = in the WTC or Lower Manhattan, 2 = in NYC, 1 = in the NYC area, 0 = outside the NYC area) and knowing someone killed by the WTC disaster (1 = yes, 0 = no). In subsequent analyses, we adjusted for the categorical variables sex, marital status, education, race/ethnicity, immigrant status, family psychiatric history, and exposure to at least one traumatic event prior to 9/11. Logistic regression was also used to assess the effect of PTSD (1 = present, 0 = absent) on other binary outcomes (other mental disorders, impairment and work loss, self-reported mental health treatment). In subsequent analyses, we adjusted for sex, marital status, education, race/ethnicity, immigrant status, family psychiatric history, exposure to at least one traumatic event prior to 9/11, proximity to the WTC on 9/11, and knowing someone who was killed by the WTC disaster. Impairment, work loss, and treatment outcomes were further adjusted for the presence of any current disorder other than PTSD (i.e., Major Depressive Disorder (MDD), GAD, PD, and/or alcohol or drug use disorder).

Because many of the outcomes in this study were relatively common (>10%), and odds ratios (ORs) are known to overestimate the relative risk (RR) in such instances, we converted all ORs and corresponding 95% confidence intervals (CIs) to RRs (regardless of the prevalence of the outcome) using the formula proposed by Zhang and Yu (1998). These RRs are always more conservative than the ORs from the logistic regression output, and provide a more accurate estimate of risk.

Linear regression was used to assess the effect of PTSD (1 = present, 0 = absent) on SF-12 scores expressed as unstandardized betas with 95% CIs. Further analyses adjusted for the same variables as the logistic regressions described above that had PTSD as the primary predictor.

We fit linear regression models to assess the effect of PTSD (1 = present, 0 = absent) on the number of outpatient visits made in the year after 9/11, controlling for the number of outpatient visits made in the year prior to 9/11. We used logistic regression to assess the effect of PTSD on the likelihood of ER visits in the year after 9/11 (1 = any, 0 = none), controlling for ER visits in the year prior to 9/11. Analysis of hospital admissions was analogous to that of ER visits.

Exploratory analysis of PTSD rates during each month of the study suggested that from the start of the study until the 1-year anniversary of 9/11 (i.e., September 11, 2002), the likelihood of PTSD gradually receded and leveled off after the anniversary. However, the number of patients with PTSD in any 1- or 2-month period was too small to allow a sufficiently powered test of trend based on these rates. Therefore, we used piecewise linear regression to test the slope of PCL-C scores across time during two periods: between study start on April 1, 2002, and the 1-year anniversary of 9/11 on September 11, 2002; and between September 12, 2002, and study end on January 16, 2003. We further assessed whether the pre-anniversary and post-anniversary trends (i.e., the two slopes) were equivalent.

All tests were two-tailed, and significance was set at 0.05. Statistical analyses were conducted with SAS software version 9.0 (SAS Institute Inc, Cary, NC).

Main findings

Sample characteristics and location during the attacks of 9/11/2001

The sample was composed primarily of low income, Hispanic patients, who were born outside of the USA and had little formal education. 69.6% of the patients were females; mean age was 51.2 (SD = 11.9) years; 55.3% had not graduated from high school; 75.9% reported an annual family income of less than $12,000; 70.0% had never married or were currently separated, divorced, or widowed, and only 20.0% of the patients reported they were paid workers; 81.1% of the sample had immigrated to the USA; 81.9% were of Hispanic origin, predominantly from the Dominican Republic (78.7%), followed by Puerto Rico (8.7%) and other Spanish-speaking countries (7.6%). Of the non-Hispanic patients, 73.2% were black. Notably, 38% of all patients reported a family psychiatric history and 62% reported pre-9/11 exposure to trauma.

The majority of the patients (78.2%) reported that they were in NYC during the 9/11 attacks and another 3.8% reported being in the WTC or in Lower Manhattan below 14th Street. More than a quarter (27.1%) reported knowing someone who was killed during the 9/11 attacks.

PTSD and sociodemographic and exposure characteristics

Seven to sixteen months after 9/11, a total of 4.7% of the sample (95% CI: 3.5–6.7%) had a positive screen for current 9/11-related PTSD (*hereafter referred to as PTSD*). PTSD was significantly related to being born outside of the USA, not being married or cohabiting, and having a family history of psychiatric disorders, and pre-9/11 trauma exposure (Table 16.1). No significant differences in PTSD were found between patients from Puerto Rico (3.0%; $n = 2/66$) as compared to the Dominican Republic (5.7%; $n = 34/600$) and to other Spanish-speaking countries (5.2%; $n = 3/58$) ($p = 0.76$; Fisher's exact test with df = 2)

Mean PCL-C scores in patients interviewed 7–12 months after the attacks ($n = 491$) significantly declined during this period ($t = -4.38$, $p < 0.0001$) (Figure 16.1). Starting at the first year anniversary (9/11/2002), PCL-C scores ($n = 439$) started to increase. We found a positive time trend ($t = 1.92, p = 0.055$). The two slopes (pre-anniversary and post-anniversary) were significantly different ($t = 3.13, p = 0.002$).

Proximity to the epicenter of the attacks was associated, but not significantly, with PTSD. A monotonic increase in the likelihood of PTSD was found: from 1.15% among patients who were outside NYC; to about 5% among patients who were in NYC/NYC area; and to 8.6% among patients who were in the WTC/Lower Manhattan area during the attacks (Table 16.2).

PTSD was more common among patients who reported that they lost a person due to the attacks of 9/11 compared to those who did not experience such loss (Table 16.2).

To test whether indirect exposure to the attacks is associated with PTSD independent of family psychiatric history and history of trauma, we examined the prevalence of probable PTSD in patients who were not directly exposed to the attacks and reported no family psychiatric history or past trauma exposure ($N = 178$). None of these participants screened positive for PTSD.

Table 16.1. Prevalence rates of current WTC-related PTSD, by patient background characteristics

Characteristic	Percentage	χ^2 (df = 1)	P value
Entire sample (N = 930)	**4.73**		
Age			
18–54 (n = 536)	5.22	0.68	0.41
55–70 (n = 394)	4.06		
Gender			
Female (n = 647)	5.41	2.17	0.14
Male (n = 283)	3.18		
Ethnicity			
Hispanic (n = 762)	5.25	2.51	0.11
Non-Hispanic (n = 168)	2.38		
Immigrant status			
Born outside of the USA (n = 754)	5.44	4.41	0.04
Born in the USA (n = 176)	1.70		
Marital status			
Separated/divorced, widowed, or never married (n = 631)	5.71	4.06	0.04
Married/cohabiting (n = 297)	2.69		
Education level			
Not a high school graduate (n = 509)	5.89	3.12	0.08
High school graduate (n = 412)	3.40		
Annual household income			
<$12,000 (n = 700)	5.14	1.50	0.22
≥$12,000 (n = 222)	3.15		
Gainfully employed			
No (n = 744)	5.11	1.17	0.28
Yes (n = 186)	3.23		
Family psychiatric history[a]			
Yes (n = 341)	8.21	15.45	<0.0001
No (n = 558)	2.51		
Any pre-9/11 trauma[b]			
Yes (n = 474)	7.38	19.49	<0.0001
No (n = 285)	0.35		

[a]First-degree family member(s) have been diagnosed with "bipolar disorder", "manic depression", "depression", "anxiety/bad nerves", and/or "alcohol/drug use problems".
[b]Data available for 759 subjects.

Psychiatric comorbidity

The majority of the patients with PTSD (79.6%) met criteria for a positive screen of one or more other mental disorder. The most frequent comorbid disorders were MD (63.6%); GAD (45.5%); and PD (18.6%) (Table 16.3). After adjustment for

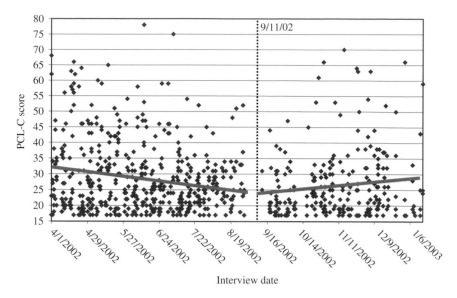

Figure 16.1 Each dot represents a PCL-C score for a single participant plotted above the date of the interview. Separate lines of best fit are shown for two periods (a) between study start on April 1, 2002, and the 1-year anniversary of 9/11 on September 11, 2002; and (b) between September 12, 2002, and study ends on January 16, 2003.

demographic and exposure covariates, PTSD remained strongly associated with each of the anxiety and mood disorders. One quarter (25.0%) of the patients with PTSD, as compared with 3.8% of those without PTSD, reported suicidal ideation at least some days during the previous 2 weeks (Table 16.3). After controlling for the presence of MDD, demographic, and exposure covariates, PTSD did not remain significantly associated with current suicidal ideation.

Impairment, functioning, and health

Significant social and family life impairment were more common among patients with PTSD than those without it (Table 16.3). Impairment in both areas remained strongly associated with PTSD after adjusting for demographic and exposure covariates and the presence of any current mental disorder.

Work loss of 1 week or more in the past month was also more commonly reported by patients with PTSD than by those without, but was not significantly associated with PTSD after controlling for demographic and exposure covariates and the presence of any current mental disorder (Table 16.3). Finally, mental and physical health-related quality of life were worse for those with PTSD than for those without PTSD (Table 16.3). The group difference in SF-12 Mental Component Summary scores remained statistically significant after controlling for demographic and exposure covariates and the presence of any current comorbid mental disorder.

Table 16.2. Rates of WTC-related PTSD stratified by type of exposure to the WTC attacks and the Crash of Flight 587

Exposure variable	PTSD+		Tests[a]			
	n	Percentage	χ^2 (df = 1)	P	Crude RR (95% CI)[b]	Adjusted RR (95% CI)[c]
Proximity to WTC during 9/11 attacks						
In the WTC or Lower Manhattan (n = 35)	3	8.57			7.45 (0.81, 42.01)	8.13 (0.71, 49.12)
In NYC (n = 692)	34	4.91	3.18[d]	0.08[d]	4.27 (0.60, 24.05)	4.15 (0.56, 24.20)
In the NYC area (n = 114)	6	5.26			4.58 (0.56, 27.82)	5.07 (0.60, 30.88)
Outside the NYC area (n = 87)	1	1.15			1.00 –	1.00 –
Loss in 9/11 and the Crash of Flight 587						
Know someone killed by the WTC disaster						
Yes (n = 252)	27	10.71	27.39	<0.0001	4.27 (2.40, 7.30)	4.46 (2.23, 8.43)
No (n = 677)	17	2.51			1.00 –	1.00 –
Loved one or someone close on Crash of Flight 587						
Yes (n = 231)	24	10.39	21.83	<0.0001	3.63 (2.06, 6.16)	3.16 (1.56, 6.12)
No (n = 699)	20	2.86			1.00 –	1.00 –

[a]RR of PTSD compared to those in the reference group (i.e., those with RR = 1.00), calculated from ORs using the following equation:

$$RR = OR/[(1 - P_o) + (P_o'OR)],$$ where P_o is the probability of PTSD among those in the reference group.

[b]Due to missing data, n = 929–930.

[c]RR is adjusted for sex, marital status (married/cohabiting vs. other); education (high school diploma: yes vs. no); race/ethnicity (Hispanic vs. black, non-Hispanic vs. white/other, non-Hispanic); born in the USA (yes vs. no); family psychiatric history (yes vs. no); and exposure to at least one traumatic event prior to 9/11 (yes vs. no). Due to missing data, n = 729–733.

[d]Mantel–Haenszel test of linear trend.

Table 16.3. Mental health diagnoses and impairment/health status among patients with and without WTC-related PTSD

Outcome	PTSD+ (n = 44)		PTSD− (n = 886)		Tests[a]	
	n	Percentage	N	Percentage	Crude RR (95% CI)[b]	Adjusted RR (95% CI)[c]
Mental disorder						
Major depressive disorder	28/44	63.64	173/880	19.66	3.24 (2.45, 3.91)	3.10 (2.06, 3.97)
Panic disorder	8/43	18.60	29/880	3.30	5.65 (2.69, 10.58)	3.96 (1.40, 9.62)
Generalized anxiety disorder	20/44	45.45	84/885	9.49	4.79 (3.23, 6.44)	3.35 (1.83, 5.35)
Alcohol or drug use disorder	6/44	13.64	66/848	7.78	1.75 (0.77, 3.59)	2.00 (0.76, 4.52)
Any of the disorders above	35/44	79.55	251/849	29.56	2.69 (2.19, 3.02)	2.56 (1.84, 3.01)
Suicidal ideation	11/44	25.00	33/881	3.75	6.68 (3.58, 11.14)	1.89 (0.71, 4.71)[d]
Impairment						
Social impairment	24/33	72.73	127/867	14.65	4.96 (3.74, 5.83)	3.68 (2.03, 5.21)[e]
Family life impairment	22/39	56.41	105/872	12.04	4.68 (3.32, 5.94)	3.53 (1.94, 5.33)[e]
Work loss						
At least 7 days lost in past month	24/32	75.00	164/566	28.98	2.59 (1.96, 3.01)	1.48 (0.76, 2.30)[e]

	n	$M \pm SD$	n	$M \pm SD$	β (95% CI)[f]	Adjusted β (95% CI)[c]
Health/functioning						
SF-12 Mental component summary	44	31.67 ± 10.22	863	46.58 ± 12.02	−14.89 (−18.51, −11.27)	−5.44 (−9.02, −1.86)[e]
SF-12 Physical component summary	44	32.63 ± 9.91	863	40.11 ± 11.43	−7.48 (−10.93, −4.03)	−3.62 (−7.63, +0.39)[e]

Mental disorders and suicidal ideation were assessed with the PRIME-MD PHQ. Impairment was assessed with the Sheehan Disability Scale; scores ≥ 7 (marked or extreme impairment) on the social and family life subscales were taken to indicate impairment. Health/functioning was assessed with the SF-12.

[a]RR for those with (vs. without) PTSD, calculated from ORs using the following equation: RR = OR/[$(1 - P_o) + (P_o \text{OR})$], where P_o is the probability of the outcome among those without PTSD.

[b]Due to missing data, $n = 892–929$, except for the "Work Loss" outcome ($n = 598$).

[c]RR is adjusted for sex; marital status (married/cohabiting vs. other); education (high school diploma: yes vs. no); race/ethnicity (Hispanic vs. black, non-Hispanic vs. white/other, non-Hispanic) ("to overcome estimation problems due to small cells, race/ethnicity was collapsed to "Hispanic" vs. "non-Hispanic" for the PD outcome); born in the USA (yes vs. no); family psychiatric history (yes vs. no); proximity to the WTC on 9/11/01 (see Table 16.2 for description of the four levels); know someone killed by the WTC disaster (yes vs. no); loved one or someone close on Crash of Flight 587 (yes vs. no); and exposure to at least one traumatic event prior to 9/11 (yes vs. no). Due to missing data, $n = 677–726$, except for the "Work Loss" outcome ($n = 519$).

[d]Adjusted also for the presence of MD.

[e]Adjusted also for the presence of at least one of the four listed mental disorders.

[f]Expected score difference for those with PTSD (lower scores denote worse health).

Mental health treatment and utilization of medical services

One-half of the patients (50.0%) with PTSD reported receiving mental health treatment and 69.8% reported taking a prescribed psychotropic medication in the last month. The most commonly reported medications were antidepressants (64.3%) (Table 16.4). A history of previous mental health hospitalization was significantly more commonly reported by patients with PTSD than those without PTSD. In logistic regression models that adjusted for demographic and exposure covariates, PTSD remained significantly associated with the use of prescribed psychotropic medications and antidepressant drug and previous mental health hospitalization.

9/11-related current PTSD was not associated with making an ER visit, being admitted to a hospital, or the number of outpatient visits made during the 12-month post-9/11 period, in either the crude or adjusted analyses.

Discussion

Nearly 5% of participants at an urban general medicine clinic screened positive for current 9/11-related PTSD approximately 1 year after the attacks of 9/11. This estimated prevalence exceeds previously reported estimates of probable PTSD (1.5%) found 6 months after 9/11 in NYC (Galea *et al.*, 2003). The high estimated prevalence of 9/11-related probable PTSD in this clinical setting (4.7%) may be related to extensive exposure to pre-9/11 trauma and family psychiatric history, as well as immigrant and marital status of this population. In a community survey in NYC conducted 6 months after 9/11, the prevalence of PTSD was the highest (15.1%) among participants who experienced four or more lifetime stressors before 9/11 (Galea *et al.*, 2003). In our clinical sample nearly 6 in 10 patients reported pre-9/11 trauma, and the rate of probable PTSD was significantly associated with exposure to pre-9/11 trauma. These findings are consistent with both community and clinical studies conducted before 9/11 (Breslau *et al.*, 1998; Bromet *et al.*, 1998; North *et al.*, 1999; Brewin *et al.*, 2000; Neria *et al.*, 2002; Norris *et al.*, 2002; Galea *et al.*, 2003).

While community studies in NYC suggested a rapid decline and diminished rates of PTSD over the 6 months after 9/11 attacks, our findings suggest that a significant proportion of this sample of NYC residents seeking primary care, continued to have PTSD associated with substantial functional impairment 7–16 months after the attacks. Similar to the pattern observed in previous studies (Galea *et al.*, 2002; Silver *et al.*, 2002) our findings indicate a steady decline in the prevalence of PTSD over time, but notably, starting at the 1-year anniversary (9/11/2002) an upward trend in PCL-C scores was observed. This finding might reflect the so-called "anniversary reaction", possibly related to the massive media coverage of the 9/11 events around the 1-year anniversary. The graphic documentaries of the

Table 16.4. Mental health treatment in the past month, and visits in the first year after WTC attacks, among patients with and without WTC-related PTSD

Outcome	PTSD + (n = 44)		PTSD − (n = 886)		Tests[a]	
	N	Percentage	n	Percentage	Crude RR (95% CI)[b]	Adjusted RR (95% CI)[c]
Mental health treatment (self-report)						
Past month						
Mental health treatment	21/42	50.00	155/882	17.57	2.85 (1.98, 3.71)	2.32 (1.37, 3.42)
Took a "prescribed medication"	30/43	69.77	155/876	17.69	3.94 (3.05, 4.63)	3.40 (2.26, 4.38)
Took an antidepressant drug	27/42	64.29	142/872	16.28	3.95 (2.97, 4.77)	3.29 (2.09, 4.42)
Took an antimanic drug	2/42	4.76	14/867	1.61	2.95 (0.67, 11.48)	2.82 (0.50, 13.51)
Took an antipsychotic drug	8/42	19.05	23/867	2.65	7.18 (3.37, 13.60)	3.12 (0.91, 9.31)
Lifetime						
Psychiatric admission	18/44	40.91	77/885	8.70	4.70 (3.06, 6.54)	3.73 (2.00, 6.00)
Health services in the year after 9/11[d]						
ER visits, any	11/23	47.83	192/467	41.11	1.24 (0.73, 1.73)[e]	0.66 (0.26, 1.32)[e]
Hospital admissions, any	19/23	17.39	375/467	19.49	0.88 (0.33, 2.01)[e]	0.48 (0.06, 2.36)[e]

(*Cont.*)

Table 16.4. (*Continued*)

	N	M ± SD	n	M ± SD	β (95% CI)[f]	Adjusted β (95% CI)[c]
Primary care visits	23	7.43 ± 3.75	467	7.58 ± 5.47	−0.72 (−2.38, +0.93)[e]	−0.11 (−2.08, +1.86)[e]

[a]RR for those with (vs. without) PTSD, calculated from ORs using the following equation:

$$RR = OR/[(1 - P_o) + (P_o \times OR)],$$ where P_o is the probability of the outcome among those without PTSD.

[b]Due to missing data, n = 909–929 for the "Mental health treatment (self-report)" outcomes, and n = 490 for the "Health services in the year after 9/11" outcomes.

Outcome	PTSD + (n = 44)		PTSD − (n = 886)		Tests[a]	
	N	Percentage	n	Percentage	Crude RR (95% CI)[b]	Adjusted RR (95% CI)[c]

[c]ORs are adjusted for sex; marital status (married/cohabiting vs. other); education (high school diploma: yes vs. no); race/ethnicity (Hispanic vs. black, non-Hispanic vs. white/other, non-Hispanic); born in the USA (yes vs. no); family psychiatric history (yes vs. no); proximity to the WTC on 9/11/01 (see Table 16.2 for description of the four levels) (to overcome estimation problems due to small cells, proximity was recoded to "In NYC" vs. "Outside of NYC" for the outcome "Took an antipsychotic drug", and proximity was omitted for the outcome "Took an antimanic drug"); know someone killed by the WTC disaster (yes vs. no); loved one or someone close on Crash of Flight 587 (yes vs. no); and exposure to at least one traumatic event prior to 9/11 (yes vs. no). Due to missing data, n = 715–727 for the "Mental health treatment (self-report)" outcomes, and n = 358 for the "Health services in the year after 9/11" outcomes.

[d]Visit data are presented for subjects who were locatable in the computerized medical records database and who were found to have made at least one visit (outpatient, emergency, and/or inpatient) prior to September 11, 2000 (i.e., a year prior to the 9/11 disaster).

[e]Adjusted also for service use during the 12 months prior to the 9/11 attacks: for ER visits, any (yes vs. no); for hospital admissions, any (yes vs. no); and for outpatient visits, the number of visits.

[f]Expected difference in number of visits for those with PTSD.

attacks entailed in this coverage, as well as detailed accounts of bereaved, evacuees, rescue workers, and witnesses might have activated or exacerbated PTSD symptoms in a significant number of individuals to either meet full diagnostic criteria in persons with a partial syndrome or trigger a new onset of PTSD. Further research is needed to clarify this finding.

Nationwide post-9/11 surveys suggest that when disaster strikes indirect exposure might be associated with PTSD (e.g., Silver *et al.*, 2002). Our findings suggest that indirect exposure to the attacks by itself was not associated with PTSD among patients who did not report pre-9/11 trauma and/or family psychiatric history. These results are consistent with disaster (North *et al.*, 1999; Norris *et al.*, 2002; Hoven *et al.*, 2005) and combat (Solomon *et al.*, 1994) studies documenting a relationship between trauma severity and PTSD.

Previous research at our clinic (Olfson *et al.*, 2000) has found high rates of MD and suicidal ideation. The current study found that a majority of participants with current probable PTSD had comorbid MDD (64%), GAD (45%), and PD (19%). PTSD is associated with significant disability (Yehuda, 2002). Many patients with chronic PTSD are not able to function in work and social activities and they remained impaired despite maintenance treatment (Marshall & Cloitre, 2000). Our study demonstrates that primary care patients who screen positive for PTSD also experience significant disability in health, social, and family functioning even after adjusting for the presence of exposure to trauma both before and during 9/11 and other mental disorders.

Findings from the general population and war veterans suggest that visits to mental health professionals and use of psychiatric drugs decreased over time following 9/11 (Galea *et al.*, 2002; Boscarino *et al.*, 2003, 2004) or were unchanged (Rosenheck & Fontana, 2003; Druss *et al.*, 2004). Findings from this primary care population suggest that while self reported use of medication increased after 9/11, the administrative records from this population indicate that PTSD is not associated with increased hospital admissions, emergency care use, or outpatient care during the first year after the 9/11 attacks. The accuracy of these self reports remains uncertain. Adults who report high levels of distress tend to report more mental health care than can be confirmed in administrative records (Rhodes *et al.*, 2002, Rhodes & Fung, 2004).

Taken together, these findings highlight the specific needs for health care associated with post-disaster psychopathology among low-income Hispanic primary care patients. Because poor and ethnic populations tend to avoid seeking (Howard *et al.*, 1996) or receiving treatment from mental health specialists (Gallo *et al.*, 1995; Leaf *et al.*, 1998), and disproportionately rely on primary care services for the provision of their mental health care (Olfson *et al.*, 1996), our findings underscore the importance of developing post-trauma care for affected individuals in general medical practices, especially when disasters strike minority communities (Lecrubier, 2004).

Limitations

The study has several limitations. First, self-report of traumatic exposure is subject to recall bias, and it is possible that some participants may have attributed PTSD symptoms to the 9/11 attacks that were actually more closely related to other traumatic events. Second, the computerized database that recorded the utilization of services of the patients in this sample is limited to Columbia University Medical Center and so does not capture services delivered by other providers. However, people in this community tend to be highly dependent on the university hospital services and therefore it is likely that the medical records provide a reasonable index of total medical care use. Third, our outcomes might be affected by the small number of patients with PTSD, which could render the results statistically unstable. However, the precise assessment of PTSD via face-to-face interview by mental health professionals, using a validated and reliable instrument, and the use of continuous scores when statistical power was limited, helped preserve statistical power. Fourth, because our survey assessed current PTSD, it undoubtedly missed patients that had 9/11 PTSD that resolved prior to survey completion who did not seek treatment. However, this sample provides an important opportunity to learn about chronic, persistent post-disaster PTSD. Last, because the study was undertaken in an urban general medical practice serving a low-income population, the findings may not be generalizable to primary care settings with different populations (Blazer *et al.*, 1985; Bruce *et al.*, 1991).

Our findings have clinical implications. Primary care patients from vulnerable populations, present in general medical settings, are likely to experience PTSD associated with long-term and clinically significant symptoms and functional impairment following large-scale events (e.g., Stein *et al.*, 2000). In order to recognize PTSD in primary care, physicians and mental health professionals need to obtain a detailed trauma history (Lecrubier, 2004; Engel, 2005). Timely interventions in patients who have been detected with exposure to trauma and manifest with PTSD symptoms in the aftermath of large scale disasters could prevent long-term, chronic morbidity.

Acknowledgements

The study reported in this chapter was supported by grants from the National Institute of Mental Health (1RO1 MHO72833-01; Yuval Neria), the National Association of Schizophrenia and Depression (NARSAD; Yuval Neria) Eli Lilly & Company (Myrna M. Weissman) and Glaxo Welcome (Adriana Feder).

REFERENCES

Andrykownsky, M.A., Cordova, M.J., Studtz, J.L.& Miller, T.W. (1998). Posttraumatic stress disorder after treatment for breast cancer: prevalence of diagnosis and use of the PTSD Check List – Civilian Version (PCL-C) as a screening instrument. *Journal of Consulting and Clinical Psychology*, **66**, 586–590.

Armenian, H., Morikawa, M., Melkonian, A., Hovanesian, Haroutunian, N., Saigh, P., Akiskal, K. & Akiskal, H.S. (2000). Loss as determinant of PTSD in a cohort of adult survivors of the 1988 earthquake in Armenia: implications for policy. *Acta Psychiatria Scandinavia*, **102**, 58–64.

Blanchard, E.B., Jones-Alexander, J., Buckley, T.C. & Forneris, C.A. (1996). Psychometric properties of the PTSD Check List (PCL). *Behavioral Research Therapy*, **34**, 669–673.

Blazer, D., George, L.K., Landerman, R., Pennybacker, M., Melville, M.L., Woodbury, M., Manton, K.G., Jordan, K. & Locke, B. (1985). Psychiatry disorders: A rural/urban comparison. *Archives of General Psychiatry*, **48**, 470–474.

Bleich, A., Gelkopf, M. & Solomon, Z. (2003). Exposure to terrorism, stress-related mental health symptoms, and coping behaviors among a nationally representative sample in Israel. *Journal of the American Medical Association*, **290**, 612–620.

Bolin, R. & Klenow, D. (1988). Older people in disaster: a comparison of black and white victims. *International Journal of Aging and Human Development*, **26**, 29–43.

Boscarino, J., Galea, S., Adams, R., Ahern, J., Resnick, H. & Vlahov, D. (2004). Mental health service and medication use in New York City after the September 11, 2001, terrorist attack. *Psychiatric Services*, **55**, 274–283.

Boscarino, J.A., Galea, S., Ahern, J., Resnick, H. & Vlahov D. (2003) Psychiatric medication use among Manhattan residents following the World Trade Center disaster. *Journal of Traumatic Stress*, **16**, 301–306.

Breslau, N., Kessler, R.C., Chico, T.H.D., Schultz, L.R., Davis, G.C. & Andreski, P. (1998). Trauma and posttraumatic stress disorder in the community: the 1996 Detroit Area Survey of Trauma. *Archives of General Psychiatry*, **55**, 626–632.

Brewin, C.R., Andrews, B. & Valentine, J.D. (2000). Meta-analysis of risk factors for post-traumatic stress disorder in trauma-exposed adults. *Journal of Consulting and Clinical Psychology*, **68**, 748–766.

Bromet, E., Sonnega, A. & Kessler, R.C. (1998). Risk factors for DSM-III-R posttraumatic stress disorder: findings from the National Comorbidity Survey. *American Journal of Epidemiology*, **147**, 353–361.

Bruce, M.L., Takeuchi, D.T. & Leaf, P.J. (1991). Poverty and psychiatric status: Longitudinal evidence from the New Haven Epidemiologic Catchment Area Study. *Archives of General Psychiatry*, **48**, 470–474.

Bruce, S.E., Weisberg, R.B., Dolan, R.T., Machan, J.T., Kessler, R.C., Manchester, G., Culpepper, L. & Keller, M.B. (2001). Trauma and posttraumatic stress disorder in primary care patients. *Journal of Clinical Psychiatry*, **3**, 211–217.

Caldera, T., Palma, L., Penayo, U. & Kullgren, G. (2001). Psychological impact of Hurricane Mitch in Nicaragua in a one-year perspective. *Social Psychiatry and Psychiatric Epidemiology*, **36**(3), 108–114.

Deykin, E.Y., Keane, T.M., Kaloupek, D., Fincke, G., Rothendler, J., Siegfried, M. & Creamer, K. (2001). Posttraumatic stress disorder and the use of health services. *Psychosomatic Medicine*, **63**, 835–841.

Dickinson, M.L., Verolin III, D.G., Dickinson, W.P. & Candib, L.M. (1998). Complex posttraumatic stress disorder: evidence from the primary care setting. *General Hospital Psychiatry*, **20**, 214–224.

Druss, B.G. & Marcus, S.C. (2004). Use of psychotropic medications before and after September 11, 2001. *American Journal of Psychiatry*, **161**, 1377–1383.

Epstein, R.S., Fullerton, C.S. & Ursano, R.J. (1998). Posttraumatic stress disorder following an air disaster: a prospective study. *American Journal of Psychiatry*, **155**(7), 934–938.

Engel, C.C. (2005). Improving primary care for military personnel and veterans with posttraumatic stress disorder: The road ahead. *General Hospital Psychiatry*, **27**, 158–160.

Fifer, S.K., Mathias, S.D., Patrick, D.L., Mazonson, P.D., Lubeck, D.P. & Buesching, D.P. (1994). Untreated anxiety among adult primary care patients in a health maintenance organization. *Archives of General Psychiatry*, **51**, 740–750.

Forbes, D., Creamer, M. & Biddie, D. (2001). The validity of the PTSD Check-List as a measure of symptomatic change in combat-related PTSD. *Behavioral Research Therapy*, **39**, 977–986.

Galea, S., Ahern, J., Resnick, H., Kilpatrick, D., Bucuvalas, M., Gold, J. & Vlahov, D. (2002). Psychological sequelae of the September 11 terrorist attacks in New York City. *New England Journal of Medicine*, **346**, 982–987.

Galea, S., Vlahov, D., Resnick, H., Ahern, J., *et al.* (2003). Trends of probable post-traumatic stress disorder in New York City after September 11 terrorist attacks. *American Journal of Epidemiology*, **158**, 514–524.

Gallo, J.J., Marino, S., Ford, D. & Anthony, J.C. (1995). Filters on the pathway to mental health care. II: Sociodemographic factors. *Psychology Medicine*, **25**, 1149–1160.

Green, B.L. (1990). Defining trauma: terminology and generic stressor dimensions. *Journal of Applied Social Psychology*, **20**, 1632–1642.

Hanson, R.F., Kilpatrick, D.G., Freedy, J.R. & Saunders, B.E. (1995). Los Angeles County after the 1992 civil disturbances: degree of exposure and impact on mental health. *Journal of Consulting and Clinical Psychology*, **63**(6), 987–996.

Howard, K.I., Corniolle, T.A., Lyons, J.S., Vessey, J.T., Lueger, R.J. & Saunders, S.M. (1996). Patterns of mental health service utilization. *Archives of General Psychiatry*, **53**, 696–703.

Kaniasty, K. & Norris, F.H. (2004). Social support in the aftermath of disasters, catastrophes, and acts of terrorism: altruistic, overwhelmed, uncertain, antagonistic, and patriotic communities. In *Bioterrorism: Psychological and Public Health Interventions*, eds. R. Ursano, A. Norwood & C. Fullerton. Cambridge, UK: Cambridge University Press.

Kessler, R.C., Sonnega, A., Bromet, E., Hughes, M. & Nelson, C.B. (1995). Posttraumatic stress disorder in the National Comorbidity Survey. *Archives of General Psychiatry*, **52**(12), 1048–1060.

Kleinman, A. (1980). Major conceptual and research issues for cultural (anthrological) psychiatry. *Culture Medicine and Psychiatry*, **4**, 3–13.

Kulka, R.A., Schlenger, W.E., Fairbank, J.A., Hough, R.L., Jordan, B.K., Marmar, C.R. & Weiss, D.S. (1990). *Trauma and the Vietnam War Generation: Report of the Findings from the National Vietnam Veterans Readjustment Study*. New York: Brunner/Mazel.

Leaf, P.J., Bruce, M.L., Tischler, G.L., Freeman Jr., D.H., Weissman, M.M. & Myers, J.K. (1998). Factors affecting the utilization of specialty and general medical mental health services. *Medical Care*, **26**, 9–26.

Lecrubier, Y. (2004). PTSD in primary care: a hidden diagnosis. *Journal of Clinical Psychiatry*, **65**, 49–54.

Leon, A.C., Olfson, M., Broadhead, W.E., Barrett, J.E., Blacklow, R.S., Keller, M.B., Higgins, E.S. & Weissman, M.W. (1995). Prevalence of mental disorders in primary care: implications for screening. *Archives of Family Medicine*, **5**, 857–861.

Litz, B.T., Keane, T.M., Fisher, L., Mark, B. & Monaco, V. (1992). Physical health complaints in combat-related post-traumatic stress disorder: a preliminary report. *Journal of Traumatic Stress*, **5**, 131–141.

Manne, S.L., Du Hamel, K., Galleli, K., Sorgen, K. & Redd, W.H. (1998). Posttraumatic stress disorder among mothers of pediatric cancer survivors: diagnosis, comorbidity and utility of the PTSD CheckList as a screening instrument. *Journal of Pediatric Psychology*, **23**, 357–366.

Marshall, R.D. & Cloitre, M. (2000). Maximizing treatment outcome in PTSD: An empirically-informed rational for combine psychotherapy with parmacotherapy. *Cement Psychiatry Reports*, **2**, 335–340.

Marshall, R.P., Jorm, A.F., Grayson, D.A. & O'Toole, B.I. (1998). Posttraumatic stress disorder and other predictors of health care consumption by Vietnam veterans. *Psychiatric Services*, **49**, 1609–1611.

Mcquaide, J.R., Pedrellui, P., McCahill, M.E. & Stein, M.B. (2001). Reported trauma, post-traumatic stress disorder and major depression among primary care patients. *Psychological Medicine*, **31**, 1249–1257.

Miranda, J., Azocar, F., Organista, K.C., Muñoz, R.F. & Lieberman, A. (1996). Recruiting and retaining low-income Latinos in psychotherapy research. *Journal of Consulting and Clinical Psychology*, **64**, 868–874.

Neria, Y., Bromet, E.J., Sievers, S., Lavelle, J. & Fochtman, L.J. (2002). Trauma exposure and post-traumatic stress disorder in psychosis: findings from a first-admission cohort. *Journal of Consulting and Clinical Psychology*, **70**, 246–251.

Neria, Y., Roe, D., Beit Hallahmi, B., Mneimneh, H., Balaban, A. & Marshall. R.D. (2005). The Al Qaeda 9/11 instructions: a Study in the construction of religious martyrdom. *Religion*. **35**(1), 1–11.

Norquist, G. & Wells, K. (1991). Mental health needs of the uninsured. *Archives of General Psychiatry*, **48**, 475–478.

Norris, F.H. (1992). Epidemiology of trauma: frequency and impact of different potentially traumatic events on different demographic groups. *Journal of Consulting and Clinical Psychology*, **60**(3), 409–418.

Norris, F.H. (2002). Disasters in urban context. *Journal of Urban Public Health*, **79**, 308–314.

Norris, F.H., Friedman, M., Watson, P., Byrne, C., Diaz, E. & Kaniasty, K. (2002). 60,000 disaster victims speak. Part 1: an empirical review of the empirical literature, 1981–2001. *Psychiatry*, **65**, 207–239.

North, C.S., Nixon, S.J., Shariat, S., Mallonee, S., McMillen, J.C., Spitznagel, E.L. & Smith, E.M. (1999). Psychiatric disorders among survivors of the Oklahoma City bombing. *Journal of the American Medical Association*, **282**(8), 755–762.

North, C.S., Tivis, L., McMillen, J.C., Pfefferbaum, B., Cox, J., Spiznagel, E.L., Bunch, K., Schorr, J. & Smith G.M. (2002). Coping, functioning, and adjustment of rescue workers after the Oklahoma City bombing. *Journal of Traumatic Stress*, **15**, 171–175.

Olfson, M., Broadhead, W.E., Weissman, M.M. Leon, A.C., Farber, L., Hoven, C. & Kathol, R. (1996). Subthreshold psychiatric symptoms in a primary care group practice. *Archives of General Psychiatry*, **53**, 880–886.

Olfson, M. & Pincus, H.A. (1996). Outpatient mental health care in nonhospital settings: distribution of patients across provider groups. *American Journal of Psychiatry*, **153**, 1353–1356.

Olfson, M., Shea, S., Feder, A., Fuentes, M., Nomura, Y., Gameroff, M. & Weissman, MM. (2000). Prevalence of anxiety, depression, and substance use disorders in an urban general medicine practice. *Archives of Family Medicine*, **9**, 876–883.

Ortega, A.N. & Rosenheck, R. (2000). Posttraumatic stress disorder among Hispanic Vietnam veterans. *American Journal of Psychiatry*, **157**, 615–619.

Ortega, A.N., Rosenheck, R., Alegria, M. & Desai, R.A. (2000). Acculturation and the lifetime risk of psychiatric and substance use disorders among Hispanics. *Journal of Nervous and Mental Disorders*, **188**, 728–735.

Penk, W.E., Rabinowitz, B., Roberts, W.R., Patterson, E.T., Dolan, M.P. & Atkins, H.G. (1981). Adjustment differents among male substance abusers varying in degree of combat experience in Vietnam. *Journal of Consulting and Clinical Psychology*, **49**, 426–437.

Perilla, J., Norris. F. & Lavizzo, E. (2002). Ethnicity, culture, and disaster response: identifying and explaining ethnic differences in PTSD six months after Hurricane Andrew. *Journal of Social and Clinical Psychology*, **21**, 20–45.

Pole, N., Best, S.R., Weiss, D.S., Metzler, T., Liberman, A.M., Fagan, J. & Marmar, C.R. (2001). Effects of gender and ethnicity on duty-related posttraumatic stress symptoms among urban police officers. *Journal of Nervous and Mental Disorders*, **189**, 442–448.

Rhodes, A.E. & Fung, K. (2004). Self-reported use of mental health services versus administrative records: Care of recall. *International Journal of Methods of Psychiatric Research*, **13**, 165–175.

Rhode, A.E., Lin, E. & Mustard, C.A. (2002). Self-reported use of mental health services versus administrative records: should we are? *International Journal of Methods of Psychiatric Research*, **11**, 125–133.

Rosenheck, R. & Fontana, A. (2003). Use of mental health services by veterans with PTSD after the terrorist attacks of September 11. *American Journal of Psychiatry*, **160**, 1684–1690.

Ruef, A.M., Litz, B.T. & Schlenger, W.E. (2000). Hispanic ethnicity and risk for combat-related posttraumatic stress disorder. *Cultural Diversity and Ethnic Minority Psychology*, **6**, 235–515.

Samson, A.Y., Bensen, S., Beck, A., Price, D. & Nummer, C. (1999). Posttraumatic stress disorder in primary care. *Family Practice*, **48**, 222–227.

Schlenger, W.E., Caddell, J.M., Ebert, L., Jordan, B.K., Rourke, K.M., Wilson, D., Thalji, L., Dennis, J.M., Fairband, J.A. & Kulka, R.A. (2002). Psychological reactions to terrorist attacks: findings from the national study of Americans' reactions to September 11. *Journal of the American Medical Association*, **288**, 581–588.

Schuster, M.A., Stein, B.D., Jaycox, L.H., Collins, R.L., Marshall, G.N., Elliott, M.N., Zhou, A.J., Kanouse, D.E., Morrison, J.L. & Berry, S.H. (2001). A National Survey of stress reactions after the September 11, 2001 terrorist attacks. *New England Journal of Medicine*, **345**, 1507–1512.

Silver, R.C., Holman, E.A., McIntosh, D.M., Poulin, M. & Gil-Rivas, V. (2002). Nationwide longitudinal study of psychological responses to September 11. *Journal of the American Medical Association*, **288**, 1235–1244.

Spitzer, R.L., Williams, J.B.W., Kroenke, K., Linzer, M., DeGruy, F.V. 3rd, Hahn, S.R., Brodys, D. & Johnson, J.G. (1994). Utility of a new procedure for diagnosing mental disorders in primary care: The PRIME-MD 1000 Study. *Journal of the American Medical Association*, **272**, 1749–1756.

Spitzer, R.L., Kroenke, K. & Williams, J.B.W. (1999). The Patient Health Questionnaire Primary Care Study Group: validation and utility of a self-report version of PRIME-MD: The PHQ Primary Care Study. *Journal of the American Medical Association*, **282**, 1737–1744.

Stein, M.B., McQuaid, J.R., Pedrelli, P., Lenox, R. & McCahill, M.E. (2000). Posttraumatic stress disorder in the primary care medical setting. *General Hospital Psychiatry*, **22**, 261–269.

Taubman-Ben-Ari, O., Rabinowitz, J.R., Feldman, D. & Vaturi, R. (2001). Post-traumatic stress disorder in primary care settings: prevalence and physicians' detection. *Psychological Medicine*, **31**, 555–560.

Vega, W.A., Kolody, B., Aguilar Gaxiola, S. & Catalano, R. (1999). Gaps in service utilization by Mexican Americans with mental health problems. *American Journal of Psychiatry*, **156**, 928–934.

Vlahov, D., Galea, S., Resnick, H., Ahern, J., Boscarino, J.A., Bucuvalas, M., Gold, J. & Kirkpatricks, D. (2002). Increased use of cigarettes, alcohol, and marijuana among Manhattan, New York, residents after the September 11th terrorist attacks. *American Journal of Epidemiology*, **155**, 988–996.

Ware Jr., J., Kosinski, M. & Keller, S.D. (1996). A 12-Item Short-Form Health Survey: construction of scales and preliminary tests of reliability and validity. *Medical Care*, **34**, 220–233.

Weathers, F.W., Litz, B.T., Herman, D.S., Huska, J.A. & Keane, T.M. (1993). The PTSD Checklist: reliability, validity, & diagnostic utility. Boston: National Center for Posttraumatic Stress Disorder.

Yehuda, R. (2002). Post-traumatic stress disorder. *New England Journal of Medicine*, **346**, 108–114.

Yang, Y.K., Yev, T.L., Chen, C.C., Lee, C.K., Lee, I.H., Lee, L.C. & Jeffries, K.J. (2003). Psychiatric morbidity and posttraumatic symptoms among earthquake victims in primary care clinics. *General Hospital Psychiatry*, **25**, 253–221.

Zhang, J. & Yu, K.F. (1998). What's the relative risk? A method of correcting the Odds Ratio in cohort studies of common outcomes. *Journal of the American Medical Association*, **280**, 1690–1691.

17

Project Liberty: responding to mental health needs after the World Trade Center terrorist attacks

Chip J. Felton, Sheila Donahue, Carol Barth Lanzara, Elizabeth A. Pease and Randall D. Marshall

Introduction

The impact of the World Trade Center terrorist attacks has no historical peacetime precedent in the USA in terms of loss of human life, magnitude of physical destruction, adverse economic consequences, and psychological distress and disorder. In this chapter, we review the literature on mental health consequences of disaster, review research findings on the mental health consequences of the 9/11 attacks, describe the large-scale response undertaken by the New York State Office of Mental Health (NYSOMH) to address the mental health needs, and, finally, summarize lessons learned and their public health implications for mental health and homeland security policy.

Historical perspective: long-term mental health impact

Disaster experts have consistently documented the persistence of mental health needs long after the disastrous event itself. The 1995 bombing of the Alfred P. Murrah building in Oklahoma City was perhaps the best-documented mass violence disaster in terms of its impact on mental disorders before the attacks of September 11, 2001. Surveys conducted in the Oklahoma City metropolitan area found that 62% of persons reported experiencing at least one of the following as a direct response to the bombing: increased alcohol use (approximately double their prior amount), increased psychological distress (approximately double their prior level), post-traumatic stress disorder (PTSD) symptoms, and intrusive thoughts related to the bombing (Smith *et al.*, 1999). The psychological effects were prominent and persisted more than a year after the disaster. Two years after the disaster, children who were geographically distant from the disaster site and did not directly experience an interpersonal loss still reported PTSD symptoms and functional impairment associated with increased media exposure and indirect loss

(Pfefferbaum *et al.*, 2000). Three years following the bombing, researchers found a large proportion of survivors, especially those seriously injured, experienced long-term physical and/or emotional problems, and continued to have an increased need for treatment of bombing-related medical conditions. The most frequently reported PTSD symptoms were "being jumpy or easily startled" and "recurring distressful thoughts of the bombing," and the most frequently utilized medical services were psychological counseling (63%) (Shariat *et al.*, 1999).

These findings are consistent with prior research indicating that mass violence of human design that causes large-scale loss of life, property loss, and widespread unemployment is associated with particularly "severe, lasting, and pervasive psychological effects" (Norris *et al.*, 2002). These findings also dramatically illustrate the need for improving public health mechanisms for providing effective counseling for the larger community and evidence-based treatment for the most symptomatic persons.

The mental health impact of the September 11th terrorist attacks

The 9/11 attacks had a nationwide impact on mental health. In the immediate aftermath of the disaster, epidemiologic surveys found widespread trauma-related mental distress in the general population. Nationally, 44% of adults and 35% of children reported one or more symptoms consistent with traumatic stress (Schuster *et al.*, 2001). Eighty-seven percent of the population was estimated to have experienced one or more emotional, cognitive, or behavioral reactions that might have interfered with functioning but would not have been disabling. Fully 13% of the population was judged to be at risk for the development of trauma-related mental disorders, defined by multiple reactions of sufficient intensity and duration to limit functioning, at least in the short term. Groups at greatest risk in this study were individuals with life-threatening exposure or severe loss related to the event and individuals with prior trauma exposure.

The mental health impact of the September 11th terrorist attacks was particularly severe for New York City residents and others living within commuting distance of the World Trade Center (Felton, 2002), with 61% of adults living within 100 miles of the disaster site reporting substantial traumatic stress symptoms (Schuster *et al.*, 2001). Because government mechanisms of disaster relief require demonstration of community need, NYSOMH conducted several needs assessments in the months following September 11th. It was estimated that 3.1 million residents of New York City and the surrounding counties would experience substantial emotional distress as a result of the disaster (NYSOMH, 2001). In December 2001, estimates based on prior research and surveys conducted by the New York Academy of Medicine indicated that over the year following September 11th, 422,000 individuals in the World Trade Center disaster area would meet diagnostic criteria for PTSD and 129,000 would seek assistance (Herman *et al.*, 2002a). The cost of treating those who would seek treatment was estimated to be $197.5 million, with 65% of the cost expected to be covered by private insurance and 35% by public/philanthropic funds (Herman *et al.*, 2002b).

Subsequent epidemiologic-style surveys confirmed and extended these initial findings. One study commissioned by the New York City Board of Education and conducted by Applied Research and Consulting in collaboration with the Columbia University Mailman School of Public Health and the New York State Psychiatric Institute (2002) assessed the mental health needs of New York City public school students 6 months after the terrorist attacks. Another included the collection and analysis of data from telephone calls to New York City's mental health information and referral hotline (1-800-LIFENET).

Two months after the terrorist attacks, 58% of respondents in a telephone survey of residents in Manhattan reported at least one PTSD symptom in the previous month (Galea *et al.*, 2002a). Of Manhattan residents south of 110th Street, 14% reported symptoms consistent with PTSD and/or current depression (8% or 67,000 people with PTSD; 10% or 87,000 people with current depression) (Galea *et al.*, 2002b). These rates were nearly twice as high as those reported in national samples prior to September 11th. Among survey respondents in Manhattan, 29% reported an increased use in cigarettes, alcohol, and/or marijuana 2 months following the World Trade Center attacks, and both depression and PTSD were more common among users of these substances who increased their use than among those who did (Vlahov *et al.*, 2002). Other researchers noted an increase in illicit drug use 3 months after the attacks (Deren *et al.*, 2002).

Three to six months following the World Trade Center terrorist attacks, symptom reactions to the attacks persisted. For about one-third of adults who exhibited symptoms consistent with PTSD and major depression within 30 days of the attacks, these disorders were still present 4 months later (Galea *et al.*, 2003). Six months following the attacks, a substantial and persistent impact on school-age youth was found throughout New York City. The Board of Education assessment conducted in March 2002 estimated that 190,000 New York City children (27%) in grades 4–12 had at least one of five mental health problems, and that the impact of September 11th was responsible for a large elevation in the number of youth with mental health problems citywide (Applied Research and Consulting, Columbia University, and New York State Psychiatric Institute, 2002). The study also found that more than two-thirds of the children with probable PTSD following the September 11th attacks had not sought mental health services. Rates for all disorders were elevated based on (non-New York City) comparison data (e.g., 11% vs. 2% for PTSD).

Twelve months following the terrorist attacks, a continued emergence of trauma-related disorders was found. Preliminary findings from a survey conducted in September 2002 by the New York Academy of Medicine uncovered new-onset World Trade Center-related PTSD, where 5% of respondents without PTSD in March 2002 met criteria for PTSD in September 2002 (Galea, personal communication, 2003). Variables that were associated with new-onset PTSD were one or more significant life stressors since 9/11/2001; being "very concerned" over being in a major city; being "very concerned" over possible exposure to chemicals in the environment, food, or water supply; and/or believing another terrorist attack in New York City is "very likely" over the next year.

Project Liberty: New York State's emergency mental health response program

The World Trade Center disaster produced an unprecedented and chaotic post-disaster environment that required the most complex emergency management response ever mounted in U.S. history. As part of this response, NYSOMH rapidly implemented "Project Liberty," the designated name of New York's federally funded disaster mental health crisis-counseling program. President Bush's designation of the New York City region and 10 surrounding counties as a federal disaster area on September 11th made the region eligible for a range of Federal Emergency Management Agency (FEMA) programs, including one specifically designed to address the short-term mental health needs of communities affected by disasters: the Crisis Counseling Assistance and Training Program (CCP). This program, which is jointly operated by FEMA and the federal Center for Mental Health Services (CMHS) of the Substance Abuse and Mental Health Services Administration (SAMHSA), funds short-term public education, outreach, and crisis-counseling services. It explicitly does not fund specialized longer-term mental health treatment.

When applying for CCP funds after a community disaster, state mental health authorities must demonstrate that existing mental health capacity is insufficient to meet disaster-related needs. The CCP has two components: the Immediate Services Program (ISP), which covers the first 60 days following a disaster declaration and the Regular Services Program (RSP), which extends the same services for an additional 9 months. NYSOMH sought and was awarded more than $155 million in federal funding for this program through FEMA. NYSOMH also received invaluable technical assistance from CMHS following the disaster declaration. Throughout the post-9/11 work, NYSOMH also had to continue its functions in overseeing and providing services to individuals with severe mental illness.

NYSOMH's role in Project Liberty was to create a functional infrastructure that made it possible for the New York City and county mental health authorities and provider agencies to deliver the widespread interventions necessary to meet the disaster-related mental health needs in their communities. As a result, Project Liberty was a massive, unprecedented, and largely successful collaboration between NYSOMH, local governments, and nearly 200 local provider agencies. Project Liberty was the single largest and most rapidly implemented public mental health program in the history of the USA.

Project Liberty goals and program principles

Project Liberty's overall goal was to reduce psychological distress that resulted from the World Trade Center attacks by providing effective, short-term, community-based disaster mental health services. An important objective was to help persons recover from their psychological reactions and regain their pre-disaster level of functioning. Consistent with the literature, the project operated on the assumption that most people's reactions to the disaster, although personally disturbing, constitute normal responses to a traumatic event that will be short term in duration.

Core program principles of Project Liberty focused on supporting healthy coping, and assisting each survivor to return to a pre-disaster level of functioning. With a community-based service delivery system, Project Liberty relied on a confluence of mental health professionals and other community workers to work together to achieve program goals. Outreach efforts were viewed as a critical element in reaching people who typically do not consider themselves as in need of mental health services following a disaster. Service providers strived to enhance cultural competence within community subgroups in order to maximize and encourage program participation.

Project Liberty delivered short-term outreach and educational-counseling services to affected individuals and groups at no cost to them. In addition, Project Liberty counselors made referrals to longer-term mental health services when necessary. The program's crisis counselors provided face-to-face disaster-related services through outreach in community settings: homes, businesses, schools, places of religious worship, recovery centers, shelters, and community centers. Populations of special concern thought to be at increased risk for post-disaster impairment included families of victims, survivors and their families, displaced individuals, emergency and recovery workers, the elderly, children, certain cultural and ethnic groups, and people with limited financial and social support resources, and/or mental illness.

Recognizing that a minority of persons demonstrated persistent and continuing difficulties as a result of September 11th, Project Liberty requested and received federal approval to offer expanded trauma-related services. Introduced in 2002, these expanded or "enhanced services" were designed to provide brief, intensive, and evidence-informed interventions to persons who have been highly affected by the September 11th terrorist attacks.

The extraordinary cultural, ethnic, and economic diversity of the disaster area presented a particular challenge to Project Liberty goals; in the end, services were noteworthy for their cultural responsiveness to the communities served. In addition to being offered in English, Spanish, and Chinese, services were provided in American Sign, Russian, Haitian Creole, Hebrew, Polish, Italian, French, Arabic, and a variety of Asian languages. Through Project Liberty's outreach model, New York State's public mental health system integrated culturally appropriate counseling services into the fabric of the community in non-stigmatizing ways that encouraged people to seek help. In New York City and the surrounding counties, Project Liberty was always accessible through a central number, the 1-800-LIFENET hotline, where Spanish and Asian language LIFENET and other linguistic and culturally competent services were also available.

Public outreach and education efforts

One of Project Liberty's primary functions was to provide public education about normal reactions to the events of 9/11 and assistance in accessing services. This model is based on the principle of psycho-education, which is a core component of evidence-based treatment for affective and anxiety disorders, including PTSD. The goal is amelioration of fears about intense emotional reactions that might compound functional disability and promotion of coping strategies that could ameliorate reactions through normal mechanisms. To this end, millions of New Yorkers were informed about free and confidential counseling services through a statewide media campaign and local-level media efforts, including information dissemination via newspapers, television, radio, subways, buses, and trains. According to the New York Academy of Medicine, awareness of Project Liberty among New York City residents survey increased more than 100% between January 2002 and September 2002, from 24% (Rudenstine *et al.*, 2003) to 53% (Galea, personal communication, 2003).

Additional Project Liberty educational outreach efforts included the distribution of more than 20 million pieces of project literature in English, Spanish, Chinese, Korean, Haitian Creole, Russian, and other languages. Large-type versions of brochures in English, Spanish, and Chinese as well as audiotapes in English and Spanish were made available for individuals who are blind or had visual impairments.

Another important vehicle for outreach and public education was Project Liberty's web site located at www.projectliberty.state.ny.us. Information in English and Spanish about project services, eligibility, access, and educational materials remains available on the site for both consumers and providers. The site has had more than 1,300,000 visits since its launch in December 2001.

Outreach to children

A special children's initiative conducted in partnership with Sesame Workshop developed a toolkit of materials and online resources to effectively reach millions of children aged 3–8 years and the adults who care for them. The project was aimed at promoting resilience and coping skills in children and providing practical strategies for parents and care providers to help their children. Materials were prepared in English, Spanish, and Chinese, and provided children with culturally appropriate lessons, skills, and tools to deal with their responses to the 9/11 attacks. The video component, which consists of four Sesame Street episodes that deal with loss, disasters, grief, and accepting differences, was shown on television as a public service and in schools.

Project Liberty also built project awareness by working collaboratively with other New York State agencies to reach special populations through their agency networks and affiliate groups. Project Liberty collaborated with the New York State departments of health, children and family services, temporary and disability assistance, aging, thruway authority, and alcohol and substance abuse.

Linking to crisis counseling via LIFENET

During the first 12–16 months following the World Trade Center attacks, the call volume at 1-800-LIFENET remained high, with approximately 4000 calls monthly, which was more than double the number of calls received monthly by LIFENET prior to September 11th. With the advent of Project Liberty television and radio advertisements, calls rose to 5300 in December 2001. From January to July 2002, Project Liberty implemented multimedia campaigns with television, radio, subway, and print media, and monthly LIFENET calls averaged close to 6000. During August to October 2002, the months surrounding the 1-year anniversary of the attacks, LIFENET averaged more than 10,000 monthly calls, which tapered to an average of 6700 calls monthly during November 2002 to January 2003. LIFENET's call volume has continued at an average of more than 6000 calls per month through September 2003, and decreased slightly to an average of 5600 calls monthly by December 2003 (Mental Health Association of New York City, 2003).

In January 2002, 9% of individuals surveyed in New York City by the New York Academy of Medicine reported that they had called or had considered calling LIFENET to find out more about Project Liberty services (Rudenstine *et al.*, 2003); by September that same year, 33% of New Yorkers reported that they had called or had considered calling, suggesting a startlingly high rate of both awareness of the program and potential need for assistance (Galea, personal communication, 2003).

Overview of Service Delivery

Between Project Liberty's inception and the end of December 2004, face-to-face counseling, education, and outreach services were provided to an estimated 1.5 million individuals in the disaster area. Nearly 740,000 individuals were served with public education, and more than 750,000 individuals received crisis counseling. Approximately 89% of those served were in New York City. By comparison, the total number of individuals served in the New York State public mental health system in 1999 was estimated to be 600,000.

Project Liberty's service volume steadily increased throughout the first 7 months of operation, with the number of counseling and educational sessions about doubling in each succeeding month, from a September 2001 start of 700 service encounters. In May 2002, monthly volume reached 41,000 sessions and that level of service was sustained over the next 14 months until August 2003 when program phase down began. Subsequently, from September through the close of most of the community-based crisis-counseling program in December, 2003 the number of sessions provided gradually declined from about 24,000 to 12,000 per month. In 2004, services continued to be offered only to the FDNY and in the New York City Public Schools. In all, nearly 923,000 counseling and education sessions were provided, demonstrating the continuing need for the program's services over more than 3 years.

In addition to the sustained volume of service provision, Project Liberty outreach efforts continued to identify and provide counseling services to new individuals previously not served by the program, even after the program had been operating for months. The anonymous nature of the service reporting data precludes knowing the number of sessions any particular individual received; however, first sessions can be distinguished from follow-up sessions, so examining the number of first-session encounters gives an indication of the proportion of services going to new service entrants. In the first year of the program, 80% of the counseling sessions were first sessions. During the second year, the number of new service entrants remained high, and nearly two-thirds (65%) of counseling sessions were first sessions. Even when phase down was occurring in the fall of 2003, half of the counseling sessions were initial sessions. During 2004 when services continued to be available only to the FDNY and in New York City Public Schools, 27% of those receiving individual or family counseling were new entrants to service.

The crisis-counseling model emphasizes active outreach and provision of services at easily accessible locations within the community. Consistent with this philosophy, only 20% of Project Liberty sessions were held at provider sites, with the remaining 80% at a variety of settings in the community. Services were provided at individuals' homes, schools, places of worship, work places, community centers, disaster recovery centers and public places such as parks, libraries, transportation stations, and shopping areas. For children, school was the most common location to receive services, with 83% of counseling sessions occurring there.

Demographic description of service recipients

Data on age group, gender, race/ethnicity, and preferred language were collected on persons receiving individual or family counseling. The majority of service recipients (72%) were adults 18–54 years of age, followed by older adults (13%) 55 years and older; 159% of services were provided to children 17 years of age or younger. Slightly more than half (53%) of crisis-counseling recipients were female. The residents of the disaster area represented a wide variety of ethnic backgrounds, cultures, races, and languages. Project Liberty made significant efforts to provide culturally appropriate outreach and service delivery to these diverse communities. Ethnic characteristics showed recipients to be 30% African American, 26% Hispanic American, 31% Caucasian, and 10% Asian/Pacific Islander. The preferred language of 20% of crisis-counseling service recipients was something other than the English. Spanish was preferred by 10% of recipients and a Chinese language by 6%; 4% expressed a preference for some other language. These other languages numbered more than 20 and included: American Sign, Russian, Haitian Creole, Hebrew, Polish, Italian, French, Arabic, and a variety of Asian languages.

High-risk groups

Nearly 45% of Project Liberty individual or family counseling was delivered to individuals who were members of groups highly impacted by the disaster or considered at elevated risk for mental distress due to past or pre-existing trauma, psychological or substance abuse problems, and/or physical disability. Among recipients of individual or family counseling, about 16,000 lost a family member or friend and 27,000 were injured, evacuated or experienced major damage to their homes as a result of the disaster. Another 51,000 were emergency workers including firefighters, police officers, and other rescue and recovery workers, accounting for approximately 10% of those receiving services. Persons who lost their jobs or were displaced as a result of the attack represented 11% of those receiving counseling. Slightly more than 72,000 persons (14%) who received crisis counseling had past or pre-existing trauma, psychological or substance abuse problems or physical disability.

Needs assessment estimates developed using FEMA criteria resulted in estimates of direct victims, rescue workers, displaced employed or unemployed and others in the general population of slightly more than 3,100,000 individuals affected. Based on this estimate, penetration rates for Project Liberty for counseling and public education were 62% for those directly impacted (including victims, rescue workers, and displaced employed or unemployed individuals), and 43% for other general populations, for an overall total penetration rate of 47%. These rates did not include the millions of additional New Yorkers who, while they did not receive face-to-face services through the program, did receive written public educational materials and mass media-based public informational messages through Project Liberty.

Reactions, symptoms, and probable disorders in service recipients

The majority of individuals (69%) receiving crisis counseling through Project Liberty reported multiple reactions and substantial distress. Reactions most commonly reported by Project Liberty service recipients include sadness/tearfulness (41%), anxiety/fear (40%), irritability/anger (28%), sleep difficulties (24%), hypervigilance (24%), intrusive thoughts or images (23%), difficulty concentrating (23%), extreme change in activity level (22%), distressing dreams (16%), and isolation/withdrawal (17%).

Recipients with "depression-like" symptom clusters included those with four or more of the following reactions: change in activity level, sadness/tearfulness, despair/hopelessness, sleep disturbances, difficulty eating, fatigue/exhaustion, difficulty concentrating, difficulty remembering things, difficulty making decisions, suicidal thoughts, or suicidal thoughts alone. Thirty percent of service recipients exhibited reactions suggestive of depression.

Another set of four items that commonly appear on brief screens for PTSD include intrusive thoughts or images, distressing dreams, hypervigilance, and emotional numbness. Recipients experiencing two or more of those reactions or hypervigilance alone are likely to be at elevated risk for PTSD. Thirty percent of individuals receiving counseling reported such reactions.

Looking at event reaction groupings suggestive of PTSD or depression, we found that nearly half (48%) of the individuals who participated in individual counseling experienced reactions consistent with one or both groups. The proportion of individuals exhibiting these more intensive reactions when beginning counseling remained substantial and also quite consistent over time, ranging between 40% and 52% when the data were examined quarterly.

Initially, in keeping with the federal CCP guidelines, Project Liberty provided only short-term counseling and public education services. Persons found to be in need of longer-term, more intensive professional mental health treatment were offered referrals to those services. Ten percent of those receiving counseling were offered such referrals. Nearly two-thirds (64%) of persons referred had event reactions suggestive of PTSD or depression. The most exhibited event reactions of persons referred for additional mental health services included: sadness/tearfulness (45%), anxiety/fear (46%), sleep difficulties (35%), irritability/anger (36%), extreme change in activity level (34%), distressing dreams (28%), intrusive thoughts or images (33%), difficulty concentrating (31%), and/or isolation/withdrawal (25%). Event reactions for individuals who were not referred for additional mental health services ranged from 15% to 41% in these areas.

Project Liberty Evidence-Informed Enhanced Services

The accumulated evidence from first-year studies of the mental health impact of September 11th and from the Project Liberty service delivery process showed that, while the project's short-term psycho-educational services were likely sufficient to facilitate a rapid return to pre-disaster functioning for the majority of individuals encountered, these services alone were not sufficient for the sizeable minority of individuals who, 1 year after the attacks, continued to experience persistent traumatic symptoms at levels resulting in substantial functional impairment.

Project Liberty service encounter data showed that nearly half (48%) of all counseling service recipients encountered in the 12 months following September 11th exhibited event reactions suggestive of PTSD and/or depression, and that the proportion of individuals exhibiting these reactions did not show a consistent pattern of decrease over time. These findings agree with evidence from a study by North *et al.* (1999) that assessed mental health after severe trauma, which suggests that up to one-third of those who develop PTSD may continue to meet full PTSD criteria 6 months after the traumatic event, and that a substantial proportion of persons may continue to suffer symptoms in the long term.

NYSOMH used this new information to expand Project Liberty services to meet the needs of more severely impacted individuals with new screening methods, a broader set of free, evidence-informed brief counseling interventions, and additional training and technical assistance to a select set of service providers. These expanded services, known as Project Liberty enhanced services, were approved by FEMA and SAMHSA in August 2002. This is the first time that such an expansion of crisis-counseling services has been authorized under an FEMA grant, and it exemplifies how federal and state agencies worked together to move the field of public health disaster response forward based on needs survey data and current evidence-based knowledge.

In implementing this new component of the CCP, NYSOMH identified a select group of qualified providers for Project Liberty enhanced services. Additionally, NYSOMH collaborated with the September 11th Fund and the American Red Cross – who partnered to fund a mental health benefit for September 11th direct victims and their families – to insure that individuals encountered through Project

Liberty would be screened for benefit eligibility, which for qualified individuals paid for all mental health treatment outside of Project Liberty. In addition to these efforts, NYSOMH reallocated $33 million in Project Liberty funds to more intensively address the serious and continuing September 11th-related mental health needs of New York City's schoolchildren.

The Child and Adolescent Trauma Treatment Services program

In the aftermath of the World Trade Center disaster, NYSOMH was greatly concerned about possible significant and lasting effects the disaster might have on children and adolescents. Previous studies from the Oklahoma City bombing had shown significant psychological distress and problems among children and adolescents exposed directly and indirectly to the bombing (Pfefferbaum *et al.*, 1999, 2000, 2001).

Through funding from SAMHSA, NYSOMH created the Child and Adolescent Trauma Treatment and Services (CATS) program, which was designed to reach children and adolescents affected by September 11th who showed severe symptoms as a result of trauma or who had not improved through existing services such as Project Liberty. CATS was a nine-site collaborative project that offered affected youths intensive, evidence-based trauma treatments provided by mental health professionals who had received specialized training from nationally recognized trauma experts. The project also provided direct outreach to school districts where a high proportion of students had been affected. Referrals for CATS services were made in a number of ways, including through Project Liberty and the LIFENET hotline.

Based on its review of the child trauma literature, CATS identified two therapies that are demonstrated to be effective with traumatized youth. The *Child and Parent Trauma-Focused Cognitive Behavioral Therapy Treatment Manual* (Cohen *et al.*, 2002), and is based on a program used extensively with sexual abuse populations and targeted toward children between 3–18 years of age who show significant emotional or behavioral difficulties after exposure to a traumatic life event, such as the September 11th disaster. The *Trauma/Grief-Focused Group Psychotherapy Program* (Layne *et al.*, 2001) is directed toward adolescents (aged 12–18 years) and was developed by members of the University of California, Los Angeles, and Trauma Psychiatry Service. This program is used in Southern California with adolescents exposed to community violence and in postwar Bosnia with severely war-exposed school students. Results from studies of the effectiveness of these treatments show significant reductions in post-traumatic and grief symptoms, improvements in grade point averages, reductions in the number of disciplinary actions, and improvements in classroom attention and concentration (Saltzman *et al.*, 2001). Both treatments demonstrate an overall decrease in impairment in addition to symptom reduction. In total, about 445 children received CATS services.

Program evaluation

NYSOMH, in collaboration with New York City, the participating counties, and academic partners, conducted a multifaceted evaluation of Project Liberty. In addition to the collection of service encounter data, information was gathered from stakeholders involved in providing and receiving crisis counseling to document issues related to the program's implementation and operation, and the needs of the communities served. Feedback from crisis-counseling recipients was sought through surveys and telephone interviews regarding their experiences, needs, and opinions on the helpfulness of Project Liberty and their satisfaction with the care received from crisis-counseling providers.

Respondent demographics for the outcome survey ($N = 352$) showed the majority as female (57%), with an ethnic breakdown composed of 53% Caucasian, 21% Hispanic, and 11% African American. Among survey respondents, 84% saw the World Trade Center attacks live or on television; 36% thought they would be injured or killed; 32% lost a family member; 23% had personal possessions damaged in the attacks; 19% were evacuated from an area due to the attacks; 22% lost a job due to the attacks; and 23% were involved in rescue efforts. The Project Liberty evaluation found that recipients rated services received highly, with percentages of "good" to "excellent" ranging from 90% to 97%, and an overall quality rating of 97%. Similarly, recipients rated the efficacy of services received highly, with an overall rating of 94% ranking "good" to "excellent." Comparison of functioning prior to the attacks to current functioning following receipt of Project Liberty services ranged from 69% to 83% as "same" or "improved" in areas for employment, school, maintaining relationships, handling daily tasks, maintaining health, and involvement in activities.

The evaluation provided useful information about program operations that assisted in decision making. It also informed disaster preparedness efforts by describing the implementation process used, identifying best practices and obstacles encountered, and based on the lessons learned, making recommendations about how to organize a mental health response in the future. Given the scope of this project, its innovations, and the unfortunate but likely need for future broad-scale responses to disasters, we believe the evaluation of Project Liberty effectiveness was critical. This also represented the first time in US history that a FEMA program was intensively evaluated for effectiveness.

In addition to the Project Liberty evaluation, CATS also conducted a number of ongoing evaluations to examine the effectiveness of its treatment intervention programs. The first examined a wide range of symptoms including anxiety, depression, overall functioning, and substance use. Data were collected at intake, treatment completion, and 3-month follow-up intervals from children and their parents. CATS also evaluated aspects of the therapeutic process that contributed to improvements in mental health outcomes. Lastly, the project studied the implementation processes associated with delivery of these evidence-based interventions in a variety of settings including schools, outpatient clinics, and community-based clinics. Understanding gained from these activities will be used to inform the implementation of evidence-based practices on a large scale.

Challenges, lessons learned, and implications for policy development

The magnitude and devastation of September 11th presented unprecedented challenges to NYSOMH in implementing Project Liberty immediately following the attack. Challenges included working in a chaotic post-disaster environment, developing protocols and infrastructures for a major new emergency public health intervention, and simultaneously preparing grant submissions for federal aid to obtain project funding. What we have learned from these challenges in developing and implementing such a large-scale program may prove valuable in future planning for community mental health disaster preparedness.

Challenges posed in development and implementation

Although it was certain that there would be major mental health implications as a consequence of the disaster, the dimensions of the need were largely unknown. The needs assessment was demanding due to the inherent difficulties in rapidly assessing the number of human deaths, injuries, and evacuations, and the physical and economic consequences following a catastrophic disaster. In addition, the use of FEMA's disaster mental health response program model, with the exception of the Oklahoma City bombing, had previously been confined to the aftermath of natural disasters in less densely populated geographic locations with less heterogeneous populations. It was necessary to adapt the model on a large scale to meet the needs of the sizeable, diverse population in a broad geographic area that included the five boroughs of New York City and 10 surrounding counties, and to reflect the fact that this disaster was caused by an intentional act of mass violence as opposed to the forces of nature.

Project Liberty's large-scale outreach effort needed to efficiently address issues including, but not limited to, contracting, staffing, training, budgeting, and informing the public of the existence and services available through Project Liberty. To meet these challenges, a variety of mechanisms were developed and implemented to sustain the infrastructure necessary to create and support effective outreach services within a short time span. These mechanisms included establishing new contracts to allow the emergency mental health funds to flow from state to local government; developing new service claim and reimbursement mechanisms; creating new service encounter reporting forms and procedures to monitor the program's geographic and demographic penetration; designing and disseminating print and electronic public education materials; creating a media campaign to inform the public about Project Liberty and its services; recruiting counseling staff to supplement existing staff; and developing curricula and providing training to thousands of mental health professionals and paraprofessionals in community outreach and disaster mental health counseling.

Such challenges required the rapid development of new expertise within the public mental health system, drawing upon the assistance of a wide range of experts from around the country. Perhaps the most dramatic challenge was a shift from a focus on severe mental illness to the mental health of the general population using a public health model. Completely new service infrastructures were built, with large-scale provision of community-based, psycho-educational services to people who might have been responding normally to an abnormal experience, but who were impaired by fears of the intensity of these reactions. Promotion of healthy coping in response to psychological trauma was also a major shift in emphasis for NYSOMH. As a result of this disaster, the residents of greater metropolitan New York may be among the best educated in the country with respect to response to psychological trauma.

The New York City and county mental health departments developed local plans of service and recruited existing mental health agencies to participate. The project assisted localities in identifying and contracting with a large number of culturally competent and specialized providers were capable of meeting the crisis-counseling needs of the affected populations, which were remarkably diverse in terms of socio-economic status, age, ethnicity, culture, language, geographic spread, and special needs. Among nearly 200 mental health agencies participating in the delivery of Project Liberty services, more than 8,000 workers were trained in outreach-based disaster mental health counseling and public education techniques.

Lessons learned

The rapid implementation of Project Liberty, within 6 weeks of the disaster, and the high volume of services delivered has demonstrates that the fundamental goal of the project was met in reaching and providing services to individuals in need, and that such services could aid in the vast majority of people returning to pre-disaster levels of functioning. However, the numerous systemic challenges with development and implementation indicated that the public mental health system, including the provider community, was not sufficiently prepared to respond to terrorism.

Responding effectively required a dramatic expansion of focus to the entire population and large-scale provision of out-of-the office, psycho-educational services that were unfamiliar to most providers, but are the essence of a public health model. Because disaster mental health has not been a central part of clinical training or public health, all programs had to be developed essentially from scratch immediately in the aftermath of the disaster. This took vast amounts of time and energy. Moreover, disaster mental health funding streams historically have not supported the brief, more intensive services needed to enable individuals with more severe and persistent traumatic reactions to return to pre-disaster functioning. We believe the new enhanced services program instigated by NYSOMH is one of our more valuable contributions to planning for large-scale post-disaster programs.

Implications for mental health and homeland security policy

Components of a comprehensive mental health terrorist-response strategy include a broad-based outreach and public education effort concerning normative reactions to trauma, and supportive counseling to respond to emotional distress. Additionally, the identification of individuals with intensive and persistent trauma reactions must be included as well as provision of appropriate interventions for populations at risk for trauma-related disorders. Last, resiliency at the individual and community levels must be enhanced to promote better preparation for and more effective responses to terrorist disaster should the need arise again.

The mental health impact of terrorism is substantial, varied and can be persistent, particularly in an environment of ongoing threats, an environment in which "the major impact of terrorism is terror." The public sector is capable of mounting a large-scale response, but to do so requires intense intergovernmental collaboration and flexibility. Since terrorism is new to us, the necessary infrastructure for an effective mental health response to terror has to be built largely from scratch; once built, government needs to support its persistence over time as a preparedness strategy. Government also needs to support continued clinical and services research concerning the mental health impact of terrorism and effective clinical and organizational interventions, as scientific knowledge remains scarce. The experience and knowledge gained in New York should be used to inform national level planning and policymaking concerning the role of mental health in homeland defense.

REFERENCES

Applied Research and Consulting, LLC, Columbia University, and New York State Psychiatric Institute (2002). Effects of the World Trade Center attack on New York City public school students: initial report to the New York City Board of Education. New York: Applied Research and Consulting, LLC, Columbia University Mailman School of Public Health, and New York State Psychiatric Institute.

Cohen, J.A., Mannarino, A.P. & Deblinger, E. (2001). *Child and Parent Trauma-Focused Cognitive Behavioral Therapy Treatment Manual*. Pittsburgh: MCP-Hahnemann University School of Medicine.

Deren, S., Shedlin, M., Hamilton, T. & Hagan, H. (2002). Impact of September 11th attacks in New York City on drug users: a preliminary assessment. *Journal of Urban Health*, **79**, 409–412.

Felton, C.J. (2002). Project liberty: a public health response to New Yorkers' mental health needs arising from the World Trade Center terrorist attacks. *Journal of Urban Health*, **79**, 429–433.

Galea, S., Resnick, H., Ahern, J., Gold, J., Bucuvalas, M., Kilpatrick, D., Stuber, J. & Vlahov, D. (2002a). Posttraumatic stress disorder in Manhattan, New York City, after the September 11th terrorist attacks. *Journal of Urban Health*, **79**, 340–353.

Galea, S., Ahern, J., Resnick, H., Kilpatrick, D., Bucuvalas, M., Gold, J. & Valhov, D. (2002b). Psychological sequelae of the September 11 terrorist attacks in New York City. *New England Journal of Medicine*, **346**, 982–987.

Galea, S., Vlahov, D., Resnick, H., Ahern, J., Susser, E., Gold, J., Bucuvalas, M. & Kilpatrick, D. (2003). Trends of probable post-traumatic stress disorder in New York City after the September 11 terrorist attacks. *American Journal of Epidemiology*, **158**, 514–524.

Herman, D., Susser, E. & Felton, C. (2002a). *Rates and Treatment Costs of Mental Disorders Stemming from the World Trade Center Terrorist Attacks: An Initial Needs Assessment*. Albany, NY: New York State Office of Mental Health.

Herman, D., Felton, C. & Susser, E. (2002b). Mental health needs in New York State following the September 11th attacks. *Journal of Urban Health*, **79**, 322–331.

Layne, C.M., Saltzman, W.R. & Pynoos, R.S. (2001). *Trauma/Grief-Focused Group Psychotherapy Program*. Los Angeles: University of California, Trauma Psychiatry Program.

Mental Health Association of New York City (2003). *LifeNet Call Tracking Database*. New York: Mental Health Association of New York City, Office of the Director of LifeNet.

New York State Office of Mental Health (2001). *Crisis Counseling Assistance and Training Program Regular Services Program Application [FEMA 1391-RD-NY]*. Albany, NY: New York State Office of Mental Health.

Norris, F.H., Friedman, M.J., Watson, P.J., Byrne, C.M., Diaz, E. & Kaniasty, K. (2002). 60,000 disaster victims speak: an empirical review of the empirical literature, 1981–2001. *Psychiatry*, **65**, 207–239.

North, C.S., Nixon, S.J., Shariat, S., Mallonee, S., McMillen, J.C., Spitzmagel, E.L. & Smith, E.M. (1999). Psychiatric disorders among survivors of the Oklahoma City bombing. *Journal of American Medical Association*, **282**, 755–762.

Pfefferbaum, B., Nixon, S.J., Krug, R.S., Tivis, R.D., Moore, V.L., Brown, J.M., Pynoos, R.S., Foy, D. & Gurwitch, R.H. (1999). Clinical needs assessment of middle and high school students following the 1995 Oklahoma City bombing. *American Journal of Psychiatry*, **156**, 1069–1074.

Pfefferbaum, B., Seale, T.W., McDonald, N.B., Brandt, E.N., Rainwater, S.M., Maynard, B.T., Meierhoefer, B. & Miller, P.D. (2000). Posttraumatic stress two years after the Oklahoma City bombing in youths geographically distant from the explosion. *Psychiatry*, **63**, 358–370.

Pfefferbaum, B., Nixon, S.J., Tivis, R.D., Doughty, D.E., Pynoos, R.S., Gurwitch, R.H. & Foy, D.W. (2001). Television exposure in children after a terrorist incident. *Psychiatry*, **64**, 202–211.

Rudenstine, S., Galea, S., Ahern, J., Felton, C. & Vlahov, D. (2003). Awareness and perceptions of a communitywide mental health program in New York City after September 11. *Psychiatric Services*, **54**, 1404–1406.

Saltzman, W.R., Pynoos, R.S., Layne, C.M., Steinberg, A.M. & Aisenberg, E. (2001). Trauma and grief-focused intervention for adolescents exposed to community violence: results of a school-based screening and group treatment protocol. *Group Dynamics*, **5**, 291–303.

Schuster, M.A., Stein, B.D., Jaycox, L., Collins, R.L., Marshall, G.N., Elliott, M.N., Zhou, A.J., Kanouse, D.E., Morrison, J.L. & Berry, S.H. (2001). A national survey of stress reactions after the September 11, 2001, terrorist attacks. *New England Journal of Medicine*, **345**, 1507–1512.

Shariat, S., Mallonee, S., Kruger, E., Farmer, K. & North, C. (1999). A prospective study of long-term health outcomes among Oklahoma City bombing survivors. *Journal of Oklahoma State Medical Association*, **92**, 178–186.

Smith, D.W., Christiansen, E.H., Vincent, R. & Hann, N.E. (1999). Population effects of the bombing of Oklahoma City. *Journal of Oklahoma State Medical Association*, **94**, 193–198.

Vlahov, D., Galea, S., Resnick, H., Ahern, J., Boscarino, J.A., Bucuvalas, M., Gold, J. & Kilpatrick, D. (2002). Increased use of cigarettes, alcohol, and marijuana among Manhattan, New York, residents after September 11th terrorist attacks. *American Journal of Epidemiology*, **155**, 988–996.

18

Mental health services support in response to September 11: the central role of the Mental Health Association of New York City

John Draper, Gerald McCleery and Richard Schaedle

When the New York City (NYC) Department of Mental Health contracted with the Mental Health Association (MHA) of NYC in 1996 to start a new program called *LifeNet*, all parties believed that this multi-cultural, 24-hour, seven-day-a-week professional crisis, information, and referral hotline would become an essential vehicle for promoting access to treatment resources around the City. In doing so, they laid the foundation for mobilizing the largest mental health disaster response in the nation's history.

In addition to expanding the hotline's geographic reach beyond the five boroughs of NYC, LifeNet's extended role has encompassed aspects of professional training and outreach to businesses and community groups; central coordination of referrals for the Federal Emergency Management Agency (FEMA) funded counseling program, Project Liberty; and administration of an innovative program, funded jointly by the American Red Cross (ARC) and the September 11th Fund (SEF), for enabling access to mental health and substance treatment for "primary victims" of the disaster.

This chapter will discuss the various roles the MHA of NYC's LifeNet has played in the post-disaster recovery, and review the many lessons learned – thus far – in this ongoing effort.

LifeNet before the disaster

Lesson 1: Before a major disaster occurs, it is a major advantage to have a behavioral health hotline that is already performing functions that are useful following a disaster on a daily basis.

The success of LifeNet's post-disaster experience resulted from its pre-disaster history. By establishing a credible presence in the community prior to September 11th – through building relationships with government agencies, law enforcement, social service provider networks, the media, and a multi-cultural public at large – LifeNet was poised to take on the broad, multi-level spectrum of challenges unfolding in the wake of this unprecedented catastrophe.

Partnering with government, agencies, and community at large

Although the MHA of NYC and its LifeNet service enjoyed a positive relationship with the State Office of Mental Health before the disaster, LifeNet's primary networks were within the NYC limits. Through its founding partnership with the City's Department of Mental Health, LifeNet built strong ties in subsequent years with the City's Department of Health, the Department for the Aging, the City's Board of Education, and the NYC Police Department. LifeNet's professional hotline service was attractive to these systems due to its promise of making mental health and substance treatment referrals a simple process.

Police officers, school counselors, hospital or clinic staff, members of the clergy, senior center workers, or anyone near a telephone could call at any time of day to anonymously seek services for themselves or someone they cared about. The majority of LifeNet's staff comprises master's level social workers, most of whom have had extensive experience in working with persons suffering from mental health or substance problems. A caller would speak to a LifeNet staff member who would listen to the problem, assess its nature and severity, and provide the caller with appropriate referrals to services from a database of over 6000 support and treatment resources. In addition, LifeNet's separate hotlines for Chinese and Latino callers (as well as a translation service for other languages) have made it easier for cultures not traditionally known to be high users of mental health care to seek services in their own language.

Although the vast majority of LifeNet's calls have been information and referral-related (99%), LifeNet is known by many as the city's "crisis hotline." The hotline has authorized linkages with the city's crisis and emergency services, including Emergency Medical Services and the City's 25 psychiatric mobile outreach teams. LifeNet has been central to all of the Department of Mental Health's disaster planning efforts, used primarily by on-site mobile outreach teams as an information and referral line for survivors needing additional support services.

Promoting awareness through public education campaigns

LifeNet has developed strong public recognition over 5 years through citywide public education campaigns and grass roots outreach activities. LifeNet joined with the Department of Mental Health and other city agencies in several major campaigns designed to reduce the stigma of mental illness and promote awareness of mental health problems. Campaigns targeted the general public as well as special populations, including seniors, adolescents, serious and persistently mentally ill persons, Latinos, and Asian-Americans. For 5 years prior to 9/11, MHA of NYC and LifeNet personnel conducted extensive multi-cultural outreach among service providers, and in schools, community centers, workplaces, faith-based organizations, and other key locations to enhance awareness of mental health concerns and promote access to treatment through the hotlines.

Call volume pre-9/11

By September 2001, LifeNet's years of outreach and public education work had yielded increasing call numbers, which had roughly stabilized at approximately 3000 calls per month over the previous 8 months. Many of LifeNet's callers (40%) had reported no previous history of seeking treatment, reinforcing our belief that this was a non-stigmatizing, highly accessible method of seeking help.

Although no disaster plan had been constructed to prepare for the events that were soon to unfold, LifeNet's high visibility, its City partnership and its ability to handle high call volume had unknowingly prepared the organization to ramp up for a broad-scale response to catastrophe. As a federally funded case study conducted by the National Center for Post-traumatic Stress Disorder (PTSD) noted in their description of New York's 9/11 mental health response:

Communication systems are a critical element of a disaster mental health response plan. "The communications infrastructure [such as LifeNet] must be something that consumers recognize, government recognize, and providers recognize as a central means of communicating about or accessing services." It is critical for this system to be in place beforehand.... A joint venture of NYC DMH and the Mental Health Association, LifeNet had relationships with government at all levels and with service providers. It was critically important, perhaps the "single most important asset in the response". (Norris *et al.*, in press)

September 11, 2001: the immediate disaster response

> *Lesson 2: When a major disaster occurs, it is important to have a vehicle to efficiently mobilize qualified crisis counselor volunteers to affected sites.*

After the planes crashed into the World Trade Center (WTC), communications around the city were severely disrupted. The toll-free phone lines in LifeNet's call center, 20 blocks north from the scene, fell silent. Outside our offices, thousands of pedestrians marched swiftly, uptown, away from the WTC Towers. When it was discovered that the toll-free lines were not working, we quickly provided our alternate phone numbers to our colleagues at the Department of Health and Mental Hygiene's (DOHMH) communications office, who relayed the information to the media. LifeNet's Director sat with his staff and reviewed post-disaster crisis counseling techniques, discussed symptoms of acute stress disorder, and prepared them for the calls we expected to come at any moment. On September 11, 2001, LifeNet had fewer calls – 16 – than on any other day in its history.

Early hotline calls were typically related to basic needs

In the days and weeks immediately following the collapse of the Twin Towers, LifeNet received a mix of calls unique to the disaster reflecting a need for basic information about missing persons, or available charitable benefits related to food, cash, and shelter. Some callers reported acute stress symptoms, such as a horrified, sleepless delivery driver who escaped Tower Ones minute just before its collapse, who had to drive his truck "over bodies and body parts" to leave the scene.

Emerging importance of coordinated mobilization of trained professionals

Beginning of September 12, 2001, through the Office of Emergency Management command center, the city and state governments called on LifeNet to identify, organize, and dispatch thousands of crisis counselors to family assistance centers, shelters, workplaces, schools, and community centers around the City. Each day, from September 12, 2001, through December 2001, LifeNet worked together with DOHMH, the State Office of Mental Health and the ARC to maximize coordination of up to 100 personnel per day at the family assistance centers. This crew formed the basis of the Trauma Resource Network, a group that continued to meet regularly for the next three years to collaborate on the delivery of long-term recovery services.

Meanwhile, LifeNet was receiving hundreds of calls from counselors, trauma experts, and disaster support teams from all over the city, state, and nation, wanting to volunteer their services. For weeks, it seemed that we received more calls from well-intentioned individuals seeking to *give* assistance than from persons actually *seeking* help. Sorting through qualifications from many hundreds of volunteers to determine fitness for deployment was often a precarious endeavor. We typically relied on major NYC mental health providers to constitute the core force of volunteers, most of whom had no previous experience in post-disaster crisis counseling. *Clearly, in planning for a mental health response to a disaster of this magnitude, it is crucial to have both procedures for credentialing qualified volunteers and coordination in place to ensure that counselors provide the support most appropriate for the situation.*

However, our greatest challenge came in responding to the scores of requests from shaken schools, community centers, and workplaces around the city seeking an outreach worker to conduct group crisis counseling. LifeNet needed to find counselors who were qualified to conduct crisis counseling and who were willing and able to go before groups in a wide variety of settings. Only a few services in the city had regular experience and training in these skills, and they were used exhaustively.

> ***Lesson 3: Following a large-scale disaster, there will be a need to expand and adjust local mental health resources to respond to persons in distress.***

Resource needs become clear

Emerging from the first 2 weeks of the disaster, we met with officials from local government and charitable foundations and recommended the following resource needs based on our experience:

- expansion of LifeNet to meet the continuing and expected growth in calls;
- extensive mobile outreach services to affected persons throughout the communities of NYC and beyond;
- greater coordination of services across agencies to reduce service duplications and identify service gaps;
- preparing clinicians for work with disaster-affected populations via "best practices" trainings;
- an ongoing public education, multi-media messaging, and outreach campaign to promote awareness of disaster-related mental health problems and access to relevant support services;
- continuing disaster planning and preparation, utilizing a centralized communications infrastructure to enable better coordination of resources.

LifeNet hotline expansion through the SEF

Parallel to the flood of volunteers was the speed and generosity in which individuals, businesses, foundations, and government agencies sought to provide financial assistance to meet the massive mental health needs of the many thousands of New Yorkers shocked and devastated by the tragedy.

During the week of September 11, 2001, The United Way of NYC – in partnership with the New York Community Trust – created the SEF, and collected over $518 million, more than $128 million of which was received within the first 2 weeks after the disaster (September 11th Fund Report, 2002). Beyond extending direct cash assistance and other immediate benefits to impacted families, the SEF determined that the need for expanding LifeNet's hotline network was its top mental health funding priority. In just over 2 weeks after the disaster, the Fund provided a grant to LifeNet to enhance its disaster response infrastructure.

In addition, the SEF allocated funds to form LifeNet's Crisis Resource Center (CRC), comprising dedicated personnel to facilitate the continuing group outreach requests and mobilization of crisis counselors. The CRC's function was two fold:

- Provide support to communities – neighborhoods, businesses, and other organizations – by coordinating and mobilizing mental health professionals to work with groups
- Equip regional mental health professionals with the skills and tools they need to serve their clients and patients after 9/11.

The CRC's initial role of mobilizing outreach to distressed groups within the community waned as Project Liberty counselors began to proactively deliver psychoeducation and outreach services throughout the New York area. However, its role in the massive, two year promotion of the SEF-sponsored trauma and bereavement treatment trainings to professionals – as will be described further in this chapter – became central to the City's response to the long-term recovery needs of 9/11-affected New Yorkers.

Aside from the services provided through the SEF's support, FEMA initially granted $22.7 million for New Yorkers to provide free crisis counseling resources through a program to be administered by the New York State Office of Mental Health (SOMH), called *Project Liberty*.

LifeNet as a centralized access vehicle for Project Liberty services

By the end of October 2001, Project Liberty service providers were positioned to provide a valuable resource for the thousands of LifeNet callers seeking referrals for crisis counseling and public education services. The New York SOMH designated 1-800-LIFENET as the central hotline to assist New Yorkers in accessing all Project Liberty sites in NYC and its 10 surrounding counties.

Project Liberty's public education campaign

Soon after the disaster, Project Liberty would embark on the most comprehensive, ongoing mental health public education and media campaign ever launched in the New York area, and the most broad-scale post-disaster mental health media campaign ever supported by the federal government. Beginning in November 2001, this campaign stretched across the city and its surrounding counties, with 1-800-LIFENET as the hotline anchoring all communications. The SOMH's Project Liberty office developed English and Spanish television and radio ads that were broadcast in neighborhoods from NYC to as far as upstate New York, New Jersey, and Connecticut. The NYC's Project Liberty Office and the DOHMH blanketed the local subways, telephone kiosks, and billboards with Project Liberty messages and LifeNet's phone number. Brochures describing common emotional, behavioral, and physiologic responses to disasters – as well as the scope of Project Liberty services and how to access them through LifeNet – were developed and distributed throughout the New York area. Web sites, newspaper ads and articles further alerted the public to these counseling services, accompanied by legions of Project Liberty outreach workers combing the communities to distribute literature and provide a supportive presence.

As Project Liberty media and outreach saturated the region from November 2001 through March 2002, LifeNet calls continued to surge upward. LifeNet's CRC worked closely with the NYC Project Liberty office, which assigned the various

Project Liberty providers to the continuing group outreach requests from LifeNet callers. But the vast majority of calls were from the many thousands of distressed individuals who were seeking services for themselves or their loved ones.

LifeNet call volume trends after 9/11

LifeNet's professional staff utilizes a customized software application that allows them to efficiently assess caller needs, manage confidential caller information, and facilitate referrals from a database of nearly 6000 services. From the aggregate data it collects, the software can instantaneously produce a variety of reports that can demonstrate geographic, demographic, and/or temporal trends in behavioral health problems reported, services needed, etc. However, because LifeNet workers are engaged in an information and referral process rather than in conducting research, they only record information about callers that is necessary for enabling an efficient referral. While blank fields in call records are common, they are not systematic, and the large sample size of calls over the years has shown general reliability in using the recorded data to measure call trends.

As noted in Table 18.1, LifeNet calls have more than doubled in volume since the disaster. The prominent trends related to LifeNet call volume have been driven by three primary, interrelated factors: *media influences; broad-scale "activating events"; and temporal distance from September 11, 2001.*

> *Lesson 4: In order to inform the public about available behavioral health resources for support following a disaster, it is vital to conduct public education campaigns linked to a central hotline to facilitate access to services.*

Media influences

Clearly, no single factor has had greater affect on LifeNet call patterns than Project Liberty's multi-media public education campaigns. From December 2001 until December 2003 when the final Project Liberty print campaign appeared in subways, LifeNet's number was publicly advertised in one or more media for 13 of the 24 months. The television ads, which were seen in much of the tri-state area primarily during 2002 (for 8 months), were the most significant media prompt to call LifeNet, as calls to the hotlines rose anywhere from 11% to 103% when they were added to the print campaign. In 2003, when only the television ads appeared in March, calls rose 40%, and returned to their pre-March levels after the ads ceased.

One Project Liberty multi-media campaign that was particularly effective in targeting a specific demographic group was designed to reach parents and adult caregivers of children who had been affected by 9/11. The importance of reaching affected youngsters was reinforced by a survey conducted by the Columbia Psychiatric

Table 18.1. LifeNet call volume

Month	2001	2002	2003
January	2978	6646[b]	6661
February	2805	5735	5488
March	3158	7857[b]	7711[a]
April	2968	5887	6393
May	3123	5037	6330
June	3341	4809	6087
July	3248	5187[a]	6353
August	3098	9057[b]	5950
September	3404	12,602[b]	6334
October	5194	8856[b]	6408
November	4647	6339	5158
December	5310[a]	7016[b]	5316
July–August 2001, monthly average = 3173			
September–December 2001, monthly average = 4639			
2003, monthly average = 6182			
2002, monthly average = 7086			

[a]Project Liberty television campaign only.
[b]Project Liberty multi-media campaign.

Institute in partnership with the NYC Department of Education, which showed that approximately one in five children in grades 4–12 in NYC-area public schools had some significant emotional problem 6 months following the disaster (Hoven *et al.*, 2002). A combined Project Liberty–LifeNet television, poster, and brochure campaign targeting children and caregivers sustained a 58% increase in calls for children under 12 years old (the campaign's primary target group) and a 44% increase in adolescent-related hotline calls (the secondary target group) from September 2002–August 2003.

In the first 6 months after 9/11, half of LifeNet's callers reported that they had never sought treatment before, a significant increase of novice users over pre-9/11 rates (41.5% with no treatment history, March 2001–August 2001). Many of these new 9/11-related treatment seekers attributed the Project Liberty media campaign as the prompt for calling the hotline.

While there were periods when print and broadcast journalists gave 9/11 intensive and extensive coverage, this type of media had little or no effect on hotline calls unless the report specifically mentioned 1-800-LIFENET. However, when such reports featured LifeNet and explicitly described the services it could offer for victims, the results could be dramatic. For example, when LifeNet was mentioned in a front-page New York Times article on 8/21/2002 describing its role in enrolling "primary victims" who were eligible for the SEF's and ARC's "mental health benefit program" (see description later in this chapter), it persuaded hundreds of callers to contact the line on that day … and for each day after for a solid week.

> *Lesson 5: Broad-scale activating events alone – such as anniversaries – are not likely to promote more mental health help-seeking unless a public education campaign is co-occurring with the event.*

Broad scale activating events

Calls to LifeNet began to exponentially increase in October 2001, well before any of the far-reaching Project Liberty ads were developed. The work of the City's DOHMH to distribute the LifeNet number to the media within a day of the attacks (and in subsequent press releases) was instrumental in creating greater public awareness of this hotline. However, the symptoms of continuing acute stress disorder and the onset of PTSD began to emerge in October, and were further activated by the alarming reports of anthrax in Florida, Manhattan, and New Jersey. At that time, it was not clear how these initial post-9/11 activating events were interfacing with the wider distribution of the hotline number to affect the first remarkable increase of calls in October 2001 (53%).

In March 2002, print and broadcast journalists from all over the world focused attention on the status of NYC and its residents in preparation for the "six-month anniversary of the September 11th attacks", a period in and of itself heretofore unfamiliar to typical post-catastrophic observances. Beams of light shot skyward in a memorial tribute from Ground Zero; a vivid French documentary filmed by a crew just blocks from the WTC on 9/11 was broadcast on a major television network; news reports replaying film of the attacks were frequently shown on networks; and Project Liberty messages appeared on television, subways, in newspaper print, and heard on the radio. While the notion of a six-month anniversary alone may not have been a sufficient "activating event", the surrounding exposure from the media clearly was: distressed callers dialed LifeNet's line in unparalleled numbers, with 37% more persons phoning in March 2002 than the previous month. As one caller in March reported:

ALL THIS MEDIA, THESE REMINDERS … IT'S KILLING ME. After the towers fell, I was digging for survivors for days – picking up body parts, fragments, different colored skin tissues, and toys. I did that for 5 days straight, moving and loading bodies, until I couldn't handle it anymore. It's made me a different person … somebody I don't recognize, somebody I don't want to be. I've lost my job … I'm drinking all the time. I can't go near the news – I get all choked up – and I smell that putrid odor from the site all the time, I see the pile, the bodies … I don't know how I'll ever get over it if I haven't gotten over it by now …

LifeNet's experience of the six-month anniversary was a small-scale preview of what could be expected when the first anniversary arrived. Prior to August 2002, the largest single number of calls to register on the LifeNet hotlines was 515 calls on the six-month anniversary of March 11, 2002 (nearly 200 calls above its previous high). In the weeks approaching the actual anniversary, LifeNet averaged nearly that number every weekday, with over 650 calls a day received the week of September 11th. On the day before the anniversary, the anticipatory anxiety levels were nearly equal to the experience of the anniversary itself. On September 10th, LifeNet registered 758 calls, and on September 11th, LifeNet realized a new peak of 761 contacts. Approximately 70% of callers were seeking services directly related to problems resulting from the 9/11 attacks (as compared to approximately 40% of callers over the past year). For that memorable month, calls occurred at four times the rate seen pre-9/11/2001.

The calls on the anniversary captured the lingering devastation of the attacks a year before, as the stories and symptoms of witnesses, evacuees, family members, rescue workers, and others were recounted in fresh, explicit detail. Several callers contacted LifeNet stating, "Today is my birthday," disturbed by how the attacks robbed them of their feeling of celebration. Almost every other caller described symptoms of post-traumatic stress (PTS), with sleep problems, flashbacks, and anxiety about their safety prominent among their concerns. Most of them received Project Liberty referrals. Simply, September 11, 2002, was apart from anything that LifeNet has ever experienced.

While broad-scale activating events have certainly occurred, their impact on LifeNet calls seems inextricably linked to accompanying media that directs distressed persons to the hotline. Following the first anniversary, Project Liberty media campaigns appeared only during December 2002 and during the war with Iraq in March 2003 (for 3 weeks). Other than those 2 months, at no other times during the past 15 months have LifeNet calls spiked in accordance with potentially activating events such as terrorist alerts, embassy bombings, and the second anniversary of the attacks.

> *Lesson 6: Help-seeking for mental health care is more pronounced beginning a month to 3 months after the disaster, continuing at higher rates for at least 2 years thereafter.*

Temporal distance from the disaster

While calls to the hotline rose within 2 weeks following the attacks, they were consistently and dramatically higher than pre-9/11 call volume beginning the third month after the disaster, continuing to date. Calls to the LifeNet hotline network rose over

98% the first year after 9/10/2001 (36,254 calls). In the second year beginning 9/11/2002, calls rose 130% over pre-9/11 rates (83,627 calls), with many calls occurring during and shortly after the first anniversary.

In Table 18.1 it is clear that in 2002 extraordinary increases in calls fluctuated with the presence of media and specific activating events, such as anniversaries. However, in 2003, LifeNet had less media presence than at any time in its 7-year history (3 weeks of television ads, 2 weeks of subway poster placements). Nevertheless, monthly call rates in 2003 virtually stabilized at levels just over double those observed for the year prior to 9/11.

The increase in calls over the second year is comparable with the help-seeking behaviors of the survivors of the 1995 Oklahoma City bombings. Nancy B. Anthony, Executive Director of Oklahoma City Community Foundation, observed that it took 2–3 years before most of the persons suffering from bombing-related psychiatric problems sought counseling (Goode & Eakin, 2002). In spite of apparent consistencies in experience, specific LifeNet data regarding the actual ratio of LifeNet 9/11 calls to non-9/11 calls in 2003 suggest a scenario different from Oklahoma City. Although overall calls have increased, the frequency of callers reporting 9/11-specific problems diminished noticeably, from 1 out of 3.6 callers in 2002 to 1 out of 5.7 callers in 2003.

Why then, have LifeNet calls gone up over time, while 9/11-specific calls decreased? Certainly, one explanation for the general call escalation must be that the Project Liberty 2002 media campaign allowed LifeNet's number to successfully penetrate public awareness, particularly within the human service culture (agencies throughout the City accounted for the overwhelming majority of referrals to the hotline in 2003). Second, it may be that the unprecedented media and outreach campaign was so potent that it prompted many more persons to seek help sooner, rather than later (as in Oklahoma City).

However, there may be a more insidious 9/11-related explanation for the higher number of calls. That is, the further we move away from the terrorist attacks, the more difficult it is for emotionally affected persons to identify 9/11 as a significant factor related to their current concern. Experts in trauma research state that many persons emotionally affected by catastrophic events tend to delay seeking professional mental health services until other crisis situations emerge, such as job loss or problems in their relationships (CDC press release, September 2002). Specifically, the accumulation of such stressful life events for persons who have been exposed to the WTC attacks have resulted in devastating psychological affects. In a survey of persons living in Manhattan, those who reported significant disaster exposure and had one major stressor (loss of a job, loved one, etc.) since 9/11 had a 4.5-fold greater incidence of PTS symptoms. Exposed individuals with more than one stressful event reported PTS symptoms had a 47 times greater frequency of PTS symptoms (Galea *et al.*, 2003).

Other trends in LifeNet call data

> *Lesson 7: Certain prominent ethnic groups – such as Asian and Latino populations – are not nearly as likely as non-minority groups to seek free behavioral health services following a disaster, even with aggressive, culturally targeted outreach efforts.*

Comparisons among the Asian, Spanish, and general LifeNet hotlines reveal some cultural differences in post-disaster help-seeking behaviors

With two well-established, culture-focused hotlines – Asian LifeNet and Ayudese (Spanish LifeNet) – adjoining the general LifeNet number for 2 years prior to the attacks, the hotline network was positioned to assist a cross-section of cultures widely impacted by the disaster. Since the catastrophe, the culture-focused hotlines have registered remarkably few calls, particularly in comparison to the general LifeNet line (see Figure 18.1) and in light of the disaster's well-documented impact on these cultural groups. Interestingly, both non-English lines showed a slight decline in calls for the first 6 months after the disaster, while LifeNet's calls nearly doubled in that same time frame.

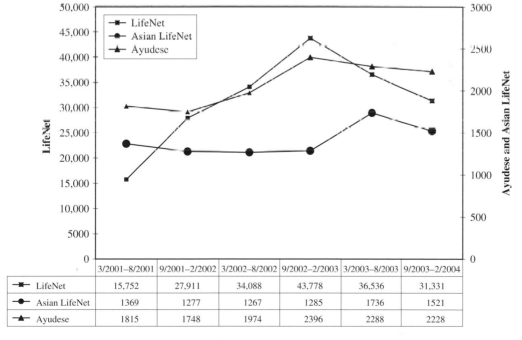

	3/2001–8/2001	9/2001–2/2002	3/2002–8/2002	9/2002–2/2003	3/2003–8/2003	9/2003–2/2004
LifeNet	15,752	27,911	34,088	43,778	36,536	31,331
Asian LifeNet	1369	1277	1267	1285	1736	1521
Ayudese	1815	1748	1974	2396	2288	2228

Figure 18.1 Growth comparison among call lines.

There are several factors that may be contributing to the little or no rates of increase among the Asian and Spanish hotlines. First, the relative absence of culture-focused Project Liberty ads (particularly for Asian ethnic groups) has had some bearing on call rates. Although all Hispanic print ads, radio commercials and outreach clearly publicized the 1-877-AYUDESE hotline number, it was not until the Project Liberty television ad was broadcast in Spanish around the first anniversary that Spanish calls began to show a marked increase (rising from a 9% increase 6 to 11 months after the attacks to a 32% increase in the fall of 2002). In all, seven separate English Project Liberty television ads were produced and rotated through several network and cable stations for a total of 27 weeks, as compared to approximately 10 weeks for the single Spanish television ad. Although more than 500,000 Asian (Chinese and Korean) Project Liberty brochures were disseminated and Asian newspapers and radio featured stories about 9/11 mental health, no Project Liberty radio, television, or subway campaigns specifically targeted the Asian community.

In spite of the comparatively limited Asian and Latino public mental health messaging by Project Liberty, there are other reasons to suspect that call rates for these hotlines would still have been lower than what was experienced on the general English-oriented LifeNet hotline. In general, treatment seeking is lower among these cultural groups, stemming from mistrust, stigma, and the tendency for these ethnic groups to first seek care through primary care or less formal sources of support, such as family, friends, clergy, and "traditional" healers (US Department of Health and Human Services Report, 2001.) The mistrust factor, in particular, has some profound relevance to the post-9/11 environment among immigrant groups, many of whom feared risking identification and deportation if they sought services advertised publicly. However, many of the 9/11-affected Asians and Latinos who have been coming forward for services have been more likely to seek assistance for basic needs such as health insurance or job training and placement (9/11 United Services Group Report, 2002).

> *Lesson 8: Anxiety disorder symptoms – such as those for PTS – will be among the most commonly reported problems for many months after the catastrophic event.*

PTS and anxiety symptoms remain the principal concerns reported by callers

In the months following 9/11/2001, LifeNet experienced exponential increases in the number of callers reporting symptoms of sleeplessness, pre-occupation with their safety and subsequent attacks, intrusive memories of the attacks, and avoidance of people, places or things that either reminded them of the disaster or portended potential risk. Some of the classic PTS symptoms such as hypervigilance – and its

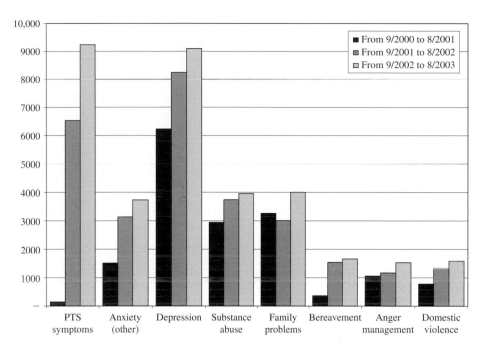

Figure 18.2 Year-to-year comparison of problems reported by LifeNet callers.

impact on both psychologic and physical health – are evident in this teacher's call to the hotline:

Every day when I get on the subway and walk down the stairs I have to prepare myself. I work at a school downtown, and had to run for my life with a few hundred kids that terrible day. Now, I spend the whole day worrying about 'what ifs' … what if an attack comes and the kids are in between periods? They know how to evacuate from a classroom, but not during passing time. What if an attack comes during recess and everyone is all spread out on the playground? I'll never be able to get them to line up, count them and run. It's all I think about. When I mention it to my co-workers, they tell me to relax and that I worry too much … I never want to be unprepared again, I just want to be ready for anything. At the end of the day, I'm relieved that another day has gone by, and nothing bad has happened. … but each day I feel worse. My stomach is in knots, my head always hurts, and when I get in my house and close the door, I break down and cry. I feel like my life has been ruined, and I feel like I'll never be able to relax again. Maybe I'm losing it …

Prior to 9/11/2001, about one of every 200 problems reported to LifeNet consisted of PTS symptoms. Six months after the attacks and beyond, 1 in 7 problems recorded for callers were consistent with one or more symptoms of PTS. Relative to the exponential increase in calls and problems reported overall in the year after the attacks, only reports of bereavement complications were disproportionately noted (322% above the prior year; see Figure 18.2 for more information).

As also noted in Figure 18.2, reports of PTS were recorded more frequently in the second year post-9/11, particularly in the months following the first anniversary. Only problems related to anger management (31%) and family conflicts (33%) rose significantly in the second year, relative to overall increases in recorded problems (20%). The growing number of post-traumatic symptom reports to the hotline is consistent with a statement made by Dr. Rachel Yehuda of Bronx Veteran's Affairs in the New York Times: "Everything we know about PTSD suggests that it takes a long time for the serious cases to make an appearance" (Goode & Eakin, 2002).

Outpatient service and Project Liberty service requests predominate

Traditionally, the most frequent service need recorded for callers to the hotline has been for mental health outpatient clinic-related needs (individual therapy, medication management, etc.). Since the disaster, requests for outpatient mental health assistance has remained the most frequent need of callers, becoming even more prominent in the months furthest away from the disaster. For example, in the 6 months *following the first anniversary* of the attacks, mental health outpatient requests have nearly doubled relative to pre-9/11 rates (Table 18.2).

Since 6 months after the attacks, LifeNet callers have been seeking more outpatient clinic services than ever before. However, following the second anniversary, outpatient clinic referrals dropped by 23.6%, particularly in the winter of 2003–2004. Interestingly, this trend reflects pre-9/11 patterns, when outpatient referrals tended to decline in the winter by over 20%. Beyond outpatient clinic needs, Project Liberty services have been the second most regularly recorded request. During its months of operation, it is likely that the Project Liberty services significantly buffered the number of referrals that would have otherwise been made to outpatient clinics.

Compared to the other common service referral categories, the relatively modest increases in substance abuse/addiction resource referrals is noteworthy. The greatest number of substance treatment service referrals occurred between 6–11 months after the disaster, but this higher rate was not sustained following the first anniversary. This trend towards a modest, short-lived increase appears consistent with findings among rescue workers engaged in the cleanup following the Oklahoma City bombing, where few new cases of substance abuse problems were seen among the workers, but significant relapses were seen among personnel with a history of problem drinking (North *et al.*, 2002).

Although LifeNet does not routinely conduct follow-up, the Robin Hood Foundation supported a project that enabled this hotline to check on the status of 9/11 callers. Beginning around the second anniversary, LifeNet began calling back 9/11-affected persons who had agreed to participate in the survey after contacting us for help approximately 3 months earlier. Of the 250 clients contacted in the first

Table 18.2. A comparison of selected service referral types pre- and post-9/11

Service types	Time periods												
	3/2001–8/2001		9/2001–2/2002		3/2002–8/2002		9/2002–2/2003		3/2003–8/2003		9/2003–2/2004	
	N	%	N	%	N	%	N	%	N	%	N	%
Mental health outpatient services	10,064	37	11,598	31	15,329	26	17,649	27	18,684	32	14,265	28
Project Liberty	0	0	3098	8	5064	9	6887	11	3069	5	841	2
Substance abuse	1632	6	1728	5	2367	4	1860	3	1888	3	2091	4
Child and adolescent	1748	6	1793	5	2691	5	3564	6	3292	6	2784	6
All 98 other services	14,050	51	18,804	51	32,654	56	34,460	53	30,829	53	30,114	60
Total	27,494	100	37,021	100	58,105	100	64,420	100	57,762	100	50,095	100

3 months of the survey, 77% had linked to services (more than half through LifeNet's referrals). Most (89%) of the persons contacted by LifeNet also reported feeling better, with the majority feeling "quite-a-bit" (31%) to "extremely better" (13%).

LifeNet's data suggests what many disaster mental health experts predicted following the events of 9/11/2001: more people would be reporting symptoms of PTS, and more people than ever would be seeking treatment to resolve mental health issues precipitated or aggravated by the disaster. Many of these persons would require more sophisticated clinical interventions than could be applied through Project Liberty encounters.

Many questions subsequently emerged for both providers and funders of post-9/11 treatment services: How do we prevent cost from being a barrier to accessing the mental health care system? Further, it was believed that many persons impacted by this disaster would not seek help if it were provided through the public mental health system. How then, do we help such persons obtain access to private practitioners? In addition, 9/11 victims have dispersed across the nation and to various regions throughout the world. How do services aimed at addressing their needs reach them where they are?

In an ambitious and extraordinary undertaking, the ARC and the SEF collaborated with LifeNet to address these concerns for many of the "primary victims" of the terrorist attacks.

9/11 Mental health and substance abuse program

Beyond the short-term assistance provided by FEMA and the private charities, both the SEF and the ARC each committed to the support of long-term recovery programs for victims. By the early spring of 2002, both groups affirmed that in some form, sustained mental health treatment should be one of the key components of their respective long-term recovery efforts.

By June 2002, it was determined that the most effective course would be for both charities to coordinate their respective plans to support mental health treatment. 1-800-LIFENET was selected as the key point-of-entry to accommodate the wide geographic distribution of potential beneficiaries, and MHA was designated to be the administrator of the enrollment process for SEF's program beneficiaries. All callers would be screened through the hotline, those who appeared to meet eligibility requirements would be conditionally enrolled, and enrollees would be subsequently contacted by either ARC or MHA benefit coordination staff to complete the process. An added advantage of using LifeNet as the "front-end" for enrollment was that LifeNet referral specialists could provide alternative referrals for callers that do not fall within the populations covered by the charity programs.

The task facing the parties was to develop a coordinated mental health program on an unprecedented scale from the ground up in a very short period of time.

Operational planning for the combined mental health benefit program took place during the period June through mid-August 2002, with the program's official launch occurring in late-August, 2002. Never before has such a broad scale, "insurance-like" program for behavioral health been developed and implemented so quickly. Our joint commitment to this extraordinary program created equally unprecedented challenges, and led to a series of critical decisions to address these concerns. The working solutions to major policy and operations questions are summarized below.

Portable benefit model chosen over grant funding

Since the victims and their families came from all over the USA and from around the world, a model based on grant-funding local mental health providers would be impractical. The alternative of an insurance-like, portable benefit program under which beneficiaries would be free to work with mental health providers of their own choosing – regardless of where they lived – was selected as the model better suited to the aims of the program.

Eligibility and division of responsibility for victim population pursuant to Mitchell plan

Neither nationality nor immigration status played any part in defining benefit eligibility. Victims from the Pentagon, WTC, and Pennsylvania disaster sites were all to be included. Under the Mitchell plan, the ARC was required to devote its resources to the following groups: the immediate families of the deceased; persons seriously injured and their families; uniformed and non-uniformed rescue and recovery workers; and displaced residents. To afford the broadest possible coverage to affected groups, the SEF supplemented this population coverage by adding categories defined as: extended families of the deceased; evacuees; persons working in the vicinity of the WTC who lost jobs or had a significant wage reduction; families of rescue and recovery workers; and school age children and their families in the vicinity of the WTC. The ARC and the SEF agreed that, when a person fell into categories covered by both charities, the ARC would assume coverage responsibility. Only a broad estimate of the total population defined by these categories has been possible, and it should also be noted that within the first 6 months of operations, several of the definitions have been expanded (most notably, the category of evacuee). Our best estimate is that somewhere between half and three-quarters of a million people may comprise the victim categories as currently defined.

Types of providers and services covered

The charities defined a comparable, but not identical benefit structure. The definition of covered services is quite detailed, compiled as a listing of industry-standard current procedure terminology (CPT) codes. Generally speaking, however, most out-patient psychotherapies, psychotropic medications and substance abuse treatment services are covered. Inpatient psychiatric and substance abuse treatment services are also covered for some groups. Persons covered by the SEF portion of the program have a dollar limit on the benefit ($3000), whereas persons covered by the ARC portion of the program have a days or sessions limit (e.g., 32 outpatient sessions or 30 inpatient days). Both charities have required that providers must either be from a licensed mental health program, or must be a licensed individual mental health practitioner in the state in which they are providing services.

Provider rate limits for services set per industry standards

The charities defined a common fee schedule for covered services that would be attractive enough to persuade most licensed professionals to accept the benefit's reimbursement as full payment. Based on aggregate insurance industry data, the final fee structure was established at the 80th percentile reimbursement level for out-of-network providers.

Interaction with other benefits or insurance coverage

This has proven to be a very complex issue. In its simplest form, the policy is that this benefit picks up where other benefits leave off. For example, if a person has mental health insurance that covers 50% of the cost of treatment, the 9/11 Mental Health and Substance Abuse Program will cover the remaining 50%, up to the limits of the program fee schedule. If the person has no insurance coverage, the Program becomes the primary payer. Both charities made the decision to contract with third party claims payment vendors to handle the actual claims submission and payment processes.

New technology developed to handle information management

There was an immediate recognition that there would be substantial information processing needs associated with an undertaking on this scale. Accordingly, MHA of NYC undertook the development of a new benefit software application system, that supported LifeNet's front-end screening, as well as enrollment process tracking, claims payment, and program evaluation activities for both charities.

Who has the program served?

Through the end of December 2003 more than 13,000 people have requested enrollment in the benefit program and have been determined to be "conditionally eligible." Conditional eligibility means that, pending submission of required documentation regarding victim status, a person appears to meet eligibility criteria, and he/she is transferred to a benefit coordinator. The benefit coordinator works with the person to confirm eligibility, answer questions about use of the benefit, and issue enrollment materials.

The monthly conditional eligibility volume is shown in Figure 18.3. As with LifeNet, the demand has been sensitive to activating events such as anniversaries

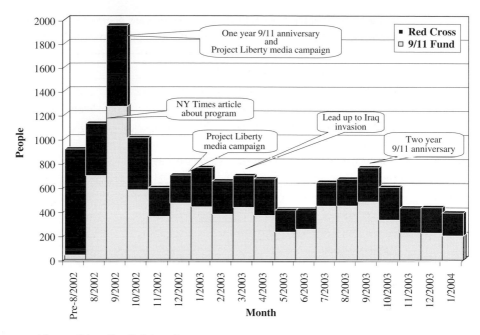

Figure 18.3 Monthly conditionally eligible callers.

and direct and indirect media coverage. The same week during which the program was launched, a very favorable article appeared on the front page of the New York Times national edition. In the next 10 days, there were nearly 1000 calls for the benefit. Although Project Liberty's extensive broadcast campaign did not mention the mental health treatment program, there was nevertheless a corresponding spike in demand each time such 9/11 campaigns was launched. LifeNet's role as the entry point for both Project Liberty and the 9/11 treatment benefit program nullified the need for the charities to spend a great deal of donor money on program advertising.

Table 18.3 shows the distribution of conditionally eligible beneficiaries by victim category for both charities combined. We note that the evacuee category is by far the largest. Originally defined as someone who evacuated a building that was damaged or destroyed, the definition of evacuee was very quickly changed to a definition with street, rather than building, boundaries because we encountered many personal accounts such as the following:

I was approximately 200 yards from the SouthTower when the plane hit. It was horrible. I ran for my life. I will never forget that moment. I have been haunted by it ever since that day. I have nightmares all the time. I can't seem to get past this.

The definition has recently been expanded yet again to encompass more extended street boundaries, based on accounts from many people whose subjective experience was that they had to run for their lives that morning. Indeed, one of the inevitable

Table 18.3. Distribution of victim categories for persons deemed conditionally eligible for the mental health benefit program

Victim category	N	%
Evacuee	3889	28.2
Displaced resident	2604	18.9
Immediate family of deceased	1613	11.7
Extended family of deceased	1169	8.5
Family of evacuee	895	6.5
Un/underemployed	748	5.4
Uniformed rescue and recovery	747	5.4
Not determined at initial screening	596	4.3
Non-uniformed rescue and recovery	495	3.6
Family of rescue and recovery	353	2.6
Family of un/underemployed	216	1.6
Family of student	145	1.1
Injured	143	1.0
Student	136	1.0
Family of injured	19	0.1
Total	13,768	100.0

difficulties in developing operational definitions for these victim categories is that wherever the lines are drawn, there are always groups of people whose personal circumstances that day placed them just outside the lines that bound the covered categories. This is particularly common with people who approach us on the basis that they have lost a job, but whose work location falls outside the boundaries that have been established for this victim category.

Table 18.4 shows this distribution of conditionally eligible beneficiaries by state. Note that international cases, most of which are managed through a separate process by the international Red Cross, are not included in these figures. Not unexpectedly, the highest demand has been from New York. New York demand has principally been from Manhattan and the other boroughs, but a zip code analysis shows that it has also been high from within a "commuting radius" of approximately 75 miles from NYC. Reflecting that this has indeed been a national tragedy, to date people from a total of 44 states and the District of Columbia have sought services under the mental health benefit program.

On a voluntary basis, beneficiaries covered by the SEF portion of the program are asked to provide information about racial/ethnic identification, using categories established by the US Census Bureau. Through December, 2001, 59.9% of the SEF enrolled beneficiaries had provided this optional information, as shown in Table 18.5.

A significant observation is that demand has been somewhat disproportionately low from the non-white victim populations for mental health services under the

Table 18.4. State distribution of conditionally eligible beneficiaries

State	%
New York	81
New Jersey	11
Connecticut	1
41 Other States	7
Total	100

Table 18.5. Ethnic/racial mix of a sample of enrolled mental health program beneficiaries

US census categories	N	%
Hispanic/Latino any race	419	17.1
Not Hispanic, one race		
White	1527	62.5
African-American	235	9.6
Asian	115	4.7
Native American	9	0.4
Hawaiian/Pacific Islander	3	0.1
Other	19	0.8
Two or more races	118	4.8
Total reporting (59.9% of enrolled beneficiaries)	2445	100.0
Not reported (40.1% of enrolled beneficiaries)	1639	

program. We have conducted focus groups with representatives of the Asian and Latino communities around this issue. As noted in the earlier section describing lower call volume among Asian and Latinos on the respective LifeNet lines, a wide variety of cultural influences (ranging from stigma, misinformation, perceived threats to immigration status, other culturally accepted alternatives for support, etc.) have affected the uptake of the benefit in these communities. In some cases, local support groups that do not have the connotation of mental health treatment are often perceived as safer, less stigmatizing, more culturally relevant alternatives than licensed mental health treatment. Nevertheless, focused outreach has had the effect of increasingly enrollment on a proportionate basis from the end of 2002 to the end of 2003.

Lessons learned in administering the 9/11 benefit program, thus far

The program is a work in progress. There are changes in eligibility criteria, covered services, covered providers, benefit limits, and approaches to outreach made on an ongoing basis. In general, we have learned that media helps enrollment, and enrollment needs remain substantial more than 2 years after the disaster. Other lessons learned more specific to this program are noted below.

Nimble, mid-course correction approaches are essential

The first lesson is that to be effective, responsive, and fair, a program such as this must be willing to make modifications based on operating experience. It is virtually impossible to imagine in advance all of the variations of individual experience and circumstances within the populations seeking services.

Programs must address diverse culture needs *vis á vis* outreach and actual services

While the effects of the disaster have been felt broadly, there is a strong, culturally determined predisposition in some groups against defining their personal experience as a mental health problem, and against seeking licensed mental health treatment as a culturally appropriate remedy for such problems. Part of the outreach effort must include community education to counteract stigma associated with mental health problems. It may also be necessary to move beyond support for traditional, licensed mental health services, to alternative modalities and providers perceived to be more natural and relevant supports by the members of some cultural communities.

Create a point-of-entry that is easily accessible

In addition, the transom must be culturally sensitive, and, ideally, have the capacity to also offer on-the-spot alternatives for those persons who do not meet program criteria. As the multi-lingual point of entry for all other 9/11 (as well as non-9/11) behavioral health programs, LifeNet has been particularly well suited to this task. By layering in a customized benefit coordination software application, it has been possible to process thousands of calls in a timely, responsive, and organized fashion. We have been able to match callers with the appropriate resources very efficiently, helping people avoid a succession of attempts at finding out where the most appropriate help might be available.

> *Lesson 9: When a large-scale disaster creates large-scale demand for mental health services, it will be critical for the clinical workforce to have the skills appropriate for responding to their needs.*

A challenge related to ensuring greater access to behavioral health care for persons emotionally troubled by the disaster has also been that of ensuring "appropriate, quality care". In the tri-state area, many providers expressed a need for more training in clinically managing the symptoms related to PTSD and complicated bereavement, so that 9/11-affected victims could receive optimal care upon entering treatment. The SEF utilized LifeNet's new CRC program to meet this vast training demand, providing support for the largest post-disaster training program for licensed mental health practitioners ever seen in the USA.

LifeNet's CRC and the SEF's training program

As noted earlier, the SEF supported the formation of LifeNet's CRC. Although its original purpose was to provide support to communities by coordinating and mobilizing mental health professionals to work with groups, its most significant role in the recovery effort was to equip mental health professionals in the region with the skills needed to serve people seeking their help in the aftermath of 9/11.

The CRC served as a clearinghouse for workshops and training in trauma and crisis counseling around the New York area. The CRC advertised this via MHA of NYC web site postings and mass faxing to the thousands of providers in LifeNet's database. In December 2001, MHA received funds from The New York Times Foundation to establish the CRC as the engine for promoting and coordinating the trauma treatment workshops offered through a consortium of local facilities with notable expertise in the field (The Consortium for Effective Trauma Treatment). Subsequently, the CRC was called upon by the SEF to administer a program designed to bring training for various evidence-based trauma and bereavement treatment approaches to thousands of metropolitan NYC area mental health professionals.

Setting up the skills training program

Since evidence-based, trauma treatment is not necessarily included in every graduate school training program, it was assumed that many mental health professionals in the surrounding area would not have the requisite skills to provide appropriate clinical interventions following such an incident of mass trauma (Ruzek, 2002). The program established the goal of training between 6000 and 7000 mental health providers in a variety of trauma-related assessment and intervention skills. MHA of NYC organized, promoted and administered more than 130 courses over an 18 month period, beginning in 2002 and continuing through 2004. The trainings were offered at no cost and were held in a variety of venues, such as mental health agencies, hospitals, and at other private facilities.

Trainings were promoted through direct mailings, faxes to mental health and substance abuse agencies in the LifeNet database, e-mails to membership lists maintained by mental health agencies who had partnered with us in the past, and through advertising in mental health trade journals. The most effective response rate resulted from direct mailings, followed by faxes to mental health and substance abuse agencies. Continuing education credits were secured for medical, psychology, social work, nurse practitioner and certified alcohol and substance abuse counsellor (CASAC) disciplines. More than 6500 area professionals have registered for these courses, with attendance for all modules averaging at over 70%. More than half of attendees are licensed social workers (16% are psychologists), and they average 13 years experience in providing clinical treatment.

The trauma training program components are summarized below:

Program	Faculty	Description
Practical Front Line Assistance and Support for Healing (PFLASH) and Practical Front Line Assistance and Support for Healing for Children (KFLASH)	A pool of local professionals with backgrounds in this area was trained by Dr. Carol North	Developed by Carol North, M.D., from the Washington University School of Medicine and Betty Pfefferbaum, M.D. from the University of Oklahoma School of Medicine, based on their research with victims of the Oklahoma City bombing in 1995 (North *et al.*, 1999). Training provided an introduction to assessment of pathologic responses, understanding outcome predictors and basic front line intervention techniques. The KFLASH version emphasized issues unique to children and adolescents
9/11 Group Therapy Training series	Instructors recruited by the American Group Psychotherapy Association	Developed by the American Group Psychotherapy Association, these 10 modules focused on group interventions that can be used with populations affected by mass violence and trauma
Prolonged Exposure Therapy	Faculty from Columbia University and the New York State Psychiatric Institute, Trauma Studies and Services	Based upon work by Edna Foa (Foa *et al.*, 2000). Focused on providing cognitive behavioral techniques for the treatment of individuals suffering from PTSD. The emphasis was on training licensed clinicians. Program included clinical demonstrations, role-plays and an advanced practice manual
Traumatic Grief	Faculty from Columbia University and the New York State Psychiatric Institute, Trauma Studies and Services	Katherine Shear, MD, from the University of Pittsburgh, developed a curriculum focused on treating complicated grief in individuals unable to progress through the normal mourning process
Trauma-Based Family Therapy	Faculty and affiliates from the Ackerman Institute for the Family	Developed by Kenneth Hardy, Ph.D and Peter Fraenkle, Ph.D, the training was built around the idea that trauma experienced by one member of the family can negatively impact the functioning of the family unit. For traumatized individuals, family response can be a source of healing and resilience, or can greatly exacerbate symptoms

Addressing "compassion fatigue"

Training programs frequently offer little in the way of follow-up activity or support to trainees, so a small pilot project was conceived to offer free support group services to clinicians. The provider community also expressed concern regarding issues of compassion fatigue, and training evaluation data collected by MHA of NYC indicated that trainees surveyed were expressing interest in attending support groups. MHA of NYC partnered with the American Group Psychotherapy Association (AGPA) to implement groups specifically for providers working with 9/11 populations. Five separate groups initially met at mutually convenient locations, on a monthly or bi-weekly basis. Qualified licensed AGPA clinicians with extensive experience in facilitating group activities led the support groups.

Although a large percentage of registered clinicians (61%) had expressed interest in attending support groups, most groups were lightly attended, and several were discontinued after a short period of time. A number of factors may have influenced this, such as the difficulty in developing freestanding support groups from scratch vs. utilizing naturally occurring groups within existing agencies settings. In addition, there may be a gap in the education of clinicians regarding their ability to recognize the need for self-help and mutual aid.

Assessing the impact of the training program

Through the training program, the SEF sought to diversify the range of skill-acquisition opportunities for clinicians, by establishing short-term training initiatives to meet the specific demands of this unprecedented event. While it is too early to assess the longer-term impact of these trainings on clinical practice, the participants have given the trainings high ratings (on 1–5 scale with 5 being outstanding, workshops have averaged an overall rating of 4.22). Further, these trainings appear to have reached 9/11-affected clients in treatment, as participants have estimated that 53% of their caseload has been impacted by 9/11.

Conclusion

A number of factors have enabled the MHA of NYC's LifeNet Hotline Network to support the massive mobilization of mental health resources in the wake of the September 11th attacks. However, a central key to LifeNet's post-disaster success was that its every-day operations (responding to persons in crisis; assessing, educating and referring troubled persons to services; working closely with government agencies and community providers; and conducting broad-scale behavioral health public education campaigns) were in place well before 9/11.

While LifeNet's pre-9/11 operations were vital to the short- and longer-term disaster response, it appears that LifeNet's current "every day" service will never look exactly as it did before 9/11. At this time, calls to the hotline continue to be more than double the volume experienced 2 years before, with many callers regularly remarking, "*I thought I would be over this by now.*" General public recognition of the service, high levels of distress, and perhaps some reduction in the stigma associated with seeking help for emotional problems may be contributing to the new base-line for this hotline's expected monthly call volume. Further, LifeNet will continue to be the front-line for enrolling eligible persons in the 9/11 mental health benefit for some years to come, ensuring that this once NYC-centered service will continue to take regular calls from 9/11-affected persons wherever they live, for as long as the benefit remains available.

As LifeNet and the ARC/SEF treatment benefit work to enhance access to care for persons with longer-term 9/11-related emotional problems, the massive SEF training program for clinicians in the tri-state area will potentially improve access to *clinically appropriate* treatment. At the very least, introducing a program rich in cognitive-behavioral lessons to a community of New York therapists traditionally steeped in psychoanalytic theory is, itself, some measure of advancement towards eclecticism in treatment methods. It is hoped that the ultimate impact of such a program – which eventually trained 5436 professionals in 18 months – will perhaps leave a legacy of broader clinician skill and preparedness for a wide variety of trauma cases in the years to come.

The need to actively promote access to readily available services following a disaster is a high priority for public mental health. A common post-catastrophe behavioral health malady, PTSD, is characterized by *avoidance*, and requires aggressive outreach measures. Project Liberty's campaign showed that an extensive media and community-based efforts are effective in drawing people from behind closed doors. However, Project Liberty's historic program closed its own doors at the end of 2003, leaving LifeNet and a handful of other 9/11-focused behavioral health programs to continue this vital long-term work.

For LifeNet and the mental health system's treatment providers who seek to directly assist 9/11-affected persons, serious challenges confront us in the months and years ahead.

As we drift further from that day in September when terrorists steered American planes into American buildings, the lives still troubled from exposure to those horrific attacks may feel increasingly disconnected from the event. Its psychologic fallout may create lower thresholds for stress, anxiety, and depression in these individuals, while blending deeper into the fabric of the overall population's experience of emotional problems, struggles with drugs and alcohol, domestic disputes, and/or work and school complications. A major task for us will be to educate the public – through both targeted and broad-scale methods – as to how catastrophic events can complicate lives even now, affecting different people in different ways, and at different times in their lives. Above all, we must find a variety of ways to inform the public that LifeNet will be here to help those who need it, whenever that may be.

Acknowledgments

Major contributors and collaborators for the development, implementation, and evaluation of Project Liberty include: Columbia University, Mailman School of Public Health; The Federal Emergency Management Agency; The Nathan Kline Institute, Center for the Study of Issues in Public Mental Health; The National Center for PTSD; The New York Academy of Medicine, Center for Urban Epidemiological Studies; The NYC DOHMH and Departments of Mental Health in 10 counties surrounding NYC; The New York State Psychiatric Institute; Mount Sinai School of Medicine, Division of Health Services Research; and the Substance Abuse and Mental Health Services Administration, Center for Mental Health Services.

REFERENCES

Foa, E.B., Keane, T.M. & Friedman, M.J. eds (2000). *Effective Treatment for PTSD: Practice Guidelines from the International Society for Traumatic Stress Studies.* Guilford Press.

Galea, S., Resnick, H., Ahern, J., Stuber, J., Kilpatrick, D., Gold, J. & Vlahov, D. (2003). Post-traumatic stress disorder in New York City after September 11. *American Psychiatric Association Annual Meeting* [Oral presentation], San Francisco, CA, May 2003.

Goode, E. & Eakin, E. (2002). Mental health: the profession tests its limits. *New York Times*, 12 September.

Hoven, C.W., Duarte, C.S., Lucas, C.P., Mandell, D.J., Wu, P. & Rosen, C. (2002). Effects of the World Trade Center attack on NYC public school students – initial report to the New York City Board of Education. Applied Research and Consulting, LLC & Columbia University Mailman School of Public Health and New York State Psychiatric Institute: New York, 2002.

Norris, F., Hamblen, J., Watson, P., Ruzek, J., Gibson, L., Pfefferbaum, B., *et al.* (in press). Understanding and creating systems of post-disaster care: A case study of New York's mental health system's response to the World Trade Center Disaster. In *Mental Health Intervention Following Disasters or Mass Violence*, eds. C. Ritchie, P. Watson & M. Friedman. New York: Guilford Press.

North, C.S., Nixon, S.J., Shariat, S., *et al.* (1999). Psychiatric disorders among survivors of the Oklahoma City bombing. *Journal of American Medical Association*, **282**(8), 755–762.

North, C.S., Tivis, L., McMillen, J.C., Pfefferbaum, B., Cox, J., Spitznagel, E.L., Bunch, K., Schorr, J. & Smith, E.M. (2002). Coping, functioning, and adjustment of rescue workers after the Oklahoma City bombing. *Journal of Traumatic Stress*, **15**(3), 171–175.

Ruzek, J.I. (2002). Dissemination of information and early intervention practices in the context of mass violence of large-scale disaster. *Behavior Therapist*, **25**(2), 32–36.

September 11th Fund (2002). One Year Later (Annual Report). New York, NY.

US Department of Health and Human Services (2001). Mental health: culture, race, and ethnicity – a supplement to mental health: A report of the Surgeon General. Rockville, MD: US Department of Health and Human Services, Substance Abuse and Mental Health Services Administration, Center for Mental Health Services.

9/11 United Services Group (2002). A study of the ongoing needs of people affected by the World Trade Center disaster. New York, NY: Mckinley & Company.

19

The New York Consortium for Effective Trauma Treatment

Randall D. Marshall, Yuval Neria, Eun Jung Suh and Lawrence V. Amsel
John Kastan and Spencer Eth
Lori Davis and Marylene Cloitre
Gila Schwarzbaum and Rachel Yehuda
Jack Rosenthal

INTRODUCTION

Randall D. Marshall

From the first chaotic days after the attacks of September 11, 2001, the co-directors of the Consortium – Marylene Cloitre, PhD, Spencer Eth, MD, Randall Marshall, MD, and Rachel Yehuda, PhD – shared a collective sense of alarm that the need for mental health services in our community would greatly exceed capacity to provide evidence-based treatment for trauma-related problems and disorders. Because federal programs almost exclusively emphasize the public health objective of restoring the general population to a semblance of normal functioning, we worried that there would not be adequate programs devoted to helping persons developing serious psychiatric disorder as a result of the attacks. Subsequent epidemiological studies (reviewed in this volume) confirmed our impression, but by the time these data were available – many months after 9/11 – we were already well underway with the project of providing intensive training to a group of clinicians at each of our centers, who could then serve as expert treatment providers, and, more importantly, clinician experts available to the community for educational programs. In sum, the Consortium was a rapidly implemented large-scale project with the overall objective of disseminating evidence-based treatments for trauma-related disorders to the greater New York community.

During the first year alone, approximately 920 patients were evaluated and treated at all sites. Treatment was provided in English, Spanish, Hebrew, German, Korean, and several Chinese dialects. Some sites developed intensive trainings for clinicians, and other focused on clinical work or other kinds of educational programs (e.g. intensive training and supervision for a small group of community clinicians). The flexibility of the Consortium was critical, in that each site could respond according to its own strengths and the needs of its local geographic community. In the first year, 201 clinicians were trained in these seminars, and training continued into the second year after the attacks. In addition, we gave more than 115 lecture-format trainings to an estimated several thousand persons. Trainees included clinicians, clergy, school personnel, human resources personnel at corporations, and lay audiences. Over the second year, all four centers continued work established by the Consortium project.

This chapter documents the process of forming the Consortium and the individual experiences and activities of each center. We hope this will prove useful to other communities attempting similar such efforts, and to dissemination researchers. Ideally, such projects could be prepared in advance, with research methodology embedded in the project. These "off-the-shelf" programs could then be made available to communities after any large-scale disaster that threatens to overwhelm capacity to provide evidence-based treatment. At present, FEMA Program templates focus only on short-term and resistence-enchancing interventions, as they are mandated.

What is clear in retrospect is that the Consortium was possible only because it was funded through philanthropy. Within a few weeks, the generosity of donors from around the world, and the visionary leadership of Jack Rosenthal at the New York Times 9/11 Neediest Fund, made it possible for us to move quickly and decisively while most other programs and efforts were still in the planning phase, including government-sponsored programs. The success of this kind of partnership in itself might serve as a model for future disaster response initiatives.

We thought it best to allow each center to speak for itself, after an introduction by our first benefactor, Jack Rosenthal, President of The New York Times Company Foundation.

Acknowledgments

We are deeply indebted to The New York Times Foundation, The Surdna Foundation Project Liberty, and The Atlantic Philanthropies for their support.

THE NEW YORK TIMES COMPANY FOUNDATION

Jack Rosenthal

On September 11, 2001, the demand side was instantly clear. The World Trade Center disaster scorched the psyche of New York. There would surely be many thousands who would soon learn firsthand about the time bombs that such a trauma can leave in the mind.

The supply side, however, was far from clear. What we at The New York Times Company Foundation asked ourselves was, would there be enough therapists, even in this, the shrink capital of the western world, sufficiently skilled in shock trauma, to meet the need? Even within a scrupulous definition of victims, it was easy to calculate that 200,000 or more people were subject to trauma – 3000 families who lost a loved one; 25,000 or so who escaped from the buildings and their families; 10,000 school kids and their families; perhaps 50,000 families which saw their livelihoods evaporate in minutes.

We didn't anticipate that 200,000 people would experience post-traumatic stress. But as Betty Pfefferbaum's research teaches, some proportion would, perhaps 15%. Were there enough therapists with advanced trauma training to handle 30,000 new patients? Our initial inquiries brought a startling answer. Not only was the answer no, but some people we consulted believed that the rudimentary treatment many therapists could offer might even be *toxic*. As we considered how best to spend the many millions that the public was contributing to our New York Times 9/11 Neediest Fund, we could see that quickly increasing the supply side, was a priority goal.

The next question was how to do that. We turned for advice to Dr. Randall Marshall at the Trauma Studies and Services Program of the New York State Psychiatric Institute at Columbia University. With appealing candor, he said, "Please understand, we're only one of several hospital-based trauma centers in the city". Others included at Mount Sinai, St. Vincent's, and Cornell Medical, which later moved to New York University. And when we asked whether the four might get together, Randall Marshall immediately set out to make it happen. Within days of 9/11, the Consortium was formed. Dr. Marshall won the eager cooperation of Dr. Spencer Eth at St. Vincent's Hospital; Marylene Cloitre, then at the New York Cornell Medical Center and now at the NYU Child Studies Center; and Rachel Yehuda, Director of the Traumatic Stress Studies Division at Mount Sinai. These four became joint directors of the Consortium and its success arises from the intelligence and extended energy each has brought to the enterprise.

One measure of success is reflected by a study Rachel Yehuda is doing that involves three categories of patients: those who were treated by therapists without specialized trauma training, those who were treated by the original 60 clinicians trained by the Consortium, and those who were treated by the hundreds of clinicians who were students of the original 60. Her initial study yields two impressions: patients of therapists without the advanced training have done much less well. And patients treated by the 500 have done just as well as those treated by the original 60. It's a satisfying indication that the training is being passed on effectively.

The comfortable collaboration of the four trauma centers in the Consortium offers a model for some potential disaster in the future, one that applies far beyond mental health. Our experience demonstrates the wisdom of creating a loose council of philanthropies, service providers, and professional associations. Such a council could convene immediately, not necessarily with the aim of tight coordination but at least to share information and goals. As Vartan Gregorian, President of the Carnegie Corporation told a group that met after 9/11, "Look, this is not coordination; this is just information, so I know that if you're giving shoeshines, I can give haircuts".

We find it at least as gratifying that the Consortium has continued its work. Its seminars continue, it has won further funding from more permanent sources of support and it daily demonstrates the mutual benefits of working as partners. We are pleased and proud to be among them.

TRAUMA STUDIES AND SERVICES, THE NEW YORK STATE PSYCHIATRIC INSTITUTE, COLUMBIA UNIVERSITY COLLEGE OF PHYSICIANS AND SURGEONS

Randall D. Marshall, Yuval Neria, Eun Jung Suh and Lawrence Amsel

Training, Treatment, and Research Team included: Steven B. Rudin, MD, Donna Vermes, BS, NPP, BC, Gretchen Seirmarco, APRN, BC, Smit Sinha, MD, Raz Gross, MD, Jaime Carcamo, PsyD, Arturo Sanchez, MD, Helena Rosenfeld, BA and Kimesha Thompson.

The first few weeks

As the primary clinical research site for the New York State Office of Mental Health (NYSOMH), our staff was immediately enveloped in an atmosphere of emergency. A few of our staff had been directly affected. Several staff members lost siblings. One lost three members of her family. Another lost an uncle who had essentially raised her from early childhood. Others lived in lower Manhattan, and were displaced from their homes. These personal losses compounded our already heightened sense that we had all been deeply and permanently affected by this tragedy, and lent urgency to all our activities for many months to follow.

The first weeks passed in a blur of long days and nights spent in helping NYSOMH develop a plan for its emergency relief services application; assisting persons at corporations and institutions that had been directly affected by the attacks; and learning as much as possible from the experience of other disaster experts through their writings and through emergency meetings.

In the first weeks, Dr. Marshall presented to the Columbia faculty on what was known about acute intervention after severe trauma. There are no medications proven effective for either reducing symptoms or preventing the development of chronic post-traumatic stress disorder (PTSD). A handful of studies suggested a cognitive–behavioral therapy (CBT) that focused on processing the trauma might be helpful, but this was by no means conclusive. No treatment study had been conducted specifically with victims of a large-scale community disaster. Most concerning, however, was the fact that almost no one in the audience had advanced training in this approach. It became clear to us at this point that our mental health community was almost certainly not going to be able to provide the latest evidence-based treatments to 9/11 victims on the scale required. As confirmation of this impression, in the first week our center had received hundreds of calls from clinicians all over the city asking for additional training in how to treat the survivors of the World Trade Center attacks.

Creating the Consortium

It was at this point that Jack Rosenthal called asking if the New York Times Foundation could help with the mental health needs of New Yorkers affected by 9/11. We felt the need was going to be too big for any single institution to handle, and turned to our colleagues for help. We met and developed a proposal based on two core principles: first, that there was likely to be an epidemic of mental health problems related to 9/11, for which our community was unprepared; second, that victims of 9/11 deserved the highest quality treatment, based on state-of-the-art research, that could be obtained anywhere in the world.

The strategy, then, was clear: we needed to enhance the expertise of our staff; be available to provide services; and devote a portion of our energies to disseminating evidence-based techniques to the larger community of mental health practitioners.

Enhancing expertise in trauma treatment

The Consortium grant allowed each center to designate core personnel who would become "trauma treatment experts". To provide rapid training to our newly expanded staff, we turned to trauma experts around the country.

Over the next several months, we invited the following experts to present to our group on trauma-related treatment issues:

- Edna Foa, "Prolonged Exposure Therapy for PTSD".
- Katherine Shear, "Traumatic Grief Treatment".
- Shirley Glynn and Kim Muesser, "Family Involvement in Recovery from Acute Trauma".
- Patricia Resick, "Cognitive Processing Therapy".
- Arieh Shalev, "Living Under Chronic Threat".
- Jonathan Davidson, "Psychopharmacological Management of PTSD".
- Bessel van der Kolk, "Complex PTSD".
- Roberto Lewis-Fernandez, Carmela Perez and Maria Astidillo, "Cultural Competence in Trauma Treatment".
- Judith Cohen, "Treating Children with PTSD".
- Marylene Cloitre, "Skills Training in Affective and Interpersonal Regulation (STAIR) as a Preparatory Stabilization Phase for the Multiply Traumatized Patient".

- Barry Krakow and Dominic Menendrez, "Treatment of Post-traumatic Nightmares".
- Tuvia Peri, "Treating Acute Stress".
- John Markowitz, "Interpersonal Psychotherapy".
- Denise Hien, "Substance Abuse in PTSD".
- Claude Chemtob, "Children with PTSD in Disaster Settings".
- Stan Rosenberg and Kim Meusser, "PTSD in Chronically Mentally Ill Patients".

We owe a tremendous debt of gratitude to the above colleagues who were willing to share their time and expertise.

Developing a focus on training

As time passed, our initial concerns were confirmed by multiple surveys demonstrating epidemic rates of new-onset PTSD-related specifically to the 9/11 attacks. At Columbia and the New York State Psychiatric Institute, we perceived a growing appreciation in the mental health community that treating these patients did indeed require special expertise, together with a genuine openness not seen before to acquiring additional clinical skills. We therefore decided to make this our special area of emphasis, and set about developing a training strategy and curriculum that could provide effective training to as many clinicians as possible in a relatively brief amount of time.

We initially made the decision that our trainings would emphasize diagnosis of trauma-related psychopathology and psychotherapy techniques, rather than psychopharmacology. This decision was based on our strong impression that the availability and effective use of medication for the treatment of chronic PTSD and major depression was widely known and appreciated, whereas evidence-based psychotherapy techniques for PTSD were known and practiced only by a small, highly specialized group, and had not yet been embraced by the general community of practitioners. In addition, we were aware that the majority of mental health service providers in the community are not physicians and thus do not prescribe medication.

Developing a state-of-the-art training program

We recognized from the outset that our training project was in essence an *educational* endeavor, not a clinical one. Although this appears obvious, it was a critical first realization, since it followed that we should turn to the educational research literature for guidance. Drs. Lawrence Amsel and Peter Jensen contributed their special expertise in educational methodology. To be effective, a psychotherapy training (as is true for any educational program) needed to specific, practical, interactive, experiential, highly engaging and able to overcome at least some trainee barriers to implementation. What, then, should such a training look like, and how could we evaluate its effectiveness?

We selected two manualized psychotherapies for our trainings: a well-studied form of CBT called prolonged exposure, developed by Edna Foa and colleagues; and a new psychotherapy for persons with the new diagnosis of Complicated Grief, developed by Katherine Shear (Shear *et al.*, 2005).

We then settled on the use of several different educational strategies that were implemented systematically to teach a series of core concepts or skills: lectures and discussion (present the concept/skill), followed by clinical case demonstration (demonstrate the concept/skill), and then individual role-play in pairs (foster discussion of the concept/foster practice of the skill). Passive learning – that is, lecturing, the mode used most widely in professional education, and the mode known to be ineffective in promoting behavioral change – had to be kept to a minimum. The other widely used mode of training – supervision – was too labor intensive, too difficult to organize quickly in the community, and insufficient for reaching large numbers of practitioners. The challenge then became the following: develop the most effective training possible that will maximize the likelihood of attendees acquiring new concepts and skills such that they could be implemented appropriately in clinical practice.

Dissemination of an evidence-based psychotherapy had never before been attempted on this scale in the setting of community disaster. As researchers, we placed a high priority from the beginning on the importance of evaluating the quality of our trainings, in an effort to further this much-neglected field of professional education in mental health. In small-scale trainings, the typical approach is to provide a training workshop, and then study the implementation of new skills in the attendees' clinical practice. This would have been logistically impossible and prohibitively expensive, however, since several hundred clinicians were to be trained in a relatively brief period of time. Instead, we opted to study the training itself, and specifically whether the training *(1) increased perceived favorableness for the therapy we were teaching and (2) increased skill level in the techniques being presented.* High ratings on both variables are necessary if attendees are going to apply the skills they are learning in clinical practice.

Our theoretical framework was derived from *motivation science* (Amsel *et al.*, this volume). The premise of our model was that, in the trainees, the motivation to alter practice patterns and incorporate new behaviors as a therapist would of necessity precede the actual behavior. Effective training, then, should *enhance motivation* to implement the skills being presented, and *reduce psychological barriers* to their implementation. These variables are measurable. We therefore attempted to study factors that would suggest a trainee is likely vs. unlikely to try out techniques learned in the training. We also attempted to anticipate barriers to using these techniques that experienced clinicians might experience, and then systematically address these barriers in the trainings. An early report of our findings is presented in this volume (Amsel *et al.*, this volume).

Results of the training project

We conducted these trainings on a weekly basis for nearly 2 years. Our trainings were attended by over 1500 licensed mental health practitioners in the greater New York area, and were funded by a number of philanthropic and government-based programs, including the New York Times Foundation; Atlantic Philanthropies; the Surdna Foundation; the September 11 Fund; and Project Liberty. We could not have functioned without the extraordinary organizational assistance of the Mental Health Association of New York City, Inc. (LIFENET).

We are proud to report that we received "superior" ratings from our attendees, with average evaluation scores between 4 (very good) and 5 (excellent) on a 5-point scale. An overwhelming majority of the attendees stated that they anticipated changing their patient care practices by incorporating the assessment and treatment techniques learned from our trainings. In addition, attendees unequivocally endorsed recommending our courses to fellow colleagues. We think this success is in part due to our taking to heart a number of early criticisms, as well as the ongoing feedback we received, and revising our trainings accordingly.

Other beneficial consequences of the Consortium project

For our center, these funds allowed us to begin immediately with a training effort that was funded for an additional 1½ years by the September 11 Fund and Project Liberty; a clinical treatment program that led to a major National Institute of Mental Health (NIMH) treatment grant for 9/11 victims with PTSD (Randall Marshall, MD, Principal Investigator); a follow up study of primary care patients in Northern Manhattan funded by NIMH and conducted in collaboration with Drs. Myrna Weissman and Mark Olfson (Yuval Neria, PhD, Principal Investigator); a Hispanic Research and Outreach Program led by Roberto Lewis-Fernández, MD with an emphasis on improving detection and treatment; a new Grief Studies program focusing on the phenomenology and treatment of Complicated Grief, and the training of clinicians to provide effective psychotherapy for these patients (in collaboration with Katherine Shear, MD). Our work and perspectives have been presented in the USA, Canada, Japan, Israel, Great Britain, the Netherlands, and France, in lecture, television, newspaper, magazine, or radio format. The opportunity to lend our own experience in the service of helping other communities has been particularly gratifying for all of us.

Conclusions

Interacting with several hundred mental health practitioners in New York City taught us a number of invaluable lessons. Perhaps the central benefit of these trainings for us was the opportunity to learn from the collective experience of these community clinicians. In a sense, these trainings functioned for us as focus groups giving us a window on the dilemmas being faced by clinicians, and the problems that 9/11 patients were facing in their recovery. Overall, we were deeply impressed by the openness and sophistication of clinicians in the New York community. Feedback about the trainings themselves was immensely useful in refining our curriculum, techniques, and educational strategy.

We witnessed firsthand the gap between the training backgrounds of most practicing clinicians, and the expertise needed to implement recent empirical findings in PTSD research. At the time of this writing, there continues to be strong interest from the community in learning these techniques. Our last 4 weeks of trainings were booked at double capacity (150 clinicians), 2½ years after the attacks.

There are many formidable barriers to dissemination of psychotherapy techniques. We believe they can be overcome, but only with a considerable amount of effort, using methodologies that are in the early development and testing phase. Traditional approaches for continuing education are embarrassingly inadequate to the task, and yet many millions of dollars are still spent annually on traditional Continuing Professional Education (CPE). Based on our preliminary work we will be studying at least three basic strategies to improve this situation. First, in creating CPE programs, we believe programs should be designed based on a scientifically sound behavior change model. Second, trainings should maximize their use of case-based material such as documentary-style video and role-play demonstration. These appear to enhance motivation and convey potential for positive outcomes much more effectively than traditional slide and lecture presentations. Third, training modules should specifically focus on how to implement the techniques, and on strategies to overcome barriers to implementation in individual practice settings.

The only way to avoid the difficulties we had to address after 9/11 is to address them before disaster occurs – through preparedness planning. The obstacles we encountered were formidable and exhausting, and many could have been addressed before the attacks. Communities should have a disaster preparedness plan that includes effective educational programs that target common disorders such as depression, PTSD, and sub-threshold fear and phobic avoidance. This is separate from, though complementary to, an acute intervention program that is typically implemented through federal guidelines.

It was particularly important to our team to effectively "translate" manual-based, CBT-derived therapy techniques into terms that psychodynamically trained clinicians would find useful. Most of us were trained in both psychodynamic and CBT therapies, and believe that both approaches have strengths and limitations. We hope we were able to convince many New York clinicians that CBT techniques, and manualized approaches in general, can be highly effective complements to psychodynamic intuition and knowledge.

ST. VINCENT CATHOLIC MEDICAL CENTERS OF NEW YORK, BEHAVIORAL HEALTH SERVICES AND NEW YORK MEDICAL COLLEGE

John Kastan and Spencer Eth

St. Vincent's Hospital in Manhattan, an academic medical center of New York Medical College, was at the center of the emergency medical and public health response to the September 11, 2001, terrorist attack on the World Trade Center (WTC). Located less than 2 miles from the site in Greenwich Village, with a clear view of the Twin Towers, the hospital's emergency room staff were ready to receive the anticipated thousands of physically injured within minutes of the first plane hitting the North Tower at 8:46 a.m. Although the anticipated medical crisis never occurred, the need for psychological interventions continues to this day, almost 2 years after September 11, 2001.

In the hours, days, and weeks that followed the WTC disaster, St. Vincent's responded to the mental health care needs of tens of thousands of people. St. Vincent's was able to mobilize immediately dozens of mental health professionals from its own inpatient and ambulatory care programs to meet the acute mental health needs of the community. Its proximity and relationship with the community permitted the hospital to provide therapists for the hundreds of people demanding urgent crisis care in a way that was impossible for less localized state and federal institutional responders, who required days and weeks to fully establish a major presence.

Because the number of physically injured survivors needing care was relatively small, for public health response purposes, the September 11th WTC terrorist attacks can be viewed primarily as a mental health disaster. In place of injured patients, thousands of emotionally perturbed people converged on the hospital. One mass of people sought information about relatives or friends who were missing in the disaster in the hope that the victim had been hospitalized unconscious and remained unidentified. Others were neighbors and visitors, all feeling an urgency to offer to help in some way. Hundreds of people arranged themselves by blood type, though the hospital lacked the capacity for so many donors. The news media also came; St. Vincent's had quickly become a favored location for roving television and radio reporters, and word of the hospital's centrality in the disaster was soon widely known in New York City and throughout the world. Other survivors, in addition to those relatively few who experienced physical injury, also came to St. Vincent's, reeling in the aftermath of the disaster and seeking a therapeutic reconnection to undo the horror and inhumanity of the violence.

Emotional distress is the normative response to catastrophic trauma. The intensity of symptoms of survivors of a disaster can be classified according to their exposure level (Cohen, 2002). The primary level consists of those with maximum exposure to the disaster (Cohen, 2002). The demographics of Manhattan predicted an unusually large number of eyewitness victims from near the WTC site (Herman *et al.*, 2002), and these survivors arrived first and continued to present for days and weeks afterwards. The secondary level consists of grieving, close relatives (Cohen, 2002). We saw fearful or grieving relatives and friends in large numbers, as they anxiously walked through the neighborhood posting pictures and descriptions of missing loved ones, in the fervent hope that theirs would be the lucky survivors found alive in the rescue operation or in a hospital. Although the population directly exposed to the WTC disaster was clustered in lower Manhattan near St. Vincent's, the grieving survivors were distributed differently. Less than half of the people killed that day lived in New York City, so that the majority of the bereaved relatives lived many miles away from the hospital. Nonetheless, many attempted to journey to "Ground Zero" or the hospital. The third level of distressed survivors consists of rescue, recovery, and medical personnel (Cohen, 2002). Although relatively few of these survivors presented immediately for crisis counseling, St. Vincent's developed outreach, crisis counseling and alternative therapy programs which ultimately reached many individuals during the ensuing months. The fourth level is the immediate community (Cohen, 2002). In addition to on-premises response, St. Vincent's developed outreach programs for school personnel and students in closest proximity to Ground Zero. The fifth level includes those in distress from media reports (Cohen, 2002). Many New Yorkers were seen for anxiety, which appeared to have been amplified by the incessant media coverage of the disaster (Ahern *et al.*, 2002).

As mentioned above, we were able to draw on a large pool of highly trained and experienced attending psychiatrists, psychiatric residents, social workers, nurses, and other health professionals, from within the St. Vincent's – Manhattan community. On the other hand, because of the proximity of St. Vincent's to the WTC site, the individuals providing the crisis mental health response were themselves deeply affected by the events of the day. Many hospital staff lived in downtown Manhattan, and many had relatives and friends who worked and lived in the WTC vicinity. Some of the St. Vincent's community were themselves killed or lost loved ones in the attack. Thus, from the beginning, there was an imperative to provide support to all hospital staff. During the first few weeks, the Behavioral Health Service, working with other departments, developed presentations that senior clinicians delivered to managers and front-line staff in both self-care and how to refer for more intensive services. We also recognized the need for additional training for clinical staff. Despite the high prevalence of a history of traumatic stressors within our patient population, post-traumatic stress disorder (PTSD) was usually not the primary diagnosis or focus of clinical attention. Hence, staff was not uniformly schooled in specific trauma treatments. Through the support of the New York Times Foundation to the Consortium for Effective Trauma Treatment, we were able to provide our staff a range of educational opportunities offered by some of the leading experts in the field. In addition, the Consortium model helped to create a community of practitioners across the four academic medical centers and the affiliated community agencies that was unprecedented. Further, its train-the-trainer approach allowed the further dissemination of knowledge to other staff and trainees throughout the medical center and to other mental health facilities.

Immediately after 9/11, St. Vincent's deployed therapists to the New York Fire Department counseling services unit in downtown Manhattan and to the public schools closest to Ground Zero. This work was facilitated by generous support received from charitable foundations and donors.

The disaster care that we were asking our staff to perform was fundamentally different than the usual inpatient and outpatient treatment they provided. Crisis oriented therapy in the immediate aftermath of a disaster and the later treatment of traumatic anxiety and depression are demanding work. First, the therapist strives to create a safe and accepting environment to facilitate emotional expression and trauma reconstruction. Then, the therapist must listen and encourage the verbalization of the painful and dehumanizing experiences of violent trauma. If the victim experienced multiple traumas over the course of a lifetime, processing all of the misery can be enormously challenging to the patient and therapist alike (Zimering *et al.*, 2003). St. Vincent's therapists understood firsthand patient comments such as: "I remember vividly the smell of the burning bodies that spread across the city. That was the most unbearable part", and "I still do not feel truly safe anywhere" (personal communications to authors).

That clinicians themselves develop symptoms as a result of caring for traumatized patients is well documented (Salston & Figley, 2003). Cumulative exposure to victims' accounts can induce negative changes in therapists' sense of self, others, and the world, especially if the therapists shared the same traumatic experience. Thus, it has been important to monitor the therapists and titrate their exposure. For example, most of the St. Vincent's clinicians who provided crisis counseling in the immediate aftermath of the attack returned to work in their assigned mental health programs, both to protect them from a cumulative trauma burden and to insure continuity of care for St. Vincent's patients already in care prior to the terrorist attack. New therapists were recruited for the crisis counseling programs funded by Federal Emergency Management Agency (FEMA) and other sources during 2002 and 2003.

It was critical that staff achieve the requisite skills and knowledge as they ventured into this personally and professionally threatening territory. The added value of the Consortium for Effective Trauma Treatment was that it established a community of trauma professionals across New York City medical centers by leveraging internal and external expertise and conferring peer support to the ultimate benefit of thousands of New Yorkers.

REFERENCES

Ahern, J., Galea, S., Resnick, H., Kilpatrick, D., Bucuvalas, M., Gold, J. & Vlahov, D. (2002). Television images and psychological symptoms after the September 11 terrorist attacks. *Psychiatry*, **65**, 289–300.

Amsel, L.V., Neria, Y., Suh, E.J. & Marshall, R.D. (this volume). Mental health community response to 9/11: training therapists to practice evidence-based psychotherapy. In *9/11: Mental Health in the Wake of Terrorist Attacks*, eds. Y. Neria, R. Gross & R.D. Marshall. Cambridge, UK: Cambridge University Press.

Cohen, R.E. (2002). Mental health services for victims of disasters. *World Psychiatry*, **1**(3), 149–152.

Herman, D., Felton, C. & Susser, E. (2002). Mental health needs in New York State following the September 11th attacks. *Journal of Urban Health: Bulletin of the New York Academy of Medicine*, **79**, 311–322.

Salston, M.D. & Figley, C.R. (2003). Secondary traumatic stress effects of working with survivors of criminal victimization. *Journal of Traumatic Stress*, **16**, 167–174.

Shear, K., Frank, E., Houck, P.R. & Reynolds, C.F. 3rd (2005). Treatment of Complicated Grief: A randomized controlled trial. *Journal of the American Medical Association*, **1**, 2601–2608.

Zimering, R., Munroe, J. & Gulliver, S.B. (2003). Secondary traumatization in mental health care providers. *Psychiatric Times*, **20**, 43–46.

NEW YORK UNIVERSITY CHILD STUDY CENTER, NEW YORK UNIVERSITY SCHOOL OF MEDICINE

Lori Davis and Marylene Cloitre

On September 11, 2001, our clinical team was situated at New York Presbyterian Hospital-Weill Cornell Medical Center on the Upper East Side of Manhattan. Like other major hospitals in the area, we waited for the scores of patients to arrive at the emergency room who were in need of medical attention and crisis intervention, but they never arrived. Our skills as mental health clinicians, however, were soon put to use.

First response: consultation, education and support of the community

In the immediate aftermath, the hospital organized an on-site response that included a telephone hotline and a 24-hour walk-in crisis center adjacent to the emergency room, where members of the community could stop by for a half an hour of time with a therapist. A multidisciplinary team of psychologists, social workers, and psychiatrists took shifts during the week and on the weekends. During the first 2 weeks post-9/11, we spoke or met with approximately 100 individuals to provide a forum in which they could speak of their experiences or express their worries about themselves and their loved ones. We provided psychoeducation about common reactions to trauma, spoke with worried family members on how to best provide support to loved ones who had been affected by the trauma, and provided referrals for treatment, if necessary.

In addition, our service provided consultation and psychoeducation about the effects of traumatic stress and the warning signs of post-traumatic stress disorder (PTSD). We visited with companies who had lost employees during the disaster, and with schools, shelters, and city mental health associations. Our team members made over 400 visits in 2 months, primarily to Ground Zero businesses. We began to hear firsthand of what had occurred downtown, not only about the deaths and destruction, but the displacement from homes and jobs.

Our largest single effort was to one corporation which had lost over 250 employees and who had been located in one of the Twin Towers. We organized around-the-clock support service and consultation for the company during the 3-month period of the rescue efforts in downtown New York. We were located in the company's temporary headquarters in a hotel approximately 30 blocks from Ground Zero. Our tasks were primarily logistical and supportive in nature. The first task was to support management in developing a system of information dissemination concerning the outcomes of daily rescue efforts. The second, and more wrenching, task was to support family members when they received confirmation of a death, or more often, when there was an absence of evidence about a loved one's death. Thirteen weeks after the attack, the mayor of New York City declared the formal transition from a rescue effort to a search effort, indicating that no further survivors were expected to be found. This formally ended our role as a support service in the rescue effort. There was a palpable shift in the needs of family members, survivors of the attack, and the community of New York as a whole.

Second response: training the mental health community

In preparation for the longer-term effects of the attack, we helped to form the New York Consortium for Effective Trauma Treatment. As our staff became adept in learning new trauma treatments, we brought these treatments into the community by providing workshops for clinicians. Additional goals of the Consortium were to evaluate factors that influenced the likelihood that community clinicians could use these treatments themselves, and to evaluate the effectiveness of manualized treatments used by expert Consortium clinicians and community clinicians for 9/11-related trauma.

Third response: implementation of mental health services

The New York Hospital – Cornell Medical College team, led by Dr. Marylene Cloitre, had as its core set of training and service clinicians a team of ten therapists, ranging in experience from 2 to 13 years (four PhDs, one PsyD, one MD, one MSW, one CSW, and two Master's Degrees in Clinical Psychology). Prior to 9/11, we worked regularly with survivors of traumatic events, and were trained extensively in assessment and treatment regarding PTSD and other anxiety disorders.

In September 2002, Dr. Cloitre was asked to create the Institute for Trauma and Stress at the New York University Child Study Center, a division created expressly to develop and test empirically based treatments, and to provide clinical services to children, adolescents, and families in the community. Many of our staff decided to join this new institute to continue our work as a team.

We noted that a large proportion of clients at our urban clinic had significant trauma histories prior to 9/11. These histories included witnessing traumatic events, being the victim of a mugging or burglary, or living through the traumatic illness or the death of a loved one, or a series of early life losses. In addition, 61% of females and 58% of males reported a history of childhood sexual and/or physical abuse or assault. In many cases, early traumas had re-ignited or exacerbated the stress reactions to the World Trade Center disaster.

Cloitre had developed and refined a treatment called Skills Training in Affective and Interpersonal Regulation (STAIR) for women who had been multiply trauma tized (Cloitre *et al.*, 2002). It consists of sixteen 1-hour sessions with a focus on learning to identify and modulate negative emotions, particularly anxiety and anger. Other facets of the treatment included targeting improvement in interper sonal functioning. The other key component of the treatment was to work with clients to process, integrate, and find meaning in traumatic memories through sys tematic narration and analysis of the memories. Dr. Cloitre's research consistently showed reductions in symptoms and improvements in the ability to tolerate nega tive distress and in interpersonal functioning.

Since many of the individuals who came to us for help after 9/11 were also mul tiply traumatized, we used this protocol frequently with the goal of adapting it for a community setting. Our site remained focused on treating the multiply trauma tized youth and adults of 9/11.

The team also provided trainings for clinicians both in the New York City com munity and in the USA who were interested in learning about the applicability of STAIR to 9/11 patients and other communities that have suffered mass violence. We reviewed the empirical evidence that supported the efficacy of the treatment, discussed its origins as a research treatment and its inception as a community treatment, conducted role-plays, and provided videotapes to illustrate how to administer the treatment. Approximately 800 clinicians have attended these trainings, which have been held at the NYU site, around the country, and as far away as Vancouver, Canada.

Characteristics of persons seeking treatment at NYU

In the first 2 years, our team screened more than 160 individuals by phone, completed over 90 evaluations for PTSD and associated disorders and symptomatology, and treated 73 patients in more than 840 sessions. Because of our proximity to downtown New York City, the demographics of our clients reflect those of that community. We have treated artists, rescue workers, therapists experiencing vicarious or secondary traumatization, teachers, journalists, homemakers, and business people; 72% of our patients have been female, and 28% of our patients have been male. It is notable that several men came forward for treatment later on, during year 2, and stated that they thought they could handle their symptoms; 73% of our clients are Caucasian, 14% are Hispanic, and 14% fall into an "other" category. The age range of our sample is 19–61 years old, with a mean age of 44 years old. Some clients had actually been in the World Trade Center and been forced to evacuate, others stood on the streets below, while other waited at home or work waiting to hear about the fate of loved ones. The details and individual stories differ, but most of our clients were similar in their struggle to make sense of their experience on 9/11.

Outcomes in the adaptation of a treatment to the community it served

Our goal was to use and adapt STAIR for a community population. To this end, we provided it more flexibly, and also integrated it with other evidence-based modules to address comorbidity such as panic disorder, generalized anxiety disorder, depression, or bereavement issues.

Preliminary review of our data at the time of this writing shows that, of the 73 individuals who received treatment at our setting, 18 completed the treatment and show a significant decrease in PTSD symptoms. Significant reductions were also seen with regard to symptoms of depression, the ability to regulate negative emotions, and overall functioning at work, school, and in relationships. Indeed, it is of special note that the effect size of the reduction in PTSD symptoms in this pilot work is greater than that obtained under randomized-controlled conditions. These data are counter to some researchers' assumptions that the effects of good treatments get diluted in the community. Rather, we have found that community applications, at least if implemented by knowledgeable clinicians can provide even greater relief than those found in highly restricted academic applications. We are now in the process of modifying STAIR for other community settings and populations of patients.

This is one important result of our treatment effort and we are profoundly grateful for the funding that has allowed us not only to provide treatment to those in need but to evaluate whether we have done any good.

About the service providers

We took special care to create a process group for our clinical team early on. Our purpose was to deal with issues such as vicarious traumatization, and to provide support and encouragement to one another as we heard heartbreaking stories of loss, and trauma narratives that rivaled one another in terms of specificity and gruesome details. Time and again, we saw how an event such as 9/11 can cause an individual to rethink his or her view of the self and the world. We were also impressed with human resilience under the worst possible circumstances.

We connected with our patients in ways that still surprise us. We were deeply moved by the ways our patients expressed themselves through art, through their words, through photographs and through poetry. Our patients' motivation to survive and to move forward in their lives despite the losses they suffered was inspiring. For many of us, this work reinforced the reasons we decided to enter a helping profession.

REFERENCE

Cloitre, M., Koenen, K.C., Cohen, L.R. & Han, H. (2002). Skills training in affective and inter personal regulation followed by exposure: a phase-based treatment for PTSD related to child-hood abuse. *Journal of Consulting and Clinical Psychology*, **70**, 10–67.

THE MENTAL HEALTH MANDATE OF SEPTEMBER 11, MOUNT SINAI SCHOOL OF MEDICINE

Gila Schwarzbaum and Rachel Yehuda

The events of September 11, 2001, and their aftermath brought into sharp focus striking gaps in our knowledge about how to deal effectively with the mental health implications of a large-scale trauma. When faced with the immediate problem of dealing with 9/11 as a crisis and the public necessity for treatment, of thousands, and possibly tens of thousands of people needing help, those gaps became immediate mandates to address. The development of the New York Consortium for Effective Trauma Treatment was extremely instrumental in helping our center conceptualize an appropriate mental health response to the events of 9/11.

Because the Traumatic Stress Studies Division at Mount Sinai School of Medicine has been a longstanding clinical treatment program in a major academic hospital and medical school in New York, we instantly felt on 9/11 that this event was going to represent a professional watershed. However, against the backdrop of horror surrounding this event, we also believed that it would provide an opportunity to learn about certain aspects in the field of traumatic stress that were still unknown to us.

The Traumatic Stress Studies Division was established in 1991, and began with a modest clinical program aimed at the treatment of post-traumatic stress disorder (PTSD) in combat veterans. Specialized Treatment Program for Holocaust Survivors and their Families was established at the Mount Sinai School of Medicine and by 1997 the Traumatic Stress Studies division had expanded to include a Psychopharmacologic Treatment Trials Program. In 1999 we opened the Women's After Trauma Care and Health Program (WATCH) and the Children's After Trauma Care and Health Program (CATCH). Thus, by September 2001, The Mount Sinai Traumatic Stress Studies Program had an established history of conducting research in connection with and providing treatment services to trauma survivors with PTSD. However, our program had been more focused on helping people deal with events that had transpired months, and usually years or even decades, prior to seeking treatment with us.

In the immediate aftermath of 9/11, it was not clear to us whether the same treatment strategies in which we had already developed confidence for use with more chronic patients would be instrumental for persons requesting treatment in the weeks and months following 9/11. In fact, at a time when almost everyone in New York City (NYC) was reeling from the effects of 9/11, it was not clear to us that we would be able to properly identify those at risk for PTSD or long-term psychopathology based on their earlier responses.

It had been clear for many years prior to 9/11 that most people exposed to trauma initially develop symptoms of PTSD, but the great majority also recover, even without mental health treatment. In fact, statistics suggested that while many people met criteria for PTSD in the first week post-trauma, only 1–25% of those exposed to natural disasters or accidents were at risk for developing PTSD. The implications of this for the events of 9/11 were that many people would at first appear very symptomatic, but ultimately, their symptoms would resolve, with or without treatment. The question was whether persons should be treated, and if so, how, during the first few weeks or months post-trauma?

Initial epidemiological studies showed that, 5–8 weeks after the attacks, a prevalence rate of 7.5% of randomly sampled subjects living south of 110th Street reportedly had developed PTSD (Galea *et al.*, 2002), with those having the most severe exposure or personal loss at higher risk than others. Initially, this caused alarm in NYC, and in our program in particular because it suggested that there would be many more persons with PTSD than could be accommodated by the current mental health system. Indeed, greater symptom severity from 1 to 2 weeks post-trauma and onwards is positively associated with subsequent symptom severity (Shalev *et al.*, 1997; Harvey & Bryant, 1998; Murray *et al.*, 2002).

One of the things we immediately recognized was that mental health response to the World Trade Center (WTC) attack could not be wholly guided by evidence-based medicine or psychology, in that the understanding of how to treat survivors in the aftermath of a disaster of such magnitude was limited. Thus, we identified the need to form the infrastructure that would gather the necessary information so that future decisions about mental health responses could be made on the basis of empirical knowledge. In working towards that goal we determined that it was time to consolidate the various programs and hire and train more staff.

In response to the terrorist attack on the WTC, our program immediately assembled a cadre of psychiatrists, psychologists, and social workers to be on call as needed as well as to enter the community and make known the availability of our clinicians to assist survivors, their families, and the community at large in dealing with this monumental tragedy. Within a short period of time we began to receive telephone calls from individuals seeking mental health services. For people who contacted us in the weeks immediately following the trauma, we encouraged them to seek natural supports, knowing that symptoms would likely decrease with time. Simultaneously, we trained residents and first-line mental health responders to understand that the most appropriate intervention was to help survivors gauge whether their symptoms were remaining the same, slowly improving, or increasing. By about 6 weeks post-trauma, we began to see patients exhibiting serious symptoms of depression and anxiety disorders.

At the time of 9/11 we were in the midst of collaboration with Dr. Edna Foa in which we were examining biological measures associated with rape victims in the context of cognitive–behavioral therapy in the treatment of these women. At the suggestion of the National Institute of Mental Health (NIMH), we submitted an administrative supplement to this collaboration for the purpose of examining the efficacy of the Brief Recovery Program (BRP) with individuals experiencing significant symptoms of PTSD after the WTC attack and comparing it to supportive counseling (SC), examining the efficacy of prolonged exposure (PE) with individuals who failed to respond to BRP or SC, examining the biological changes over the course of both treatments and at follow up, and learning and implementing the BRP and PE models as developed and utilized by Dr. Foa, for the treatment of recent victims with severe PTSD symptoms and with chronic PTSD, respectively.

The training provided through the New York Times Consortium (Consortium) enabled the immediate establishment of such a treatment protocol with different therapeutic options. Through the New York Times Consortium, our clinicians were offered numerous training programs to further educate them with respect to interventions determined to be highly useful in treating patients affected by the WTC. Further, in some cases, arrangements were also made to have ongoing clinical supervision of diagnostic assessment and psychotherapy that took place both in-person and by telephone conference. Thus, patients treated in our program were able to receive either exposure therapy or SC by clinicians whose training supported their skills in these protocols.

As not all callers seeking treatment from our program were eligible for inclusion in the research study, it quickly became clear that a third treatment option was needed to serve those patients who although did not meet inclusion criteria, were in need of trauma treatment services. We therefore established the treatment as usual (TAU) arm of the study, which also served as a basis for comparing the Consortium trained therapists with those who were providing TAU and were being trained and supervised within our program.

Patients seen within our program through any of the treatment options underwent periodic evaluations throughout treatment in order to assess progress and to determine whether additional treatment was necessary. Upon completion of the treatment sessions, referral for further treatment was made if indicated. Additionally, our program has performed both 3- and 6-month follow-up evaluations for each patient so that longer-term progress could be monitored as well.

With respect to CATCH, the Consortium has enabled our program to expand its direct treatment services to children and adolescents who were impacted by the events of 9/11 and continue its community services. CATCH's WTC-related activities began in the immediate aftermath of the attack as its clinicians worked with the Disaster Psychiatry Outreach Program to staff the Family Relief Center set up by the Red Cross to serve victims of 9/11. The Division of Child and Adolescent Psychiatry and CATCH personnel were involved in counseling the families of the Cantor-Fitzgerald and Aeion Corporations. Immediately following the WTC attack, our staff also conducted widespread outreach to both the NYC public school system and private schools and has continued to work with school-based mental health service providers in order to assist them in helping their students cope with the disaster. This effort has been implemented through off site seminars as well as through programming at the schools themselves. Initiatives have also extended to mental health workers at higher-education facilities. Further, CATCH was and continues to be involved in a variety of other activities in an effort to raise the social consciousness about effective trauma treatment for children and adolescents. It has developed an affiliation with and provided consultation and guidance to SOS, a social action-based organization originating with synagogue-based intervention that plans to further expand. CATCH consulted with Sesame Street Workshop to assist in planning episodes of Sesame Street and other multimedia features aimed at addressing some of the issues associated with the WTC attack. Also developed for widespread distribution, was a Parent and Teacher Trauma Information Brochure, in question and answer format. The CATCH program contributed trauma-related information to the Mount Sinai Hospital and Mount Sinai

School of Medicine web sites and continues to develop a web site in conjunction with the Traumatic Stress Studies program at Mount Sinai. Finally, CATCH has been the subject of WTC media coverage in both articles and interviews, hopefully highlighting the importance of seeking effective trauma treatment for symptomatic children and adolescents.

Through research initiatives established through CATCH, our program further pursues its mission of establishing infrastructures to gather information that can inform future trauma treatment response as well as provide the necessary treatment. Together with the Jewish Board of Family and Child Services (JBFCS), we have secured funding through the NIMH to provide for the establishment of a partnership between CATCH and JBFCS to systematically develop a collaborative field research organization that integrates laboratory-based clinical research with field trials of clinical interventions. The collaboration is aimed at screening trauma in children and youths and at evaluating the efficacy of trauma-focused treatment for children and youths served by JBFCS. This initiative is in response to a federal call for proposals to establish partnerships between academic medical centers and community service agencies, a collaboration that clearly is aligned with our mission.

Beyond these activities, The Mount Sinai Traumatic Stress Studies Program has been offering seminars as well as supervision within Mount Sinai for staff and voluntary faculty members and has been actively engaged in educating other NYC mental health treatment providers with respect to effective evaluative and treatment services in the wake of the events of 9/11. Such treatment providers include clinicians practicing in community settings, school psychologists, social workers and counselors, teachers, and clinicians in private practice. And as part of our educational mission, our program has provided consultation to other agencies who offer mental health services such as the Jewish Board of Family and Children Services, in order to help them in their outreach and treatment efforts.

The Mount Sinai Traumatic Stress Treatment Program has been the subject of widespread media coverage in both recent articles and interviews, highlighting the importance of seeking effective trauma treatment for symptomatic adults and children. Our program's efforts in this regard have enabled us to be called upon as a useful resource for other mental health professionals seeking guidance-based upon our expertise in the area of trauma treatment.

CONCLUSION

Randall D. Marshall

The process of both coping with and responding to 9/11 proved to be a grueling but remarkable lesson in the difficulties of enhancing community services after a major disaster. The logistical impediments to creating a multisite collaboration under super-accelerated, crisis conditions taught us the critical importance of disaster preparedness planning within and across institutions, government, and philanthropy.

We are deeply indebted to trauma experts across the country and around the world for their participation in our program. On short notice, every expert we contacted made themself available to provide training to our newly expanded staff, and thereby enhanced mental health services in the greater New York area. This outpouring of generosity in a time of profound crisis made a deep impression on all of us.

Over the course of the year, our collaboration developed to have a number of strengths. Our geographic distribution around Manhattan facilitated accessibility to the community; our differing institutional emphases (e.g. research vs. services oriented) proved to be complementary. Our ability to operate semi-autonomously made it possible for each team to respond rapidly, drawing on their individual strengths of infrastructure and personnel.

Our effort would not have been possible without the willingness of Jack Rosenthal to adopt mental health as a critical area of focus for the New York Times Foundation. Although the data has since amply validated this decision, it was a risky and largely intuitive commitment in the first weeks after the attacks. Other funding sources were largely unavailable in the immediate post-disaster setting for mental health services and research, including research funds from NIMH. It is gratifying to see that this problem is now being recognized at both the local and national level.

Research is desperately needed in the area of interventions after community disaster. Rates of serious mental disorder have been well studied and described after numerous different kinds of events, but our knowledge base becomes grossly deficient when the practical questions arise as to what should be done to assist these persons and repair the damage done to a community in the wake of disaster. In the interim, of course, communities must still respond as best they can when disaster occurs. We hope that the documentation of our efforts serves other communities in some way in the aftermath of future disasters.

20

Evaluation and treatment of firefighters and utility workers following the World Trade Center attacks

JoAnn Difede, Jennifer Roberts, Nimali Jayasinghe
and Pam Leck

The tragic events of September 11, 2001 put the resources of the American people to the test like no other event in US history. The world watched as people came together from all walks of life, from all parts of the country, to clear up the ruin that the terrorists had left behind in lower Manhattan. At the time of the attacks, we found ourselves in the unique position to lend our psychological expertise in the field of trauma to two distinct groups called upon, by profession, to respond to the devastation: the New York Fire Department (FDNY), and employees of Consolidated Edison (Con Edison), the utility company responsible for providing New York City with electricity, gas, and steam. We had a prior history with both of these groups via the primary author's role as liaison between the Weill Cornell Medical College Department of Psychiatry and the New York Presbyterian Hospital (NYPH) Burn Center for the past 15 years. Our involvement with these specific groups stems most basically from the fact that people in these positions undergo trauma via work-related accidents and injuries and require evaluation and treatment for the psychological sequelae of trauma. It was these facts that left us in a position to organize the evaluation and treatment post-disaster, on a scale we had never imagined, to two populations that had never previously been so massively traumatized.

In this chapter we share what we have learned about how these two populations were effected by their exposure to the terrorist attacks and their aftermath. Before discussing the psychological effects of their involvement with the disaster, it is important to give the reader a picture of what the individuals that make up these populations endured in the fall of 2001. Like us, the firefighters and Con Edison employees were responding to the disaster from their areas of expertise. The firefighters were there to respond to an emergency, put out a fire, and rescue its victims, followed by a long period of recovery of human remains. Con Edison employees were there to shut off energy sources potentially feeding the fire, followed by restoring gas, steam, and electric power to lower Manhattan. Due to the nature of their jobs each of these sub-populations of what are commonly referred to in the literature as "disaster relief workers" (DRWs), came from different backgrounds to perform different duties. What they share is the fact that they were called in their line of duty to work at the World Trade Center (WTC) site for extended periods. Following, we will discuss some of the distinct features of the exposure endured by these sub-populations.

Con Edison employees were exposed to the site to varying degrees (Con Edison, 2002). Approximately 3800 workers responded to the need for stopping and recovering service in the minutes and days following the attack, often undertaking tasks that were life-threatening and witnessing horrific carnage. Some were working near the site as the events took place, others responded immediately from different locations, and others arrived days or weeks after the event. One general pattern of exposure was to arrive the day of 9/11 and work 12–16-hour shifts for about 1 month, some with a few days off, others working straight through. Physical stress resulted from working long hours for countless days, often wearing heavy protective clothing and respirators that had to be removed to speak or eat. Psychological stress resulted in part from working in a potentially dangerous environment amidst tremendous devastation and loss of human life. Many employees describe their first time to the site, staring at the six-story pile of rubble, in disbelief that all that was before them was twisted steel and dust – no desks, no computers. They walked by medical units set up to help survivors, only to notice the cots were empty. Additionally, many employees either grew up or currently lived in communities that suffered multiple losses of both rescue workers and civilians who were known in their communities as the little league coach, the store owner's daughter, the neighbor's son, etc. Their distress was compounded by concern for their health (primarily regarding what they were breathing in) and a sense of helplessness that they could not do more.

The firefighters endured different types and degrees of exposure to the attacks, both in their line of duty and in their social lives (New York City Fire Department, 2002). Responding to the attacks as they were happening many saw people hurling from the top floors of the Trade Center Towers, and also may have had to flee from the Towers as they crumbled. During and after the attacks they were occupied in desperate attempts to rescue and recover their brethren. Fundamental to understanding the exposure of FDNY to the attacks is the significance of the social network that permeates their work and personal lives. Taking into account the fact that their line of duty puts them in a position to regularly face possible injury and death, it is no surprise that firefighters live in a culture of "brotherhood." Each of the 343 firefighters who died as a result of 9/11, left not only their own families grieving, but left their close knit community in mourning as well. Some firefighters we worked with made their final eye contact with lifelong friends as they headed into the Trade Center Towers. In addition, the firefighter's exposure to the attacks seemed to only worsen after the towers fell and the site was cleaned up. There were a nightmarish string of events they were yet to endure: hearing their deceased brother's voices on the 9/11 tapes released by the *New York Times*, being notified as remains of their brothers were recovered, or actually finding the remains themselves, attending an endless number of memorial services and funerals. The aforementioned events were endured through a fog of physical and emotional exhaustion.

As shown above, as well as being described in the literature, disaster workers can be confronted with a variety of situations in the course of their efforts that challenge their physical and emotional functioning (Paton, 1997; Young *et al.*, 1998; National Center for Post-traumatic Stress Disorder, NCPTSD, 2001a). Emanuel and Ursano (1999) delineate four potential hazards of disaster work: (1) "psychological stressors," such as risking injury or death, gruesome or disturbing experiences, and isolation from primary social network; (2) "physiological stressors," such as heavy physical exertion, lack of sleep, and poor nutrition; (3) "occupational stressors," such as conflicts between personal and organizational needs and role confusion; and (4) "organizational stressors" such as concerns about personal safety and limits of ability to rescue.

This chapter will focus on our efforts to evaluate and treat both groups of DRWs. Following a brief summary of the scientific literature, we will discuss our experience in establishing a screening and evaluation program for DRWs post-9/11, providing empirical data as well as clinical observations garnered from our programs.

Post-traumatic stress disorder and DRWs

Disasters come in the form of natural events, such as earthquakes; accidents or technological failures, such as airplane crashes; and human-generated incidents, such as terror attacks (NCPTSD, 2001c). Such disparate events share a common feature – the swift, most often unanticipated, infliction of harm and damage (Neufeldt & Guralnik, 1989). Communities recovering from the aftermath of disasters may have to come to terms with members' threatened or actual injury and loss of life, disruption of social relations and networks, loss of property and resources, and increased uncertainty about the future (NCPTSD, 2001c).

A recent review of articles based on studies of 80 disasters worldwide point to five key outcomes of disaster on individuals and communities: (1) "psychological problems," such as post-traumatic stress disorder (PTSD), major depressive disorder (MDD), and generalized anxiety disorder (GAD); (2) "non-specific distress;" (3) "health problems," such as somatic complaints, increased substance use, and sleep disruption; (4) "chronic problems in living," such as increased interpersonal, occupational, and financial stressors; and (5) "psychosocial resource losses," including reductions in perceived social support and social embeddedness (NCPTSD, 2001c).

The bulk of empirical support for these outcomes is drawn from research on direct victims. However, communities depend for their recovery on the efforts of diverse groups of disaster workers – search and rescue personnel; fire and safety personnel; medical personnel; police, security, and investigators; clergy, mental health, and social service providers; elected officials; volunteers; and the media (Young *et al.*, 1998). In the past two decades clinicians and researchers have begun to appreciate the risk of trauma to disaster workers (Wright *et al.*, 1990). The section below outlines findings regarding the evaluation and treatment of disaster workers in the industrialized world.

Assessment of disaster workers

Assessment of the negative psychological sequelae of disaster work is a complex endeavor. In a recent review of studies conducted in both the industrialized and industrializing world, Norris *et al.* (2002) concluded that disaster workers are less at risk for distress than direct disaster victims. They estimated that 42% of studies of direct victims revealed at least severe distress, but put the figure at 13% for studies of disaster workers.

Clinicians and researchers have hypothesized that persons who choose emergency work as an occupation are likely to be resilient, that disaster organizations select resilient workers, and training enables disaster workers to cope with disaster conditions (e.g., Moran & Colless, 1995; Young *et al.*, 1998; North, 2002). For instance, disaster workers are thought to be characteristically independent, self-confident, and strong (Young *et al.*, 1998). They use problem-solving and suppression of emotions to effectively manage disaster situations (Moran & Colless, 1995). Certainly, it is necessary to acknowledge that many workers derive satisfaction from their efforts and report positive outcomes (Raphael *et al.*, 1983–1984; Hytten & Hasle, 1989; Moran & Colless, 1995; Young *et al.*, 1998; NCPTSD, 2001a). Negative stress reactions may be an inevitable but transitory aspect of disaster work (Young *et al.*, 1998; NCPTSD, 2001a).

Nevertheless, there is converging evidence from diverse studies that a significant proportion of disaster workers are at risk for enduring distress. This appears to hold true for responders to a wide range of incidents, from natural disasters (McFarlane, 1986, 1988; Marmar *et al.*, 1996), to accidents and technological failures associated with mass casualties (Taylor & Frazer, 1982; Raphael *et al.*, 1983–1984; Durham *et al.*, 1985; Ersland *et al.*, 1989; Fullerton *et al.*, 1992; Ursano *et al.*, 1995). Of most relevance, enduring distress occurs as a consequence of human-generated disasters (Jones, 1985; Harvey-Lintz & Tidwell, 1997; Sims & Sims, 1998); most notably war (McCarroll *et al.*, 1995) and terror attacks (North *et al.*, 2002a; Rosenczweig *et al.*, 2002).

Studies have revealed rates of generalized distress and poor mental health reaching 37% in samples of disaster workers (Taylor & Frazer, 1982; Raphael *et al.*, 1983–1984; Jones, 1985; Duckworth, 1986; McFarlane, 1986, 1988; Ersland *et al.*, 1989); and researchers have identified rates of PTSD ranging from 9% to 35% (Durham *et al.*, 1985; Duckworth, 1986; Marmar *et al.*, 1996; Harvey-Lintz & Tidwell, 1997; Marmar *et al.*, 1999; North *et al.*, 2002b; Rosenczweig *et al.*, 2002). Many studies suggest that a significant subset of disaster workers may experience sub-syndromal levels of PTSD symptoms (Wilkinson, 1983; Duckworth, 1986; Ursano *et al.*, 1995). Major depression and GAD are also common responses to disaster (NCPTSD, 2001c). McFarlane and Papay (1992) found that some 77% of Australian volunteer fire-fighters who responded to a natural disaster and developed PTSD had other conditions, most commonly depression. It is only in rare cases (Hytten & Hasle, 1989; Alexander & Wells, 1991; Renck *et al.*, 2002) that researchers conclude that workers are unaffected by disaster exposure.

What is the course of post-traumatic stress and other distress reactions among disaster workers? Some studies have documented acute distress among disaster workers within 4 months of disaster (e.g., Fullerton *et al.*, 1992; McCarroll *et al.*, 1995; Ursano *et al.*, 1995; Weiss *et al.*, 1995; Rosenczweig *et al.*, 2002). Other studies have identified significant rates of PTSD among workers 5 months to several years post-disaster (e.g., Jones, 1985; McFarlane, 1986; Harvey-Lintz & Tidwell, 1997; Marmar *et al.*, 1999). Most notably, a few longitudinal studies reveal that while symptoms may diminish somewhat over time, distress tends to be chronic in 9%–14% of individuals (e.g., McFarlane, 1986, 1988; Marmar *et al.*, 1999).

Besides revealing patterns of distress in disaster workers, studies also highlight some features of disaster work that may put DRWs at elevated risk for negative outcomes. Some limited evidence suggests that the greater the number of stressors a worker encounters, the greater will be his or her distress. For instance, researchers have found that those involved in gruesome or disturbing work, such as body handling, may experience significant levels of distress (Taylor & Frazer, 1982), higher levels than those not involved in such work (McCarroll *et al.*, 1995). Researchers have also found that workers reporting psychological stressors, such as life threat; physiological stressors, such as food and sleep deprivation; and occupational stressors, such as confusing orders, are more likely to develop PTSD reactions (Marmar *et al.*, 1996). Furthermore, workers who report high levels of dissociation or strong emotional reactions during disaster operations may be at risk for PTSD symptoms (Weiss *et al.*, 1995; Marmar *et al.*, 1996).

Certainly, these studies indicate the importance of assessing disaster workers for clinically significant negative psychological reactions. However, there are limitations to this body of evidence. Studies to date have relied primarily on self-report data, an approach that, while cost-effective, may lead to an under-identification of symptoms.

Given that disaster workers value the display of strength and mastery, and may have reservations about people outside of their sub-culture (Young *et al.*, 1998), self-reports may be unduly influenced by social desirability and other such effects. Few researchers employ in-person interviews (Taylor & Frazer, 1982; Sims & Sims, 1998; North *et al.*, 2002a, b) or conduct their studies in the workplace (e.g., Marmar *et al.*, 1996; Harvey-Lintz & Tidwell, 1997; North *et al.*, 2002a, b).

Treatment of disaster workers

As a significant proportion of disaster workers are at risk for clinically meaningful and potentially chronic distress, there is a clear need for empirically validated treatments. However, there is a paucity of research in this crucial area.

Psychological debriefings have become the standard of care for disaster survivors, especially those in the disaster worker community (NCPTSD, 2001a). Typically, debriefings involve time-limited, small group discussions held within days of the disaster experience. It is argued that debriefings serve as a stress management tool by providing for emotional release, cognitive restructuring of the disaster experience, development of social support, education about trauma reactions, and identification of symptomatic individuals (Armstrong *et al.*, 1991; Shalev, 1994). However, the effectiveness of debriefings has recently been hotly debated and empirical research on the issue is equivocal (Jenkins, 1996; Kenardy *et al.*, 1996; Nurmi, 1999; Fullerton *et al.*, 2000). (As we did not begin our interventions with either group until several weeks post-9/11, we do not discuss the role of debriefings in either group.)

Expert treatment guidelines recommend that cognitive-behavioral treatment (CBT) with an exposure component be the first-line intervention for PTSD (Foa *et al.*, 1999). In a recent review of the extant research, Rothbaum and colleagues write that some 12 controlled studies have documented positive outcomes for exposure treatment (Rothbaum *et al.*, 2000). Such treatment commonly includes relaxation training, imaginal exposure of the trauma memory, *in vivo* exposure to trauma-related stimuli, and cognitive restructuring. It aims to provide systematic desensitization of traumatic effects and cognitive reprocessing of pathogenic meanings, allowing the survivor to tolerate memories of the events without emotional flooding or rigid avoidance, and to restore more realistic views of self, others, and the world.

While no controlled trials involving disaster workers have yet to be reported in the literature on terrorism, recent case reports (Tolin & Foa, 1999) and controlled studies have been extended to include emergency service personnel dealing with non-disaster-related trauma reactions, yielding promising results. Two controlled studies of police officers diagnosed with PTSD following work-related critical incidents demonstrated that participants in psychotherapy incorporating CBT (Gersons *et al.*, 2000) or eye movement desensitization and reprocessing (EMDR) intervention

(Wilson *et al.*, 2001) showed significant remission of PTSD symptoms. Finally, while no exposure therapy treatment studies have focused their attention exclusively on disaster workers, Gillespie *et al.* (2002) included disaster workers in a study of the effectiveness of exposure therapy in treating survivors of a terrorist bombing in Northern Ireland. Both civilians and DRWs showed clinically significant levels of improvement in post-traumatic stress and depressive symptoms.

Organizational interventions

Some in the disaster community have called for organization-based intervention strategies to address the strains and challenges disasters pose for workers (Paton, 1997; Dunning, 1998; Smith, 2001). Dunning (1998) points out that organizations are often under-prepared to address their needs for a variety of reasons. First, since disasters are considered uncommon, there is little incentive for organizations to prepare for such occurrences. Second, organizational resources are often strained by disaster response, leaving little available for addressing worker strain. Third, organizations often hold the view that "stress can bring out the best in a worker" (p. 286) and thus, does not need to be addressed. However, both in the immediate aftermath and recovery period, peers and supervisors can be in a unique position to provide support and respond to workers' needs (Paton, 1997; Dunning 1998). For instance, supervisors can be trained to identify symptoms of stress so that workers can be given any needed respite from duties (Dunning, 1998). There is an increasing call for organizations to implement programs that train workers about normal reactions to disaster and stress reduction techniques (Dunning, 1998; Smith, 2001) prior to such an event.

Summary

The empirical literature underscores the paucity of research on DRWs, especially compared to civilian trauma populations. Many questions remain regarding the public health significance of multiple exposures to life-threatening events to DRWs. The dearth of treatment studies is compelling given the rates of PTSD and related problems in these civil servants. The following section describes our efforts to establish a program to evaluate and treat DRWs, using the extant literature as a guide for our efforts.

The Weill Cornell Disaster Relief Screening and Treatment Program

Our empirical data and observations stem from a breadth of involvement with disaster relief populations post-9/11 as well as a longstanding history with these and other trauma populations. The firefighters and some of the Con Edison workers became part of National Institute of Mental Health (NIMH) funded controlled clinical trials comparing the efficacy of various psychological interventions including CBT, exposure therapy, virtual reality enhanced exposure therapy, and supportive psychotherapy. In response to Con Edison's involvement at the disaster site, a special psychological screening program was set up in conjunction with a mandatory medical screening organized by their Occupational Health Department. In the end, we will evaluate 3800 utility workers and a percentage of those will also be treated for the psychological sequelae of trauma. As of this writing, we have completed over 2300 evaluations on site at the Con Edison Occupational Medicine Department. In addition, 100 utility workers and firefighters have been treated in our clinical program, while an additional 20 utility workers, 15 firefighters, and 17 civilians have completed or are currently engaged in research treatment protocols.

Establishing the screening program

Inherent in organizing services in the aftermath of a disaster is the need to act quickly, at a pace that modern bureaucracies are not typically prepared to accommodate. Our mandate was to organize the screening program for 3800 workers within about 6 weeks. We sought advice from trauma experts around the country and drew on previously formulated guidelines in establishing our screening program. According to general guidelines developed by the NCPTSD, "disaster screening should address past and current psychiatric and substance abuse problems and treatment, prior trauma exposure, pre-injury psychosocial stressors, and existing social support. Event-related risk factors should also be assessed, including exposure to death, perception of life-threat, and peri-traumatic dissociation" (NCPTSD, 2001a).

Following these guidelines, all participants in our clinical and research programs were evaluated with structured clinical interviews and widely used, well-validated self-report measures (Difede *et al.*, 2004). The structured interviews included completion of an exposure questionnaire developed for this project, the clinician-administered PTSD scale (CAPS) (Blake *et al.*, 1990), selected modules of the structured clinical interview for the *Diagnostic and Statistical Manual for Mental Disorders-IV* (DSM-IV) (SCID) (First *et al.*, 1997) and a traumatic history interview.

All of the psychologists working on the project were trained to conduct the CAPS and SCID. Some had several years experience conducting evaluations and treatment of trauma patients, administering structured clinical instruments and using standardized treatment protocols with trauma populations. Each clinician, regardless of their seniority, met weekly with the program director for supervision.

Clinical presentation of the DRW common symptomatic presentations

Approximately 15% of the 519 Con Edison employees met criteria for PTSD and 23% met criteria for sub-threshold PTSD. Sub-threshold was defined as meeting criteria on two of three symptom clusters. Fifty-three percent of the total sample had a history of prior trauma. Participants who reported having prior trauma were more likely to be diagnosed with both PTSD, or sub-threshold PTSD, as well as major depression.[1]

The most common self-reported symptoms for both Con Edison employees and firefighters were anger, irritability, difficulty falling asleep, difficulty staying asleep, and distress at reminders. While many participants found the anger, irritability, and sleep problems compelling, and a primary motive to seek treatment, the distress at reminders was not. Most expected this distress and perceived it as a normal reaction to an overwhelming event, compounding the task of the clinician faced with persuading the worker of the need for treatment. As many DRWs persisted in the view that the symptoms were expectable reactions to overwhelming trauma, we tried to focus on the relationship between their symptoms and functional impairment to motivate them for treatment. By doing so we were able to remove the focus from a discussion of whether or what might be considered "normal" and emphasize the adverse impact the symptoms were having on their quality of life and their ability to function in their social and vocational roles.

There were two common presenting profiles for the Con Edison employees.[2] There were those with PTSD from direct exposure to the attack or prolonged exposure to the recovery site; and those who did not have direct or prolonged exposure, who nevertheless technically met diagnostic criteria for PTSD. Perception of imminent life threat appeared to be a critical difference between these groups. Those in the latter group generally did not perceive imminent threat to themselves, endorsed different symptoms than those in the direct exposure group, and most notably lacked the anxious-arousal component generally associated with PTSD.

Those with PTSD from direct exposure usually presented with anxiety, irritability, and sleep problems (i.e., sleep latency and continuity, as their most common complaints; Difede *et al.*, 2004). Those in this group usually had direct and prolonged exposure to the attack beginning on September 11, 2001, as illustrated by Mr. G., a Con Edison employee. He responded within minutes of the attack, with sufficient time to observe the towers fall. His usual responsibilities included responding to emergencies and assessing safety factors. Thus, he had the burden of knowing his

---

[1]Since our research with firefighters is not epidemiological, we cannot offer data on rates of PTSD in this group.

[2]Since our research with firefighters is not epidemiological, we do not offer impressions of common presenting profiles.

decisions would affect the safety of his employees and the community. Mr. G. lived in a community in the city that is home to countless firefighters, police, and Con Edison employees. He grew up in the same neighborhood where he currently resided and was a well-respected community leader. As a consequence of his stable community ties, he knew countless men who died at the WTC on September 11, 2001, many of them since their childhood. Upon presentation, he was anxious and tearful. He chose to accept treatment because he recognized that he could no longer control his irritability. He accepted the argument that he would be more effective in his quest to help others if he was able to accept treatment for himself, and in so doing serve as a role model to others who could benefit from treatment.

The second group technically met criteria, but generally did not report anxious-irritability as among their chief complaints, nor did they usually have direct or prolonged exposure to the site. This second group was characterized by having indirect exposure, current life stressors, and often a prior psychiatric or trauma history. Those who fell into this group usually met symptom criteria by strongly endorsing one re-experiencing ("B") symptom: distress at reminders; two or three avoidant ("C") symptoms: avoiding reminders, avoiding thoughts and emotions, social withdrawal; and two arousal ("D") symptoms: difficulty sleeping (though without the sleep continuity component), and difficulty concentrating. Though not terribly specific, those in this classification would best be described as generally distressed. Often there were suggestions of a habitual way of perceiving and coping with life stressors that was maladaptive. Take for example, Mr. P. who had been out sick for close to a month at the time of the attacks. He had no direct exposure to the site until visiting there one time months later. His indirect exposure came from numerous colleagues sharing their stories with him as their union representative. This individual had numerous life stressors (coping with a chronic health condition, longstanding marital problems) as well as a significant trauma history. The events of 9/11 served as a catalyst to exacerbate the emotional distress that he was already experiencing. During the screening he endorsed all symptoms for PTSD as well as major depression. He reported the greatest distress from frequent crying spells, depressive irritability, trouble falling asleep and early morning awakening. He became distressed at reminders of the attacks; however, this distress generalized across many issues, including reminders of past traumas. Once in treatment it became clear that the experience he was undergoing, rather than to focus on the content of his traumatic life goal of treatment, would be to teach him how to better identify, tolerate, and modulate the intense emotional experiences, including his indirect exposure to 9/11.

The distinction between these two groups is an important public health issue as it has implications for both screening and interventions post-disaster as well as pre-disaster education and training. For example, those in the "generally distressed" group were pre-morbidly more vulnerable, suggesting a need for specific preventative interventions targeted to those DRWs with a trauma and psychiatric history.

Co-morbid diagnoses

Co-morbidity of major depression and substance abuse with PTSD have been well documented (Kessler *et al.*, 1995; Jacobsen *et al.*, 2001). Our empirical data, as noted above, as well as our clinical observations are consistent with this literature.

Among the Con Edison employees depression was, not surprisingly, more common among those with a pre-morbid trauma history or with additional life stressors. About 5% met criteria for major depression (Difede *et al.*, 2004). Among firefighters, the picture was further complicated by bereavement. Most firefighters experienced multiple and extensive losses. A typical example, Mr. F. had been a firefighter for 20 years. Ten men from his firehouse (who he had known from 7 to 20 years) were killed, including his two best friends. Individuals with loss this extensive were not uncommon and often appeared numb. Survivor's guilt was common, especially for officers who wished that they could take the place of younger men, who had left wives and young children behind.

Regarding substance abuse, many DRWs are not likely to readily reveal the nature or extent of their use due to the consequences of substance abuse in the workplace. However, substance use, especially alcohol use, is a frequent problem in DRWs. One not uncommon presentation among the Con Edison employees were Vietnam Veterans who had been sober for a decade or longer, now presenting with a relapse, or an overwhelming urge to drink with the risk of imminent relapse. These stories were especially poignant as many described battling with alcohol or other substances after their return from Vietnam, achieving sobriety and social stability, only to be confronted with these demons again as the price of working at the WTC site.

Substance abuse is a particularly thorny problem to address both because work-related consequences are severe, and use of alcohol, in quantities far greater than are commonly accepted in other social venues, are common. For individuals with substance abuse, it is a challenge to remain sober when one's peers are not. And it is perhaps even more extraordinary to be able to walk away from those friends, as a step on the path to sobriety, when one relies on them at work and play, especially after a catastrophic event, such as the attack on the WTC.

Though the prevailing clinical wisdom is to engage the patient in a plan to quit their substance use, premature adoption of this strategy may lead to treatment failures (Ouimette *et al.*, 1998). It was our impression, in working with both groups, that as undesirable as the excessive alcohol consumption was, we would have lost many to further treatment if we had been insistent on an immediate sobriety plan because we did not have an adequate substitute to offer that would ease their suffering. Many refused to consider psychotropic medication as a palliative measure, despite our urging. There is some debate in the clinical literature as to how to approach the dual problem of PTSD and substance use. Recent evidence suggests that the PTSD should be treated concurrently. Otherwise, if the substance problem is ignored, any gains made in the treatment hour might be mitigated by substance abuse. If the substance abuse is treated first, the patient is likely to relapse because their PTSD symptoms, such as intrusive imagery, are cues for drinking (Najavits, 2002).

In principle, we agree with the approach of treating PTSD and substance abuse concurrently. Otherwise, the priority treatment of one disorder may be undermined by the other one, as discussed above. However, while we favored this approach as our guiding principle for treatment planning, in practice it was often quite difficult to implement. Working individually with each patient, we often started by targeting whichever symptoms were most distressing to the patient. Often, diminishing one symptom made it possible to target others. For example, a bereaved firefighter acknowledged he was drinking more in order to tolerate the immensity of his grief and had no interest in curbing his alcohol use. Treatment then focused on his grief and once he began to feel some relief, he came to his therapist for help to reduce his alcohol use. The necessary steps to reduce his substance use were then assessed and implemented. However, another patient was impacted by a discussion of how alcohol use was increasing his panic symptoms. He decided to begin by reducing his alcohol intake and found that this diminished the frequency and intensity of his panic. In time he was ready to directly discuss his trauma.

Common problems consequent to trauma and PTSD

In addition to endorsement of re-experiencing, avoidance and hyperarousal symptoms, the diagnosis of PTSD includes an evaluation of the social, occupational, and subjective distress, that is Criterion E (First *et al.*, 1997). The following section describes the most common complaints reported to us. Generally, these complaints were consistent with the extant literature on PTSD. However, there were problems in each area that were idiosyncratic to each population.

Effects on cognitive appraisal

Cognitive theories of PTSD suggest that exposure to information during a trauma that is contradictory to one's fundamental beliefs may be associated with PTSD symptoms (McCann *et al.*, 1988). Thus, a cognitive framework may be of heuristic value in explaining the relationship between the DRW's subjective experience and their PTSD symptoms. Research also suggests that appraisal of fundamental beliefs is affected by terrorism (Difede *et al.*, 1997). Following 9/11 we found that there were a common set of cultural beliefs and cognitions among the DRWs that were deeply affected. The DRW's fundamental beliefs regarding themselves (invulnerability, immortality), the world (predictability, controllability, and safety), and others (trust, safety, and isolation) that had shaped their lives had been shattered. Specifically, we found that themes of "the world is a dangerous place" and "I am a failure" (common to trauma survivors in general) manifest in unique ways in each of the sub-populations as described below.

The ethos of the FDNY can be understood by the statement "we run in, when others run out." New York City firefighters are renowned for their fearlessness. It was this ethos that had members of the FDNY running up the stairs in the tallest skyscraper without a thought to their own safety. Those who survived generally had their world assumptions shattered, precipitating existential crises. Cognitive theories suggest that disconfirmation of pre-existing world assumptions may be associated with PTSD (McCann *et al.*, 1988). Many firefighters reported feeling as if the world was a dangerous place and as if they had failed. These were dissonant thoughts for men accustomed to being in control. Most reported feeling bewildered and embarrassed by the changes in their cognitive appraisal of themselves and their relation to the world, adding shame to the list of painful feelings to be mastered. From an existential perspective, their very preparedness to confront danger appeared to underlie their vulnerability to PTSD, as their self assumptions regarding efficacy, mastery, and fearlessness were called into question.

In contrast, most Con Edison employees, outside of the Emergency/Safety Division, were not trained to confront disaster scenarios. Hence, they did not usually have a self-concept that included preparedness and fearlessness in the face of danger. Their symptoms generally did not seem to be as closely related to a disconfirmation of their sense of self-efficacy. Instead, themes in cognitive appraisal seemed to focus more on "the world is a dangerous place" with an overestimation of future harm risk.

A common theme for both groups was a profound sense of helplessness. However, this helplessness appeared to be related to different cognitions for each group. For the firefighters, it was associated with the thought of "I am a failure" for being unable to meet expectations of saving the lives of their brethren and the civilians entrusted to them. For the Con Edison employees, the helplessness turned on the cognition, "the world is a dangerous" place. Many of the Con Edison workers were fathers[3] who expressed the fear that they were unable to protect their children and spouses from an increasingly dangerous world.

---

[3] The sample is 98% male.

Effects on interpersonal lives

The symptoms of PTSD are known to be associated with interpersonal conflict. Studies suggest rates of marital conflict leading to divorce at about 9% and impairment of close relationships as high as 40% (North *et al.*, 1999). Domestic violence is not uncommon (Mechanic *et al.*, 2000). Among firefighters and Con Edison workers, two commonly reported problems were elevated conflict with supervisors at work and exacerbation of pre-existing marital problems. Participants frequently reported that the interpersonal problems were more troubling than the PTSD symptoms.

Participants also frequently complained about changes in sexual functioning. Not surprisingly, many reported being confused and embarrassed by this problem. Some were scared because they interpreted their decreased interest in sex to mean that they were no longer interested in their partner. Others, feeling isolated after the attacks, craved more intimate contact with a partner who had become distant. Either way, sexual problems were cited as a frequent cause for the rapid deterioration of intimate relationships. We found that a frank discussion, that included the sexual partner, of the effects of PTSD on sexuality, often attenuated the discord. It is a notable omission that current interviews and self-report measures for PTSD do not address sexual feelings and performance; nor do manualized, empirically validated treatments address this essential area of human functioning.

Effects on work performance

Work performance is affected by trauma, and may lead to either temporary or permanent disability. Studies of firefighters after the Oklahoma City bombing suggested that work performance was impaired in 83% of those with PTSD (North *et al.*, 2002a). Problems with work performance were compounded for firefighters and the Con Edison workers. The nature of their work requires them to repeatedly confront potentially life-threatening situations that may evoke memories of the WTC attack. This was especially true of the firefighters.

The decision to stop working either temporarily, by going on "light duty," or permanently due to PTSD is often fraught with many emotional as well as bureaucratic entanglements. The decision to retire or take disability presents unique challenges, especially among firefighters, who generally derive a substantial part of their identity, including the challenge and reward of saving lives, and social community, from their work. Light duty, though a necessary therapeutic strategy for many, itself became a stressor, though of a much lower order of magnitude. Many DRWs meet their family budget by supplementing their income through overtime, which is usually not available while on light duty. Hence, light duty was potentially both a psychological and financial stressor; while making the decision to retire as a consequence of a disability, especially a psychiatric one, presented unprecedented challenges that often became a topic of therapy.

Treatment and the therapeutic alliance

In the following section we will describe aspects of treatment that we found to be either particularly challenging or idiosyncratic to working with DRWs. All workers were treated with empirically validated treatments for PTSD using CBT plus exposure therapy as the first line of treatment, where clinically indicated. We used a manualized treatment approach, adapting a manual previously developed through our research with burn patients (this study included non-WTC DRWs). If the worker did not respond, or if in our clinical judgment this approach was not clinically indicated, deviations from our protocols, including the use of virtual reality exposure therapy (Difede & Hoffman, 2002) and cognitive processing therapy (Resicke & Schnicke, 1993), as previously applied to PTSD following terrorism (Difede & Eskra, 2001) were implemented. Although workers were provided treatment through different administrative venues (i.e., treatment studies, treatment programs, private practice), the content of treatment was generally comprised of a set of empirically validated techniques tailored to each individual case. Our treatment approach can be described as one in which both therapist and patient are active participants utilizing the following techniques both during and between sessions: *in vivo* and imaginal exposure, cognitive restructuring, relaxation exercises (including controlled breathing and guided imagery), anger management, sleep hygiene, and psychoeducation. About 20% of our patients were placed on psychotropic medication; however, pharmacotherapy was recommended for a much greater percentage of participants than accepted. Referrals were offered, in accordance with Expert Consensus Guidelines for PTSD, whenever there was evidence of functional impairment, impaired quality of life, or sleep disturbance, of moderate to severe intensity (Foa *et al.*, 1999).

An active approach

We find the active as well as interactive nature of our treatment approach to be indispensable with DRWs, and it is evident from the start of the evaluation process. During the screening process it was not uncommon for the clinician to find the employee endorsing symptoms of PTSD or major depression, only to minimize or even deny any subjective distress. We have come to understand this minimization to involve, in part, the "pull yourself up by the bootstraps" mentality common to both populations. "I may not be sleeping, and my marriage may be on the rocks, but I'm able to do my job, so I must be okay." The clinician is then faced with the task of selling the treatment to someone stating that there is nothing wrong. We have found that certain tactics work best in these types of situations: (1) concretely matching the proposed treatment to the individual's particular situation and symptoms (e.g., how treatment could help to improve sleep, driving over the bridge to work without panicking, or ease marital distress), (2) framing treatment as stress management *training* wherein they will be active participants vs. psychological *treatment*, which many envisioned as a forum to complain about their problems and accomplish little else, (3) emphasizing the "training" as means to help them regain a sense of control in their lives, and (4) sharing our experience in successfully treating other DRWs. Anticipating some resistance to treatment in the Con Edison employees, we set up the treatment program to make it as likely as possible for employees from this particular population to receive treatment. To this end, employees are allowed to attend treatment during work hours, which has been a popular option.

As we have already noted, DRWs, especially the firefighters, often have a very active, mastery-focused style of coping. We capitalized on this to engage participants in particular aspects of the treatment, such as creating and completing homework assignments. For example, a critical component of the treatment for PTSD is to derive an *in vivo* hierarchy of situations the individual is avoiding, for example, talking to the wife of a deceased brother, and then to gradually approach the situation with the final goal of mastery. Most often, if the individual clearly understood the rationale of such activities and then helped create their particular assignment, motivation to follow through and complete it, as well as continue in treatment was high.

However, this active coping style did not preclude difficulties in initial engagement in treatment. DRWs with a "pull yourself up by your bootstraps" mentality who predominantly endorsed avoidant and numbing symptoms of PTSD were a noteworthy challenge. During the first session, such an individual usually stated that he had no idea why he was referred for treatment, but he was curious enough to come to the first session, and perhaps even felt he was owed something for what he went through at Ground Zero. So there he was reporting that everything was fine, stating that he copes by trying not to think about his experience, and he has no real problems from working at the site. It is imperative that the therapist does not collude with the combination of avoidance and numbing symptoms coupled with the habitual stance of self-sufficiency, and send the patient on their way. It is not uncommon for therapists new to trauma work to report to their supervisor that their patients with this presentation seem to be "just fine."

The following example will serve to illustrate the potential for colluding with avoidant and numbing symptoms, as well as the use of an active approach to treatment. Mr. W responded to the site on the night of the attacks, to help map out the shutting off of fuel potentially feeding the fires at the site. During his first session he reported that everything was basically fine and he did not know why he had been referred for treatment. He was proud of his work at Ground Zero and felt he was having no related problems. He had lost interest in most activities outside of work, but attributed this to age. He made vague mention of his wife complaining that he was forgetting more than usual at home. The therapist's job at this point was to inquire more in depth about his experience working at the site. As he began to share his story, recounting in detail, he began to cry and become visibly anxious when talking about having to run from other buildings that were potentially collapsing. Within a few weeks the patient was engaged in exposure therapy. As expected, his hyperarousal symptoms increased before diminishing as he processed his trauma experience piece by piece. Toward the end of treatment, therapist and patient together looked for ways for him to become more active in his life. During his final session, he proudly displayed pictures of the antique car he had begun working on again.

Useful modifications to the therapeutic stance

In addition to the overall active nature of our approach, there are modifications to a traditional therapeutic stance that we have found to be indispensable. These modifications can perhaps best be understood as stemming from the fact that these patients are both trauma survivors and also inhabit the sub-culture of DRWs; the latter of which fosters particular styles of relating that will inevitably impact the therapeutic relationship. As trauma survivors, DRWs are not different from other groups of trauma survivors in regards to: (1) feeling more emotionally and physically vulnerable as a result of the traumatization and (2) coping with feelings of being isolated and disengaged. As a result, these individuals will need to establish a therapeutic alliance where they feel safe revealing their vulnerability as well as experience a genuine connection with the therapist. To these ends we find that the primary issue is navigating the gulf between the world of the therapist and that of the DRW with the aim of establishing a useful working alliance.

The therapist must first acknowledge the gulf between the world of the DRW and the world of the therapist in order to navigate it. The DRW may be wondering how they can ever expect a person holed up in an office with books and diplomas to possibly help someone like themselves who is usually busy saving lives or keeping the city in power. Furthermore, they may wonder if the therapist will be tough enough to tolerate hearing the details of their work and their trauma. We have found that essential to establishing a connection with DRWs is allowing oneself to become genuinely curious and educated about their day-to-day work lives. We have also found humor to be indispensable. The worlds of firefighters and Con Edison employees are filled with bantering and "bust your chops" kinds of humor. Engaging in this bantering with patients can go far in establishing a working alliance.

Finally, therapists working with DRWs can expect to be asked a host of personal questions in the patient's attempt to establish a working relationship with their therapist. Frequently, patients inquired about our experiences on 9/11, as well as about more general areas of our lives. Perhaps the most helpful way to think of these questions are as attempts to figure out if you are going to be able to help them with the trauma. What can be most useful to keep in mind when establishing the therapeutic alliance, is that underneath the humor, the personal inquiries, the tests of fortitude, is a search for reassurance that the therapist can be trusted to guide them through a vulnerable time.

Conclusions

The empirical data and clinical observations resulting from our evaluation and treatment of the FDNY and Con Edison employees following 9/11 are, for the most part, consistent with the extant literature on trauma. Our data, which suggests that up to one-quarter of the DRWs met criteria for PTSD, highlights the importance of establishing mandatory screening programs for DRWs. It also underscores the importance of conducting controlled clinical trials for the treatment of PTSD in these groups, so we can better learn how to address their unique treatment needs. The data further suggests a need to develop prevention and education programs that occur as a routine part of on-the-job training; idiosyncratic to each population.

Many observers, both disaster relief personnel and those caring for them post-9/11, have noted the widespread reluctance of these personnel to seek treatment. Many DRWs who sought treatment in one of our programs told us of several friends and colleagues at their firehouse or in their workgroup that needed help, but would not seek it. Reasons cited included the stigma, misunderstanding of PTSD and of the treatment, and feared negative impact on career advancement. Our patients frequently asked for our advice as to how to motivate their friends to seek appropriate help. Though anecdotal, these stories were poignant reminders of the impediments to care for our city's disaster relief personnel.

Both our data and experience lead us to speculate on the potential benefits of educating disaster relief personnel about the effects of trauma and the nature of treatment, as a preventative measure. Perhaps if such education was part of training, beginning as a probationary DRW, rates of seeking help following traumatization might increase. Such training would not only provide necessary information and skills, but also convey that the organization takes the potential effects of trauma encountered in disaster relief work seriously. In addition, training might help to ameliorate the stigma of mental health treatment as well as the feared implications for career advancement. The goals could vary from a simple psycho-education program about trauma and its effects to a preventive stress inoculation program that introduces DRWs to the concepts involved in treatment before it is needed. Because DRWs generally engage in mastery as a coping style, are action oriented, and look to help others, such a program would likely meet with the most success if it was offered as training, rather than treatment, and framed as an active process that will both allow them to help themselves and others.

Though our current state of knowledge precludes prevention of the cascade of psychobiological events that occurs when a person perceives imminent threat to their life, the growing literature on the long-term consequences of trauma suggests that a concerted effort to ameliorate the effects is imperative. Preventive education campaigns, mandatory screenings, and early intervention programs are essential to addressing these public health problems. It is critical that public officials and organizational representatives of the diverse groups of DRWs work in concert with the clinical research groups with expertise in trauma to allocate necessary funding and design programs for each disaster relief group before the next disaster. It is our hope that our program, both its successes and failures, may serve as one guidepost. Finally, we are grateful to those who entrusted us with their care for the privilege of serving them.

REFERENCES

Alexander, D.A. & Wells, A. (1991). Reactions of police officers to body-handling after a major disaster. A before-and-after comparison. *British Journal of Psychiatry*, **159**, 547–555.

Armstrong, K., O'Callahan, W. & Marmar, C.R. (1991). Debriefing Red Cross disaster personnel: the multiple stressor debriefing model. *Journal of Traumatic Stress*, **4**, 581–593.

Blake, D.D., Weathers, F.W., Nagy, L.M., Kaloupek, D.G., Klauminzer, G., Charney, D.S. & Keane, T.M. (1990). A clinician rating scale for assessing current and lifetime PTSD: the CAPS-1. *The Behavior Therapist*, **13**, 187–188.

Con Edison (2002). ConEdison's response to the World Trade Center Attack. Available at http://m020-w1.coned.com/PublicIssues/pi_wtc-reponse.html. Accessed 12/08/03.

Difede, J. & Eskra, D. (2001). Cognitive processing therapy for PTSD in a survivor of the WTC bombing: a case study. *Journal of Trauma Practice*, **1**, 155–165.

Difede, J. & Hoffman, H. (2002). Use of virtual reality exposure therapy to treat PTSD following the WTC attack. *Cyberpsychology*, **5**, 529–535.

Difede, J., Apfeldorf, W., Cloitre, M., Speilman, L. & Perry, S. (1997). Acute psychiatric responses to the explosion at the World Trade Center: a case series. *Journal of Nervous and Mental Disease*, **185**, 519–522.

Difede, J., Weathers, F., Jayasinghe, N., Leck, P., Roberts, J., Kramer, M. & Crane, M. (2004). Psychiatric consequences of the World Trade Center attack in a sample of utility workers. *American Psychiatric Association Annual Meeting*, New York, NY, May 2004.

Duckworth, D. (1986). Psychological problems arising from disaster work. *Stress Medicine*, **2**, 315–323.

Dunning, C. (1998). Intervention strategies for emergency workers. In *Mental Health Response to Mass Emergencies: Theory and Practice (Psychosocial Stress Series, No. 12)*, ed. M. Lystad. New York, NY: Brunner/Mazel, pp. 284–307.

Durham, T.W., McCammon, S.L. & Allison Jr., E.J. (1985). The psychological impact of disaster on rescue personnel. *Annals of Emergency Medicine*, **14**, 664–668.

Emanuel, R.J. & Ursano, R.J. (1999). Integrative group therapy with disaster workers. In *Group Treatments for Post-traumatic Stress Disorder*, eds. B.H. Young & D.D. Blake. Ann Arbor, MI: Brunner/Mazel, pp. 51–74.

Ersland, S., Weisaeth, L. & Sund, A. (1989). The stress upon rescuers involved in an oil rig disaster. "Alexander L. Kielland" 1980. *Acta Psychiatrica Scandinavica*, **80**(Suppl. 355), 38–49.

First, M.B., Spitzer, R.L., Williams, J.B.W. & Gibbon, M. (1997). *Structured Clinical Interview for DSM-IV (SCID)*. Washington, DC: American Psychiatric Association.

Foa, E.B., Davidson, R.T. & Frances, A. (1999). Expert consensus guideline series: treatment of posttraumatic stress disorder. *Journal of Clinical Psychiatry*, **60**(Suppl. 16), 5–76.

Fullerton, C.S., McCarroll, J.E., Ursano, R.J. & Wright, K.M. (1992). Psychological responses of rescue workers: fire fighters and trauma. *American Journal of Orthopsychiatry*, **62**(3), 371–378.

Fullerton, C.S., Ursano, R.J., Vance, K. & Wang, L. (2000). Debriefing following trauma. *Psychiatric Quarterly*, **71**(3), 259–276.

Gersons, B.P.R., Carlier, I.V.E., Lamberts, R.D. & van der Kolk, B.A. (2000). Randomized clinical trial of brief eclectic psychotherapy for police officers with posttraumatic stress disorder. *Journal of Traumatic Stress*, **13**, 333–347.

Gillespie, K., Duffy, M., Hackmann, A. & Clark, D.M. (2002). Community based cognitive therapy in the treatment of posttraumatic stress disorder following the Omagh bomb. *Behaviour Research and Therapy*, **40**, 345–357.

Harvey-Lintz, T. & Tidwell, R. (1997). Effects of the 1992 Los Angeles civil unrest: post traumatic stress disorder symptomatology among law enforcement officers. *Social Science Journal*, **34**, 171–183.

Hytten, K. & Hasle, A. (1989). Fire fighters: a study of stress and coping. *Acta Psychiatrica Scandinavica*, **80**(Suppl. 355), 50–55.

Jacobsen, L.K., Southwick, S.M. & Kosten, T.R. (2001). Substance use disorders in patients with posttraumatic stress disorder: a review of the literature. *American Journal of Psychiatry*, **158**, 1184–1190.

Jenkins, S.R. (1996). Social support and debriefing efficacy among emergency medical workers after a mass shooting incident. *Journal of Social Behavior and Personality*, **11**, 477–492.

Jones, D.R. (1985). Secondary disaster victims: the emotional effects of recovering and identifying human remains. *American Journal of Psychiatry*, **142**(3), 303–307.

Kenardy, J.A., Webster, R.A., Lewin, T.J., Carr, V.J., Hazell, P.L. & Carter, G.L. (1996). Stress debriefing and patterns of recovery following a natural disaster. *Journal of Traumatic Stress*, **9**, 37–49.

Kessler, R.C., Sonnega, A., Bromet, E., Hughes, M. & Nelson, C.B. (1995). Posttraumatic stress disorder in the National Comorbidity Survey. *Archives of General Psychiatry*, **52**, 1048–1060.

Marmar, C.R., Weiss, D.S., Metzler, T.J., Ronfeldt, H.M. & Foreman, C. (1996). Stress responses of emergency services personnel to the Loma Prieta earthquake interstate 880 freeway collapse and control traumatic incidents. *Journal of Traumatic Stress*, **9**, 63–85.

Marmar, C.R., Weiss, D.S., Metzler, T.J., Delucchi, K.L., Best, S.R. & Wentworth, K.A. (1999). Longitudinal course and predictors of continuing distress following critical incident exposure in emergency services personnel. *Journal of Nervous and Mental Disease*, **187**, 15–22.

McCann, I.L., Sakheim, D.K. & Abrahamson, D.J. (1988). Trauma and victimization: a model of psychological adaptation. *Counseling Psychology*, **16**, 531–594.

McCarroll, J.E., Ursano, R.J. & Fullerton, C.S. (1995). Symptoms of PTSD following recovery of war dead: 13–15-month follow-up. *American Journal of Psychiatry*, **152**, 939–941.

McFarlane, A.C. (1986). Long term psychiatric morbidity after a natural disaster: implications for disaster planners and emergency services. *Medical Journal of Australia*, **145**, 561–563.

McFarlane, A.C. (1988). The longitudinal course of posttraumatic morbidity: the range of outcomes and their predictors. *Journal of Nervous and Mental Disease*, **176**(1), 30–39.

McFarlane, A.C. & Papay, P. (1992). Multiple diagnoses in posttraumatic stress disorder in the victims of a natural disaster. *Journal of Nervous and Mental Disease*, **180**, 498–504.

Mechanic, M.B., Uhlmansiek, M.H., Weaver, T.L. & Resick, P.A. (2000). The impact of severe stalking experienced by acutely battered women: an examination of violence, psychological symptoms and strategic responding. *Violence Victims*, **15**, 443–458.

Moran, C. & Colless, E. (1995). Positive reactions following emergency and disaster responses. *Disaster Prevention and Management*, **4**(1), 55–61.

Najavits, L.M. (2002). *Seeking Safety: A Treatment Manual for PTSD and Substance Abuse*. New York, NY: Guilford Press.

National Center for Post-traumatic Stress Disorder (2001a). Disaster rescue and response workers. 9/14/01. Available at http:/www.ncptsd.org/facts/disasters. Accessed 12/08/03.

National Center for Post-traumatic Stress Disorder (2001b). The range, magnitude, and duration of effects of natural and human caused disasters: a review of the empirical literature. 10/04/01. Available at http://www.ncptsd.org/facts/disasters. Accessed on 12/08/03.

Neufeldt, V. & Guralnik, D.B. (1989). *Webster's New World Dictionary* (3rd ed.). New York: Prentice Hall.

New York City Fire Department (2002). McKinsey report. Available at http://nyc.gov.html.fdny/html/mck_report/index.shtml. Accessed 12/08/03.

Norris, F.H., Friedman, M.J., Watson, P.J., Byrne, C.M., Diaz, E. & Kaniasty, K. (2002). 60,000 disaster victims speak: Part I: An empirical review of the empirical literature, 1981–2001. *Psychiatry: Interpersonal and Biological Processes*, **65**, 207–239.

North, C.S. (2002). Trauma anonymous. *Fire Chief*, June 1.

North, C.S., Nixon, S.J., Shariat, S., Mallonee, S., McMillen, J.C., Spiznagel, E.L. & Smith, E.M. (1999). Psychiatric disorders among survivors of the Oklahoma City bombing. *Journal of the American Medical Association*, **282**(8), 755–762.

North, C.S., Tivis, L., McMillen, J.C., Pfefferbaum, B., Cox, J., Spitznagel, E.L., Bunch, K., Schorr, J. & Smith, E.M. (2002a). Coping, functioning, and adjustment of rescue workers after the Oklahoma City bombing. *Journal of Traumatic Stress*, **15**, 171–175.

North, C.S., Tivis, L., McMillen, J.C., Pfefferbaum, B., Spitznagel, E.L., Cox, J., Nixon, S., Bunch, K.P. & Smith, E.M. (2002b). Psychiatric disorders in rescue workers after the Oklahoma City bombing. *American Journal of Psychiatry*, **159**(5), 857–859.

Nurmi, L.A. (1999). The sinking of the Estonia: the effects of critical incident stress debriefing (CISD) on rescuers. *International Journal of Emergency Mental Health*, **1**, 23–31.

Ouimette, P.C., Brown, P.J. & Najavits, L.M. (1998). Course and treatment of patients with both substance use and posttraumatic stress disorders. *Addictive Behaviors*, **23**, 785–795.

Paton, D. (1997). Training disaster workers: promoting well being and operational effectiveness. *Disaster Prevention and Management*, **5**, 11.

Raphael, B., Singh, B., Bradbury, L. & Lambert, F. (1983–1984). Who helps the helpers? The effects of disaster on rescue workers. *Omega: Journal of Death and Dying*, **14**(1), 9–20.

Renck, B., Weisaeth, L. & Skarbo, S. (2002). Stress reactions in police officers after a disaster rescue operation. *Nordic Journal of Psychiatry*, **56**(1), 7–14.

Resicke, P. & Schnicke, M. (1992). Cognitive processing therapy for sexual assault victims. *Journal Consulting and Clinical Psychology*, **60**, 748–756.

Rosenczweig, C.C., Kravitz, J. & Delvin, M. (2002). The psychological impact of helping in a disaster – the New York City experience, September 11th, 2001. *Academic Emergency Medicine*, **9**, 502-a.

Rothbaum, B.O., Meadows, E.A., Resick, P. & Foy (2000). Cognitive-behavioral therapy. In *Effective Treatments for PTSD*, eds. E.B. Foa, T.M. Keane & M.J. Friedman. New York: The Guilford Press, pp. 60–83.

Shalev, A.Y. (1994). Debriefing following traumatic exposure. In *Individual and Community Responses to Trauma and Disaster: The Structure of Human Chaos*, eds. R.J. Ursano, B.G. McCaughney & C.S. Fullerton. Cambridge, UK: Cambridge University Press, pp. 201–219.

Sims, A. & Sims, D. (1998). The phenomenology of post-traumatic stress disorder: a symptomatic study of 70 victims of psychological trauma. *Psychopathology*, **31**, 96–112.

Smith, R.L. (2001). Coping with catastrophe, *Fire Chief*, December. Available at http://firechief.com/ar/firefighting_coping_catastrophe/index.htm. Accessed 12/08/03.

Taylor, A.J.W. & Frazer, A.G. (1982). The stress of post-disaster body handling and victim identification work. *Journal of Human Stress*, **8**, 4–12.

Tolin, D.F. & Foa, E.B. (1999). Treatment of a police officer with PTSD using prolonged exposure. *Behavior Therapy*, **30**, 527–538.

Ursano, R.J., Fullerton, C.S., Kao, T.C., Bhartiya, V.R., *et al.* (1995). Longitudinal assessment of posttraumatic stress disorder and depression after exposure to traumatic death. *Journal of Nervous and Mental Disease*, **183**, 36–42.

Weiss, D.S., Marmar, C.R., Metzler, T.J. & Ronfeldt, H.M. (1995). Predicting symptomatic distress in emergency services personnel. *Journal of Consulting and Clinical Psychology*, **63**(3), 361–368.

Wilkinson, C.B. (1983). Aftermath of a disaster: the collapse of the Hyatt Regency Hotel skywalks. *American Journal of Psychiatry*, **140**, 1134–1139.

Wilson, S.A., Tinker, R.H., Becker, L.A. & Logan, C.R. (2001). Stress management with law enforcement personnel. A controlled outcome study of EMDR versus a traditional stress management program. *International Journal of Stress Management*, **8**, 179–200.

Wright, K., Ursano, R., Bartone, P. & Ingraham, L. (1990). The shared experience of catastrophe: an expanded classification of the disaster community. *American Journal of Orthopsychiatry*, **60**, 35–42.

Young, B.H., Ford, J.D., Ruzek, J.I., Friedman, M.J. & Gusman, K. (1998). *Disaster Mental Health Services: A Guide for Clinicians and Administrators.* Menlo Park, CA: Department of Veterans Affairs.

21

The World Trade Center Worker/Volunteer Mental Health Screening Program

Craig L. Katz, Rebecca P. Smith, Robin Herbert, Steven M. Levin and Raz Gross

The traumatic exposure

The dramatic effect of the pictures notwithstanding, the physical and mental effects of being at "Ground Zero" were described by many "Ground Zero workers" as only able to be understood through direct experience of it. The site occupied 16 acres in lower Manhattan, with buildings grouped around a 5-acre central plaza. The site is bounded by Vesey Street on the north, Church Street on the east, Liberty Street on the south, and West Street on the west, about three blocks north of the New York Stock Exchange. The Twin Towers were 110 stories, 1353 feet (412 meters) tall. In total, there were about 10,000,000 square feet of rentable space. About 50,000 people occupied the buildings. There were 43,200 square feet (4020 square meters) – about an acre of rentable space – on each floor. The seven buildings were made up of 95% air by volume, and contained 13 million square feet of space. Commercially, the seven-story mall beneath the World Trade Center (WTC) was America's third most heavily trafficked mall (Tomasky, 2003). In the aftermath of 9/11, the site continues to be an object of much interest, discussion and meaning for droves of visitors.

Whatever else "Ground Zero" may have been, it was also the workplace for a large number of workers and volunteers. In addition to the firemen and policemen whose volunteer, rescue, and recovery efforts have been chronicled in the media, "Ground Zero" also provided employment for at least 50 other professions, as well as a host of volunteers. Estimates of the number of people involved in the volunteer, rescue, recovery, and salvage effort at "Ground Zero" range from 18,000 to 35,000 (CNN.com. January 28, 2002; Herman *et al.*, 2002), of which firemen and policemen comprised a minority. In addition to the 343 lives lost from the New York City Fire Department, and the 37 and 23 lives lost from the Port Authority and New York City Police Departments (NYPD), respectively, there were 152 members of the building trades unions who were killed when the WTC collapsed. The New York Medical Examiner reported that in the recovery effort, "Ground Zero workers" found more than 18,000 body parts, and had issued 1932 death certificates. The protracted nature of the recovery effort is illustrated by the fact that in the month of March 2002 as many as 3000 body parts were discovered (Kugler, 2002). By the completion of the salvage, recovery, and cleanup process on May 30, 2002, 1.8 million tons of debris had been removed from the disaster site (WTC web site). The scale of contributions made by building tradesmen and women and construction workers was clearly enormous from a physical as well as a political and social perspective.

Estimates of the short-term psychiatric consequences of 9/11 have been described previously in local and national subsets of the general population (Schuster *et al.*, 2001; Ahern *et al.*, 2002; Galea *et al.*, 2002a, b). Additionally, increases in tobacco, alcohol, and marijuana consumption were reported in the general population in New York and surrounding states (Melnik *et al.*, 2001; Vlahov *et al.*, 2002). In Galea *et al.* (2002a) among 1008 individuals contacted through random digit dialing, 111 of 877 interviewed stated they had been involved in the WTC rescue efforts. Their rates of probable post-traumatic stress disorder (PTSD) and depression were 16.2% and 14.1%, respectively, compared to average prevalence rates in this group of 7.5% and 9.7%. While the association between involvement in rescue effort and depression did not attain statistical significance, the association with PTSD was significant at $p < 0.03$. Ahern *et al.* (2002) did not report results in this subgroup about whether reported exposure to TV images of 9/11 was associated with increased risk of PTSD or MDD (major depressive disorder) symptoms in this group.

In a needs assessment conducted by the Department of Epidemiology of the Mailman School of Public Health at the request of the New York State Office of Mental Health in October 2001, the potentially affected population from the attacks on the WTC' was divided into four groups: 10 surrounding counties of NY; New York City; Manhattan below 110 street; and the WTC population (Herman *et al.*, 2002). The category of "rescue workers" comprised one of four sub-categories of a larger "WTC population." The number of rescue workers was estimated at 17,859. The authors focused on PTSD because they hypothesized that the effect on PTSD had generally been greater than on other measured disorders. Because of a dearth of data on the exposures of the rescue workers, the risk of PTSD was estimated as 24%, which represented an average of 34% for those who were extremely exposed and the rate of 14% reported for Oklahoma City rescue workers (North *et al.*, 2002).

Mental health sequelae in relief and recovery workers

The psychiatric literature contains a range of findings to confirm the likelihood of mental health sequelae among the relief and recovery workers participating in disaster response. Wright *et al.* (1990) advanced the concept of a disaster community as a group of people and organizations affected by disasters arrayed in concentric rings around the direct victims. Service and support providers to the disaster scene are placed in the third and fourth rings, following only next of kin, and were deemed to be subject to significant, but potentially overlooked, psychological distress as a result of their work. The diversity of disasters investigated in the psychiatric literature, while each different from one another and of course from the unique circumstances of 9/11, also appears relevant in anticipating the mental health impact of Ground Zero on those who worked there. Many comprehensive reviews of this literature are available elsewhere; some relevant aspects of the literature are briefly discussed below.

Among specific populations of disaster workers, firefighters have probably been the best characterized from the perspective of mental health. McFarlane (1986) followed 459 firefighters who were exposed to the Ash Wednesday bushfires in Australia and found rates of likely PTSD to be as high 30% 29 months after the incident. A descriptive report of firefighters involved in either a mass casualty air disaster or special missions work found four common types of stress response: identification with victims, feelings of helplessness and guilt, fear of the unknown, and physiological reactions (Fullerton *et al.*, 1992). Of the factors deemed relevant to these experiences, clear role training and preparation were considered crucial. This seems especially prescient with regard to 9/11, as the magnitude and scope of what ultimately became known as Ground Zero clearly overwhelmed and challenged prior preparations by firefighting departments. Others have likewise commented on the psychological impact of situation and role uncertainty among disaster workers (Paton, 1989). In a related vein, the perception of relative success may bear on firefighters' ability to cope with the stress of their efforts in response to disasters such as massive hotel fires (Hytten & Hasle, 1989).

With regard to other disaster workers, Raphael *et al.* (1983) examined 95 rescue personnel involved in the Granville rail disaster in Australia. Of the 95 subjects, 77 (81%) found the experience to be stressful. Five sources of stress were identified as especially prominent: feelings of helplessness, the magnitude of the disaster, the sight and smell of dead bodies, the anguish of relatives, and the pressurized work environment. All of these factors appear directly relevant to 9/11. In a study of Amsterdam police officers involved in serious shooting incidents, 46% were found to have met criteria for PTSD at some point since the event (Gersons, 1989). Thirty-five percent of police officers involved in a massive fire at a 1985 soccer stadium were found to be likely psychiatric cases based on the General Health Questionnaire (GHQ) while another 9% were determined to be serious cases (Duckworth, 1986). Five months after assisting victims of an apartment building fire, 74% of on-site responders spanning rescue, police, fire, and medical personnel reported at least one symptom of PTSD and 28% had four or more symptoms consistent with mild-to-moderate stress (Durham *et al.*, 1985).

Among persons who handled remains in Operation Desert Storm, inexperience with body handling and extent of exposure to bodies, including number of bodies, correlated with intrusive and avoidant symptoms of PTSD (McCarroll *et al.*, 1993). Of special concern with regard to 9/11, identification with the deceased may be a particular risk factor for the development of PTSD among those handling the dead (Ursano *et al.*, 1999). Studies of other populations involved in public safety work have included those of medical students (Kent, 1991) and of social workers (Hodgkinson & Shepard, 1994), both of which detail significant levels of distress among higher-risk individuals (based on disaster and individual characteristics) and the need for adequate support for this issue. A recent survey of New York City medical students involved in the various roles in response to 9/11 detected high levels of emotional distress among those who were least supervised (Katz *et al.*, 2002b).

Workers involved in the rescue and recovery work at Ground Zero thus were likely exposed to a number of elements and factors known from the literature to lead to psychiatric or psychological sequelae, including high exposure to a massive catastrophe (where exposure includes loss of colleagues, personal injury, and physical proximity to the sights and scenes of Ground Zero), work in chaotic circumstances for which prior training seemed wholly inadequate, and likely intense identification with the dead. Although PTSD has been the primary *Diagnostic and Statistical Manual of Mental Disorders, Fourth Edition* (DSM-IV) diagnosis evaluated in the aforementioned studies and can thus be predicted as a likely mental health consequence for the Ground Zero workers attending the Mount Sinai Selikoff Center for Occupational and Environmental Medicine (COEM) Program, other common problems that have been found in the wake of disasters among the general population include major depression, generalized anxiety disorder, and substance abuse/dependence (Katz *et al.*, 2002a). These could be anticipated in the Ground Zero workers as well.

Experiences of salvage, volunteer, and rescue workers at Ground Zero

While it is nearly impossible to generalize about the experiences of individual members of each of the occupations represented in the WTC Recovery and Cleanup Effort (WTCRCE), there are nonetheless some general comments, which may have implications for understanding worker and volunteer experiences, both positive and negative, which have been described.

Motivations for being at the site

In addition to the volunteers who generously gave of their time at "Ground Zero," there were also workers who were contractually obligated to work at "Ground Zero," or at the Staten Island Landfill to which debris was brought. Among paid workers who were not contractually obligated to participate in the WTCRCE, economic pressure to work may have impacted their experience, particularly those workers from vulnerable populations (e.g., undocumented asbestos workers).

Dosing: degree and type of exposures

The degree and intensity of exposure to the site can be conceived of in a number of different ways. In previous investigations of the psychiatric impact of disasters, proximity, number of lives lost or extent of property damaged have been predictors of subsequent distress (Katz et al., 2002b; Norris et al., 2002). On the most concrete level, measurement of duration of time spent at "Ground Zero" (total time spent, number of consecutive days spent there, number of hours spent each day) provides one estimate of an exposure. On another level, there is the type of work done – digging for bodies could be more distressing than rigging lighting fixtures. Many different individuals described months spent sifting through rubble looking for the remains of victims. However, for some affected individuals, being prevented from participating in the recovery effort and being assigned instead to security or to administrative work might plausibly be a source of considerable distress. It could be conceived of as an "exposure" to disaster-related disempowerment and frustration.

Identification with the victims

Identification with deceased victims in a disaster has been described previously as a mechanism through which exposure to the dead leads to disease and symptoms in disaster workers (Ursano et al., 1999). Among the "Ground Zero workers" were many who had lost family, friends, colleagues, or members of their communities on 9/11. Given the nature of this disaster and the substantial representation of rescue workers among the victims, the potential for identification with victims was obviously quite high for those belonging to, for example, police and fire departments. However, substantial number of building tradesmen and carpenters were killed as well. And, other workers/volunteers who did not have direct connections, either personal or professional, to particular disaster victims, nonetheless could experience highly personal identifications with victims.

Subjective individual experiences of the site

Individuals will have different reactions to the site, ranging from those who saw it as "sacred ground – a memorial" to those who described it as "really just a construction site." Variations in the experience of being a worker or a volunteer likely stem from various intrapsychic factors, including both issues of motivation, and the conscious and unconscious personal meaning of the event (Katz & Nathaniel, 2002). Objective and profoundly subjective interpretations of the manifest horror of Ground Zero are relevant to the emotional impact of the WTCRCE. Of importance, of course, are perceptions of the clarity, meaning, and impact of one's role in the rescue/recovery effort. Some individuals may even have found that their work in the WTCRCE revealed to them personal capacities and resources of which they had previously been unaware.

Complex effects on support networks

For some patients, such as members of NYPD and retired firemen, the disaster resulted in clear and catastrophic disruptions of significant sources of support, such as the loss of significant number of colleagues and friends. However, the experiences of community and loss were multidimensional. Some retired firemen and policemen reported their distress coming in waves. First, they experienced the devastation of the initial losses of comrades. When the site closed on May 30, 2002, however, they experienced a second loss – the loss of a community and of a place to go to work with colleagues, a place to collectively mourn, and finally, a loss of a connection to those who were killed. It may be that studies that have defined "dose" of disaster exposure in terms of lives lost may also be indirectly measuring a disaster-induced diminution in the level of social support (Katz *et al.*, 2002b).

Development of the Mental Health Screening Program

The WTC Worker/Volunteer Mental Health Screening Program (MHSP) arose as a module within a broader 9/11-related medical screening program, the WTC Worker/Volunteer Medical Screening Program. Organized and administered by the Mount Sinai-Irving J. Selikoff COEM, this unique medical screening program was funded by the National Institute of Occupational Safety and Health (NIOSH), a federal agency within the Centers for Disease Control (CDC). NIOSH focuses on work-related injury and disease.

The medical directors of the COEM secured over $11 million in NIOSH funding to provide medical screenings of individuals who worked or volunteered at the WTC site after 9/11. These screenings were primarily focused on identifying the degree of persistent upper and lower airway disorders/dysfunction in individuals who were eligible for participation in this program based on how soon and how long they were present at the WTC site after the 9/11 attacks. The CDC funding permitted the screening of 8500 such individuals by the COEM.

During the initial period, beginning July 16, 2002, workers were eligible to participate in the program if they satisfied three criteria. First, they needed to have been worked and/or volunteered within (a) the site perimeter bounded by Chambers Street, Broadway, Rector Street, and the Hudson River; (b) the Staten Island Landfill; or (c) barge loading piers. Second, they needed to have been present on-site for at least 24 hours between 9/11/2001 and 9/14/2001 in addition to having spent a minimum of a total of 10 days on-site in September 2001. Third, they needed to have performed rescue, recovery, debris cleanup, and related support services. These criteria were revised effective August 15, 2002, to allow participation by workers present on-site for at least 24 hours between 9/11 and 9/14, and also those who had spent a minimum of 80 hours on-site in September 2001. Subsequent revisions in the stringency of these criteria have been considered. Federal employees, New York City firefighters, and New York State employees are covered by other medical screening programs and therefore were not eligible for this program. However, a number of retired firemen and retired New York State employees had volunteered on the site. They were therefore eligible for the screening.

In total, 6500 workers/volunteers were scheduled for evaluations at the Mount Sinai Medical Center in New York City, whereas an additional 2000 workers/volunteers would be seen at various collaborating sites in New York and nationally. The COEM would administer this massive program via its several organizational "cores" – administration, medical, outreach/exposure, and data management. The outreach/exposure core, in particular, was to play a central role in communicating with various trade unions and other entities which played a role in the WTC response, capitalizing and building on the COEM's longstanding relationship with many of these unions. Through such relationships, union members would be encouraged to attend the medical screening program. The outreach core was operational months in advance of the start of the screening program in July 2002, working together with the other cores to identify and schedule eligible patients.

Beyond the broad awareness of what was felt to be the immense psychological impact on 9/11, several factors led to the eventual incorporation of a mental health component in the medical screenings. First, during a pilot study for the medical screening program in February 2002, 97 ironworkers who had assisted at the WTC site for at least one of the 4 days beginning with 9/11/2001 and for at least 3 more days thereafter were evaluated; 68% reported at least one significant and persistent symptom of PTSD (J. Moline, Communication, June 1, 2002). Second, the clinical observations of the COEM clinicians in seeing patients from the WTC response suggested abundant emotional needs. Finally, NIOSH indicated the need for collection of psychological information about the programs' participants, although it did not provide specific funding for this purpose.

The COEM thus sought the assistance of the Mount Sinai Department of Psychiatry to address the mental health needs of the screening programs' participants. The Department of Psychiatry, through its affiliation with Disaster Psychiatry Outreach (DPO) as well as other efforts, had already provided extensive assistance to the community after 9/11. DPO is a non-profit organization devoted since 1998 to providing psychiatric care to all people affected by disasters and to promoting research and education in support of its overriding clinical mission. DPO's volunteer psychiatrists, many of them from Mount Sinai, had specifically provided assistance to over 3000 workers and volunteers at the WTC site in the first 2 months after the 9/11 attacks (McQuistion & Katz, 2001). This assistance consisted of largely informal support to what usually remained anonymous individuals working amid the pile. The COEM program was a natural opportunity to provide more formal help to this same population.

With the request from the COEM to the Department of Psychiatry coming in late winter of 2002, there existed a narrow window in which to organize, fund, and staff a mental health program in time for the scheduled July 2002 start date of the medical program. Neither DPO nor the Department of Psychiatry had the internal resources to accomplish this. At the time, the possibility of funding from Project Liberty, the crisis counseling program funded by the Federal Emergency Management Agency, was uncertain and was also based on a retrospective model of funding that posed fiscal challenges for starting the program.

Thankfully, DPO had previously been in communication with the Robin Hood Foundation, a New York City based foundation that works to eradicate inner city poverty. Expanding its mission in the face of 9/11, the Robin Hood Foundation raised a sizable amount of funds after 9/11 for the purpose of disaster relief. They had communicated an interest in funding direct mental health services to otherwise under-served populations in the New York City area. When DPO approached the foundation with the hope of providing such services to what has indeed traditionally been the under-served population of disaster workers, the Robin Hood Foundation agreed to review a proposal. Just a month after receiving this proposal, the Robin Hood Foundation's 9/11 Relief Fund granted a nearly $1 million grant to Mount Sinai and DPO to establish the WTC Worker/Volunteer MHSP. Notification of the award came just weeks before the intended start of the screening program.

Program design

A major challenge in designing the MHSP, as in the broader medical screening program, lay in how to conduct informative and ideally therapeutic evaluations of thousands of individuals in the course of what was already a busy visit to the medical screening program. Approximately 50 patients were forecast to attend the program up to 6 days per week for nearly a year. Moreover, their medical screening consisted of a number of stations, namely physical exposure assessment, physical examination, blood-work, chest radiograph, and pulmonary function tests. Where and when could mental health be addressed without overly burdening the patients and the staff?

Ultimately, the evaluations were conceptualized as occurring in two steps: (1) completion of a self-administered mental health questionnaire; and (2) clinical evaluations by mental health professionals of those patients who "screened in" based on the answers they gave to the questionnaire. This format was chosen for a number of reasons. First, it was felt that formal diagnostic evaluation via a structured clinical interview of all program attendees would be too time-consuming and too staff intensive. Second, it was felt that an overly structured interview would jeopardize the development of a therapeutic alliance with this group. Finally, relying on self-report screening instruments seemed like a very efficient way to capture an abundance of mental health information that could be readily counted on to determine the likelihood that any one individual would benefit from an in-person evaluation by a mental health professional.

The initial design of the screening process was relatively simple. Based on prior writings of DPO (Katz *et al.*, 2002a) the GHQ was selected as an instrument used previously in post-disaster investigations that could provide ready information on the likelihood of an individual's having a psychiatric disorder and that has also been shown to be predictive of PTSD (Goldberg & Hillier, 1979; McFarlane, 1986; Gregg *et al.*, 1995; McFarlane *et al.*, 1997). The GHQ consists of a set of questions aimed at discriminating between the general class of psychiatric patients and all other individuals. The 28-item version of the GHQ, the GHQ-28, is distinguished from the other versions in that it has four sub-scales, reflecting somatic symptoms, anxiety symptoms, social dysfunction, and depressive symptoms (Goldberg & Hillier, 1979). Because of this additional feature, it was chosen for use in the MHSP as an efficient way to collect multidimensional psychological information about the patients.

Although the GHQ-28 offers the advantage of sub-scales, it is unclear how to operationalize them, since the GHQ-28 was not designed to arrive at psychiatric diagnoses. The initial plan involved having the MHSP clinicians arrive at diagnoses based on their interviews with the patients and whatever information the GHQ-28 could provide. This plan was reviewed by what was a nascent Scientific Advisory Team consisting of senior medical staff from the COEM, the Medical Director and Senior Psychiatrist of the MHSP, and a consulting epidemiologist from Columbia University. It was then concluded that the screening questionnaire could, and should, be expanded to offer diagnostic assessment in a way that was not overly burdensome for either the patients or the patient flow within the program. The hope was to render the questionnaire as efficiently informative in establishing likely diagnoses as possible, apart from the issue of general "caseness."

Based on the prior disaster mental health literature, the diagnoses of foremost concern were PTSD, major depression, and alcohol abuse/dependence, although there is some debate about the pervasiveness of the latter problem post-disaster

(Katz *et al.*, 2002b). The PTSD Symptom Checklist (Blanchard *et al.*, 1996) was selected for patient administered assessment of PTSD. The Cutdown Annoyed Guilty Eye Opener (CAGE) Alcohol Questionnaire was chosen for determination of likely alcohol problems (Ewing, 1984). These were both chosen for their brevity and for being well known for their use in a range of settings. For example, the PTSD Checklist (PCL) has been found to have utility in the primary-care setting (Stein *et al.*, 2000). The Patient Health Questionnaire (PHQ) was chosen for evaluation of major depression (Spitzer *et al.*, 1999). This was done for two reasons. First, the PHQ was designed for the detection of mental illness in medical settings. Second, the PHQ has modules for other disorders, including panic disorder and generalized anxiety disorder, and given the focus on respiratory complaints in the medical evaluation, these were both felt to be relevant to the worker/volunteer population being served in the screening programs. Thus, the PHQ modules for major depression, panic disorder, and generalized anxiety disorder were incorporated into the screening questionnaire.

Finally, the questionnaire was modified to include non-diagnostic information that was believed relevant to the disaster mental health issues of the WTC Workers/Volunteers. A modified Sheehan Disability Scale was added in order to ground the patients' symptom self-reports in a measure of psychosocial function/dysfunction (Leon *et al.*, 1997). In a related vein, a number of items were borrowed from the Diagnostic Interview Schedule/Disaster Supplement of Carol North (North *et al.*, 1999). In particular, sections on the occurrence of stressful life events since 9/11, so-called secondary stresses, and the presence of symptoms of emotional disturbance in patient's children were added in order to round out the social picture of the screening program participants. Likewise, in order to capture the large role that perceived social support plays in post-disaster coping (Katz *et al.*, 2002b), a table of questions addressed those people who provided important or disappointing support to the patient post-9/11.

The questionnaire ultimately grew to nearly 200 questions over 11 pages and was found to take about 15–20 minutes to complete. In order to enhance the likelihood of patients' completing the screening survey, it was decided that they would receive the packet along with other orientation paperwork when they first arrived for their screening. As non-clinical mental health staff would be responsible for collecting and scoring the mental health questionnaire, a scoring protocol was designed for their use that incorporated pre-established thresholds for the GHQ-28, PCL, the three PHQ modules, and the CAGE alcohol survey. A patient was designated as having "screened in" for a clinical interview with a mental health clinician if they crossed the thresholds on any or all of these components. In addition, any indication of severe problem(s) with psychosocial function on the Sheehan Disability Scale was also considered a trigger in and of itself for a fuller clinical evaluation.

Alone among all of the symptoms in the questionnaire, an endorsement of any degree or frequency of suicidal thinking on the GHQ-28 or PHQ was also considered a reason for "screening in."

In order to assist the mental health screening coordinator and staff to manage the heavy influx of patients amid the hectic flow of the overall screening program, a color system was established. "Green" patients did not screen in based on their surveys and were not referred to a mental health clinician unless they asked for this service or were referred based on the clinical impressions of the occupational medicine staff. "Yellow" patients were those who exceeded the thresholds on any one or more of the pre-established triggers but who did not endorse suicidality. A subcategory of these patients was identified that consisted of patients who not only screened in on one of the diagnostic instruments but who also endorsed severe problems with psychosocial function. Finally, "red" patients were those patients who indicated any degree of suicidality. These last patients were to be accorded a high degree of priority and were to be seen by one of the mental health clinicians as early in the screening process as possible.

The clinical interview was designed to be a semi-structured interview that would permit the completion of the Clinical Evaluation Record. The goals of this interview were many. First, they were meant to be therapeutic or at least supportive experiences for the program participants, many of whom may never have spoken to a mental health professional before. Some may not have even had the prior chance to tell their story about 9/11. Second, the interviews had the parallel goal of assessing the accuracy of the screening instruments in detecting emotional/psychological problems in a given patient. Did a patient in fact have the problems identified by the screening questionnaire? Third, the clinicians had the related task of determining if such problems were present, did they necessitate referral for ongoing care and attention? If so, they provided the patient with a referral.

The Clinical Evaluation Record encompassed a number of sections and, supplemented by the screening questionnaire, was designed to permit a thorough psychiatric evaluation of patients that took approximately 1 hour. The opening section included a detailed review of patients' exposure to the WTC site, including the amount of time spent there, the nature of their role, and a review of disturbing aspects of their experience. This element of their exposure was not included in the self-report questionnaire, as it was felt to be potentially too emotionally laden. In addition, it was intended to serve as a springboard for patients' construction of a potentially therapeutic personal narrative about their experience.

Subsequent sections of the Clinical Evaluation Record prompted the clinician to review a patient's answers to the GHQ-28, PTSD Symptom Checklist, PHQ, and CAGE alcohol survey. All of these sections were open-ended with the exception of the alcohol section, which prompted the interviewer to administer the AUDIT survey for alcohol use disorders if the patient had screened in on the CAGE questions (Rumpf *et al.*, 2002). Such structure was incorporated into the interview in order to reduce the likelihood of a patient's minimizing their alcohol use. Questions about illicit drug use in various time frames since 9/11 were also included at this point. Other sections reviewed the details of the various domains of patients' psychosocial functioning, namely those of family/relationships, work, and recreation. Finally, the Clinical Evaluation Record incorporated questions regarding past psychiatric history, utilization of psychiatric services post-9/11, trauma history, and family history. It concluded with a traditional mental status examination, diagnostic conclusions, and plans for referral for any relevant treatment. Conclusions included clinicians' opinion of the degree to which psychiatric and psychosocial problems were related to 9/11.

The initial version of the Clinical Evaluation Record was largely open-ended. That is, although it prompted clinicians to address important topics, it generally made provision for only open-ended recording of replies and was intended as the basis for a thorough and meaningful clinical interview and record and not as an epidemiological tool. This emphasis was explicitly chosen in order to make what may have been many patients' first contact with mental health professionals as comfortable and "non-clinical" as possible within the limits of the necessary information required for clinical decision-making. However, several months into the program, the Clinical Evaluation Record was modified to include many more close-ended questions in order to render the information collected in the interviews more uniform as well as susceptible to statistical analysis. This was done at the recommendation of the Scientific Advisory Team, which had by then coalesced into a collection of experts in epidemiology, statistics, trauma, and psychiatric research from the Mount Sinai School of Medicine, Columbia University, and New York University. It was felt that the interview could be an opportunity to learn a considerable amount of epidemiological information without sacrificing the quality of the experience for the patients. MHSP clinicians were thus retrained in the use of this revised record.

Operation of the MHSP

On each day of the MHSP, three social workers and one psychiatrist were on hand to meet with patients who screened in based on their responses to the self-administered questionnaires. This level of staffing was calculated based on an expectation of an approximately 50% rate of screening in, a figure arrived at from an averaging of the rates of various psychiatric disorders post-disaster (Katz *et al.*, 2002b) and an appreciation for the high exposure which many of the workers/volunteers endured at the WTC site. Clinicians were to see patients in turn. Where possible, "red" patients were referred to the psychiatrist. Otherwise, the social workers were encouraged to review difficult cases with the on-site psychiatrist, including requesting in-person consultations prior to arriving at dispositions for certain patients. In brief, the psychiatrist was present to provide a high level of oversight on appropriate cases but otherwise was to work alongside of the social workers in seeing patients as they arrived. It was expected that many patients' problems would not be of an acuity requiring a psychiatrist. A senior social worker served as the Clinical Director of the MHSP, providing additional off-site supervision to the social workers. The Medical Director of the MHSP supervised the staff psychiatrists.

Due to the rapidity with which the mental health program was conceived and funded, design and implementation phases of the project were intermingled. While the shortage of office space for the mental health team posed an initial obstacle, it facilitated the development of familiarity and collegiality with the medical team. This ultimately intensified formal and informal collaboration with the medical team in the development of procedures and in a unified approach to the patients. Much collaborative planning centered on maintaining the "flow" of patients through the necessary medical and mental health portions of their visit. The mental health team did not end up being ghettoized, or relegated to a back room. The presence of informal bonds and easy physical access to mental health professionals permitted informal conversation and case consultation, resulting in the development of innovative strategies for intervention with and follow-up on patients. Without question, by being situated within the medical program, the accessibility and credibility of the mental health program was markedly enhanced in the eyes of patients who were not otherwise necessarily seeking mental health services as their primary agenda at the WTC Medical Screening Program.

Individual patient visits took between 2.5 and 4 hours. Nearly all patients have completed the self-report questionnaires, a situation that has been helped by developing Spanish and Polish language translations. After the completion of self-administered mental health questionnaires, patients were all initially interviewed by nursing staff as the first step in their medical evaluation. However, these assessments were a key aspect of many of the successful mental health evaluations and referrals. Nursing staff were often able to identify and support individuals in significant distress and intervene rapidly. For some such patients, immediate evaluation by a member of the mental health screening team diminished their distress and permitted them to complete the rest of the medical screening in greater comfort. There were some extremely distressed patients who, despite their difficulties, were initially reluctant to meet with a member of the mental health staff. In such cases, nursing staff frequently facilitated the mental health evaluation process.

The multidisciplinary approach allowed clinicians to individualize approaches to patients. The valuable different perspectives afforded by multidisciplinary collaboration were well represented in this program's conceptualization and functioning. There were six essential facets of the evaluation process: recruitment/administrative, nursing, medicine/allied health, psychiatric and social work. However, each facet was in turn a composite. "Medicine" involved physicians with specializations in occupational medicine, internal medicine, and pulmonology. "Social work" involved clinical professionals with a range of backgrounds from pure clinician psychotherapists to non-clinical entitlements specialists. "Mental health" encompassed social workers and psychiatrists. Medical staff might initiate discussions about emotions with the patients whereas mental health staff could get involved in addressing the combined medical and mental health follow-up needs of the patients.

While it might seem that mental health professionals or nurses would be the most likely to be able to solicit or facilitate open discussion of mental health issues, for many patients, the key connection was made with another member of the team. Some patients reported that undergoing a structured facts-based interview about the extent and nature of their physical exposures and symptoms helped them to think through and process their experiences, sometimes arriving at an openness toward talking about mental health issues that was new for them. For others, the physician taking the history and physical was the initiator of what may have been the patient's first discussion of mental health issues with a physician. Indeed, the sensitivity with which non-mental health clinicians in the program broached the topic of mental health with their patients often proved to be a crucial linchpin in facilitating their comfort with meeting with mental health staff.

A major goal of the MHSP was to refer patients in need for ongoing mental health care. With the exception of the Division of Traumatic Stress Studies within the Department of Psychiatry, a research division specializing in trauma, limited resources were initially available at the Mount Sinai Medical Center. Thus, under the supervision of the senior social worker, the MHSP clinicians gradually developed a resource manual for 9/11-related mental health services in the New York City metropolitan area. In addition, they developed a working knowledge of other quality mental health services, whether trauma or disaster-related or not, across the region. These included employee assistance programs and providers supported by employee insurance plans. Much of this knowledge was acquired by trial and error. To inform this process, all MHSP clinicians maintained a computerized Referral Log by which they could track information pertinent to patients who needed referrals, including where they were referred; whether they made the initial appointment; and whether the patient was satisfied enough with the treating clinician or facility to plan to continue under their care. Clinicians were expected to try to make initial appointments for patients and to follow-up regarding their adherence with planned treatment within a clinically appropriate time frame. This level of involvement was mandated due to concerns about treatment adherence rates among a population that may not have been mental health treatment seeking in the first place.

Midway through the work of the MHSP, additional funding was obtained by the Department of Psychiatry and the COEM to provide on-site treatment for 9/11-related psychiatric and medical needs of workers/volunteers from the WTC site, respectively. The latter funding also included support for a psychiatrist. Support to the Department of Psychiatry came from two sources, the Substance Abuse and Mental Health Service Administration of the US Government and Project Liberty, the Federal Emergency Management Agency's 9/11 crisis counseling program. The COEM was granted an award for a "Health for Heroes" program from the Bear Sterns Foundation in New York City. Together, these grants laid the basis for a treatment complement to the MHSP, designated the Mental Health Intervention Program (MHIP).

The MHIP included psychiatrists and social workers who were fortuitously located next door to the MHSP, a design anticipated to enhance treatment adherence for those MHSP patients willing to return to Mount Sinai for their mental health care. The same Medical and Clinical Directors jointly administered the MHSP and MHIP, thereby permitting the development of an efficient referral mechanism. In addition, this structure gave MHSP clinicians some opportunity to provide some treatment of their own, while the MHIP clinicians occasionally rotated into the MHSP. Treatment at the MHIP was clinically based.

Although the Robin Hood Foundation made it possible via the MHSP to have on-site mental health staff at the WTC Worker/Volunteer Medical Screening Program, the medical screening program in fact encompassed consortia sites in occupational medicine around the USA. These sites were to serve workers from around the USA who had taken part in the rescue and recovery activities at the WTC site. None of these sites had made provision for mental health staffing of their programs, whereas it was an expectation of the CDC that they collect information about both the medical and psychological condition of their patients. The COEM thus issued to them the MHSP screening questionnaire. Detailed instructions in how to score the survey were disseminated, as was general information about how non-mental health clinicians could manage psychiatric issues arising in the occupational medicine setting. MHSP staff made themselves available by phone and pager as much as possible to address clinical concerns that arose at these sites in the course of their trying to identify and meet the 9/11-related mental health needs of patients without the benefit of on-site mental health professionals. A training CD-ROM that included specific training information in both occupational medicine and trauma/disaster psychiatry was developed at Mount Sinai and disseminated to these sites.

Preliminary findings

At the time of writing, the phone bank responsible for conducting outreach efforts has placed over 65,000 telephone calls and arranged for the screening of nearly 5000 workers/volunteers from the WTC site. In addition to the high rates of persistent upper and lower airway disease found in these patients, nearly 60% of all of these patients have "screened in" on the mental health surveys. This proportion has been remarkably consistent from the outset of the program, suggesting little diminution in the psychological consequences of 9/11 for disaster responders despite the passage of time. A nearly identical percentage of the program attendees have then undergone an evaluation with one of the mental health clinicians – not everyone who screened in agreed to meet with the mental health staff while some who did not screen in were nonetheless referred.

Preliminary data on the first group of participants was reported in the Morbidity and Mortality Weekly Report (MMWR), published by the CDC in September 2004 (Smith *et al.*, 2004). The 1138 program participants included in the analysis were predominantly male (91%) and non-hispanic white (58%), with a median age of 41 years (range: 21–74 years). Non-hispanic blacks and hispanics accounted for 11% and 15% of the population, respectively. Participants had sustained a median of 966 hours (range: 24–4080 hours) of exposure (approximately 4 months of 8-hour workdays) to the WTC site. During July 16–December 31, the majority of participants (51%) met criteria for a clinical mental health evaluation on at least one screening questionnaire. Symptoms of depression, panic, and generalized anxiety were each reported by approximately 6% of participants. Nearly 10% reported at least one item on the CAGE Questionnaire. The Sheehan Disability Scale indicated that the top three emotionally related disabilities were problems with social life (15%), work (14%), and home life (13%). On the PCL, approximately 20% of participants reported symptoms meeting the thresholds for PTSD. The diagnosis of PTSD requires both a characteristic pattern of symptoms and impaired functioning or substantive clinical distress relative to a qualifying trauma. Among program participants, sufficient exposure to qualifying traumatic events was assumed and not assessed; however, despite meeting threshold by symptom count on the PCL, approximately one-third (32%) did not meet the criteria for both pattern of symptoms and impaired functioning or substantive clinical distress. Application of the diagnostic criteria reduces the proportion considered to have PTSD from 20% to 13%. Of the 1138 participants, only 36 (3%) reported accessing mental health services before participating in this program.

Over 20% of all patients (or approximately half of all patients who screen in) appear, upon clinical examination, to need and accept referral for ongoing mental health services, whether through the MHIP or outside of Mount Sinai.

Compilation of the Referral Logs of the clinicians at the 3-month mark revealed an adherence rate of 38% of referred patients made their first scheduled follow-up appointment.

Case examples

Beyond the objective data, the MHSP is a service-oriented program meant to address the emotional needs of the thousands of relief/recovery workers who assisted in the disaster response at Ground Zero. In the stories of these individuals lies the richness and humanity of the program. The following vignettes capture the range of such personal narratives and how the MHSP has become interwoven therein:

(1) J. is a 42-year-old married but separated white male. He had worked as a fireman until 2 years before September 11, 2001 when an injury necessitated his early retirement. He had supported himself on the income from a bar he had inherited from his father. The bar was located several blocks from the WTC. The patient reported a normal childhood, with attainment of all milestones normally. He complained of feeling like something of a "black sheep," having siblings that were more successful than he was. He was a Viet Nam veteran, who had served for 8 months, having been discharged after having been shot twice in the chest. He admitted to having had "occasional disturbing memories and dreams," about Viet Nam, but denied other PTSD symptoms. He admitted to a long history of significant alcohol use dating back to his teenage years, as well as non-medical use of multiple prescription and illicit drugs. He described one brief psychiatric hospitalization secondary to cocaine abuse 20 years previously, from which he had fully recovered.

On the morning of 9/11 J. made his way down to the a firehouse near the WTC, talked his way in, picked up boots, a coat and a bullhorn, and went to work. He reported having spent 29 days on the site and claimed to have worked mostly on "bucket brigade" (for collecting and evacuating debris and remains).

He reported the onset of increased alcohol consumption almost immediately after beginning to volunteer on the site, partly, he said, "as a social community thing" and partly as self-medication. He noted sleep disturbance and increased irritability within "a few months."

By the time he reported for screening, he had become separated from his wife, was not working, and become preoccupied with "day trading," which he later described as "compulsive gambling." On self-administered questionnaires, he reported symptoms consistent with PTSD, major depression and alcoholism. He reported having lost 3 cousins, 3 fellow Viet Nam veterans, more than 31 friends on 9/11. J. reported having sought out mental health treatment at Project Liberty in Rockland County several months previous to the evaluation and having been seen three times, after which he reported being told by his counselor "I think you'll be fine, but if you are not, ... call this hospital."

During his screening visit, he reported feeling a strong antipathy toward talking with any mental health professional. J. said he felt antagonistic, contemptuous, and fearful. He described several experiences that mitigated these feelings: first of all, the patience of the nurse he saw first, including her kindness and willingness to talk with him despite the fact that "I was being difficult." He also described seeing a picture of her grandson eating birthday cake, with a great deal of joie de vivre as "softening me up." He was initially openly contemptuous of the mental health professional with whom he initially met, but decided "I may as well trust you;" because the professional, a psychiatrist, had withstood some testiness from him and remained concerned.

Ultimately, the patient was admitted for a short psychiatric hospitalization for detoxification, stabilization on medications, and the initiation of marital and individual counseling. The patient stayed in the hospital for a week, and thereafter continued with substance abuse treatment, medication, and marital counseling. He did relapse once but re-initiated treatment.

(2) R. is a married South Asian 50-year-old operating engineer who was evaluated in the fall of 2002. He described working at a church near the site of the former WTC on the morning of September 11, 2001. He was outside the church, talking with a supervisor when they heard the explosion of the first plane hitting the building, and saw people and debris falling from the buildings. They assumed a pilot of a small plane had lost control of it and crashed into the building. As they were discussing it, they heard the second plane overhead and saw it crash into the building. They then realized the city was under attack. Their church had a preschool, and their immediate reaction was to move the hundred or so preschool children and their teachers into the basement of the church. After the first building collapsed, they decided to evacuate the children and teachers. After walking the children and teachers southward to safety, R. returned to secure the church. He was there when the second building collapsed. The power went out in the church, and there was no light. When R. made his way out of the church, he encountered several people covered with gray dust, some of whom were bleeding from cuts, none of whom appeared badly injured, all of whom were "terrified, very shook up." He assisted them in walking to safety in the same direction in which he had helped evacuate the children and their teachers.

R. was clinically evaluated as a result of reaching threshold scores on self-administered questionnaires measuring symptoms of PTSD, panic disorder, and generalized anxiety disorder. Despite the preponderance of relatively intense symptomatology, he presented to his clinical evaluation without apparent distress. He acknowledged the debilitating effect of the symptoms he had endorsed, and stated that the irritability, difficulty concentrating, and numbness were the most problematic symptoms. "I feel stressed and on guard always. I have difficulty feeling satisfied or focusing on things. I know I love my family, but it is still hard to be around them. This is the biggest problem." He described a significant decrease in his libido, which exacerbated his worries about the way he was relating to his wife. He also endorsed flashbacks and nightmares, which had lessened from their initial frequency of occurring several times a day to once a week. He described prominent avoidance symptoms. "If something about 9/11 comes on TV, I have to leave." His initial and middle insomnia had not improved. He felt that he had been very seriously affected by his symptoms, but did not seek mental health treatment because "I didn't think it would help. The union did send me a letter offering it, though."

Despite the negative impact of his symptoms on his life, R. felt very positively about his experiences on 9/11 and rather than feeling disempowered or like a victim, he felt vindicated by the choices he had made to stay at the site and help others. "After I secured the church, and came outside and saw the devastation, I was very shook up. I sat down and thought of my family, and thought I would never see them again." I thought, "Well, I am finished now, it's over for me," and I began to cry. Then I stopped. I stood up and said, "Well, if it is over for me … I may as well help as many people as I can." He said he felt very proud of what he had done. "If I had run, as many did, … I don't know how I could live with myself. When I think of it, I feel sad for those who died, but so happy that I was able to help some people."

He agreed with the evaluating clinician's recommendation that he accept treatment to decrease his symptoms, and accepted a prescription antidepressant medication, with a rapid and significant remission of symptoms.

(3) L. is a 47-year-old single Latina mother of three children who worked as an asbestos cleaner at "Ground Zero" from September 11, 2001, until February 2003. She was evaluated in August 2002, after scoring above the threshold for PTSD symptoms on the self-administered questionnaire. An immigrant from a country in Central America, she had grown up with significant adversity; her mother and father were both alcoholics, and her father had committed suicide when she was 3 years of age. She denied any mental health history, and was functioning at a high level at the time of the evaluation, working fulltime, caring for her children and taking courses in night school. She admitted to both feeling isolated and feeling avoidant of social contact. "I have friends but I do not call."

L. had sustained intense exposures to the events of 9/11. In addition to her work as an asbestos cleaner, she also had witnessed the collapse of the second building after exiting a train station nearby. Part of her work as an asbestos cleaner at "Ground Zero" had involved potential risk to her own life. Several days after 9/11, she was cleaning on the 42nd floor of a building near "Ground Zero" which was thought to be unstable. The building was emergently evacuated. She was afraid she was about to lose her life, and cannot remember the details of how she escaped the building. Surprisingly, this episode does not figure in the flashbacks and nightmares from which she continues to suffer daily. Rather, the flashbacks concern the suffering of others. "The flashbacks are about the families who will never find the bodies and never know what happened – I have clear memories of the dogs finding bodies at the site, never from close up, but from far away, as I saw it … that suddenly come into my head, without a reason. It makes me feel more sad than frightened now, although my heart beats fast and my breathing is hard when I remember this." The symptom which most upsets her is her profound sadness in thinking of the families of the victims. She also described weariness and exhaustion from trying to simultaneously present a cheerful exterior to her children, while trying to minimize contact with them because she felt "always sad and distant … numb. The panic, not so much now."

She describes a strong relationship with her family physician, who had been very concerned about her, telling her " when I saw him a few months ago, he knew I was not OK … he gave me medicine. I did not take it because I do not like medicine … I did not tell him this because he would worry." L. did agree with the interviewer that she was suffering and asked if she could return for treatment. However, she did not show up for her first appointment and did not return repeated calls and letters.

Conclusion

The MHSP has provided an unprecedented opportunity to offer mental health evaluation and assistance to a population whose medical and emotional needs previously have been too often overlooked amid the competing priorities of recovery from past disasters. Following in the wake of the tragedy of 9/11, this carefully calibrated program has enabled mental health professionals to offer whatever they can to an astounding number of individuals whose work or volunteerism directly exposed them to the events of 9/11 in New York City. A constellation of factors has made this possible, including the wisdom and generosity of funders; the collegiality of colleagues in occupational medicine; and the willingness of the workers/volunteers themselves to open up their lives and stories for examination. While providing an important opportunity for mental health professionals to help and learn in a way they have never done before, the MHSP's lasting legacy will ideally lie in the impact it has on the thousands of people it has sought to help.

REFERENCES

Ahern, J., Galea, S., Resnick, H. & Kilpatrick, D. (2002). Television images and psychological symptoms after the September 11 terrorist attacks. *Psychiatry*, **65**, 289–300.

Blanchard, E.B., Jones-Alexander, J., Buckley, T.C. & Forneris, C.A. (1996). Psychometric properties of the PTSD Checklist (PCL). *Behavioral Research and Therapeutics*, **34**, 669–673.

Duckworth, D.H. (1986). Psychological problems arising from disaster work. *Stress Medicine*, **2**, 315–323.

Durham, T., McCammon, S. & Allison, E. (1985). The Psychological impact of disaster on rescue personnel. *Annals of Emergency Medicine*, **14**, 664–668.

Ewing, J.A. (1984). Detecting alcoholism: the CAGE questionnaire. *Journal of the American Medical Association*, **252**, 1905–1907.

Fullerton, C.S., McCarroll, J.E., Ursano, R.J., Wright, K.M. & Ingraham, L.H. (1992). Psychological responses of rescue workers: fire fighters and trauma. *American Journal of Orthopsychiatry*, **62**, 371–378.

Galea, S., Ahern, J., Resnick, H., Kilpatrick, D., Bucuvalas, M., Gold, J. & Vlahov, D. (2002a). Psychological sequelae of the September 11 terrorist attacks in New York City. *New England Journal of Medicine*, **346**, 982–987.

Galea, S., Resnick, H., Ahern, J., Gold, J., Bucuvalas, M., Kilpatrick, D., Stuber, J. & Vlahov, D. (2002b). Posttraumatic stress disorder in Manhattan, New York City, after the September 11 terrorist attacks. *Journal of Urban Health*, **79**, 340–353.

Gersons, B. (1989). Patterns of PTSD among police officers following shooting incidents: a two dimensional model and treatment implications. *Journal of Traumatic Stress Studies*, **2**, 247–257.

Goldberg, D.P. & Hillier, V.F. (1979). A scaled version of the General Health Questionnaire. *Psychological Medicine*, **9**, 139–145.

Gregg, W., Medley, I., Fowler-Dixon, R., Curran, P., Loughrey, G., Bell, P., Lee, A. & Harrison, G. (1995). Psychological consequences of the Kegworth air disaster. *British Journal of Psychiatry*, **167**, 812–817.

Herman, D., Felton, C. & Susser, E. (2002). Mental health needs in New York State following the September 11 attacks. *Journal of Urban Health*, **79**, 322–330.

Hodgkinson, P. & Shepard, M. (1994). The impact of disaster support work. *Journal of Traumatic Stress*, **7**, 587–600.

Hytten, K. & Hasle, A. (1989). Fire fighters: a study of stress and coping. *Acta Psychiatrica Scandinavica*, **80**, 50–55.

Katz, C.L. & Nathaniel, R. (2002). Disasters, psychiatry, and psychodynamics. *The Journal of the American Academy of Psychoanalysis*, **30**, 519–529.

Katz, C.L., Gluck, N., Maurizio, A. & Delisi, L.E. (2002a). The medical student experience with disasters and disaster response. *CNS Spectrums*, **7**(8), 604–610.

Katz, C.L., Pellegrino, L., Pandya, A., Ng, Anthony & Delisi, L.E. (2002b). Research on psychiatric outcomes subsequent to disasters: a review of the literature. *Psychiatry Research*, **110**, 201–217.

Kent, G. (1991). Reactions of medical students affected by a major disaster. *Academic Medicine*, **66**, 368–370.

Kugler, S. (2002). Recent surge of remains found at WTC – official WTC death toll near 2,830.

Leon, A.C., Olfson, M., Portera, L., Farber, L. & Sheehan, D.V. (1997). Assessing psychiatric impairment in primary care with the Sheehan Disability Scale. *International Journal of Psychiatry and Medicine*, **27**, 93–105.

McCarroll, J.E., Ursano, R.J. & Fullerton, C.S. (1993). Symptoms of posttraumatic stress disorder following recovery of war dead. *American Journal of Psychiatry*, **150**, 1875–1877.

McFarlane, A.C. (1986). Long-term psychiatric morbidity after a natural disaster. *The Medical Journal of Australia*, **145**, 561–563.

McFarlane, A.C., Clayer, J.R. & Bookless, C.L. (1997). Psychiatric morbidity following a natural disaster: an Australian bushfire. *Social Psychiatry and Psychiatric Epidemiology*, **32**, 261–268.

McQuistion, H.L. & Katz, C.L. (2001). The September 11, 2001 disaster: some lessons learned in mental health preparedness. *Emergency Psychiatry*, **7**, 61–64.

Melnik, T., Adams, M., O'Dowd, K., Mokdad, A., Brown, D., Murphy, W., Giles, W. & Bales, V. (2001). Psychological and emotional effects of the September 11 attacks on the World Trade Center – Connecticut, New Jersey, and New York. *Morbidity and Mortality Weekly Report*, **51**(35), 784–786.

Norris, F., Friedman, M., Watson, P., Byrne, C., Diaz, E. & Kaniasty, K. (2002). 60,000 disaster victims speak: Parts 1 and 2. *Psychiatry*, **65**(3), 207–260.

North, C., Nixon, S.J., Shariat, S., Mallonee, S., McMillen, J.C., Spitznagel, E. & Smith, E. (1999). Psychiatric disorders among survivors of the Oklahoma City bombing. *Journal of the American Medical Association*, **282**, 755–762.

North, C., Tivis, L., McMillen, J.C., Pfefferbaum, B., Spitznagel, E., Cox, J., Nixon, S., Bunch, K. & Smith, E. (2002). Psychiatric disorders in rescue workers after the Oklahoma City bombing. *American Journal of Psychiatry*, **159**, 857–859.

Paton, D. (1989). Disasters and helpers: psychological dynamics and implications for counseling. *Counseling Psychology Quarterly*, **2**, 303–321.

Raphael, B., Singh, B. & Bradbury, L. (1983). Who helps the helpers? The effects of a disaster on the rescue workers. *Omega*, **14**, 9–20.

Rumpf, H., Hapke, U., Meyer, C. & Ulrich, J. (2002). Screening for alcohol use disorders and at-risk drinking in the general population: psychometric performance of these questionnaires. *Alcohol and Alcoholism*, **37**, 261–268.

Schuster, M., Stein, B., Jaycox, L., Collins, R., Marshall, G., Elliott, M., Zhou, A., Kanouse, D., Morrison, J. & Berry, S. (2001). A national survey of stress reactions after the September 11, 2001 terrorist attacks. *New England Journal of Medicine*, **345**.

Smith, R.P., Katz, C.L., Holmes, Herbert, R., Levin, S., *et al.* (2004). Mental Health Status of World Trade Center Rescue and Recovery Workers and Volunteers – New York City, July 2002–August 2004. *Morbidity and Mortality Weekly Report*, **53**, 812–815.

Spitzer, R.L., Kroenke, K., Williams, J.B. & the Patient Health Questionnaire Primary Care Study Group (1999). Validation and utility of a self-report version of PRIME-MD *Journal of the American Medical Association*, **282**, 1737–1744.

Stein, M.B., McQuaid, J.R., Pedrelli, P., Lenox, R. & McCahill, M.E. (2000). Posttraumatic stress disorder in the primary care medical setting. *General Hospital Psychiatry*, **22**, 261–269.

Tomasky, M., *New York Review of Books*, NYREV, Inc. New York, May 1, 2003.

Ursano, R.J., Fullerton, C.S., Vance, K. & Kao, T.C. (1999). Posttraumatic stress disorders and identification in disaster workers. *American Journal of Psychiatry*, **156**, 353–359.

Vlahov, D., Galea, S., Resnick, H., Ahern, J., Boscarino, J.A., Bucuvalas, M., Gold, J. & Kilpatrick, D. (2002). Increased use of cigarettes, alcohol and marijuana among Manhattan, New York residents after the September 11 terrorist attacks. *American Journal of Epidemiology*, **155**, 988–996.

Wright, K.M., Ursano, R.J. & Bartone, P.T. (1990). The shared experience of catastrophe: an expanded classification of the disaster community. *American Journal of Orthopsychiatry*, **60**, 35–42.

22

Child and adolescent trauma treatments and services after September 11: implementing evidence-based practices into complex child services systems

Laura Murray, James Rodriguez, Kimberly Hoagwood and Peter S. Jensen

Introduction

The September 11th attacks were an act of terrorism beyond what the USA had ever experienced, and represented a challenging venue for mental health professionals to respond to. Previous studies of the effects of terrorism on children largely centered on examination of frequent exposure to violence, such as war. The Oklahoma City bombing was one of the first investigations of how terrorism affects children who live in a country relatively free from large-scale acts of violence. The number of lives lost in this act were large and research results indicated far-reaching ripple effects and delayed responses. Interestingly, data from Oklahoma also demonstrated that television exposure appeared to be a significant risk factor in the development of Post-traumatic Stress Disorder (PTSD) symptoms (Pfefferbaum *et al.*, 1999; Pfefferbaum *et al.*, 2001). Although data such as these are useful in guiding the response to September 11th, there remains a grave dearth of information on how to respond to children in the aftermath of terrorism.

The destruction of the World Trade Center (WTC) was massive, and the damage shattering on the heavily populated island of Manhattan and surrounding boroughs. Early screening efforts showed that as many as 75,000 children (10.5%) had symptoms that were predictive of PTSD (Hoven *et al.*, 2002, Board of Education Study). In addition, high percentages of children presented with other psychiatric symptoms predictive of a range of disorders, including depression (8.4%), anxiety (12.3%), agoraphobia (15.0%), separation anxiety (12.3%), and conduct disorder (10.9%). These findings were compatible with previous research on children's responses after acts of terrorism. For instance, it is known that the long-term effects of terrorism most often include high rates of unremitting PTSD in children (Ayalon, 1993; Desivilya *et al.*, 1996; Trappler & Friedman, 1996; Almqvist & Brandell-Forsberg,

1997; Elbedour *et al.*, 1999). Children who do not develop PTSD are considered at-risk and may develop other significant behavioral and developmental difficulties (Ayalon, 1982; Macksoud *et al.*, 1993; March, 1999; Cohen *et al.*, 2000). Studies have demonstrated that children and adolescents can display a wide range of symptomatology in response to a trauma including repetitive play, nightmares, somatic complains, clingy behavior, difficulty concentrating, irritability, aggressive behavior, or regressive behavior (Vogel & Vernberg, 1993; Vernberg & Varela, 2001). In addition, youth who have experienced trauma may display only partial symptomatology of a disorder (Giaconia *et al.*, 1995) or present with comorbid disorders such as depression, anxiety, substance abuse, or behavioral problems (Breslau *et al.*, 1991; Goenjian *et al.*, 1995). This diversity of presentation makes it difficult to recognize, diagnose, and treat trauma in youth populations. Regardless of the presentation, exposure to trauma can significantly interfere with the normal developmental trajectory and have a negative impact on children's overall emotional and behavioral adjustment.

Given our knowledge about the effects of trauma on children and initial data on NYC schoolchildren, one major concern that emerged was the woefully low rates of therapeutic treatment or counseling services available to or used by students. The Board of Education Study data suggests that highly impacted children and youth were not receiving mental health services. For example, two-thirds of children with elevated PTS symptomatology had not sought or received mental health services from a school counselor or outside mental health provider. This led to the development of numerous projects within the New York City (NYC) area, specifically addressing the needs of children and adolescents.

The governmental mental health response to the disaster was substantial. The Federal Emergency Management Agency (FEMA) responded almost immediately with funds to provide funding to state and local agencies as well as private mental health organizations to provide professional mental health counseling services to victims of the disaster (see Felton and colleagues this volume for a more detailed description of the response). These mental health funds were used to finance Project Liberty, a massive public health initiative to address the mental health needs of individuals regardless of age, affected by the WTC disaster. These services were opened to anyone in the general public requesting them and were based on a brief crisis counseling model that depended largely on paraprofessionals and/or mental health professionals with limited training in disaster or trauma counseling. These FEMA funded projects incorporated a service activity log which is a one-page data management tool designed to document each service encounter made in the delivery of Project Liberty services. The log has sections for demographic data, characteristics of the clients relative to the WTC disaster, and documentation of the type of services provided. Characteristics of the clients being seen include event reactions and risk categories. Event reactions document psychological, behavioral, cognitive, and emotional reactions reported by the clients regarding the WTC disaster. Risk categories document various types of exposure to the WTC disaster, such as loss of family members, being related to a disaster worker (e.g., fireman, policeman, emergency medical therapists), or being directly exposed. Figure 22.1 shows the level of Project Liberty service utilization by children and youth from 6 to 17 years of age since October 2001, soon after the disaster. The data indicates an upward trend in the utilization of services by children and youth in the Manhattan, Brooklyn, Queens, and the Bronx, with the highest levels of service utilization in the Bronx. Low and even utilization is shown in Staten Island and Nassau County. The service utilization indicates a fairly common pattern across the NYC area, except for a substantial spike in service utilization in the Bronx in July of 2002. Also, the Bronx maintains very high service utilization over and above the other boroughs, most significantly, more so than Manhattan. Though service utilization has decreased, there continues to be high service utilization 2 years post-WTC disaster.

Data from these service activity logs was also used to create categories of individuals who are heavily impacted and extremely at-risk. Heavily impacted individuals are defined as those experiencing any of the three event reactions considered most distressing and consistent with depressive and PTS symptomatology, including experiencing extreme changes in activity levels, sadness and tearfulness, despair or

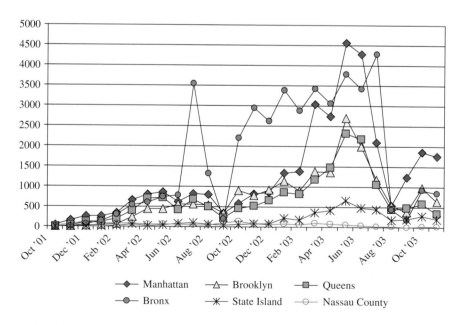

Figure 22.1 Project Liberty Service utilization youth: 6–17 years.

hopelessness, or sleep or eating disturbances since 9/11. Tier-1 children and youth are those considered most at-risk by virtue of their exposure to one or more of certain risk factors such as experiencing the loss of a family member, being injured in the attack, or living in a home damaged by the attack. Table 22.1 shows that the percentage of heavily impacted children and youth remains consistent across the boroughs ranging from 39% to 45%. This data suggests that event reactions tend to be fairly stable regardless of geography. Unlike the rates of children and youth categorized by their own subjective experience of the events, the rates of children who are considered at-risk by specific exposure factors tend to be quite variable by borough. Percentages of children and youth at-risk range from a low of 4% (the Bronx) to a high of 54% (Staten Island). This data highlights the need for ongoing services, along with services that address youth experiencing more severe reactions. Data clearly indicates that a significant proportion of the population affected by a terrorist event, particularly children, suffer long-lasting distress and impairment unlikely to be mitigated by a crisis intervention approach alone (Trappler & Friedman, 1996; Almqvist & Brandell-Forsberg, 1997).

In addition to the funds from FEMA, the Substance Abuse and Mental Health Services Administration (SAMHSA) provided modest funding to provide and evaluate outcomes associated with the delivery of evidence-based treatments (EBTs) for children and youth experiencing significant distress and/or mental illness associated with the WTC disaster. The SAMHSA funds were used to develop the Child and Adolescent Treatment Services Consortium (CATS). CATS represents a ground-breaking effort to treat youth, post-disaster, by implementing evidence-based trauma treatments across all five NY boroughs. This chapter will focus on the efforts of CATS as an example of responding to the needs of children in the aftermath of September 11th.

Table 22.1. Profiles of children and youth ages 6–17 years for the period from September 2003 to April 2004

Borough	Total initial visits	Heavy impact (%)	Tier-1 (%)
Manhattan	3621	37	13
Brooklyn	2683	36	8
Queens	2617	36	10
Bronx	4231	41	4
Staten Island	176	41	20
Nassau County	141	50	27
Totals	13,469	38	9

CATS overview

The CATS project was developed to put into place the highest quality evidence-based practices (EBP) on screening, assessment, treatments, and services, and to develop a rigorous outcome evaluation that would enable expansion of knowledge on optimal practices and examination of service delivery context variables (e.g., organizational and structural factors) that may affect the delivery of evidence-based trauma treatments. The specific goals of CATS include:

(1) to deliver these EBTs to children and adolescents experiencing distress associated with the 9/11 terrorist attack;

(2) to evaluate the effectiveness of the treatments for a diverse population;

(3) to evaluate aspects of the therapeutic process that contribute to improvements in mental health outcomes; and

(4) to evaluate implementation processes associated with delivery of these evidence-based interventions in a variety of settings (e.g., schools, outpatient clinics, community-based clinics).

The CATS consortium is a network of seven community–academic partnerships (see Table 22.2) in the NYC area that offer a range of therapeutic services in various settings, including inpatient and outpatient psychiatry, community-based mental health programs, and school-based health/mental health clinics. The CATS target

Table 22.2. CATS implementation sites

Partnership site	Specific settings
Jewish Board of Family and Children's Services/Mount Sinai Medical Center	University neighborhood High School, Stuyvesant High School, PS 83, Bicultural and Bilingual Middle School, JHS 117, TAG Program, PS 38, PS 108, Manhattan Center High School
New York University Child Study Center/ Bellevue Hospital Center	Pediatric emergency room/Child Psychiatry
North Shore–Long Island Jewish Health System/Catholic Charities of Long Island	Referrals from all school in Districts 25 and 27 (Queens) Nassau County
Lutheran Medical Center/Sunset Park Family Health Center Network	PS 24
New York–Presbyterian Hospital/Alianza Dominicana	PS 4, PS 128, PS 152, and PS 173, IS 52, IS 164, IS 136, and IS 143, George Washington HS
Safe Horizon/North Shore–Long Island Jewish Health System	Borough Assistance Centers
St. Vincent's Catholic Medical Center	Lower Manhattan Schools

population is children or adolescents from ages 5 to 21 years with an identified psychiatric disorder *or* children or adolescents with significant functional impairments who reside in the geographic area included in the Presidential Disaster Declaration issued subsequent to September 11 (the 5 Boroughs of NYC and 10 surrounding counties: Nassau, Suffolk, Westchester, Orange, Rockland, Putnam, Dutchess, Sullivan, Ulster, and Delaware).

Modeling evidence-based service delivery post-disaster

In responding to children and adolescents in the aftermath of September 11, it was important to balance what the scientific literature recommended against the reality of post-disaster work, including the need to move quickly. Specifically, CATS was designed to put the process of moving from efficacy to effectiveness to implementation to the test (see Figure 22.2).

Efficacy studies refer to a class of research that typically includes manualized treatments that have been tested under tightly controlled conditions with random assignment, and that use highly trained therapists, often graduate students who receive intensive supervision. This is considered the "gold standard" within the scientific realm but rarely fits within the context of the real world. Effectiveness studies typically involve the testing of a treatment or service protocol under conditions that more closely approximate practice settings. This requires the use of system employees (e.g., school counselors, private practitioners) as therapists, performance of the intervention under highly naturalistic conditions, and provision of supervision by the investigator team. Effectiveness research also stresses the significance of variables such as practitioners (e.g., attitudes towards adoption of treatment, training programs), service delivery (e.g., community-based, clinic-based), and organizational (e.g., culture and climate wherein treatments are delivered) (Hoagwood *et al.*, 2001; Schoenwald & Hoagwood, 2001). Thus, the most valid questions about the how, why, and with whom psychotherapy works may be best

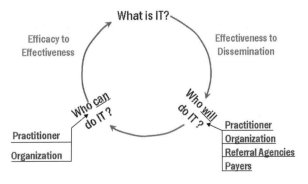

Figure 22.2 Where transportability questions arise (Schoenwald & Hoagwood, 2001).

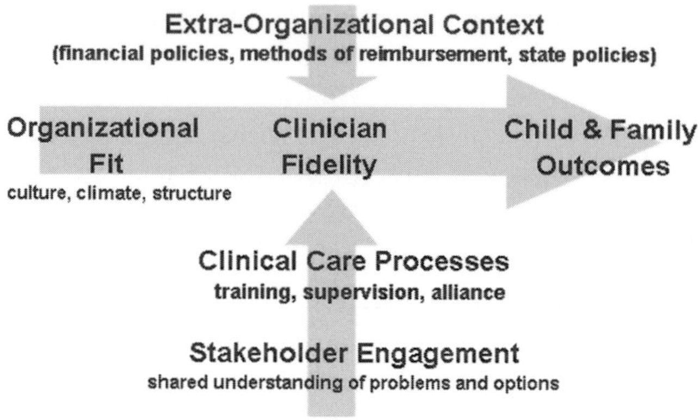

Extra-Organizational Context
(financial policies, methods of reimbursement, state policies)

Organizational   Clinician   Child & Family
Fit   Fidelity   Outcomes
culture, climate, structure

Clinical Care Processes
training, supervision, alliance

Stakeholder Engagement
shared understanding of problems and options

Figure 22.3   Implementation model for effective treatment and service transportability.

evaluated in the real world, rather than with exclusively recruited samples in laboratory conditions.

The implementation model that guides the evaluation of the project – the Implementation Model for EBP – is included in Figure 22.3.

The key elements of this implementation model include its interactive and multidimensional focus: to achieve improvement in outcomes, attention to a broader array of organizational and systems factors are needed. The organizational context issues will be assessed directly. Therapeutic processes including alliance and adherence to the EBP model will be measured and assessed continuously throughout the delivery of therapy. Stakeholder input has been part of the process of this evaluation design throughout, as the major consumer groups not only reviewed the applications that were selected, but continue to function as ongoing advisors on key aspects of the evaluation. In addition, focus groups with stakeholders is part of the evaluation design and will inform the final analysis. These factors may affect therapist behavior, which become mediating variables, influencing changes in alliance with clients or adherence to protocol. The CATS project developed its evaluation plan within these frameworks as its starting point. Working closely with a scientific advisory board and all participating sites, the best assessment measures, treatments, and research design were determined.

Assessment

Based on the most current literature, CATS developed a thorough assessment package assessing for a wide range of symptomatology including post-traumatic symptoms, anxiety, depression, externalizing behaviors, overall functioning, and substance use (see Table 22.3). This battery was designed to examine the diverse presentation of symptoms post-disaster as well as evaluate the effectiveness of trauma

Table 22.3. Child/youth and parents/caretaker assessments in the CATS project

Informants	Domain	Instruments	Length and time/mode of administration	Reported psychometrics
Children and youth	Anxiety	Multidimensional Anxiety Scale for Children (MASC) (March et al., 1997)	39 items 15 minute questionnaire	Sub-factor alphas range from 0.60 − 0.85. Total score alpha = 0.90
	Depression	Children's Depression Inventory (CDI) (Kovacs, 1981) for school-age children	27 items 15 minute questionnaire	High Cronbach's Alpha for clinic youth (alpha = 0.89).
		Beck Depression Inventory (BDI) (Beck et al., 1961) for adolescents	21 items 5–10 minute questionnaire	High internal consistency, especially for student samples (alphas range from 0.82 to 0.92)
	Post-traumatic stress	PTSD Reaction Index – Child Version (Pynoos et al., 1998)	47 items 15 minute questionnaire	Alphas range from 0.67 (Hyperarousal) to 0.92 (Avoidance). Total score alpha = 0.87
		PTSD Reaction Index – Adolescent Version (Pynoos et al., 1998)	49 items 15 minute questionnaire	Alphas range from 0.67 (Hyperarousal) to 0.92 (Avoidance). Total score alpha = 0.87
	Traumatic bereavement	UCLA Trauma Psychiatry Service Grief Inventory *	13 items 5 minute questionnaire	NA
	Exposure to WTC	Developed specifically for this project to assess different types of exposure to WTC	32 items 10 minute questionnaire	NA
	Substance use	Personal Experience Screening Questionnaire (PESQ) (Winters, 1991) for adolescents only	41 items 10–15 minute questionnaire	Alphas >0.90 across community and juvenile offender samples.
	CATS adjustment survey	Developed specifically for this project to assess anger, somatic complaints and services history	31 item 5–10 minute questionnaire	NA

(continued)

Table 22.3. (Continued)

Informants	Domain	Instruments	Length and time/mode of administration	Reported psychometrics
Parents	Therapeutic alliance	Child/Youth Therapeutic Alliance Scale (Youth–TAS) (Doucette & Bickman, 2002)	30 items 5–10 minute questionnaire	Reliability alphas >0.90 for parent, child, and clinician versions.
	Symptom severity	Symptom Screening Index (Doucette & Bickman, 2002)	30 items 5–10 minute questionnaire	Reliability alphas >0.90 for parent, child, and clinician versions. Low correlations with CBCL for youth version.
	Functioning	Behavioral and Emotional Rating Scale (BERS) (Epstein & Sharma, 1998)	24 items 5–10 minute questionnaire	Subscale and total score Alphas range from 0.79 to 0.90. Test-retest >0.84. Correlated with CBCL>.
	Externalizing behavior	Strengths and difficulties questionnaire – Child version (Goodman, 2000)	24 items 5–10 minute questionnaire	Subscale correlations with the Rutter questionnaire range from 0.78 to 0.88.
		Behavior assessment System for children (BASC) (Reynolds, 1999)	32 items 10 minute questionnaire	Good internal consistency (Alphas range from high 70s to low 90s). Median inter-rater reliability = 0.71.
	Symptom severity	Symptom screening index (Doucette & Bickman, 2002)	30 items 5–10 minute questionnaire	Reliability alphas >0.90 for parent, child, and clinician versions. High correlations with CBCL for parent version
	Post-traumatic stress	UCLA PTSD reaction index– Parent/Caregiver version (Pynoos *et al.*, 1998)	48 items 15 minute questionnaire	
	Therapeutic alliance	Therapeutic Alliance Parent/ Caregiver (Doucette & Bickman, 2002)	30 items 5–10 minute questionnaire	Reliability alphas >0.90 for parent, child, and clinician versions

Shaded areas indicate instruments that will be administered at intake. Non-shaded areas are instruments that will be used during treatment.

*Only administered if a child has suffered a loss.

treatment. This complete assessment battery is being collected from children and their parents at intake, 3-, 6-, and 12-month follow-up. CATS is also evaluating aspects of the therapeutic process that contribute to improvements in mental health outcomes, such as therapeutic alliance and engagement procedures. It has been suggested that both of these characteristics are necessary for any treatment to be successful (e.g., Szapocznik et al., 1988; 1997; Cohen & Mannarino, 2000). This data is collected at intake, and tracked approximately every other week during treatment. Finally, CATS is evaluating the implementation processes associated with delivery of these evidence-based interventions in a variety of settings (e.g., schools, outpatient clinics, community-based clinics). Evaluation of variables such as clinician attitude and organizational culture and climate is being collected at intake, and concurrently every other session. This information will help offer direction to future national initiatives to better implement effective EBP on a large scale.

Implementation obstacles: measurement tools

Some obstacles were experienced in the development of measures to be used in the CATS evaluation. First, there is currently no consensus on the best assessments to use with traumatized youth, especially with younger children between 5 and 8 years of age. In assessing children, there is usually significant reliance placed on parents and other significant adults to report symptomatology. Unfortunately, research shows that parents are poor reporters of children's trauma related symptoms (Achenbach 1990; Achenbach et al., 1991). Parents and other adults such as teachers often assume that children are resilient and that their reactions to disasters are transitory and fleeting. Adults may also underestimate a child's problems and not realize to what extent their child is distressed (e.g., Saylor et al., 1997; McNally, 1998; Silverman & La Greca, 2002). By school age, children generally report higher levels of post-disaster distress than parents report for them (Earls et al., 1988; Belter et al., 1991). Thus, recent research has demonstrated the importance of asking children directly about their post-disaster reactions rather than relying exclusively on parent or teacher report, or using such reports as the primary information. The measures selected for use in recent studies reflect an increasing focus on child self-report of PTSD, with less emphasis on parent-completed measures. Another challenge specific to trauma assessment in youth is that there is no one typical presentation seen in children. As stated previously, children can present with a diverse range of symptoms and/or impairments. Finally, one of the major symptoms clusters of post-traumatic responses includes avoidance. This often precludes a child from admitting or endorsing items that suggest any difficulties. Preliminary CATS data does show an influx of children that endorse very few items on the assessment measures, yet are showing significant trauma symptomatology.

Treatment

Despite the understood negative effects of trauma on youth, there is little empirical research on the efficacy of treatments. Manualized cognitive–behavioral therapies (CBT) have received the most empirical support, although many still lack repeated randomized clinical trials. CBT approaches to trauma have been tested most rigorously with sexual abuse populations (e.g., Cohen & Mannarino, 1996; Stauffer & Deblinger, 1996), and have been shown to be effective. Some researchers have examined the effectiveness of various trauma treatment manuals with different populations (e.g., war trauma or single-incident trauma) without randomized controlled trials (e.g., Goenjian *et al.*, 1997; March *et al.*, 1998; Saltzman *et al.*, 2001). Studies such as these report positive outcomes including reductions in anxiety and PTSD symptomatology.

After a literature review, two specific treatment manuals were chosen for the CATS project; one that focuses on children (6–12 years) and one that is directed towards adolescents (12–18 years). *Cognitive–Behavioral Therapy for Traumatic Bereavement in Children Treatment Manual* (Cohen *et al.*, 2001) was developed in response to 9/11, and based on a manual used extensively with sexual abuse populations (e.g., Cohen & Mannarino, 1996; Stauffer & Deblinger, 1996). This CBT intervention was effective in decreasing post-traumatic stress symptoms and externalizing symptoms in sexually abused children (Deblinger *et al.*, 1990). Cohen and Mannarino (1996, 1998) conducted two studies of sexually abused children, comparing CBT to non-directive supportive therapy. Children provided with trauma-focused CBT showed significantly greater improvement in PTSD symptoms, sexually inappropriate behaviors, and internalizing and externalizing symptoms. These differences were sustained at 1-year follow-up (Cohen & Mannarino, 1997). In a study with older children (ages 7–14 years), trauma-focused CBT also resulted in significant improvement in depression and social competence (Cohen & Mannarino, 1998). The *Trauma/Grief-focused Group Psychotherapy Program* (Layne *et al.*, 2002) was developed by members of the University of California at Los Angeles (UCLA) Trauma Psychiatry Service and used in Armenia following the 1988 earthquake (Goenjian *et al.*, 1997), in southern California with adolescents exposed to community violence (Layne *et al.*, 2001), and in post-war Bosnia with severely war-exposed school students (Layne *et al.*, 2001). Results from these studies show significant reductions in post-traumatic and complicated grief symptoms, improvements in grade point averages, reductions in the number of disciplinary actions, and, by teacher report, improvements in classroom attention and concentration (e.g., Saltzman *et al.*, 2001). Both treatment manuals demonstrate effectiveness in decreasing impairment, in addition to symptom reduction.

The training of clinicians and supervisors within all of the CATS sites on these treatment models was a high priority for the project. In January of 2003, approximately 45

CATS staff members were trained in each of the EBTs selected. The manual developers, Cohen *et al.* (2001) and Layne *et al.* (2002), nationally recognized experts in the field of trauma, each trained for two full days on their respective trauma treatment manuals. The training included background information, a review of literature on the efficacy and effectiveness of the specific model, didactic training on the manual, extensive role-plays of the techniques, and question/ answer periods. After the initial training, CATS clinicians were encouraged to pick up a training case. At the end of April, the manual developers returned for another full day "booster training" during which sites were encouraged to present cases and raise their questions or concerns. A second set of full 2-day trainings will be offered in September of 2003 for any new CATS staff, and as a refresher for CATS clinical supervisors. Additionally, all CATS clinical staff will participate in one more full-day "booster training" at the end of the year. For the clinical treatment protocols, the supervisors at each site have received weekly, high-level clinical consultation on the manuals and CATS cases with the treatment developers. The clinical training director on the project consults with each clinician and supervisor on a weekly basis, serves as liaison to the treatment developers, and provides case-specific consultation as needed to ensure that the treatment models are followed with fidelity.

Implementation obstacles: engagement, outreach, recruitment

Given the nature and symptom presentation of typical trauma reactions, it is common for children and their families to avoid dealing with their difficulties. Additionally, research shows that there are numerous barriers to involvement in child mental health interventions. First, the population of NYC is comprised of many families falling under a "triple threat condition" characterized by poverty, single-parent status and stress. It is also well-known that many concrete obstacles, such as time, transportation, child care, and competing priorities, can be a barrier to adequately providing mental health services. Finally, negative attitudes about mental health, or previous negative experiences with mental health institutions also complicate the outreach process. Stigma is a well-documented obstacle within the field of mental health services and presents as a constant challenge to clinicians. Often, it is designated by families as a reason to not seek services and/or not follow through with treatment. The stigma of "needing mental health services" is further complicated by one of the primary symptom categories of trauma – namely avoidance. In addition, research shows 40–60% families may drop out of services before their formal completion (Kazdin *et al.*, 1997) and that children from vulnerable populations are less likely to stay in treatment past the first session (Kazdin, 1993). Mounting evidence suggests that the most vulnerable child populations in terms of seriousness of presenting problems or complexity of social situation are less likely to be retained beyond the first mental health session (Armstrong *et al.*, 1984;

Russell *et al.*, 1987; Wahler & Dumas, 1989; Miller & Prinz; 1990; Bui & Takeuchi, 1992; Cohen & Heselbart, 1993; Kazdin & Mazurick, 1994). Rates of service usage are particularly low for children residing in low-income, urban communities (Griffen *et al.*, 1993).

In order to combat these barriers, CATS sites are also participating in engagement strategy training. This training was developed and delivered by Dr. Mary McKay and includes a systematic process of clarifying the needs of the child and family, addressing the families' concerns (how long, location, whom with), working through perception of services and "helpers" (relationship with teachers, previous therapy experiences, kids and parents), and getting the family help for their concrete obstacles. Research has shown that applying simple but specific engagement intervention strategies can have a significant effect on initial show rates and service participation. In research with low-income urban families seeking mental health treatment, 72% of parents receiving telephone engagement strategies attended initial sessions compared to only 45% of families getting normal intake services (McKay *et al.*, 1999). Other studies have indicated that telephone engagement intervention was associated with 50% decrease in initial show rates and a 24% decrease in premature terminations (Szapocznik, 1988, 1997).

To improve retention of youth and families within the evaluation protocol, the CATS project enlisted the consultation of Dr. McKay to train intake teams at each of the sites. Each engagement team (typically consisting of a project coordinator, clinicians, and intake staff who field calls related to CATS referrals) attended a one-day training in the basics of engagement strategies. Follow-up consultation visits by Dr. McKay and her training team have been conducted at each site to identify site-specific barriers to recruitment and retention, to trouble-shoot these obstacles, and to develop site-specific engagement strategies to deal with them.

Implementing obstacles: training

Implementing evidence-based interventions (e.g., trauma treatment manuals and systematic outreach efforts) has also presented some challenges. In order to effectively transport these models to real-world settings, manuals have to demonstrate a certain amount of flexibility to deal with different populations, diverse symptom presentations, and varying organizational systems. It was quickly realized that there was a need for ongoing consultation from both our treatment and outreach experts to problem-solve independently at different sites. For example, some sites access populations wherein the parents are largely inaccessible. In addition to different client populations, implementation has had to incorporate differences among staff. For instance, some staff were previously trained in CBTs while others were learning this model for the first time. Across all sites, implementation efforts included not only the challenge of who *can* conduct the interventions, but also who *will* conduct them (refer back to Figure 22.2). Altering a system or a method of treatment often meets with resistance so it was important to address this and obtain buy-in from all levels of the organizational structure.

Overview of data collection

Families, children, or youth referred to the CATS provider sites are first provided with an intensive phone engagement intervention (McKay *et al.*, 1996) to identify and overcome obstacles to service delivery. The process of engagement is critical to research recruitment and service utilization. In the course of engagement, the needs of the child are assessed and screening is completed for WTC and exposure and trauma related symptomatology. Following engagement and screening parents and children or adolescents are invited to come in for consent and assessment. After obtaining informed consent from parents and assent of minor children, the CATS assessment battery is completed.

As previously stated, the assessment battery is intended to assess a wide variety of symptoms. Parent reports of functioning and impairments are obtained in addition to child and adolescent report data. Based on inclusion criteria from the baseline assessment, children and youth are offered either: (a) the developmentally appropriate trauma focused CBT or (b) a treatment as usual condition which may include a referral to a more appropriately focused treatment (e.g., substance abuse). Regardless of whether children and youth receive the trauma focused CBT or treatments as usual, follow-up assessments occur at 3-, 6- and 12-months after baseline.

During the course of treatment dimensions of the clinical care process is also being assessed. Therapeutic alliance, therapist adherence to the treatment and symptom severity are obtained throughout the course of treatment for children and youth receiving the trauma-focused CBT. Data is obtained by a combination of child and youth, parent and clinician report data. Clinician data is also being collected throughout the project to assess a number of key dimensions to service delivery and implementation of EBTs. These include the therapeutic techniques and strategies that clinicians feel most comfortable with, their attitudes about EBTs, supervision, training and consultation, and their perceptions of the organizational culture and climates in which they work.

Data report

One vital challenge for CATS was obtaining the necessary Institutional Review Board (IRB) approvals from the State Office of Mental Health. Once all CATS providers obtained IRB approval, recruitment began. A total of 445 children and adolescents were assessed as eligible for CATS treatment. This section describes the measures of WTC exposure and PTSD symptomatology used, and some overall profiles of the current sample of subjects. Based on current completed assessments ($n = 445$), 190 (42.7%) were male, 255 (57.3%) were female, and the mean age of participants was 11.54. All of these participants were CATS eligible, based on the inclusion criteria of endorsement of at least one item on the WTC Exposure Survey and a score of 25 or greater on the UCLA Reaction Index. Table 22.4 shows the demographic characteristics of the sample and indicate that the children and youth receiving trauma treatments are predominantly male, young, Hispanic and from low-income families.

Measures

- *WTC exposure.*   The WTC Exposure Survey is a 24 item inventory of experiences related to the WTC attack. Seventeen items cover a wide variety of ways that children or youth could have been exposed, including:
  (1) direct exposure (e.g., being physically hurt),
  (2) interpersonal exposure (e.g., knowing someone else who was at the WTC),
  (3) loss (e.g., knowing someone who died as a result of the WTC),

Table 22.4. Socio-demographics for CATS children and adolescents

Total N	445
Gender	Female = 255 (57.3%)
	Male = 190 (42.7%)
Ethnicity	White = 46 (10.3%)
	Black = 66 (14.8%)
	Hispanic = 272 (61.1%)
	Other = 36 (8.1%)
	Missing = 25 (5.6%)
Age	Average = 11.54
	Range = 5–19
Income	$7,000 = 96 (21.6%)
	$7,000–$14,999 = 106 (23.8%)
	$15,000–$29,999 = 60 (13.5%)
	$30,000–$44,999 = 34 (7.6%)
	$45,000–$59,999 = 39 (8.8%)
	>$60,000 = 51 (11.5%)
	Missing = 59 (13.2%)

(4) secondary adversity (e.g., being displaced),

(5) media exposure (e.g., learning about the attack from TV, radio or the worldwide web). In addition, seven items assess symptomatology and functioning relative to 9/11 (e.g., Since 9/11, do you find it harder to do your school work?).

- PTSD.   The UCLA PTSD Reaction Index for Diagnostic and Statistical Manual of Mental Disorders (DSM)-IV (Pynoos et al., 1998) is designed to assess for exposure to a variety of traumatic events and PTSD symptoms in children and adolescents. The PTSD Index comes in three version: a Child version (7–12), an Adolescent version (13 and over), and a Parent version developed to complement the child's report. It is a self-report inventory keyed to DSM-IV Criteria: 13 questions assess exposure to a variety of traumatic events, 7 questions assess Criterion A aspects of the traumatic event, 5 questions assess the child or youth's subjective experience of the event during or just after the traumatic event, and 22 items (20 for children) assess for the frequency of self-reported DSM-IV PTSD symptoms. The instrument has good validity with alpha coefficients ranging from 0.67 (Hyperarousal) to 0.92 (Avoidance), and a total score alpha coefficient of 0.87.

Table 22.5 shows the average UCLA Reaction Index scores and subscale scores for the sample of children and youth receiving CATS treatment. The total severity mean score of 36.61 approached the established cut-off score of 38 that has high reported sensitivity and specificity of detecting PTSD (Steinberg et al., 2004). The data suggests that CATS sites recruited subjects who generally had moderately high levels of trauma-related symptomatology but included numerous subjects with levels of symptomatology beyond the range of probable PTSD diagnosis. The trend was for adolescents to score higher than young children. In order to meet DSM-IV Criteria for traumatic exposure only one A1 and one A2 item needs to be endorsed. Subjects recruited for CATS averaged three A1 and A2 criteria. Youth in CATS also reported exposure to multiple traumatic events with an average of three events endorsed on the traumatic events inventory of the reaction index. Youth in CATS were also exposed to the WTC disaster in a variety of ways.

Table 22.5. Reaction index scores: Baseline severity and sub-criteria scores

Criteria	n	Mean	SD
Re-experiencing	445	11.46	4.07
Avoidance	445	13.33	5.08
Hyper-arousal	445	11.81	3.43
Total Severity	445	36.61	9.36

Table 22.6. WTC Exposures

	n	Mean	SD	Range*
CATS	433	3.02	1.52	0–7
Comparison	142	2.67	1.32	0–7

*Includes a category for youths who report changes in behavior and functioning since 9/11.

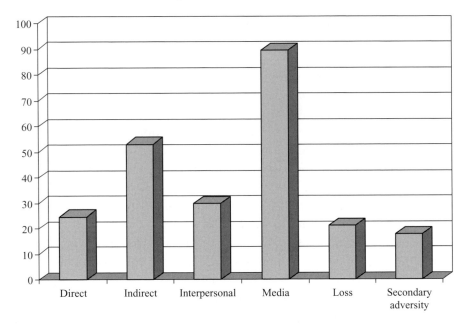

Figure 22.4 WTC exposure.

WTC exposure ranged from 0 to 7 discrete types of exposure to the disaster on the WTC exposure inventory. Table 22.6 shows the average number of WTC exposures experienced by children and youth receiving the CATS interventions and a non-equivalent comparison group of youth with lower levels of traumatic symptomatology. The average numbers of WTC exposures was 3.02 for children receiving the CATS intervention which did not differ significantly from the comparison group sample of children and youth.

Figure 22.4 shows the various types of WTC exposure for those children and youth in the CATS treatment intervention group. Among the CATS subjects, the most common type of exposure was media (e.g., "After the attack, how much time did you spend learning about the attack from TV?"), followed by witnessing aspects of events of the WTC indirectly (e.g., "Did you smell the smoke from the WTC buildings at any time after the September 11th attack?).

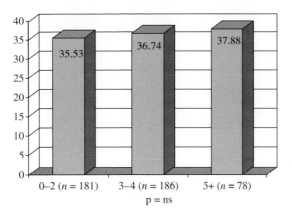

Figure 22.5   Reaction Index severity × WTC exposure.

The criteria for inclusion into the CATS treatment protocol were set broadly so as to allow the project to capture and provide services to youth experiencing trauma reactions for a variety of traumatic exposures. Youth for whom WTC was the index event for their trauma symptomatology could be recruited along with youth for whom a traumatizing event other than WTC was the source of their traumatic reactions. This was done in the belief that children without direct WTC exposure or for whom the WTC disaster was not the index event for their distress could nonetheless experience trauma symptomatology associated with the WTC. Thus, an important question to answer in this project is the degree of association between WTC exposure and PTSD symptomatology. Figure 22.5 shows the PTSD Reaction Index scores for children and youth grouped by low, medium, and high exposure to the WTC disaster as determined by number of types of exposures. As this figure indicates, PTSD Reaction Index severity scores increase relative to a greater number of WTC exposure events among children and youth.

Conclusions

The city-wide mental health response to September 11th has been robust and has touched the lives of at least 900,000 persons (Felton *et al.*, this volume). However, epidemiological studies clearly indicate that a significant proportion of the population affected by a terrorist event, particularly children, suffer long-lasting distress and impairment unlikely to be mitigated by a crisis intervention approach alone (Trappler & Friedman, 1996; Almqvist & Brandell-Forsberg, 1997). Although many initial programs were developed, logs collected in connection with those demonstrated an ongoing need for services. CATS was designed to address the ongoing and severe effects this act of terrorism had on children and adolescents. The design of CATS was crafted to test the move from efficacy to effectiveness to implementation within a post-disaster venue. This is a vital step for disaster work which requires rapid mobilization of a large number of mental health providers. Many of these clinicians may have only minimal training in trauma-specific treatment, and even fewer will have training in EBTs. Therefore, developing a method of moving scientific-based treatments to the front lines in an effective and efficient manner is much needed. The CATS project followed an implementation model that accounts for the multidimensional nature of implementation work. In addition to putting into place the highest quality EBP on screening, assessment, treatments, and services, CATS also developed a rigorous outcome evaluation. The evaluation will render invaluable information about the effectiveness of youth trauma treatments and specialized outreach efforts with a diverse population, performed by community providers. Additionally, the evaluation provides the opportunity to scientifically evaluate the implementation method, examining the many surrounding variables (e.g., organizational and structural factors) that may affect service delivery.

Although the initial data report is very preliminary and represents only a small number of youth, it raises important points. First, data supports the need for a project such as CATS. Youth in many areas of NYC are considered "at-risk" for many reasons such as poverty, single-parent homes, or living in a violent neighborhood. Due to these factors, it is likely that 9/11 exacerbated the post-trauma symptomatology that these youth present with due to another trauma. In fact, the population that CATS is serving has experienced multiple traumas. Second, the data show that there are children and adolescents who are experiencing distress due to trauma. This means that there are children who cannot sleep, are having difficulty in school, may be acting out, or are very anxious and fearful. Years of research clearly states that difficulties in childhood can significantly disrupt a child's developmental trajectory and create a vicious cycle of future and more severe impairments. Repeatedly, the take-home message is: Intervene early. The best place to start is by helping our youth. In the aftermath of disasters, it is vital that we provide youth with the highest quality of care in order to mitigate future mental health problems. These services cannot be provided by experts alone, but rather by the providers within the communities themselves.

Since September 11th, a major objective of the United States was to become better prepared for disasters. This preparedness needs to be mobile to fit with the nature of traumatic disasters. Thus, one of the most important lessons that can be learned in responding to children and adolescents in the aftermath of September 11th is the process of implementing quality treatments for our youth. In the future, this will serve to direct the response procedures and, hopefully, provide more efficient and effective help.

REFERENCES

Achenbach, T.M. (1990). "Comorbidity" in child and adolescent psychiatry: categorical and quantitative perspectives. *Journal of Child & Adolescent Psychopharmacology*, **1**(4) 271–278.

Achenbach, T.M., Howell, C.T., Quay, H.C. & Conners, C.K. (1991). National survey of problems and competencies among four- to sixteen-year-olds: parents' reports for normative and clinical samples. *Monographs of the Society for Research in Child Development*, **56**(3), Serial No. 255.

Almqvist, K. & Brandell-Forsberg, M. (1997). Refugee children in Sweden: post-traumatic stress disorder in Iranian preschool children exposed to organized violence. *Child Abuse and Neglect*, **21**, 351–366.

Armstrong, H., Ishiki, D., Heiman, J., Mundt, J. & Womack, W. (1984). Service utilization by Black and White clientele in an urban community mental health center: revised assessment of an old problem. *Community Mental Health Journal*, **20**, 269–280.

Ayalon, O. (1982). Children as hostages. *Practitioner*, **226**, 1773–1781.

Ayalon, O. (1993). Posttraumatic stress recovery of terrorist survivors. In *International Handbook of Traumatic Stress Syndromes*, eds. J. Wilson & B. Raphael. New York: Plenum Press, pp. 855–866.

Beck, A.T., Ward, C.H., Mendelson, M., Mock, J. & Erbaugh, J. (1961). An inventory for measuring depression. *Archives of General Psychiatry*, **4**, 561–571.

Belter, R.W., Dunn, S.E. & Jeney, P. (1991). The psychological impact of Hurricane Hugo on children: a needs assessment. *Advances in Behaviour Research and Therapy*, **13**(3), 155–161.

Breslau, N., Davis, G.C., Andreski, P. & Peterson, E. (1991). Traumatic events and posttraumatic stress disorder in an urban population of young adults. *Archives of General Psychiatry*, **48**, 216–222.

Bui, C. & Takeuchi, D. (1992). Ethnic minority adolescents and the use of community mental health care services. *American Journal of Community Psychology*, **20**, 403–417.

Cohen P. & Heselbart, C. (1993). Demographic factors in the use of children's mental health service. *American Journal of Public Health*, **83**, 49–52.

Cohen, J.A. & Mannarino, A.P. (1996). A treatment outcome study for sexually abused preschool children: initial findings. *Journal of the American Academy of Child and Adolescent Psychiatry*, **35**, 42–50.

Cohen, J.A. & Mannarino, A.P. (1997). A treatment study of sexually abused preschool children: outcome during one year follow-up. *Journal of the American Academy of Child and Adolescent Psychiatry*, **36**(9), 1228–1235.

Cohen, J.A. & Mannarino, A.P. (1998). Interventions for sexually abused children: initial treatment findings. *Child Maltreatment*, **3**, 53–62.

Cohen, J.A. & Mannarino, A.P. (2000). Predictors of treatment outcome in sexually abused children. *Child Abuse and Neglect*, **24**(7), 983–994.

Cohen, J.A., Berliner, L. & March, J.S. (2000). Treatment of children and adolescents. In *Effective Treatments for PTSD: Practice Guidelines from the International Society for Traumatic Stress Studies*, eds. E.B. Foa & T.M. Keane. New York: Guilford Press, pp. 106–138.

Cohen, J.A., Mannarino, A.P. & Deblinger, E. (2001). *Child and Parent Trauma-focused Cognitive Behavioral Therapy Treatment Manual.*

Deblinger, E., McLeer, S.V. & Henry, D. (1990). Cognitive behavioral treatment for sexually abused children suffering post-traumatic stress: preliminary findings. *Journal of the American Academy of Child and Adolescent Psychiatry*, **29**(5), 747–752.

Desivilya, H., Gaal, R. & Ayalon, O. (1996). Long-term effects of trauma in adolescence: comparison between survivors of a terrorist attack and control counter-parts. *Anxiety, Stress, and Coping*, **9**, 1135–1150.

Doucette, A. & Bickman, L. (2002). *Therapeutic Alliance Scale: Therapist-TAS, V5.0.* Memphis,TN: Center for Mental Health Policy at Vanderbilt University.

Earls, F., Smith, E., Reich, W. & Jung, K.G. (1988). Investigating psychopathological consequences of a disaster in children: a pilot study incorporating a structured diagnostic interview. *Journal of American Academy of Child and Adolescent Psychiatry*, **27**, 90–95.

Elbedour, S., Baker, A., Shalhoub-Kevorkian, N., Irwin, M. & Belmaker, R. (1999). Psychological responses in family members after the Hebron massacre. *Depression and Anxiety*, **9**, 27–31.

Epstein, M.H. & Sharma, J.M. (1998). *Behavioral and Emotional Rating Scale: A Strength-Based Approach to Assessment.* Austin, TX.: PRO-ED.

Giaconia, R.M., Reinherz, H.Z., Silverman, A.B., Pakiz, B., Frost, A.K. & Cohen, E. (1995). Traumas and posttraumatic stress disorder in a community population of older adolescents. *Journal of the American Academy of Child and Adolescent Psychiatry*, **34**, 1369–1380.

Goenjian, A.K., Pynoos, R.S., Steinberg, A.M., Najarian, L.M., Asarnow, J.R., Karayan, I., Ghurabi, M. & Fairbanks, L.A. (1995). Psychiatric comorbidity in children after the 1988 earthquake in Armenia. *Journal of American Academy of Child and Adolescent Psychiatry*, **34**, 1174–1184.

Goenjian, A.K., Karayan, J., Pynoos, R.S., Minassian, D., Najarian, L.M., Steinberg, A.M. & Fairbanks, L.A. (1997). Outcome of psychotherapy among early adolescents after trauma. *American Journal of Psychiatry*, **154**, 536–542.

Goodman, R., Ford, T., Simmons, H., Gatward, R. & Meltzer, H. (2000). Using the strengths and difficulties questionnaire (SDQ) to screen for child psychiatric disorders in a community sample. *British Journal of Psychiatry*, **177**, 534–539.

Griffen, J., Cicchetti, D. & Leaf, P. (1993). Characteristics of youths identified from a psychiatric case register as first-time users of services. *Hospital and Community Psychiatry*, **44**, 62–65.

Hoagwood, K., Burns, B.J., Kiser, L., Ringeisen, H. & Schoenwald, S.K. (2001). Evidence-based practice in child and adolescent mental health services. *Psychiatric Services*, **52**(9), 1179–1189.

Hoven, C.W., Duarte, C.S., Lucas, C.P., Mandell, D.J., Cohen, M., Rosen, C., Wu, P., Musa, G.J. & Gregorian, N. (2002). Effects of the World Trade Center Attack on NYC Public School Students – Initial report to the New York City Board of Education. Columbia University Mailman School of Public health-New York State Psychiatric Institute and Applied Research and Consulting, LLC. New York City.

Kazdin, A.E. (1993). Adolescent mental health: prevention and treatment programs. *American Psychologist*, **48**(2), 127–140.

Kazdin, A. & Mazurick, J. (1994). Dropping out of child psychotherapy: distinguishing early and late dropouts over the course of treatment. *Journal of Consulting and Clinical Psychology*, **62**, 1069–1074.

Kazdin, A.E., Holland, L. & Crowley, M. (1997). Family experience of barriers to treatment and premature termination from child therapy. *Journal of Consulting and Clinical Psychology*, **65**, 453–463.

Kovacs, M. (1981). *Rating scales to assess depression in school-aged children.* Acta *Paedopsychiatrica*, **46**, 305–315.

Layne, C.M., Pynoos, R.S., Saltzman, W.R., Arslanagic, B., Black, M., Savjak, N., Popovic, T., Durakovic, E., Music, M., Campara, N., Djapo, N. & Houston, R. (2001). Trauma/grief focused group psychotherapy school-based postwar intervention with traumatized Bosnian adolescents. *Group Dynamics: Theory, Research and Practice*, **5**(4), 227–290.

Layne, C.M., Pynoos, R.S. & Cardenas, J. (2001). Wounded adolescence: School-based group psychotherapy for adolescents who sustained or witnessed violent injury. In *School Violence: Assessment, Management, Prevention*, eds. Shafii, M. & Shafii, S.L., pp. 163–186.

Layne, C.M., Saltzman, W.R. & Pynoos, R.S. (2002). *Trauma/Grief-Focused Group Psychotherapy Program.* Provo, Utah: Brigham Young University.

Macksoud, M., Dyregrov, A. & Raundalen, M. (1993). Traumatic war experiences and their effects on children. In *International Handbook of Traumatic Stress Syndromes*, eds. B.Raphael & J.P. Wilson. New York: Plenum Press, pp. 625–633.

March, J. (1999). Assessment of pediatric posttraumatic stress disorder. In *Posttraumatic Stress Disorder: A Comprehensive Text*, eds. P.A. Saigh & J.D. Bremner. Needham Heights, MA: Allyn & Bacon, pp. 199–218.

March, J.S., Parker, J.D., Sullivan, K., Stallings, P. & Conners, C.K. (1997). The Multidimensional Anxiety Scale for Children (MASC): factor structure, reliability, and validity. *Journal of the American Academy of Child and Adolescent Psychiatry*, **36**, 554–565.

March, J.S., Amaya-Jackson, L., Murray, M.C. & Schulte, A. (1998). Cognitive behavioral psychotherapy for children and adolescents with posttraumatic stress disorder after a single incident stressor. *Journal of the American Academy of Child and Adolescent Psychiatry*, **73**, 585–593.

McKay, M., Nudelman, R., McCadam, K. & Gonzales, J. (1996). Evaluating a social work engagement approach to involving inner-city children and their families in mental health care. *Research on Social Work Practice*, **6**(4), 462–472.

McKay, M., Quintana, E., Kim, L., Gonzales, J. & Adil, J.A. (1999). Multiple family groups: an alternative for reducing disruptive behavioral difficulties of urban children. *Research on Social Work Practice*, **9**, 414–428.

McNally, R.J. (1998). Measures of children's reactions to stressful life events. In *Children of Trauma: Stressful Life Events and Their Effect on Children*, ed. T. W. Miller. Madison, CT: International Universities Press, pp. 29–42.

Miller, G. & Prinz, R. (1990). Enhancement of social learning family intervention for childhood conduct disorder. *Psychological Bulletin*, **108**, 291–811.

Pfefferbaum, B., Nixon, S.J., Krug, R.S., Tivis, R.D., Moore, V.L., Brown, J.M., Pynoos, R.S., Foy, D. & Gurwitch, R.H. (1999). Clinical needs assessment of middle and high school students following the 1995 Oklahoma City Bombing. *American Journal of Psychiatry*, **156**, 1069–1074.

Pfefferbaum, B., Nixon, S., Tivis, R., Doughty, D., Pynoos, R., Gurwitch, R.H. & Foy, D. (2001). Television exposure in children after a terrorist incident. *Psychiatry*, **64**, 202–211.

Pynoos, R.S., Rodriguez, N., Steinberg, A.M., Stuber, M. & Frederick, C. (1998). UCLA PTSD Reaction Index for DSM IV (Revision 1), UCLA Trauma Psychiatry Program, Los Angeles, CA.

Reynolds, C.R. & Kamphaus, R.W. (1998). *Behavioral Assessment System for Children.* American Guidance Services, INC. Circle Pines, MN.

Russell, M., Lang, M. & Brett, B. (1987) Reducing dropout rates through improved intake procedures. *Social Casework*, **68**, 421–425.

Saltzman, W.R., Pynoos, R.S., Layne, C.M., Steinberg, A. & Aisenberg, E. (2001). Trauma/grief focused intervention for adolescents exposed to community violence: results from a school-based screening and group treatment protocol. *Group Dynamics: Theory, Research and Practice*, **5**, 291–303.

Saylor, C.F., Belter, R. & Stokes, S. (1997). Children and families coping with disaster. In *Handbook of Children's Coping*, eds. S.A. Wolchik & I.N. Sandler. New York: Plenum Press, pp. 361–383.

Schoenwald, S. & Hoagwood, K. (2001). Effectiveness, transportability, and dissemination of interventions: what matters when? *Psychiatric Services*, **52**(9), 1090–1097.

Silverman, W.K. & La Greca, A.M. (2002). Children experiencing disasters: definitions, reactions, and predictors of outcomes. In *Helping Children Cope with Disasters and Terrorism*, eds. A.M. La Greca & W.K. Silverman. Washington, DC: American Psychological Association, pp. 11–33.

Stauffer, L.B. & Deblinger, E. (1996). Cognitive behavioral groups for nonoffending mothers and their young sexually abused children: a preliminary treatment outcome study. *Child Maltreatment*, **1**, 65–76.

Steinbery, A.M., Brymer, M.J., Decker, K.B. & Pynoos, R.S. (2004). The University of California at Los Angeles Post-truamatic stress disorder Reaction index. *Curr. Psychiatry Rep*, **6**(2), 96–100.

Szapocznik, J., Perez-Vidal, A., Brickman, A.L., Foote, F.H., Santisteban, D.A., Hervis, O.E. & Kurtines, W.H. (1988). Engaging adolescent drug abusers and their families into treatment: a strategic structural systems approach. *Journal of Consulting and Clinical Psychology*, **56**, 552–557.

Szapocznik, J., Kurtines, W., Santisteban, D.A., Pantin, H., Scopetta, M., Mancilla, Y., Aisenberg, S., McIntosh, S., Perez-Vidal, A. & Coatsworth, J.D. (1997). The evolution of structural ecosystemic theory for working with Latino families. In *Psychological Interventions and Research with Latino Populations*, eds. J. Garcia & M.C. Zea. Boston: Allyn & Bacon.

Trappler, B. & Friedman, S. (1996). Posttraumatic stress disorder in survivors of the Brooklyn Bridge shooting. *American Journal of Psychiatry*, **153**, 705–707.

Vernberg, E.M. & Varela, R.E. (2001). Posttraumatic stress disorder: a developmental perspective. In *The Developmental Psychopathology of Anxiety*, eds. M.W. Vasey & M.R. Dadds. New York: Oxford University Press, pp. 386–406.

Vogel, J.M. & Vernberg, E.M. (1993). Children's psychological responses to disaster. *Journal of Clinical Child Psychology*, **22**, 464–484.

Wahler, R. & Dumas, J. (1989). Attentional problems in dysfunctional mother-child interactions: an interbehavior model. *Psychological Bulletin*, **105**, 116–130.

Winters, K.C. (1991). *Personal Experience Screening Questionnaire Manual*. Los Angeles: Western Psychological Services.

23

Relationally and developmentally focused interventions with young children and their caregivers in the wake of terrorism and other violent experiences

Daniel S. Schechter and Susan W. Coates

Introduction

The terrorist attacks of September 11, 2001, made mental health professionals keenly aware of the need for relationally and developmentally focused interventions for traumatized young children and their families with greater urgency than ever before. Healthcare providers, educators, the media, and politicians were barraged by questions about parents who were concerned about the effects of this very public political violence on their young children, whether or not they were directly affected by the attacks.

Those young children who were directly affected by the attacks in New York or who witnessed the crashing of the two passenger planes into the World Trade Center (WTC) and the toppling of the Twin Towers were many in number: over 3000 children lost a parent, thousands of children attending schools and day-care centers near Ground Zero directly witnessed the attacks. Additionally, untold millions of children around the world watched the attacks repeatedly on TV. Children worldwide were reported to suffer from nightmares following the events of 9/11, and for weeks had difficulty concentrating in school (Hoven *et al.*, 2003).

Historical overview of understanding trauma in a relational context

One of the most important observations which has informed our current relational view of child traumatic stress came from the study by Anna Freud and Dorothy Burlingham (1943). They noted the following during the London Blitz of World War II: "The war acquires comparatively little significance for children so long as it only threatens their lives, disturbs their material comfort, or cuts their food rations. It becomes enormously significant the moment it breaks up family life and uproots the first emotional attachments of the child within the family group. London children, therefore, were on the whole much less upset by bombing than by evacuation to the country as a protection from it." (Freud & Burlingham, 1943).

It is hard to recall now how startling the foregoing observation was at the time. Indeed, it was so novel that its full import could not be integrated into the field. What Freud and Burlingham had discovered went beyond the awful facts of the London blitz: it was the child's separation from the mother that was traumatic.

Two years after Freud's and Burlingham's observations, David Levy (1945) observed that the impact of hospitalization on children separated from their parents was so devastating that it resembled combat neurosis. This was at a time when public health policy still dictated that the child be dropped off by their parents, who had no further role to play in their treatment. In the USA, Levy was the first person to recognize both the parent's role in moderating the child's experience of trauma and to study its impact systematically. Moreover, he was the first person to develop short-term desensitization techniques for treating the traumatized child (Levy, 1939).

The full realization that a prolonged separation from the mother was inherently traumatic for a child had to wait for the work of Bowlby in England. Bowlby and Robertson's deeply moving film entitled *A Two-Year-Old Goes to Hospital* helped improve the fate of hospitalized children all over the Western world (Bowlby *et al.*, 1952; Bretherton, 1995, p. 50).

This first wave of clinical research on trauma in children established the importance of the mother's physical presence or absence in emotionally and behaviorally moderating the impact of trauma on the child. The second wave begun in 1975 focused on the mother's role in emotionally and behaviorally mediating the transmission of trauma from one generation to the next. Fraiberg, Adelson, and Shapiro's famous paper, "Ghosts in the Nursery," remains a classic contribution to the understanding of trauma as it occurs intergenerationally within a relationship (Fraiberg *et al.*, 1975).

A third wave of trauma research in children began about 10 years ago with a focus on the developmental and psychobiological factors that contributed to individual differences in intensity and pervasiveness of posttraumatic stress disorder (PTSD) and that make it move or less likely for trauma to be transmitted across generations (Schechter *et al.*, 2004; Scheeringa *et al.*, 2004; Yehuda *et al.*, 2005).

Manifestations of PTSD in children

Children were once thought to experience only transient stress in the wake of traumatic events (Gurwitch *et al.*, 1998). Advances in the nosology of psychiatric disorders led to confirmation of clinical observations that PTSD also occurred in children with a similar duration of symptoms and course as found in adults. The classic triad of PTSD symptoms: reexperiencing, numbing/avoidance and hyperarousal, occur in young children just as in adults (Scheeringa & Zeanah, 1995;

Schechter & Tosyali, 2001; Coates *et al.*, 2003; Schechter *et al.*, 2003; Scheeringa *et al.*, 2003). The youngest case of PTSD reported to date is of a 3-month old described by Gaensbauer (1982) that noted "hypervigilance, exaggerated startle, as well as various forms of dysregulation (i.e., distress to the point of vomiting), irritability, and withdrawal in generalized form as well as in response to specific states." As in adults the range of severity is relative both to the type, duration and frequency of traumatic exposure. Several large studies (Breslau *et al.*, 1999; Yehuda *et al.*, 2001) have demonstrated that traumatic stress in childhood and, even more so, PTSD in childhood are risk factors for PTSD in adulthood. Chronic life-stress has been shown to interact with genetic vulnerability so as to contribute to the development of adult depressive disorders as well (Caspi *et al.*, 2003).

While systematic long-term studies capable of clarifying the significance of the different symptomatic presentations in children and adults are lacking, descriptive studies have been influential in the development of diagnostic criteria for young children (Scheeringa *et al.*, 2003). Increased separation anxiety, exacerbated specific fears (e.g., of the dark, car noises, or other separation-associated and/or trauma-associated features), regressive behavior (e.g., increased need for pacifier or bottle), somatoform complaints, and analogues of adult PTSD symptoms such as those clustering in the general categories of reexperiencing the event, avoidance, and arousal have all been noted for children 1-year old and older (Gurwitch *et al.*, 1998; see Table 23.1.).

Among infants and toddlers, increased irritability and disruptive behavior, exacerbation of startle responses and other manifestations of disregulation of affect, sleep, and feeding, along with, transient loss of milestones (such as bowel/bladder control or speech and language competence), and disorganization of attachment behavior have been reported (Scheeringa & Zeanah, 1995).

Reexperiencing the traumatic event(s) for preschoolers and school-age children may involve repetitive play in which themes of the traumatic event are expressed (Terr, 1987; Gaensbauer, 1995a). Automatic-appearing, rigidly repetitive activity that lacks the sense of fun or creative spontaneity and lacks symbolic abstraction inherent in normative play are hallmarks of posttraumatic play (Terr, 1987; Coates & Moore, 1997). Such compulsive forms of play or reenactment of the trauma may, depending on the child and his/her developmental capacities, concretely resemble the traumatic event and/or may be displaced in content, yet contain the affective tone, rhythmicity, or other more abstract features of the event(s) or associated details.

Posttraumatic reenactment play can lead to disorganization and obfuscation of meaning-making in the absence of a caregiver who is able to tolerate trauma-associated effects and who is able to reflect on the play's potential meanings. The traumatized caregiver's distress around posttraumatic play may lead to initiation of a referral.

Pathognomonic of PTSD is avoidance of trauma-associated memory traces and/or associated affects in the afflicted individual. In the case of young children, avoidance

Table 23.1. PTSD symptoms in young children

Reexperiencing
Posttraumatic play or non-play activity/gestures
Recurrent recollections of the traumatic event
Repeated nightmares
Distress at exposure to reminders of the trauma
Features of a flashback

Avoidance
A numbing of responsiveness in a child
Increased social withdrawal
Restricted range of affect
Avoidance of exploration
Avoidance of trauma-associated individuals, places, or associated stimuli
Avoidance of separation
Fear of something bad happening again

Hyperarousal
Night terrors
Difficulty going to sleep
Repeated night waking
Significant attentional difficulties
Hypervigilance
Exaggerated startle response
Increased irritability or disorganization of play

Other symptoms
Fears not present before the traumatic event
Aggression or agitation not present before the traumatic event
Sexualized behavior not present before the traumatic event
Temporary loss of previously acquired developmental skills
Decrease or constriction in play

---

behaviors will depend on developmental capacities such as that of gross motor abilities (Schechter & Tosyali, 2001). For an infant up to the age of 12 months, subtle aversion of gaze, or turning of the head, have been observed in reaction to traumatic triggers and frightening caregivers (Beebe & Lachmann, 1994). Marked anxiety reactions to strange situations in the 6–12-month period may be noted, with more active attempts to get away from traumatic reminders as the child learns to walk and run.

Avoidance behaviors in young children may take on extremes of generalization perhaps due to developmentally based limitations in cognitive capacities. Preschool children who experienced windows being blown out in their day-care center while in the adjacent building to that which was destroyed in the Oklahoma City bombing would go out of their way to avoid walking near windows in their subsequent schools for some time (Gurwitch *et al.*, 1998). While social withdrawal, numbing and other dissociative or internalizing symptoms have been observed in very young children, it is thought that children below the age of 4 years may more noticeably exhibit separation anxious clinging (i.e., avoidance of separation), and externalizing behaviors such as tantrums (Scheeringa & Zeanah, 1995; Thomas, J.M. & Guskin, K.A. 2001; Gaensbauer, 1995b; Gurwitch *et al.*, 1998).

Several authors (Levy, 1939; Gaensbauer, 1995a; Scheeringa *et al.*, 2003) have noted that observational assessment and treatment of children with PTSD most often requires a structuring of play so as to permit gradual therapeutic exposure within a supportive, controlled setting to the traumatic events that the child will otherwise avoid due to the PTSD during free-play. The degree to which a child avoids traumatic themes during free-play coupled with a detailed history of their peritraumatic dissociative response and degree of associated dysregulation may be the most important factors in assessing the severity of the condition (Pfefferbaum *et al.*, 2001; Scheeringa *et al.*, 2003).

In terms of the hyperarousal symptom-cluster of PTSD, traumatized children often have difficulties paying attention, and have increased hypervigilance and startle responses, in addition to difficulty falling or staying asleep. Their disturbances of arousal may well take the form of increased irritability and temper tantrums over minor events.

Contemporary models of PTSD in young children: relational PTSD

Trauma researchers that have studied young children have found that the *Diagnostic and Statistical Manual for Mental Disorders, Fourth Edition* (DSM-IV) definition for PTSD as involving actual or threatened death or serious injury, or a threat to the physical integrity of self or other has considerable limitations if one considers the very young child's perspective (American Psychiatric Association, 1994). A preschooler who hears his traumatized mother's shrieks after hearing news of her partner's death may fear separation from his/her mother as she becomes emotionally unavailable due to her grief, even when there is no tangible threat to self or other. Analogous to "shared psychotic disorder" or folie a deux, shared or "relational" PTSD has been proposed as an alternative construct for thinking about trauma in young children who are so thoroughly dependent on their primary caretakers for their feelings of safety (Scheeringa & Zeanah, 2001). In their model of relational PTSD, Scheeringa and Zeanah consider various ways the care-giving relationship mediates and moderates childhood PTSD symptomatology.

They hypothesized the following models. In the Moderating Effect Model, the child is traumatized directly by an event, but the "mother's relationship with the child (including her ability to read his/her cues and respond effectively to his/her needs) affects" or moderates the degree to which the child will become symptomatic. The mother's behavior either amplifies or helps contain the child's traumatic reaction. In the Vicarious Traumatization Model or what one could also call the Mediation Model the mother has experienced a trauma and the child has not. In this situation the impact of the trauma on the mother impinges on her relationship with her child altering her responsiveness and thus mediates the child's development of symptoms. In the Compound Effect Model the mother and the child are both traumatized and each exacerbates the symptomatology of the other (Scheeringa & Zeanah, 2001).

In an effort to improve the nosology for infants, toddlers, and preschool-age children, Zero to Three: National Center for Infants, Toddlers and Families (1994) has developed the following diagnostic criteria for traumatic stress disorder. While the diagnoses in the Zero to Three classification system are currently under reconsideration for revision (Emde *et al.*, 2004), the following criteria for Traumatic Stress Disorder remains more developmentally specific for infants and young children than the DSM-IV. For a review of developmentally specific symptom criteria (see Table 23.1).

The traumatic event (i.e., DSM-IV PTSD "Criterion A") must also be considered from a developmental perspective: for example, falling off a bed will not be traumatic for a healthy teenager; whereas for an infant or handicapped young child, such an experience may seem life threatening. For any age, however, there are events like being a passenger in a crashing car, being attacked by an animal, or being raped that are likely to be traumatic. Having any of these experiences more than once, is more likely to result in sustained PTSD than being traumatized once (Breslau *et al.*, 1999). Terr had put forth a simple distinction between isolated traumatic exposures or "Type I" traumas such as a traffic accident or natural disaster, and chronic repeated exposures or "Type II" traumas, the latter associated with child maltreatment or chronic illness (Terr, 1987). A recent review of studies of single-event traumas has supported the need for further research of this distinction (Wiedenmayer, in press).

Relationship between parental and family functioning and child outcome

In an ongoing study involving assessment of parents and children (via parental report and direct observation) who were ages birth to 5 years on September 11, 2001, and living near and/or within viewing distance of the Twin Towers, preliminary analyses have shown that as many as 96% of preschool age children experienced one PTSD symptom and 35% met DSM-IV for PTSD and diagnostic classification (DC): 0–3 criteria for Traumatic Stress Disorder (Klein *et al.*, 2003). While parental data from this study are still pending, in several prior studies where the family and child were both evaluated, a significant relationship has been found between "poorer maternal or family functioning" and worse child outcomes (Cornely & Bromet, 1986; Laor *et al.*, 1997; Yehuda *et al.*, 2001). Koplewicz and colleagues found that following the first WTC bombing in 1993, parents who had greater severity of PTSD had children with more PTSD and disaster-related fears than children of parents with less or absent PTSD (Koplewicz *et al.*, 2002).

In a study by Laor *et al.* (1997) of the impact of scud missile attacks on Israeli children, where effects were studied separately for ages of 3, 4, and 5 years, a strong relationship between family functioning and child outcomes was found in children ages of 3 and 4 years but not at age of 5 years. Thus younger children appeared to be more affected by the state of their parents.

Scheeringa and Zeanah (1995) attempted to determine which kinds of trauma best predicted severity of PTSD in children under age of 4 years and found only one factor, "trauma that occurred when there were threats to the child's caregivers."

In a separate study, Pynoos and colleagues found that after a traumatic event mothers who tried to avoid being confronted with reminders of the trauma and who were in numb emotional states that restricted their capacity for closeness, were unable to help their children process the experience of trauma (Pynoos *et al.*, 1995). These studies show that mother's presence is not enough. For mothers and other caregivers to serve as a "protective shield" to their child in the face of trauma they need to be emotionally present as well (Lieberman *et al.*, 2005).

The importance of the mother's emotional accessibility to her child after the experience of a traumatic event was dramatically underscored by the impressive findings from a survey conducted at the New York Academy of Medicine after 9/11 (Stuber *et al.*, 2002). They found that children whose parents did not know how their child responded after 9/11 were 11.1 times more likely to have behavior problems at ages of 6–11 years and 4.0 times more likely at ages of 12–17 years. Parents who cannot keep their child's experience in mind after a traumatic event have more behaviorally disturbed children and this effect is nearly 3 times greater in younger children than in adolescence (Stuber *et al.*, 2002). This important study brought into stark relief the fact that in the wake of a trauma caused by an external catastrophic event, a child's response, especially the young child's response depends on the nature of their parent's relatedness to them after the trauma.

Guidelines for working with children after acute disaster

Based both on the research findings reviewed above and our clinical observations at the Kids Corner of the Family Disaster Relief Center at Pier 94 in the months following 9/11 (Schechter *et al.*, 2001; Coates *et al.*, 2003), and consonant with those developed by Robert Pynoos and colleagues as psychological first aid after traumatic events (Pynoos & Nader, 1988). We devised a set of guidelines for clinicians working with young children and their caregivers in the wake of disasters similar to that of the attacks of 9/11. Before describing those guidelines, we would like to place the work that informed our recommendations in a context of the space and time in which our work occurred.

Psychological mooring: clinical work at the Kids Corner at Pier 94

While as clinicians we are able to hold in mind the minimum requirements or "frame" that our work with patients requires, the setting for our interventions within this frame following a disaster is in many ways as unpredictable as the disaster itself. The setting for our work after the events of 9/11 was Pier 94, which remains a vast aluminum-sided hangar-like structure on the Hudson River on the West side of Manhattan. The Family Assistance Center at this site (which was needed because of limitations of space at the original site at the Lexington Avenue Armory) was set up by the New York City Mayor's Office to expedite provision of services to families who had lost a family member, jobs or housing as a consequence of the events of 9/11. Dozens of temporary booths served as the workstations for representatives of numerous federal state and city agencies as well as the Red Cross Disaster Relief Services and private agencies.

Mental health workers stood available to those presenting for these services as those often grieving individuals completed their grim business of providing forensic evidence for identifying remains and completed forms related to entitlements. There were translators and chaplains, cafeterias and lounges, and as has been mentioned the central informal memorial of the "Walk of Bears" or teddy bears sent with comforting messages from the children of Oklahoma City – a city that had also experienced a massive terrorist attack.

This setting facilitated a positive transference to the whole Family Assistance Center. Even though clinicians took shifts and, therefore, did not work in an ongoing way with any one individual or family, there was a sense that the next clinician on duty would continue the therapeutic work of those who had gone before them in a collective effort, and often with the help of an informal verbal sign-out at the changing of the shift. This context was particularly important because we observed that it influenced the trust and confidence with which families approached us at the "Kids' Corner."

"Kids Corner" at Pier 94 was founded within the first weeks after the events of 9/11 by Desmond Heath and several other child psychiatrists under the auspices of Disaster Psychiatry Outreach (DPO) that provided mental health services on site at Pier 94 as well as at Ground Zero. Kids Corner was located centrally at Pier 94 and was easily visible so that families could leave their children and easily check back in-between visits to various Family Assistance agencies. Parents also came to seek advice, talk about their predicaments around parenting while grieving, and to be with their children in a place that offered respite from the stress of the fulltime demands of children who were already distressed.

Kids Corner was the size of a small classroom, and had an adjoining carpeted family consultation area with comfortable sofas. It had a block-building and toy area, equipped especially with toy fire engines, police cars, and rescue vehicles to facilitate children's expression of trauma-related feelings, thoughts, and memories with an emphasis on repair and restoration. Clinicians monitored the quantity and quality of the toys so as to ensure that the environment would not be over stimulating. There was a crafts and painting table, which also promoted older children's working and talking together. It was especially meaningful and consoling for children to see their signed artwork mounted all around the walls of the Kids Corner, knowing that others similarly affected would see them. Snacks and children's books for a range of ages were always available.

Clinical contact with children was often no more than a single visit but the child's stay might be for 2–3 hours duration because of the freedom for parents to drop off children while using the Family Assistance Center services. Some children were brought back over consecutive days or for several weekends in a row. Follow-up by the volunteer clinicians at the Kids Corner was often no more than a sometimes successful attempt to reach the family by phone to see how they were faring.

While families seen by mental health professionals at Pier 94 were offered mental health referrals through an outside agency for subsequent treatment if needed or requested – and were given that agency's phone number, the mental health agencies within the Family Assistance Center did not permit clinicians volunteering at Pier 94 (including at the Kids Corner) to continue working with families outside of their volunteer role in that setting. This prohibition was intended to maintain, as much as would be possible, equal opportunity for mental health treatment to all-comers if they were motivated to pursue it.

One could argue that at least for some affected families, ongoing intervention with the therapists who engaged, assessed, and worked with them closest to the time of the disaster might provide a stronger overall treatment experience. On the other hand, the degree of organization required to fairly distribute case-loads with attention to geographical convenience, triaged urgency, fees, therapist availability, treatment of individual vs. multiple family members, competing bids to treat the same families by different therapists, perceived rejection by families if not accepted by an on-site clinician, etc., would likely have exceeded the already overextended administrative capacity of the on-site mental health agencies at the Family Assistance Center. Further thought might be applied to these issues in preparation for future disaster work.

That being said, within the constraints in which we did work, we tried to be available and responsive to children and caregivers without being intrusive, guided by the hope that the presence of understanding adults would provide a safe space where, as a first step, children's overwhelming feelings of pain, shock, loss, anguish, anger and fear could be expressed in a containing atmosphere to thoughtful, available staff. Often we and other clinicians were providing ordinary human acknowledgment and recognition for very difficult experiences, and often with few words. Interventions on Pier 94 were of course often spontaneous though clinically and developmentally informed responses to the moment. After reflecting on what we had been doing at Kids Corner, we formulated the following clinical guidelines.

Guidelines for working with caregivers and young children after disaster strikes

These guidelines are useful as a first response to traumatic events. These guidelines are reproduced here with minor revisions (Coates *et al.*, 2003, p. 35–38).

Guidelines for children

The following guidelines apply to children:

Listen

Some children spontaneously want to talk about what they or their parents and other family members are going through with a sensitive listener from outside the family. Here acknowledging the reality of trauma and loss is implicit in simply listening.

Clarify

Children who wish to talk can be helped to make sense of their feelings and to find words to name emotions. Finding words promotes containment, the development of symbolic representation and the capacity for self-regulation. Clarification of affects and events helps toward the restoration of a coherent narrative. It is important to follow the child's lead, to avoid probing exploration, responding only to what the child spontaneously introduced, in order to support containment of overwhelming feelings.

Facilitate

It is important to facilitate children's symbolic expression in play and in art projects by being supportively interested and available to observe or join play or to talk with them while they use art and crafts materials.

Support the capacity to imagine repair

Robert Pynoos (2001, personal communication) described key moments in the crisis intervention after the bombing in Oklahoma City when he helped children to imagine reparative possibilities. When a session ends with a child who has relived the trauma by telling about it or representing it in play or drawings, this may retraumatize the child, unless the session ends by helping the child imagine some way of repairing or healing the damage. It is important to help younger children to think about how their family and community will take care of them.

Support attachment bonds

In cases of loss a parent and for children who are ready to do this one can provide support for the child's identification with or internalization of the attachment to the lost family member by actively facilitating the child's need to remember and talk about their lost loved one.

Guidelines for parents

The following guidelines apply to parents:

Contextualize the parents' reactions

Contextualize the parents' reactions, by helping them to understand that their fears, anxieties and flashbacks are understandable reactions in the context of an extremely traumatic event.

Support the child's surviving attachment relationships

Support the child's surviving attachment relationships by helping parents to understand the child's feelings and by facilitating communication between them. Help parents recognize how much their children understand about the events all around them. Help parents, family members and friends to be more accessible by answering children's questions directly and honestly without providing more information than children need.

Clarify

Help parents to make sense of their children's perplexing and disturbing expressions and behavior. For example, help parents understand and make meaning of the feelings being expressed through children's repetitive dramatic play, traumatized drawings, dreams or nightmares that parents often have difficulty making sense of and find upsetting. Some parents are frightened or became angry with their children for their increased clinginess, tantrums, and aggression. Parents sometimes are afraid that these reactions are signs of lasting damage and future pathology. It can be difficult for parents to see these reactions as expectable responses to a situation of great insecurity. Parents' anxiety or anger in turn makes the child more frightened of losing them, and so more demanding or aggressive. It is important to help parents answer both the direct and indirect questions that children raise while protecting children from exposure to adult conversations. In this way, the adult's reflective function can be reengaged so that they can begin to understand their child's experience.

It is also important to encourage families to try to return to ordinary daily life and customary routines as soon as possible.

In highly public traumatic events such as occurred on September 11, 2001 we encourage parents to turn off the TV and not expose children to endless repetitions of images of the traumatic event, as supported by research findings following the Oklahoma City bombing (Pfefferbaum *et al.*, 2003).

Case illustrations

In the two case vignettes that follow: each preschool-age child was suffering from nightmares after the 9/11 attack. Maria was seen soon after 9/11 in the Kids Corner at Pier 94 and Abbey was seen 5 months later in a private practice setting.

The case of Maria

Maria had settled at our play-table with some crayons and paper while her father, Mr. P, waited to speak to a benefits counselor at an adjacent booth. He had lost his job as a cook because of the WTC attack. Maria a 3-year old Hondurian girl was left in the Kids Corner by her father while he explored available benefits after he lost his job as a cook at the WTC. Her mother was at home with her younger brother. Since 9/11 Maria had had nightmares and slept in the bed with her parents because she was too frightened to sleep by herself.

Maria began to scrawl intently in bright overlapping reds, yellows, and black. She readily told us that she was drawing the buildings that "fell and burned," adding that she had seen this on TV. Maria said her father had escaped from the WTC, as the buildings collapsed. She said her father's lungs had been filled with smoke so that he could hardly breathe. While her father was running from the WTC to get home, burning pieces of the building fell on him and burned his arms. She added loudly, "He has marks from the fire on his arms!"

Mr. P. came over to check on his daughter while waiting for some forms to be processed. Dr. Schechter asked father about the events his daughter had described. He was surprised. "I was not anywhere near the WTC," he said and added incredulously, "She told you I was there?" Mr. P. had indeed been employed as a cook at Windows on the World (hence the old burn scars from splattered grease on his arms), but he had exchanged the breakfast shift with a colleague the week prior to the attack. On the morning of 9/11, while his daughter had stayed home with her mother, Mr. P. went out to do some errands in Manhattan, but he was nowhere near the WTC.

Dr. Schechter enquired of the father as to how he was doing. The father, a young man, slight and soft-spoken, wanted to downplay any troubles of his own. It took two or three further gentle probes for him to reveal that he was profoundly distressed by the loss of his co-workers at Windows on the World. He struggled with feeling responsible for having switched shifts and also because he had found work at the WTC for some of his friends. His agonizing survivor-guilt took the form of feeling obliged to vividly imagine how his friends had died: the fire, the smoke, and what they had felt. He also had nightmares from which he awakened several times a night, leaving him to ruminate over their deaths by himself, as he thought, in the dark.

After father spoke, Dr. Schechter exclaimed, "So your daughter is drawing your dreams!" Indeed, Mr. P. appeared shocked that his daughter's drawings and fantasies (perhaps also her nightmares) so closely resembled his own nightmares; he had not discussed them with her. He went on: "Every night when I close my eyes, I see all my co-workers trapped in the smoke and burning up, and there's nothing I can do to save them." His eyes welled with tears as he said: "I guess I'm lucky. It could have been me there. But I miss all of my friends. I am sorry for the guy who took my place. I pray for his family."

This conversation that began in Spanish between Dr. Schechter and Maria's father, continued in English and was carried on within earshot of Maria, sometimes intentionally including her.

After this, Maria turned to drawing a picture of her school, a low rectangle with many windows and doors. She emphasized that there were as many doors as windows, and counted them. A co-therapist from the Columbia University Parent–Infant Program faculty Elsa First remarked that perhaps she meant that there were many openings, many ways to get out of the school so that it would be safe if there were a fire. When asked if she meant her preschool was safe, Maria replied, "Yes."

In sum, both Mr. P. and his daughter were confused about what each other had in mind. Mr. P. did not expect that his daughter would assume that he was a hero-survivor of the WTC as she had presented him to Dr. Schechter. He was so preoccupied with his job-loss and mourning of his co-workers, that it had not occurred to him that his daughter would not understand what his actual experience was on 9/11 unless he explained it to her – and in so doing, contain her anxiety. Maria, on the other hand, resonated with his guilty fantasies but lacked connection with her father's actual experience on 9/11.

Neither parent had been available to Maria on this day that created such insecurity for her. She had not been helped to understand what was going on in the mind of the other. Father and daughter were each attempting to make sense of the trauma in relative isolation. This resulted in their regulating their negative affect individually at the expense of mutual regulation and understanding, which they began to recover through interaction with the two Parent–Infant Program co-therapists.

Dr. Schechter gave the family a referral network phone number and we asked father for his permission to make a follow-up call. He agreed. As promised, Dr. Schechter called the following week. Dad answered and spoke of how his daughter and infant son were busy at play. Since our meeting, he reported, the little girl's symptoms had subsided though she still needed to sleep in her parents' bed. He also said that his own symptoms were better, he was receiving benefits, and he was hopeful that he might get another job. He had not felt the need to bring his daughter back to the Kids' Corner and had no plans to seek further evaluation or treatment for himself, wife, or children at the time of the follow-up. Further follow-up was unfortunately not feasible for many of the families seen at the Family Disaster Relief Center due to lack of manpower, funding, and foresight. A preplanned systematic follow-up mechanism to crisis intervention in the aftermath of future disasters would be desirable from the authors' point of view.

The case of Abbey

Ms. A and her 2-year-4-month-old daughter were at Ground Zero on 9/11 when the first plane attacked the Twin Towers. Since 9/11 Abbey was having difficulty sleeping including having frequent night awakenings and night terrors, and recurrent recollections of the events of 9/11. Ms. A did not get help at first when Abbey was 2-year-4-month old but waited for 5 months after the terrorist attack to get help for herself and for her daughter who was then 2-year-9-month old. Since 9/11 she and Abbey had been suffering from symptoms of PTSD. Ms. A was suffering from flashbacks triggered by the sound of planes, fire engines and police cars as well as exposure to any images on TV of the Twin Towers burning or falling.

On 9/11 Ms. A was in the plaza between the Twin Towers pushing Abbey in her green stroller to her preschool classroom on the first floor of Tower 1 when the first plane hit. The mother immediately panicked, grabbed Abbey and swung her up in the air while she was still strapped into her stroller. Both were exposed to what she said was an indescribably hideous loud sound followed by debris falling everywhere. Ms. A thought "it was the end of the world," that "we had been hit by a nuclear bomb." She ran to safety in a nearby building. After a massively traumatic day she returned home in the evening. Ms. A's experience of terror was so great that she would not open the door to her home for over a week even to get her mail at the front door. Several weeks later after things begin to calm down a little bit she found a new school for Abbey that to Ms. A's relief Abbey took to immediately. She adjusted without apparent anxiety and went off eagerly to join the other children. Despite continuing to have severe PTSD after 6 weeks, Ms. A went back to work.

At the time of her first appointment with Dr. Coates, Ms. A reported that she was so traumatized on 9/11 that she had no memory of Abbey's reactions that day. Nor had she noticed whether Abbey's play has been affected since her experience on that day. Some time after 9/11 Ms. A bought a new blue stroller to replace the green one that she had abandoned at Ground Zero. Whenever Abbey saw the new stroller she got very upset and said over and over again, "green stroller, rocks falling, terrible, terrible, terrible."

During Dr. Coates' first session with Ms. A, a plane flew overhead and was then followed by the sound of a fire engine. Ms. A startled, turned white, looked frightened and began to weep. She said that this was typical of the constant flashbacks that she had had since 9/11 and that they were triggered whenever she heard a plane overhead. Hearing a fire engine afterwards only made things worse. She said she had tried to put the whole experience behind her but had been unable to.

Dr. Coates met Abbey in a second session. Abbey was an adorable spunky little girl who easily made herself at home, exploring the play materials and talking to Dr. Coates' readily. In about the middle of the session her mother left the room to take a cell-phone call. After a minute or so Abbey went to the waiting room to check on her mother and finding her there came right back to the playroom to resume her activities. She discovered some small blocks about 3 inches long by about ¼ of an inch thick. She began to build two towers with the blocks, building them higher and higher until they fell down". She closely monitored Dr. Coates' face and must have registered her uneasiness about what she was doing because she was worried that Abbey might retraumatize herself. Abbey looked startled when the blocks fell down and looked at Dr. Coates to check her reaction. Dr. Coates said with a little smile on her face, "boom they fell down". In a pause in which she seemed to not know what to do Dr. Coates said, "shall we build them up again?" With great eagerness Abbey began to build them up again and Dr. Coates asked her if she would like to push them over or if she might like her to push them over for her. She became animated and asked Dr. Coates to do it. Dr. Coates built another tower, narrating as she did it asking her whether she wanted Dr. Coates to knock it over. She nodded her head enthusiastically. Then Abbey began to build them by herself over and over again knocking them down in a very animated way. Dr. Coates picked up a few blocks and gently dropped them on the floor from a height of about 2 inches. She had in mind the fact that on 9/11 Abbey had experienced debris falling from the sky some of it landing on her head. Abbey immediately imitated Dr. Coates and began picking the blocks up higher and higher into the air dropping them becoming more animated with squeals of "glee."

Dr. Coates looked over at her mother and saw tears in her eyes. She said, "I can't believe that she can remember all this." Dr. Coates asked her how it made her feel? She said, "I can't bear the sound of the noise of the blocks clinking, it makes me think of the crash." Dr. Coates explained to her that this was her daughter's way of working through and mastering her own experience of trauma just the way she was trying to do by talking to her own therapist. Dr. Coates said, "Abbey needs your help," and invited her to come join in and actively help Abbey build towers and knock them down. Dr. Coates asked her to let Abbey take the initiative and let her be the director of her own story: let her decide who would build up the blocks and who will knock them down. She played with her daughter building and knocking down towers until the session was over. At the end of the session Ms. A asked Dr. Coates where she could buy these small blocks in my neighborhood so that she could take them home to help her daughter.

As they were leaving Dr. Coates' office, Ms. A heard some very soft footsteps in the apartment above and had a startle reaction to it. Abbey then became very anxious about the sound. Ms. A noted that she needed to try to keep her startle reactions in check because she noticed that Abbey was beginning to have anxious reactions in response to her own startle reactions.

Both Maria's and Abbey's reaction to 9/11 illustrates the way that young children's reactions to trauma is closely linked to their parents own reactions. In the case of Abbey and her mother each traumatized the other, thereby illustrating Scheeringa and Zeanah's relational PTSD model of "compound effect." Given how unbearable Ms. A found it to witness Abbey reenacting her 9/11 experience in Dr. Coates' office, it seems likely that she avoided and shut out Abbey's ongoing experience since 9/11 much in the same way that Maria's father had done in his grief and while experiencing intense survival guilt. During this time of great threat and disorganization neither Maria's father nor Abbey's mother were able to reflect upon their child's experience and keep their child's experience in mind. Once they were in the presence of a third who could help them contain their own experience each parent became able to take in their child's experience.

Discussion

One might ask how the interventions described would lead to such impressive results so rapidly. As has been described elsewhere by the authors (Coates *et al.*, 2003; Schechter, 2003a), the very young child's unmodulated outpouring of negative affect has the power to render accessible in the parent, her own repressed, dissociated, or otherwise posttraumatically avoided feeling states. The maternal drive to repair the wounds of past traumas, to experience the mutual regard with her present child, and to protect future generations from experiencing the traumas that she has known are all positive motivators for change within the safety of a safe and reflective therapeutic relationship. Rapid change within the parent–child relationship in the wake of trauma can be stimulated by therapeutic techniques that directly address posttraumatic avoidance and dissociation.

Clinician guided video feedback (Schechter *et al.*, 2003; Schechter, 2003a), a tool frequently used with caregivers in parent–infant psychotherapy, as well as guided exposure through play with young children (Gaensbauer, 1995a; Scheeringa *et al.*, 2003) are examples of such techniques that can induce rapid integration of avoided and dissociated negative affects and trauma-associated cognitions. More established PTSD-directed psychotherapies such as cognitive behavioral techniques for adults involving prolonged exposure, are only now being explored in relation to effects on parenting behavior (Schechter, 2003b) as well as in modified form for young school-age children (Scheeringa, 2003, personal communication).

The cases discussed above also clearly illustrate the principle supported by research findings (Egeland *et al.*, 1988; Scheeringa & Zeanah, 1995; Lyons-Ruth & Block, 1996; Schechter *et al.*, in press), that trauma and its sequelae must be considered particularly for young children and caregivers in a relational and developmental context. Attachment when secure and organized can be a source of resilience in the face of trauma or, when insecure and disorganized, can be a vehicle for the exacerbation of trauma's effects as well as transmission of those effects across generations. When the primary caregiver is herself a source of trauma, alarm, or massive failure of protection over the course of the relationship, disturbances of the attachment relationship itself begin to overlap with PTSD (Hinshaw-Fuselier *et al.*, 1999).

Relationally and developmentally informed community interventions post-9/11

Implications for intervention therefore involve both treatment of trauma-associated psychopathology as well as bolstering and stimulating recruitment of social affiliation and reflectiveness within socially supportive relationships (Schechter, 2003a).

Several community-based projects in Israel and, more recently, in the USA have attempted and/or are attempting to integrate knowledge of attachment theory, child development, trauma studies, community systems, and public policy.

Lahad has developed a "Community Stress Prevention Center" (CSPC) in Kiryat Shmona, Israel (Lahad, 2003) that involves mental health professionals working with preschool teachers in small groups to enable these teachers to work with parents and young children. The primary goals of the CSPC are to: (1) build capacity for resilience within the preschool community; (2) impart general disaster preparedness (i.e., learning how to use and tolerate gas masks); and (3) create a holding environment for preschool staff and the children it serves.

Lahad has presented a thoughtful relationally based, developmentally attuned approach to community disaster preparedness involving staff, preschoolers and parents, the latter via education and support groups (Lahad, 2003). He has trained mental health professionals to train preschool staff to become attuned to their own strengths and vulnerabilities around trauma, as well as to locate the strengths and address the vulnerabilities in the preschoolers and their caregivers.

Within the preschool environment, Lahad's team promotes positive associations to underground disaster shelters, and a sense of familiarity and predictability. His team does this by routinely having children celebrate birthday parties in the shelters. An identical set of toys and materials to that in the classroom is kept in the shelter. Lahad and his team also have created child-friendly coloring books with stories that use what might otherwise involve frightening disaster preparedness materials such as gas masks and other protective gear. Preschool staff build relationships with the preschoolers so that the children can anticipate specific individuals who will be monitoring them in times of crisis and exercise a rehearsed team approach.

While Lahad and colleagues have focused on primary prevention, Laor and colleagues have recently described "principles of systemic intervention" within disaster-struck communities (Laor *et al.*, 2003). The key principles of this approach include the following:

- Early risk assessment that reaches as many new parents and families with preschool-age children as possible and that involves user-friendly, reliable, and sensitive screening tools.
- Systematic broad-scale outreach programs no later than 1–3 months after the disaster to address a range of needs of disaster-struck families with young children.
- Clinical triage protocols to match risk groups with appropriate intervention programs for preschoolers and their families. Clinicians therefore need to be familiar with the various relevant systems that are affected and activated by a disaster (i.e., concrete food and housing provisions, paramedic teams, social services, religious and other community non-profit agencies).

The Early Trauma Treatment Network (ETTN) of the National Child Traumatic Stress Network under the direction of Alicia Lieberman is a consortium of early childhood mental health specialists from across the USA who joined together in the wake of 9/11 to develop better family- and community-based interventions for traumatized families with young children. Programs consulting with the ETTN at sites across the country are studying available interventions and reporting their outcomes. The ETTN is furthermore studying available models in other countries such as those described above in Israel. Largely based on these efforts, the ETTN has already developed the first of a series of practice guidelines: namely, a book that describes recommended treatment of traumatic bereavement in infancy and early childhood (Lieberman *et al.*, 2003).

Conclusion

In conclusion, we now know that the events of September 11, 2001, affected both infants and young children and their caregivers. The intentional interpersonal violence of the terrorist attacks on that fateful day, particularly with their high visibility in New York City – and via the media, across the globe, fractured assumptions of safety in the homes of many parents and young children.

Research has supported the notion that violence exposure is one of the most potent deregulators of psychophysiology. Those most affected by the events of 9/11 were those with very high direct exposure to the attacks via presence at or very near to Ground Zero or experience of a loved one's death. Severe avoidance symptoms such as numbing at the time of or shortly after the event (i.e., peritraumatic dissociation) in the case of the caregivers and/or child, as well as presence of prior history significant for early trauma in the caregivers and/or child's life, are risk factors for the development of PTSD (Pfefferbaum *et al.*, 2001) and its transmission across generations (Yahyda *et al.*, 2005).

To be available for the mutual emotion regulation that a very young child needs for social-emotional development, the caregiver must be able, more often than not, to have the presence of mind to think about what might be going on with their child and to feel for their child's experience. Interventions that enhance the ability of caregivers to recover their presence of mind – which is so often disrupted by trauma, are therefore essential and require further research.

Promoting relationships that enhance this needed ability to think about and feel for what is going on in their own mind and that of their young child become primary goals of prevention and intervention efforts across the board. Relationships can thus provide healing in the wake of violent trauma at best, and at worst, in the absence of this reflective capacity, can render individuals more vulnerable to the adverse effects of trauma, and even increase intergenerational risk for subsequent traumatization.

Enhancing sensitive and reflective relationships and promotion of help- and support-seeking before, during, and after traumatic events is a goal that unites peridisaster trauma treatment efforts for very young children and caregivers at the individual, parent–child, family and larger community systems levels.

In summary, decreasing violence exposure (i.e., promoting safety), fully treating trauma-associated psychopathology in the family, and increasing resilience by strengthening relationships that support reflective care-giving are three essential components of preventive and intervention work with preschoolers and their families in the wake of terrorism, war, and other violent experiences.

REFERENCES

American Psychiatric Association (1994). *Diagnostic and Statistical Manual of Mental Disorders, Fourth Edition (DSM-IV)*. Washington, DC: American Psychiatric Press.

Beebe, B. & Lachmann, F.M. (1994). Representation and internalization in infancy: three principles of salience. *Psychoanalytic Psychology*, **11**, 127–165.

Bowlby, J., Robertson, J. & Rosenbluth, D. (1952). A two-year-old goes to the hospital. *Psychoanalytic Study of the Child*, **7**, 82–94.

Breslau, N., Chilcoat, H.D., Kessler, R.C. & Davis, G.C. (1999). Previous exposure to trauma and PTSD effects of subsequent trauma: results from the Detroit Area Survey of Trauma. *American Journal of Psychiatry*, **156**(6), 902–907.

Bretherton, I. (1995). The origins of attachment theory: John Bowlby and Mary Ainsworth. In *Attachment Theory: Social, Developmental and Clinical Perspectives*, eds. S. Goldberg, R. Muir & J. Kerr. Hillsdale NJ: The Analytic Press, p. 50.

Caspi, A., Sugden, K., Moffitt, T.E., Taylor, A., Craig, I.W., Harrington, H., McClay, J., Mill, J., Martin, J., Braithwaite, A. & Poulton, R. (2003). Influence of life stress on depression: moderation by a polymorphism in the 5-HTT gene. *Science*, **18**, 386–389.

Coates, S.W. & Moore, M.S. (1997). The complexity of early trauma: representation and transformation. *Psychoanalytic Inquiry*, **17**, 286–311.

Coates, S.W., Schechter, D.S. & First, E. (2003). Brief interventions with traumatized children and families after September 11. In *September 11: Trauma and Human Bonds*, eds. Susan W. Coates, Jane Rosenthal & Daniel S. Schechter. Hillsdale NJ: The Analytic Press, pp. 23–49.

Cornely, P. & Bromet, E. (1986). Prevalence of behavior problems in three-year-old children living near Three Mile Island: a comparative analysis. *Journal of Child Psychology and Psychiatry*, **27**, 489–498.

Egeland, B., Jacobvitz, D. & Sroufe, L.A. (1988). Breaking the cycle of abuse. Child Development, **59**(4), 1080–1088.

Emde, R., Guedeney, A., Wright, H., Fenichel, E. &Wise, B. (2004). *Diagnostic classification of 0–3 results of clinical trial, user survey, and a preliminary revision*. Paper presented at the *World Association of Infant Mental Health*, Melbourne, Australia.

Fraiberg, S., Adelson, E. & Shapiro, V. (1975). Ghosts in the nursery. *Journal of the American Academy of Child and Adolescent Psychiatry*, **14**, 387–421.

Freud, A. & Burlingham, D. (1943) *Children in War*. New York City: Medical War Books.

Gaensbauer, T. (1995a). Therapeutic approaches to posttraumatic stress disorder in infants and toddlers. *Infant Mental Health Journal*, **16**(4), 292–305.

Gaensbauer, T. (1995b). Trauma in the preverbal period. *Psychoanalytic Study of the Child*, **50**, 122–149.

Gaensbauer, T.J. (1982). The differentiation of discrete affects: a case report. *Psychoanalytic Study of the Child*, **37**, 29–66.

Gurwitch, R.H., Sullivan, M.A. & Long, P.J. (1998). The impact of trauma and disaster on young children. *Child and Adolescent Psychiatry Clinics North America*, **7**(1), 19–32.

Hinshaw-Fuselier, S., Boris, N.W. & Zeanah, C.H. (1999). Reactive attachment disorder in maltreated twins. *Infant Mental Health Journal*, **20**, 42–59.

Hoven, C.W., Mandell, D.J. & Duarte, C.S. (2003). Mental health of New York City public school children after 9/11. In *September 11: Trauma and Human Bonds*, eds. Susan W. Coates, Jane Rosenthal & Daniel S. Schechter. Hillsdale, NJ: The Analytic Press, pp. 51–74.

Klein, T.P., Devoe, E. & Miranda, C. (2003). *Impact of the World Trade Center disaster on young children at Ground Zero*. Paper presented at the *Biennial Meeting of the Society for Research in Child Development*, Tampa, Florida.

Koplewicz, H.S., Vogel, J.M., Solanto, M.V., Morrissey, R.F., Alonso, C.M., Abikoff, H., Gallagher, R. & Novick, R.M.D. (2002). Child and parent responses to the 1993 World Trade Center bombing. *Journal of Traumatic Stress*, **15**(1), 77–85.

Lahad, M. (2003). *The Integrative Model of Coping and Resiliency*. Paper presented at the *Annual Meeting of the International Society of Traumatic Stress Studies*, Chicago, Illinois.

Laor, N., Wolmer, L., Mayes, L.C. & Gershon, A. (1997). Israeli preschool children under scuds: a 30-month follow-up. *American Academy of Child and Adolescent Psychiatry*, **36**, 349–356.

Laor, N., Wolmer, L., Spirman, S. & Wiener, Z. (2003). Facing war, terrorism, and disaster: toward a child-oriented comprehensive emergency care system. *Child and Adolescent Clinics North America*, **12**, 343–361.

Levy, D. (1939). Release therapy. *American Journal of Orthopsychiatry*, **9**, 713–736.

Levy, D. (1945). Psychic trauma of operations in children and a note on combat neurosis. *American Journal of Diseases of Children*, **69**, 7–25.

Lieberman, A.F., Compton, N.C., Van Horn, P. & Ghosh Ippen, C. (2003). *Losing a Parent to Death: Guidelines for The Treatment of Traumatic Bereavement in Infancy and Early Childhood*. Washington, DC: Zero to Three Press.

Lieberman, A.F., Padron, E., Van Horn, P. & Harris, W.W. (2005). Angels in the nursery: the intergenerational transmission of benevolent parental influences. *Infant Menta Health Journal*, **26**(6), 504–520.

Lyons-Ruth, K. & Block, D. (1996). The disturbed caregiving system: relations among childhood trauma, maternal caregiving, and infant affect and attachment. *Infant Mental Health Journal*, **17**, 257–275.

Pfefferbaum, B. (2003). Media exposure in children one hundred miles from a terrorist bombing. *Annals of Clinical Psychiatry*, **15**(1), 1–8.

Pfefferbaum, B., Doughty, D.E., Reddy, C., Patel, N., Gurwitch, R.H., Nixon, S.J. & Tivis, R.D. (2002). Exposure and peritraumatic response as predictors of posttraumatic stress in children following the 1995 Oklahoma City bombing. *Journal of Urban Health*, **79**(3), 354–363.

Pfefferbaum, B., Seale, T.W., Brandt, E.N., Pfefferbaum, R.L., Doughty, D.E. & Rainwater, S.M. (2003). Media exposure in children one hundred miles from a terrorist bombing. *Annals of Clinical Psychiatry*, **15**(1), 1–8.

Pynoos, R.S. (2001). Personal communication to S. Coates, November 3, 2001.

Pynoos, R.S. & Nader, K. (1988). Psychological first aid and treatment approach to children exposed to community violence: research implications. *Journal of Traumatic Stress*, **1**(4), 445–473.

Pynoos, R.S. Steinberg, A.M. & Wraith R. (1995). A developmental model of childhood traumatic stress. In *Developmental Psychopathology, Vol. 2: Risk, Disorder and Adaptation*, eds. D. Cicchetti & D.J Cohen. New York: Wiley.

Schechter, D.S. (2003a). Intergenerational communication of maternal violent trauma: understanding the interplay of reflective functioning and posttraumatic psychopathology. In *September 11: Trauma and Human Bonds*, eds. Susan W. Coates, Jane Rosenthal & Daniel S. Schechter. Hillsdale, NJ: The Analytic Press, pp. 115–142.

Schechter, D.S. (2003b). Maternal PTSD and interactive behavior with very young children (Abstract). *Computerized Retrieval of Information on Scientific Projects (CRISP)*, National Institutes of Health, Bethesda, Maryland.

Schechter, D.S. & Tosyali, M.C. (2001). Posttraumatic stress disorder from infancy through adolescence: a review. In *Anxiety Disorders in Children and Adolescents: Epidemiology, Risk Factors, and Treatment*, ed. C.A. Essau & F. Petermann. New York: Brunner-Routledge, pp. 285–322.

Schechter, D.S., Coates, S.W. & First, E. (2001). Observations from New York on Young Childrens' and their Families' Acute Reactions To the World Trade Center Attacks. *Bulletin Zero to Three*, **22**(3), 9–13.

Schechter, D.S., Kaminer, T., Grienenberger, J.F. & Amat, J. (2003). Fits and starts: a mother–infant case study involving pseudoseizures across 3 generations in the context of violent trauma history. *Infant Mental Health Journal*, **24**(5), 510–528.

Schechter, D.S., Zeanah, C.H., Myers, M.M., Brunelli, S.A., Liebowitz, M.R., Marshall, R.D., Coates, S.W., Trabka, K.T., Baca, P. & Hofer, M.A. (2004). Psychobiological dysregulation in violence-exposed mothers: salivary cortisol of mothers with very young children pre- and post-separation stress. *Bulletin of the Menninger Clinic*, **68**(4), 319–337.

Schechter, D.S., Coots, T., Zeanah, C.H., Davies, M., Coates, S.W., Trabka, K.T., Marshall, R.D., Liebowitz, M.R. & Myers, M.M. (2005). Maternal mental representations of the child in an inner-city clinical sample: violence-related posttraumatic stress and reflective functioning. *Attachment and Human development*, **7**(3), 313–331.

Scheeringa, M.S. (2003). Personal communication to D. Schechter, December 10, 2003.

Scheeringa, M.S. & Zeanah, C.H. (1995). Symptom expression and trauma variables in children under 48 months of age. *Infant Mental Health Journal*, **16**, 259–270.

Scheeringa, M.S. & Zeanah, C.H. (2001). A relational perspective on PTSD in early childhood. *Journal of Traumatic Stress*, **14**, 799–815.

Scheeringa, M.S., Zeanah, C.H., Myers, L. & Putnam, F.W. (2003). New findings on alternative criteria for PTSD in preschool children. *Journal of the American Academy of Child and Adolescent Psychiatry*, **42**, 561–570.

Scheeringa, M.S., Zeanah, C.H., Myers, L. & Putnam, F.W. (2004). Heart period and variability findings in preschool children with posttraumatic stress symptoms. *Biological Psychiatry*, **55**(7), 685–691.

Stuber, J., Fairbrother, G., Galea, S., Pfefferbaum, B., Wilson Genderson, M. & Vlahov, D. (2002). Determinants of counseling for children in Manhattan after the September 11 attacks. *Psychiatric Services*, **53**(7), 815–822.

Terr, L.C. (1987). Childhood psychic trauma. In *Basic Handbook of Child Psychiatry*, Vol. 5, ed. J.D. Noshpitz. New York: Basic Books, Inc, pp. 262–762.

Thomas, J.M. & Guskin, K.A. (2001). Disruptive behavior in young children: What does it mean? *Journal of the American Academy of Child & Adolescent Psychiatry*, **40**(1), 44–52.

Wiedenmayer, C.P. (2004). Adaptations or pathologies? Long-term changes in brain and behavior after a single exposure to severe threat. *Neuroscience and Biobehavior Review*, **28**(1), 1–12.

Yehuda, R., Halligan, S.L. & Grossman, R. (2001). Childhood trauma and risk for PTSD: relationship to intergenerational effects of trauma, parental PTSD, and cortisol excretion. *Developmental Psychopathology*, **13**, 733–753.

Yehuda, R., Engel, S.M., Brand, S.R., Seckl, J., Marcus, S.M. & Berkowitz, G.S. (2005). Transgenerational effects of posttraumatic stress disorder in babies of mothers exposed to the World Trade Center attacks during pregnancy. *Journal of Clinical Endocrinology and Metabolism*, **90**(7), 4115–4118.

Zero to Three: National Center for Infants, Toddlers, and Families (1994). *Diagnostic Classification: 0–3 (DC: 0–3)*. Washington, DC.

Washington, DC

24

The mental health response to the 9/11 attack on the Pentagon

Elspeth Cameron Ritchie, Willis Todd Leavitt and Sandra Hanish

The views expressed in this article are those of the authors and do not reflect the official policy or position of the Department of the Army, the Uniformed Services University of the Health Sciences, the Department of Defense or the US Government.

Introduction

The prominent images of September 11, 2001, focus on the World Trade Center falling, the firemen digging through the rubble, and the grieving in New York City. The crash of the plane in Pennsylvania has been immortalized by the brave actions of the passengers, and the enduring and inspiring "Let's Roll" battle cry. The story of the plunge into the Pentagon of the third plane, and the immediate valiant response of the workers there, is less well known.

The medical and mental health personnel provided a superb and relatively comprehensive response to the disaster in Northern Virginia. Yet that story was dwarfed by the larger tragedy in New York. This chapter hopes to highlight the work at the Pentagon and the surrounding community.

Shortly after two airplanes smashed into the World Trade Center on the morning of September 11th, the American Airlines 77 plane hit the south side of the Pentagon. Those in the affected wedge heard a boom, and depending on how close they were, saw, smelled, and heard smoke and fire. Many had to struggle to get out through fireballs of jet fuel and dense smoke. Some even scrambled over the burning plane to safety. Many returned numerous times to aid others. Others tried to get back in, but could not, because of the intense raging fire.

After a relatively brief period of time, everyone requiring medical assistance was treated or referred for further care. Within hours, it became apparent that the dead were many and the wounded were few – though some of the wounded were very seriously burned and injured. The responses thus turned to two missions: 1) to find and identify the remains; and 2) to provide mental health support to the survivors, rescue workers, family members of the victims, and other affected personnel.

One hundred and eighty-nine people were killed in the crash, to include Pentagon personnel, the airplane passengers and crew, and the five highjackers. Several offices were especially hard hit, including the Army's Deputy Chief of Staff for Personnel, and the Navy's Command Center. It would have been the biggest terrorist event on American soil since Oklahoma City, if not for the World Trade Center tragedy that morning.

This chapter outlines an overview from the authors' experiences, and incorporates what they learned from others. The first author wrote the first section, and the latter two authors the second section. Interested readers are referred to a supplement to *Military Medicine* containing almost 30 articles, from some 70 authors, which are drawn on here (Ritchie & Hoge, 2002; Ritchie & Stokes, 2002). Vignettes are used to illustrate, but identifying details have been masked, so that no identities will be revealed. Some of the lessons learned are highlighted; others are implicit in the text.

Teams and individuals from the Services (Army, Navy, Air Force, and Marines), Department of Defense (DoD), the Red Cross, the National Center for Post Traumatic Stress Disorder (NCPTSD) from the Department of Veterans Affairs (VA), and many others provided assistance. Hundreds of mental health personnel, chaplains, mortuary affairs personnel and others worked around the clock for weeks. Although some of the immediate responders were recognized with medals and by the media, many others were not. These authors want to acknowledge all their contributions.

As is true in most disasters, the mental health needs came in phases: immediate, short-term, and long-term. The responses were also calibrated, and will be described thus in this chapter. The literature on disaster psychiatry is, fortunately or not, growing exponentially and has been extensively reviewed elsewhere. Thus a review will not be repeated here (NIMH, 2002; Norris *et al.*, 2002).

Part I: The immediate response

September 11, 2001

The Pentagon is nestled by the Potomac in Northern Virginia, flanked by numerous office buildings in Crystal City, with Arlington Cemetery sloping up a hill behind it. Built on 34 acres of land in 1943, the 6,500,000 square feet of office space has 17½ miles of corridors. Five concentric interior "rings" surround a central courtyard. It houses 24,000 personnel, and another 16,000 work in buildings near or adjacent to that building. Of the 24,000, approximately 10,000 are military and another 10,000 are DoD civilian employees; the rest are contractors.

The incoming plane ploughed into the southwest side of the Pentagon, going through almost four of the building rings. It did not penetrate through to the courtyard. Shortly after the crash, fire and black walls of smoke billowed into the air. Smoke rapidly filled the corridors in that side of the building.

Many of those in the far side of the Pentagon did not even feel the crash. All quickly learned of the event however: the entire building was immediately evacuated. The childcare center, just outside the north side, was also emptied. Staff members described putting four infants in each crib, rolling the cribs out across the parking lot, then picking them up over the concrete barriers. They relocated further outward a total of five times, with the flames and smoke billowing behind them. Finally, later that day, the children were reunited with their parents.

Northern Virginia fire and rescue crews responded first. The immediate medical response was a mission to evacuate and treat the wounded. Initially, most of the severely injured were brought to the central courtyard. They were immediately airlifted to local hospitals, including the burn unit at the Washington Hospital center. Only a few were brought to local military hospitals. Several times there were reports of other planes approaching, and the rescuers needed to vacate the crash site for fear of more plane bombs.

The flames were put out with a deluge of water, which caused further extensive damage. The crash site was immediately secured. Law enforcement agencies, engineers, chaplains, the Red Cross, and numerous other agencies set up tents there to house their operations. Route 27 or Washington Boulevard, which runs next to the Pentagon, was closed off. Medical facilities for the first responders and the morgue were set up there.

Each branch of the military service hosts a major hospital in the Washington DC area: Walter Reed Army Medical Center (WRAMC), National Naval Medical Center (NNMC or "Bethesda"), and Malcolm Grow Medical Center (MGMC) at Andrews Air Force Base. Immediately following news of the attack, the hospitals implemented their respective disaster plans and team procedures for providing emergency medical and mental health care. Assets from other military facilities, including Ft. Myers, Ft. Belvoir, Bolling Air Force Base, and Keesler Air Force Base also joined the effort.

Chaplains and mental health personnel were immediately deployed both to the crash site, and to the DiLorenzo Health Care Clinic in the Pentagon. The fire at the crash site was put out within hours, but the building continued to smoke for days. Thus the site remained hot and hazardous.

The DiLorenzo Clinic, on the north side of the Pentagon building, quickly became the operations center for the medical and mental health response throughout the building and the site. Fortunately the clinic had recently rehearsed their disaster plan in a scenario that featured a plane slamming into the building (Geiling, 2002). Communications between the site and the clinic were difficult, as the walk took at least 20 minutes, cell phones do not work well in the Pentagon, and radios were not immediately available.

> *Lesson Learned: Numerous chaplains and mental health personnel went to the crash site, instead of planning for the ripple effect on the community. Anecdotally, one heard that "you could not move without tripping over a chaplain". The rescue workers, in general, were absorbed and motivated by their task, and often felt like they did not need a formal "debriefing". On the other hand, as body parts were brought out, the chaplains prayed over the remains, and many found that helpful (Edmondson, 2002; Powers, 2002).*

The days and weeks after the attack

A wide variety of activities commenced the day after the attack. The bulk of the mental health personnel were deployed to the Pentagon itself. Group sessions were offered at the crash site, in the workplace, and in the DiLorenzo Clinic. Many workplaces had been destroyed, so often sessions were conducted in makeshift office spaces. Individuals were seen at the clinic and the crash site on a walk-in basis. Group interventions ("debriefings") were offered on a regular basis at the health clinic, crash site, and in work areas. (See below under "Therapeutic Activities" for more details.)

Wounded individuals were first treated primarily in civilian local hospitals. The severely burned came to Washington Hospital Center. The psychiatry consult liaison service from Walter Reed worked with many of the hospitalized wounded (Wain *et al.*, 2002). Others were seen in their local emergency rooms and referred to mental health if needed.

Special efforts were needed to coordinate interventions, both between the Services, and between DoD, the VA, the Red Cross, local governments, and other agencies. Conference calls were initiated by the first author for four afternoons following the attacks. E-mail was used extensively. This mechanism helped reduce unnecessary over-lap and minimized gaps in areas of need (Ritchie & Stokes, 2002; Ritchie & Hoge, 2002).

> *Lesson Learned: The departments in the hospitals all had their own alert roster, which did not reach across disciplines or hospitals. In addition, the hospitals set up their own emergency control centers, the numbers of which were not known to other facilities. (Ritchie & Stokes, 2002; Ritchie & Hoge, 2002). The importance of having alert rosters, which are known across the different hospitals, became apparent.*

Army and Air Force personnel principally operated out of the DiLorenzo Clinic. The bulk of Navy personnel who had been located in the Pentagon were relocated to the Navy Annex, which is a large building overlooking the Pentagon. Thus the Navy mental health team concentrated their efforts there (Grieger & Lyszczarz, 2002). The Air Force also developed a separate operations center, for reaching Air Staff personnel located nearby (Rowan, 2002).

The impact on the daycare center was extremely disruptive. It was closed for the next 10 days. (Children therefore had to endure not only the sights and smells of the bombing but also their location and change of caretakers.). Their parents were working long hours, in preparation for war. Two children lost their mothers. Many parents decided not to send their children back there, out of fear of future attacks. Therefore the staff did not know whether they would have a workplace to return to. Child psychiatrists, first from Children's Hospital and then from Walter Reed, worked with the staff and children there (Black & Morris, 2002).

> *Lesson Learned: Each shift of mental health workers arrived highly moti-vated, and each planned a strategy. Unfortunately the plans thus changed with each shift. It was initially unclear as to who really was in charge of the whole effort (Tarpley, 2002). Communication was problematic. (Communi-cation problems are common during disasters.)*

From other disasters, it was clear that many would not go into a mental health clinic, but would respond to outreach. Military mental health has a strong tradi-tion of operating within the workplace (Artiss, 1963). Thus outreach to the entire Pentagon was undertaken a few days after the attack. Fortunately this effort was supported at the highest levels of command.

By the fifth day, maps showing the sections of the Pentagon were pasted on the walls of the conference room in the Wellness Center in the health clinic. Teams of two walked through these areas to make contact, distribute a specially developed flyer, and to help people become aware of the services that could be provided. This proved to be a challenge, as the building is full of blind alleys and secured spaces.

The Employee Assistance Program, located in the Civilian Occupational Clinic (part of the DiLorenzo Clinic), provided treatment and referrals to civilian employees (Thomas, 2002). Civilian employees and contractors, not officially eligible for military health care, were encouraged, but not required, to participate in both individual and group interventions (again a decision made at the highest levels of command).

Many people officially assigned to the Pentagon work in adjacent offices in Northern Virginia, such as in Crystal City, and the Hoffman and Skyline Buildings. In addition, organizations whose offices were destroyed were relocated to buildings such as the Taylor Building and the Navy Annex. Within a week group and indi-vidual assistance was also offered to all these locations.

Vignettes

During a group session a muscular handsome captain appeared very perturbed. Eventually he said that he felt guilty that he had followed the orders to evacuate, rather than gone in to rescue others, as he thought that some of his co-workers may have been still alive when he left. During the session he learned that his efforts would have been fruitless. He seemed much less upset after the session.

A group session was held in an adjacent building with people assigned to the Pentagon but relocated because of the ongoing renovation. Because they were not in the affected building, several of the workers felt left out of the whole process of grieving. They had also lost many of their long-term colleagues: "20 of my friends are dead, but I don't know when the memorial services are".

Several civilian employees came for assistance who were spooked by the sounds of safes being unloaded – they thought it was another bomb. After learning that treatment was free and easily available, they reappeared often with symptoms and situations that clearly pre-dated the 9/11 attack. (It became problematic to continue psychiatric treatment or prescribe medication for civilians, since they were technically not eligible for long-term military care.)

The Family Assistance Center

Each Service (Army, Navy, and Air Force) initially set up their own Family Assistance Center. However, the day following the event, a tri-service DoD Family Assistance Center was set up at the Sheraton Hotel in Crystal City, near the Pentagon. There was theoretically to be a center for airline passengers organized at Dulles Airport, but as the airline agencies were in such disarray, the services were moved to the hotel, a wise decision. This was organized and staffed by DoD personnel, and provided services to the family members of all the victims.

This DoD Family Assistance Center provided a wide range of services to the families of victims. The general in charge briefed twice daily on the status of the rescue, then recovery effort. Each family had assigned to them a casualty assistance care officer (CACO), who stayed with the family to help them negotiate all financial issues and other issues related to sudden death. Personnel from the Office of Victims of Crime of the Department of Justice, the Red Cross, the Federal Emergency Management Agency, and the different Service relief agencies offered assistance. There was a robust presence from chaplains, medical and mental health assets (including child psychiatrists), and volunteers. Pet therapy was also available.

Hundreds of family members gathered at the hotel over the next month. The ballroom, the main briefing room, became a shrine. Pictures and other mementos were set up all around the walls. To watch the children play in the room and the hotel, not yet truly realizing the loss of a parent or grandparent, was very poignant.

A team from the NCPTSD (part of the VA) drove non-stop from California to join this effort. They primarily worked with the staff of the assistance center, to help them process their work with the victim's families. Many of these staff had lost friends in the attack, but still worked continuously with the families for the following month. The VA counselors paid special attention to the hotel staff as they knew of the severe stress on ancillary staff through working with other disasters (Huleatt *et al.*, 2002; Ruzek, 2002; Thomas-Lawson, 2002).

The Armed Forces Institute of Pathology (AFIP) was responsible for the care and identification of the remains. They also had a presence at the hotel, collecting DNA swabs from family members, and informing them of the identification process (Wagner & Kelly, 2002). Family members appeared to benefit by assisting in that process.

Some disputes arose over who could be buried in Arlington Cemetery, and the disposition of unidentified remains. Great pains were used to ensure that none of the remains of the highjackers were mixed with those of the victims for burial. However, in many cases, remains were identified over a period of time, and it was not always apparent whether further remains should be returned to the families. (Since then the military has developed a form to ask the family their wishes as to what should be done if further remains are located.)

A memorial service was held on the north side of the Pentagon on October 11, 2001. Initially there were only to be eight seats per family member of the victim, which caused some anger for those with larger families wanting to attend. However, staff lobbied for more seats, and these were provided.

It was a beautiful morning service, with a full moon high in the morning sky. President Bush and other notables spoke. Meanwhile, many mental health volunteers from the local community were available to help those family members who requested assistance.

> *Lesson Learned: Numerous volunteers offered to help. However, it was difficult to verify their credentials. Again this is an issue common to many disasters. The Pentagon security immediately became extremely tight. Because of their lack of military identification they could not gain access. However, they were very gainfully employed at the Family Assistance Center. After the immediate crisis, much discussion was held on how to provide an easily available, centralized database for assessing credentials. This issue is still not resolved, either here or throughout the country.*

After the service the Family Assistance Center was closed, and a smaller one re-opened nearby. The casualty officers continued to work with the nuclear families. Those who lived in other parts of the country were provided with information about Red Cross and other assistance in their local communities.

The Red Cross helped to coordinate efforts between governmental and non-governmental agencies and volunteers. The American Psychological Association picked up that function after the departure of the visiting Red Cross workers. At those meetings, representatives from the federal government, different local governments (DC, MD, VA), different professional associations, and local hospitals and military members met to exchange information. These meetings continued over the next year, and participants exchanged valuable information related to the anthrax attacks (Dodgen *et al.*, 2002). The informal network helped during the anthrax attacks in October 2002.

Therapeutic activities

A variety of therapeutic activities were initially employed. Individual supportive therapy was offered, again both in the clinic and as part of the outreach. Usually the group intervention activities were tailored to the group and their particular situation. The term "debriefing" was used for the group meeting, but seldom was a formal "Critical Incident Stress Debriefing" or "CISD" utilized. Groups were run several times daily in the DiLorenzo Clinic, both for specific workplaces and for walk-ins.

Meetings in the workplace often focused on "repairing the organizational fabric". A common theme emerged: few people would come to the clinic to be "debriefed" or for therapy, but many were very willing to talk in their office or on "coffee rounds".

All mental health disciplines were represented in the effort to include psychiatric nurses and occupational therapists. Individual supportive therapy was offered, again both in the clinic and as part of the outreach. Chaplains provided spiritual and therapeutic services, both through individual and group work, and through memorials and remembrances in the workplace. Fortunately, there is a long tradition of chaplains and mental health working side by side in the military, and chaplains were well incorporated in the initial mental health response (Powers, 2002).

Special mention should be made of the work provided to members of the Old Guard. Those young infantry soldiers, stationed at nearby Ft. Myers, are normally responsible for providing support for funerals and at the Tomb of the Unknown Soldier. After 9/11, they were responsible for entering the smoking hole in the Pentagon and clearing debris. Mental health workers provided information about dealing with dead bodies before they began, and were given a chance to discuss their experiences in the mental health tent at the end of each shift.

Lesson Learned: In general, both command and soldiers were receptive to the briefings. However, long "debriefings" provided at the end of a long shift were not always welcomed. Invitations for smoking cessation classes were definitely anathema.

Similarly individual contact and group meetings were offered to other personnel at the crash site, including first responders, the criminal investigative services and mortuary affairs. These personnel were, in general, seasoned professionals, and did not seek out counseling – although they were perhaps comforted by the aid offered there.

An Army team, working at the Hoffman Building, was concerned because many workers who had been displaced there expressed a fear of going back into the Pentagon. They performed a "group desensitization", whereby they first brought workers back together in buses to initially view the crash site, then had them view photos of their old offices, before offering them a chance to go back in and reclaim their personal effects. (Waldrep & Waits, 2002).

A mental health team also was present at Dover Air Force Base, where the task of identifying remains was centralized. The regular staff of experienced forensic pathologists and other forensic scientists from AFIP was augmented with more junior X-ray and dental technicians. The team working there drew in the experience of more senior staff to help more junior members with coping with the grisly business. Apparently one of the hardest details was sorting through personal effects, including family pictures and wedding jewelry (Peterson *et al.*, 2002; Wagner & Kelly, 2002).

Issues about stigma and research

Great efforts were taken to reduce the stigma of receiving mental health counseling. In large part, this was done through the workplace interventions, where everyone was encouraged to participate. Confidentially was stressed. Charts were not opened unless it was clear that a psychiatric illness was present.

The research community in the military wanted to do research on the physical and psychological effects of the trauma. As is true in many disasters, leadership was worried about the impact of "having clipboards shoved in the faces of those who have lost their loved ones". Eventually the decision was made to do surveillance, rather than research *per se*.

Lesson Learned: It is critical to have an Independent Review Board (IRB) approved plan for doing research on disaster survivors prior to an event. Recently the National Institute of Mental Health (NIMH) has tackled issues of informed consent and ethics, but no "off the shelf" protocol has emerged at the time of this writing.

Part II: The long-term response: Operation Solace

The US Army Surgeon General, Lieutenant General James B. Peake, assembled his behavioral health consultants in psychiatry, psychology, social work, and other fields, to develop a comprehensive behavioral health outreach program, Operation Solace (OPSOL). Military planners identified those persons at high risk for the development of behavioral health-related problems as were persons injured in the attack, the next of kin or family members, work colleagues of injured or deceased personnel, emergency responders, Casualty Affairs Officers, other Pentagon personnel, and the National Capital Region (NCR) at large.

The program had these objectives: to provide behavioral health services for active duty service members, Pentagon employees, and family members; to minimize the long-term behavioral health impacts of the Pentagon attack; and to learn from the Pentagon attack to better prepare the Army Medical Department for future terrorism responses.

During the 3 week long planning effort, the behavioral health consultants considered the lessons learned from the April 1995 Oklahoma City Murrah Federal Building domestic terrorist bomb attack due to the many parallels between it and the Pentagon terrorist attack (Hoge, *et al.*, 2002). Since the study of adult survivors in the immediate blast area in Oklahoma City showed that 45% met satisfied criteria for a post-disaster psychiatric disorder, and that 34.3% had post-traumatic stress disorder (PTSD) (North *et al.*, 1999), planners estimated that as many as 2000 Pentagon personnel located in the impacted wedge might develop PTSD or other significant behavioral health problems. Within the whole NCR, over 13,500 beneficiaries were anticipated to require behavioral health care, resulting in 54,000 sessions or visits (Hoge, *et al.*, 2002).

Activities of OPSOL: challenges and solutions

The following information describes the OPSOL/Pentagon Stress Management Team: its development and implementation. References to OPSOL in this discussion imply the Pentagon Stress Management Team.

Military planners assumed that, unless specific corrective measures were taken, OPSOL would suffer from the same obstacles impeding routine access to behavioral health care.

Availability

Before 9/11 the Pentagon did not have a dedicated behavioral health clinic to address the needs of military personnel. In order to seek help, service members had to travel to behavioral health clinics in local military treatment facilities or medical centers. An Employee Assistance Program for civilian employees is located in the

Pentagon and many DoD-leased buildings to provide assessment, crisis counseling, brief treatment, referral and consultation services. Due to the inconvenient locations of behavioral health care clinics, service members often chose not to pursue evaluation and treatment during the workday.

The lack of worksite-based behavioral health care was the first and foremost obstacle that OPSOL faced. Within the first week after the attack, a temporary command center was developed in the Wellness Clinic of the DiLorenzo Health Clinic, as previously described. From there, during the following 3 months, over 90 military behavioral health professionals and chaplains spread throughout the Pentagon to conduct group stress debriefings, individual sessions, and psycho-educational classes for the 25,000 DoD personnel. From December 2001 to the present time, OPSOL was staffed by two Army psychiatrists, one psychiatric clinical nurse specialist, two administrative specialists, and five to nine clinical social workers.

Due to water, smoke, and structure damage, many Pentagon offices were relocated to outlying DoD-leased buildings in the immediate area. Displaced personnel were considered a high risk for the development of behavioral health symptoms given their probable proximity to the attack site. The displacement of nearly 4,000 personnel made it difficult for OPSOL to track office relocations, especially during the heightened state of security concerns following the attack. The development of a close working relationship with the Pentagon's Building Management helped OPSOL identify the dates and destinations for office relocations.

In the aftermath of the attack, Pentagon personnel, whose emotional resources were nearly depleted, reported that fatigue and fear made it difficult to travel for behavioral health care – even to the Pentagon's clinic. Similarly, accounts from injured survivors highlighted their difficulties in just getting to their worksite. During this time span, the DC Metro station was undergoing renovation. This created an additional, unforeseen stressor to Pentagon personnel. It was not unusual to hear "I'm exhausted before I even get to my desk".

Travel to the Pentagon was more emotionally laden than ever before due to lingering concerns of terrorist acts. DC Metro riders were keenly aware of the similarities between the attack site and subway environment. The ordinary rough-and-tumble of subway travel evoked powerful memories of the attack. The vacillations in light, the noise, the crowds, and the strangers, all contributed to feelings of vulnerability, suspicion, fear and unease. Extraordinary events, such as subway cars temporarily losing power or internal lights, immediately triggered a cascade of fears.

OPSOL specifically chose convenient and discrete locations within the workplace to minimize customer discomfort and anxiety. The main office is now located in a major thoroughfare on the second floor of the Pentagon, which was easily accessible to incidental traffic. The Wellness Clinic served as the primary hub of OPSOL clinical services in the DiLorenzo Clinic. The Wellness Clinic's emphasis on monitoring

> **Vignettes**
>
> One employee reported having attacks of diarrhea everyday for months. She routinely brought in a change of clothes for those days when she could not make it to the nearest restroom. She did not stop coming to work or riding the DC Metro. Over time her symptoms subsided.
>
> A captain reported that a Metro experience sent him into the building to immediately seek out his support group of other injured office-mates in order to discuss an experience that had immediately triggered a series of flashbacks to 9-11. He stated, "I'm sure that I looked just fine, but I was 'jello' on the inside."

health maintenance helped to deflect stigma commonly attached to behavioral health services. Later, quality improvement surveys of OPSOL customers revealed that convenient location was the leading reason for seeking OPSOL services.

Perception

Military planners were likewise concerned that potential stigma-related fears, both real and imagined, could result in an obstacle to timely identification of emerging stress reactions and to corrective interventions. In general, employees associate negative consequences to seeking behavioral health care (Lawton, 1988).

Among Americans, less than one out of every four persons needing care actually seeks help for behavioral health issues (Epidemiological Catchment Area Survey, 1980). Among military service members, the 1998 Department of Defense Health Survey of Health Related Behaviors revealed that less than 20% of active duty respondents believed that behavioral health care was safe for their careers (Department of Defense Survey of Health Related Behaviors, 1998).

Personnel fear potential humiliation, vulnerability, and discrimination. They worry about jeopardizing their security clearances, flight statuses, command opportunities, and career progressions (Porter & Johnson, 1994). Others are concerned that their leadership authority will be eroded if their situation were discovered (Kahn, 1993). The leading concern for most military service members is the documentation of mental health interventions in their medical records, which could haunt them throughout the rest of their careers.

Their concerns are not necessarily baseless. Confidentiality is limited for military service members. Like their civilian counterparts, military clinicians are legally obligated to notify authorities for specific self-reports made by their patients (e.g., abuse of children, threats to kill others). Confidentiality is limited under the following circumstances: (1) potential risk to national security; (2) abuse of alcohol, use of illegal drugs, or misuse of prescribed medications; (3) inability to meet mission requirements; and (4) command directed mental health evaluations (Department of Defense Directive 6490.1, 1997). In reality, for the vast majority of service members seeking care, confidentiality is very rarely broached, but that is not the perception.

To overcome to the problem of negative perception, OPSOL developed a policy limiting documentation only to those cases when medication was prescribed, when a condition satisfied criteria for a serious clinical disorder within the Diagnostic and Statistical Manual for Mental Disorders IV, or when legally mandated. The shorthand version of this policy, "no names; no social security numbers," was widely advertised throughout the defense community.

Limiting documentation kept OPSOL fundamentally in a "combat stress control" mode of functioning, characterized by supportive, psycho-educational, and stress management interventions, without documentation. The trappings of traditional behavioral health care, such as diagnoses and treatment plans, were avoided whenever possible. For personnel needing clinical interventions, OPSOL referred them to community- or military-based providers. In addition, OPSOL established a behavioral health clinic, staffed by an Army psychiatrist within the DiLorenzo Clinic, to provide onsite clinical evaluations and treatment.

Although this policy proved successful in skirting the negative perceptions by Pentagon personnel, there was an unforeseen twist. In hindsight, some personnel wished for documentation to establish the extent of their emotional pain and suffering to strengthen their compensation claims through the Victims' Compensation Fund.

It has been recognized that the policy of limiting documentation further hinders research opportunities. Given the urgency of the situation and the potential for large numbers of casualties, OPSOL planners decided to sacrifice future research potential for the immediacy of accessible, de-stigmatized care.

Care delivery model

When designing OPSOL, military planners created methods to circumvent obstacles inherent in the traditional medical care. Although working to establish collaborative relations, traditional medicine emphasizes the identification and treatment of disease. Persons seeking consultation are encouraged to identify with the role of "patient". The care provider is the authority figure, and the patient passively accepts recommendations and guidance. The emphasis on disease and patient-status potentially increases exposure to unnecessary procedures, prolongs symptoms, and creates a sense of disability and limitation.

Additionally, traditional medicine inherently waits for self-recognized symptoms to surface before care can take place. A person may delay seeking appropriate care due to unconscious denial, failure to recognize the symptoms as warranting medical attention, failure to recognize the symptom as having an emotional cause (e.g., somatization), or stigma-related fear. Delays in seeking care among Pentagon personnel were common.

> **Vignette**
>
> One lieutenant colonel sought care for significant PTSD symptoms approximately 18 months after the attack. The precipitant for seeking care was an inappropriate outburst at his superior in public. He reported considerable relief in learning from OPSOL staff members that his condition was treatable and that help was readily available.

If asked, active duty personnel presenting for treatment often acknowledged that they were there because of spouse and/or child pressures secondary to their significant behavioral changes within the family constellation. Individual tolerance for a significant number of symptoms remained quite high.

To offset the medical paradigm, OPSOL implemented methods to engage personnel in a partnership on behalf of their own care. OPSOL attempted to de-emphasize the authoritarian role of the care provider, and de-pathologize responses to trauma by avoiding diagnoses. Health-risk communications were carefully managed through interactive, educational dialog between OPSOL staff members and symptomatic contacts. This proved to be a narrow tightrope to walk: too much information was perceived as threatening or intimidating while too little appeared to have minimal impact on perception of the problem.

Psycho-education focused on normal responses to traumatic events, methods of symptom self-monitoring, and individual goals for symptom-tolerance. Resources were provided for symptoms that interfered with family and/or work functions.

OPSOL endorsed the hypothesis that the more safe and in control a Pentagon employee felt, the more likely he/she would seek care. To encourage that degree of control and safety, OPSOL opened itself to delivering care in unconventional settings embedded within the workplace, such as the cafeteria, hallway, office space, window alcoves, courtyard benches, and coffee bars. Thus, a typically social environment was used to provide structure to the interaction.

A surprising amount of privacy was afforded as personnel clearly were very used to avoiding interactions that appeared to be a "meeting". Only one employee actually evidenced emotional upheaval "in public". This was seen as a therapeutic indicator. Likewise, the duration of meetings was contact-driven, and driven by the needs of the individual (e.g., tolerance, available time, and competing appointments).

Key to outreach and surveillance was the practice of "therapy-by-walking-around" (Milliken *et al.*, 2002). Rather than wait for Pentagon personnel to come to OPSOL, therapy-by-walking-around brought OPSOL staff members into offices of the Pentagon and outlying buildings. This served several functions, it: (1) provided immediate access to a behavioral health care provider for individual, group, and command consultations; (2) provided ongoing surveillance of the emotional climate within the workplace; (3) offered onsite support for the supervisor and employees; and (4) enhanced trust and rapport between office personnel and the assigned OPSOL staff member through repeated visits.

The OPSOL staff member's familiarity helped to guide future supportive interventions and referrals. An additional long-term benefit of initial "debriefings" was the formation of small, informal office support groups which continued to meet spontaneously over several months. As one civilian stated, "These guys in green (battle-dress uniforms) came thru and pulled us all together at the table and talked to us about what had happened. After that, we just felt freer to talk among ourselves".

OPSOL faced the difficult challenge of providing care to Pentagon personnel who needed to simultaneously clean up, relocate, heal, and go to war. Regression and decompensation were not options available to this population. Interventions were founded in supportive and solution focused psychotherapy techniques, thereby fortifying ego strengths, and encouraging utilization of environmental supports and resources.

The long-term results of OPSOL are not easily retrievable, partly because of the deliberate efforts made to maintain strict confidentiality. As of December 2003, OPSOL records show that it has made contact with over 83,000 military and civilian personnel and surviving family members. Over 188 group debriefings, 100 support group sessions, and 224 psycho-educational classes have been conducted. OPSOL maintains supportive interventions to 1022 high-risk individuals.

OPSOL also provides traditional clinical care in the DiLorenzo TRICARE Health Clinic. A chart review revealed that 249 patients had been evaluated and treated by OPSOL from 9/11/01 to 12/31/03. Of these 249 patients, the charts of 55 (22%) patients contained intake documentation indicating that they attributed the 9/11 terrorist attack to their need for seeking mental health care. Of these 55 patients, men accounted for 28 patients (51%) and women accounted for 27 patients (49%). PTSD (29%) and Depressive Disorders (22%) represented the two leading primary diagnoses within this population. Of these 55 patients, 18 (33%) are still in treatment with OPSOL providers.

Table 24.1 shows the demographic and diagnostic results based on the analysis of those Operation Solace's 9/11/01-related patient population.

There have been no known suicides or other major adverse events among impacted personnel.

Table 24.1. Operation Solace 9/11/01-related patients

	#	% of 55 Patients
Demographic category		
Men	28	51
Women	27	49
Military	48	87
Civilian	7	13
Primary diagnoses		
Adjustment disorder	2	4
Anxiety disorder (excluding PTSD)	4	7
Bereavement	2	4
Depressive disorder	12	22
No diagnosis	11	20
Other diagnoses	8	15
PTSD	16	29

Psychological sequelae

As mentioned above, formal research was very difficult to do in the aftermath of the attack. However, a survey published recently by researchers from the Uniformed Services University sheds some light on the degree of disability 7 months after the attack. An electronic questionnaire was administered via Internet. Although the response rate was low (11%) for a number of reasons, the findings are interesting. Most respondents (70%) saw, heard, felt or smelled the aircraft, the explosion or the resultant fire. However only 14% of respondents met the criteria for probable PTSD. The respondents were all employed at the time of the survey, and neither use of mental health interventions nor level of disability was assessed. (Grieger *et al.*, 2003).

The authors conclude, "This study may represent a 'best case' scenario of the psychological consequences of a terrorist attack in the United states. The sample was taken from a group of highly educated, employed, socially supported individuals, many of whom had warfare skills and had survived previous traumatic events without negative sequelae." (Grieger *et al.*, 2003).

Conclusion

The tragedy of September 11, 2001, has shaken and traumatized the country. Subsequent anthrax and sniper threats, as well as combat operations in Iraq and

Afghanistan, have turned the issue from a single, awful, acute event to a series of chronic stressors. The response from mental health and chaplain personnel from the Department of Defense to the Pentagon tragedy was comprehensive and immediate. Mental health workers and chaplains provided immediate services to first responders, Pentagon personnel, wounded victims and mortuary affairs workers. The casualty offices provided additional ongoing support to family members of the victims. Challenges did arise, however, as different agencies integrated in providing services.

As a result of the combined efforts of OPSOL and sister military and civilian agencies, the Pentagon community continues on its healing journey. Though the majority of this population remains resilient and steadfast, even at 2 years after the attack survivors continue to come forward with delayed recognition of grief, anxiety, and/or depression.

There are critical research needs to be addressed. What is the burden of the disability caused by the attack? Were our interventions successful? Since we are unlikely to be able to put the traumatized populations into randomized clinical trials, how do we measure the effectiveness of our interventions? Nevertheless, even without solid data on the evidence of effectiveness, we think that the mental health response to the attack on the Pentagon was robust, guided by the literature, and one to be proud of.

REFERENCES

Artiss, K.L. (1963). Human behavior under stress: from combat to social psychiatry. *Military Medicine*, **128**, 1011–1015.

Black, N. & Morris, J. (2002). The child and adolescent psychiatrist in the Pentagon response. *Military Medicine*, **167**(Suppl. 4), 79–80.

Department of Defense Directive 6490.1 (1997). Command Directed Mental Health Evaluations.

Department of Defense Survey of Health Related Behaviors (1998).

Dodgen, D., LaDue, L.R. & Kaul, R.E. (2002). Coordinating a local response to a national tragedy: community mental health in Washington, DC after the Pentagon attack. *Military Medicine*, **167**(Suppl. 4), 87–88.

Edmondson, M.W. (2002). Professionalism, honor and respect on September 11th: a historical view of the initial response and recovery mortuary team. *Military Medicine*, **167**(Suppl. 4), 6–7.

Geiling, J.A. (2002). Overview of command and control issues: setting the stage. *Military Medicine*, **167**(Suppl. 4), 3–5.

Grieger, T.A. & Lyszczarz (2002). Psychiatric responses by the U.S. Navy to the Pentagon attack. *Military Medicine*, **167**(Suppl. 9), 26–30.

Grieger, T.A., Fullerton, C.S. & Ursano, R.J. (2003). Posttraumatic stress disorder, alcohol use, and perceived safety after the terrorist attack on the Pentagon. *Psychiatric Services*, **54**(20), 1380–1382.

Hoge, C.W., Orman, D.T., Robichaux, R.J., Crandell, E.O., Patterson, V.J., Engel, C.C., Ritchie, E.C. & Milliken, C.S. 2002. Operation Solace: overview of the mental health intervention following the September 11, 2001 Pentagon attack. *Military Medicine*, **167**(Suppl. 9): 44–47.

Huleatt, W.J., LaDue, L., Leskin, G.A., Ruzek, J. & Gusman, F. (2002). Pentagon Family Assistance Center inter-agency mental health collaboration and response. *Military Medicine*, **167**(Suppl. 4), 68–70.

Kahn, J.P. (1993). Executive distress: organizational consequences. In *Mental Health in the Workplace: A Practical Psychiatric Guide*, ed. J.P. Kahn. NY: Van Nostrand Reinhold.

Lawton, B. (1988). The EAP and workplace psychiatric injury. *Occupational Medicine State of the Art Review*, **3**,695–706.

Milliken, C., Leavitt, W.T., *et al.* (2002). Principles guiding implementation of the Operation Solace plan: "Pieces of PIES," therapy by walking around, and care management. *Military Medicine*, **167**(Suppl. 4), 48.

National Institute of Mental Health (2002). Mental health and mass violence: evidence-based early psychological intervention for victims/survivors of mass violence. *A Workshop to Reach Consensus on Best Practices*. NIH Publication No. 02-5138, Washington, DC: US Government Printing Office.

Norris, F., Watson, P., Byren, C., Diaz, E. & Kaniasty, K. (2002). 60,000 disaster victims speak, Part I: an empirical review of the empirical literature, 1981–2001. *Psychiatry*, **65**, 207–239.

North, C.S., Nixon, S.J., Shariat, S., Mallonee, S., McMillen, J.C., Spitznagel, E.L. & Smith, E.M. (1999). Psychiatric disorders among survivors of the Oklahoma City bombing. *Journal of the American Medical Association*, **282**, 755–762.

Porter, T.L. & Johnson, W.B. (1994). Psychiatric stigma in the military. *Military Medicine*. **159**, 602–605.

Peterson, A.L., Nicolas, M.G., McGraw, K., Englert, D. & Blackman, L.R. (2002). Psychological intervention with mortuary workers after the September 11 attack: The Dover Behavioral Health Consultant Mode. *Military Medicine*, **167**(Suppl. 4), 83–86.

Powers, R. (2002). Help in troubled times: Chaplain comments concerning Operation Noble Eagle. *Military Medicine*, **167**(Suppl. 4), 17–18.

Ritchie, E.C. & Hoge, C.W. (2002). The mental health response to the 9-11 attack on the Pentagon. *Military Medicine*, **167**(Suppl. 4).

Ritchie, E.C. & Stokes, J. (2002). Perspectives on coordination from the Office of the Assistant Secretary of Defense/Health Affairs. *Military Medicine*, **167**(Suppl. 4), 31–33.

Rowan, A.B. (2002). Air Force critical incident stress management outreach with Pentagon staff after the terrorist attack. *Military Medicine*, **167**(Suppl. 4), 33–35.

Ruzek, J.I. (2002). Providing "brief education and support" for emergency response workers: an alternative to debriefing. *Military Medicine*, **167**(Suppl. 4), 73–75.

Tarpley, A.A. (2002). A perspective on the Air Force's mental health response to the Pentagon. *Military Medicine*, **167**(Suppl. 4), 26–30.

Thomas, M.O. (2002). New priorities in evacuation training based on the Pentagon experience. *Military Medicine*, **167**(Suppl. 4), 22–23.

Thomas-Lawson, M., Whitworth, J., Doherty, J. The role of leadership in trauma response: Pentagon family assistance center. *Military Medicine*, 71–73.

Wain, H.J., Grammar, G.G., Stations, J.J. & Miller, C.M. (2002). Meeting the patients where they are: consultation-liaison response to trauma victims of the Pentagon attack. *Military Medicine*, **167**(Suppl. 4), 19–21.

Waldrep, D. & Waits, W. (2002). Returning to the Pentagon: the use of mass desensitization following the September 11, 2001 attack. *Military Medicine*, **167**(Suppl. 4), 73–75.

Wagner, G.W. & Kelly, C.C. (2002). Operation Noble Eagle: forensic and psychosocial aspects of the Armed Forces Institute of Pathology's response to the September 11 Pentagon attack. *Military Medicine*, **167**(Suppl. 4), 81–82.

25

Learning lessons from the early intervention response to the Pentagon

Brett T. Litz

Ritchie and colleagues should be congratulated for their work at the Pantagon on and after September 11, 2001, for their useful and rich depiction of that horrific day, and its aftermath, and for the various mental health activities provided to victims, the traumatically bereaved, first responders, and graves registration personnel. In order to appreciate the demands placed on Ritchie and colleagues, any mental health professional need only to ask themselves what they would have done on 9/11, and what they are prepared to do if a mass violence event were to occur in their work setting or vicinity and they are called on to plan, implement, or assist in providing mental health services to victims, workers, and their families. There is no doubt that mental health professionals, public health officials, and individuals responsible for planning disaster mental health and terrorism responses in employee assistance programs and various work systems and organizations have much to gain by absorbing the information provided by Ritchie and colleagues.

The authors describe the enormous difficulties and exigencies of deriving a work-ing, good-enough mental health response plan that would be amenable or tolerable to the military culture, and to the unique work culture at the Pentagon for civilians and families of employees and military personnel directly and indirectly exposed to the attack on 9/11. The decisions made about resources, the content and process of the interventions provided, and who and where they would provide them were arguably about as good as could be expected, given the state of knowledge in disaster mental health and the unprecedented nature of 9/11 terror.

Because we don't know how best to meet the immediate, acute, and long-term needs of individuals exposed to terror and the aftermath of terror, it is critical to learn as much as possible from the events that unfolded in the hours, days, and months that followed the attacks. Working in conditions of great emotional upheaval and uncertainty, some decisions about early mental health intervention were extraor-dinarily valuable and prescient and bear repeating, while others may have wasted resources or may have been inappropriately timed or implemented. Because most people are heroically resilient in the face of extraordinary trauma and loss – they recover on their own for a variety of reasons (King *et al.*, 2003) – the field needs randomized-controlled trials to determine the efficacy of secondary prevention interventions for victims of terrorism. However, it is very difficult, but not impossible, to conduct planned randomized trials after disaster (Gray & Litz, 2003; Litz & Gibson, in press). As a result, we need to learn as much as possible after the fact. What follows is a series of comments and suggestions to assist in accomplishing this goal, using the very helpful information provided by Ritchie and colleagues as an embarking point.

What happened and how can we maximize the lessons learned?

A first and critical step is to describe accurately and in an unbiased fashion what was decided and planned and what was implemented at every stage (immediately afterwards, in the days that followed, and to the present), at every level of care planned. We need to appreciate the struggles, pitfalls, conflicts, and the errors in decision-making, as well as the apparently effective strategies. In effect, we need to be uncompromising, objective *Monday morning quarterbacks*. We need to ask: "how were decisions made;" "what assumptions about recovery from trauma were used;" "what model of care was employed and why;" "what was actually implemented and how do we know;" "how were needs assessed;" "how accessible were various services?" Ritchie and colleagues appreciate the value of describing these facets of the post-attack mental health response. Unfortunately, they rely exclusively on their own subjective perceptions and inferences about the service delivery planning process the plans themselves, and the value of various features of the services provided (and the manner in which it was provided). In the spirit of the ideal Monday morning quarterbacking exercise, we need someone outside the Pentagon and the military to describe the planning process, the plans, and their effectiveness in a variety of different domains. This in no way suggests that Ritchie and her colleagues in their chapter and other published accounts have not been forthcoming or would shy away from sharing this information, it only suggests that there are state-of-the-art social science methods of evaluating organizational behavior that should be brought to bear in order to maximize the lessons learned from the attack on the Pentagon.

With respect to describing what took place immediately after the plane crash, it appears from Ritchie's and colleagues' account that chaplains and a variety of mental health professionals converged on the scene at what must have been a time of panic and confusion. No doubt these people wanted to help in whatever way they could to secure the area and assist the wounded as would any able person in such a time of need. As described by Ritchie and colleagues, it appears that just like in New York City on 9/11, there were many impromptu acts of heroism, large and small at the Pentagon. There must have been many people at the crash site that witnessed great horror and were experiencing all possible combinations of shock, panic, and despair. There must have also been many emergency services personnel (and individuals with no formal training with similar roles) who also experienced horror, helplessness, and the various strains of helper and rescue roles. If these individuals were secure from harm and they had no physical health care needs or severe fatigue, in an ideal world, any *naturally unmet* emotional need would be attended to as soon as possible, *if so desired*. It would be instructive to appreciate the tacit assumptions that motivated and guided the emotional support provided at the Pentagon in the immediate trauma context. Too often, in the crisis intervention and grief counseling arenas, it is assumed that immediate emotional sharing, support, and validation are necessary and sufficient to achieve secondary prevention goals (Litz *et al.*, 2002). The field is at best unclear about what to label this kind of emotional support, what it should entail, who should provide it, what the goal is, and most importantly how to identify individuals who want it. The worst case would be to assume that individuals need it when they don't want or need it (e.g., they may need respite from engaging on any level, they may need to be left alone, they may get what they need on their own terms in the natural environment) and to consider this kind of help necessary in the face of any number of more pressing needs (e.g., the need for information). It is of note that chaplains, by virtue of their garb and their special role in the culture, for some would be instantly unmistakable as possessing a unique ability to provide comfort and support in a time of despair. In the immediate aftermath of trauma, it is very rare to be able to readily identify individuals who are indeed specially prepared and readily acceptable to provide immediate emotional support and comfort.

In order to learn from what took place in the immediate context, we need answers to the following questions: Did mental health professionals "converge" on the scene to any greater degree than any other able person? Did they have special access early on? Were chaplains experienced as uniquely approachable? What was the implicit model of care employed by mental health professionals – what assumptions guided their work? Was there a common model? Were there instances of intrusive interventions? To what extent did individuals with prior relationships or by virtue of their common trauma provide a comforting presence to one another and was this any more or less useful than the comforting presence of a mental health professional?

In many respects, the same questions apply to all mental health interventions provided at every stage described by Ritchie colleagues. As time passed and safety needs were no longer pressing, it is especially important to ascertain, if possible, what planners and clinicians assumed about what victims and their families needed. Ritchie and colleagues described a surveillance study conducted at the

Pentagon, which is unprecedented in this context, *but how were these data used to guide mental health care decisions about resources, intervention types, targets, and methods?* Were these data ever used to assist decision-making? If not, why? In large-scale disasters and mass violence events, anonymous population surveillance can be employed as a critical first step in preparing a meaningful and focused mental health response. It is typically assumed that mental health needs are paramount and pressing and services are needed and desired, but this is an empirical question that has never been addressed.

It seems that Ritchie and colleagues (and others) struggled with at least two key issues that are emblematic of conflicts that exist in the field and thus should be underscored and expanded upon. First, throughout their chapter, Ritchie and colleagues use vague, equivocating terms to describe the mental health needs of victims and the interventions provided by professionals. They appeared unwilling to formalize secondary prevention goals and methods of achieving these goals. For example, the word debriefing was put in quotations, and the vague terms "sessions," "group sessions," and "briefings" were used to describe interventions. They stated that *critical incident stress debriefing* or *CISD* was used seldom, but failed to specify why this was the case and what was used in its place. The authors used the rather vague term "behavioral health problems" as the targets for interventions at all levels. The terms *trauma, acute stress,* and *post-traumatic stress disorder (PTSD),* and other forms of specifically trauma-linked problems were conspicuously absent. This lack of specificity may reflect a degree of self-consciousness and conflict in the field of early intervention for trauma. On the one hand, this is perhaps the way it should be: mental health providers and decision makers should circumscribe and constrain their early intervention efforts and they should not pathologize psychological responses to terror that will likely abate without any formal intervention. This is especially warranted because there is a grossly insufficient conceptual or empirical base to appeal to for decisions about care, *the large majority of victims and emergency services personnel do not require services,* and there is no consensus method of screening for those most at risk for developing severe PTSD and thus in need of early secondary prevention interventions (Litz & Gray, 2003). On the other hand, the lack of specification makes replication virtually impossible (e.g., "group sessions were held at the crash site"). Also, it would be instructive for the field to appreciate if the planners did not know what interventions to recommend, or that CISD was the only viable game in town even though there is no evidence to support its use, or that supportive counseling, although not serving a secondary prevention function, was seen as an important service to provide, and so on. The question that arises is: what should well-intentioned mental health professionals prepare to do within organizations affected by mass violence in the future, given the state of the field?

The other generic issue Ritchie and colleagues faced is the concern about stigma and the need to find a way of using the work setting and organization to promote recovery and provide care without overly blurring the boundaries between worker and helper, work setting and therapeutic setting, and helper and supervisor/manager. These issues appear to have been handled with great care at the Pentagon. However, it would be surprising that the measures taken to reduce stigma, maintain confidentiality, and maintain professional boundaries did not fail in some circumstances. If that is true, these are important lessons to be learned. For example, since group sessions were provided to co-workers, how do we know whether this may have created undue vulnerability or avoidance? How can we know if some individuals avoided talking to an *Operation Solace* counselor at the water cooler because of stigma or embarrassment – how confidential could these "sessions" truly have been? The points made by Ritchie and colleagues regarding the need to label counseling and advice giving as something other than formal psychotherapy, the need to not medicalize problems that may not reflect psychopathology, the need to do very creative outreach, and the need to highly circumscribe the roles of counselors are very well taken and cogent, especially with respect to work cultures such as the military and the emergency services (fire, police, etc.). On the other hand, it appears that *Operation Solace* counselors made a lot of contacts and provided a lot of care. How can we know what constituted a substantive or sufficient contact, what services were delivered, and whether they were associated with any degree of effectiveness? We can't rely solely on individuals who developed this form of care or on individuals who provided it to answer these questions. The question is: Should this form of care be recommend as a form of early intervention again? If so, why? Perhaps the most important lesson to be gleaned from these efforts is that some form of quality monitoring, validity checking, and anonymous follow-up outcome evaluation is necessary. This is one of the unfortunate burdens of clinical decision-making and planning in a field that sorely lacks an evidentiary base.

An additional objective in this post-event analysis is to find ways of asking consumers of services to share their experiences in a way that elicits the most unbiased, critical, yet informative data. To reiterate, because most people adjust well, *on their own, post-hoc*, uncontrolled research of this nature cannot answer questions about *the efficacy* of interventions. If you ask people whether they are doing better, chances are they are. If you infer from this information that victims and helpers are doing better because they received some sort of intervention, this would be a gross error. In addition, if you can't specify what was done to help people (i.e., if it is not replicable), and if the interventions were highly variable in content, process, and length, it is similarly impossible and inappropriate to infer causal links between what was done and outcome. On the other hand, there is important qualitative information from care providers and consumers that will be useful and still can be collected in the aftermath of the mass violence crash at the Pentagon on 9/11. We can gather correlational evidence that can give us some important clues about effectiveness and clarify important questions for future controlled research.

One method of achieving this goal is to conduct focus groups, with the overarching goal of gathering bottom-up, phenomenological data about how care was delivered, perceived, and taken (e.g., whether it was experienced as useful and why this was the case). These focus groups would need to be conducted by professionals outside the Pentagon. Creating a comfortable and open atmosphere is essential. Focus group participants would be encouraged to amplify and build on comments from other focus group members to generate a more comprehensive discussion of the nuances and complexities of putatively therapeutic contacts and its impact on the coping process. Special attention would need to be paid to concerns about stigma, confidentiality, and professional boundaries in the work setting.

Transcripts of the focus groups would need to be coded using reliable schemes. Themes and exemplars of themes would be generated. This method would generate very rich qualitative information about how people coped with the aftermath of their experiences on and after 9/11 and how they experienced the care they received. It seems highly likely that we would learn a great deal about what victims and emergency services personnel needed over time, how they coped, how they appraised the services provided, and whether they experienced the care as useful.

Final remarks

The events that unfolded after the attack on the Pentagon to meet the anticipated mental health needs of victims were well presented by Ritchie and colleagues. However, many questions were unaddressed and many lessons are still to be learned. We can't assume that preexisting models of care are valid, we can't know what victims need, we need quality monitoring, and there is much we can glean after the fact by interviewing decision-makers and planners, counselors, and consumers.

Because no consensus model or framework existed, Ritchie and others at the Pentagon did the right thing: They provided the least intrusive level of care possible and assumed that most people were not at risk for severe post-traumatic adjustment problems. If they threw up their hands, succumbed to the lack of evidence, and did nothing structured at various post-crash stages, they would have been condemned. On the contrary, they assumed that some contact was better than none, and they probably assumed that non-intrusive, supportive, and information-based interventions would reduce stigma and get people on the right track to get the formal sustained care they need, when this was indicated. This is an empirical question that can be addressed: Were victims who received brief interventions via *Operation*

Solace more likely to seek formal professional trauma-focused treatment than those who did not take part in such interventions?

More than anything what becomes evident from Ritchie's and colleagues' rich overview of the mental health response to the attack on the Pentagon after 9/11 is that the early intervention field needs a parsimonious, evidenced-based model of care that can be flexibly applied, relative to the scope of an event and the resources available at every post-disaster stage. Secondary prevention is critical because of the individual and societal costs associated with chronic PTSD and other physical and mental health problems implicated by exposure to severe trauma (Kessler *et al.*, 1995). We need to recognize the need to provide formal secondary prevention interventions to those who need it and we need much more research to identify mechanisms of risk to pinpoint screening methods. We need to disaggregate palliative, supportive, brief interventions from formal secondary prevention interventions, which require sustained therapy at a point in which victims can participate actively in a process of learning, reframing, and implementing a plan of action, as occupational, interpersonal, and self-care demands emerge over time (Litz & Gray, 2002, 2003). We have argued that the former type of early intervention should be labeled *psychological first aid* – a term first used by Beverly Raphael (Raphael, 1977). Psychological first aid is designed to provide information, emotional support, and a human presence during a time of great anguish, confusion, despair, and helplessness. Psychological first aid is not a time when event processing is promoted and it respects the tremendous range of human response to tragedy (i.e., there is no single index of healthy response). It does not serve a formal secondary prevention function, but it should reduce stigma and trigger help seeking down the line.

The good news is that there is sufficient evidence to recommend cognitive–behavioral therapy as the guiding framework for formal secondary prevention interventions (Bryant *et al.*, 1998). However, these interventions require training, adherence, time and effort on the part of the victim, and evaluation of process and outcome. These factors can be a hindrance, but they should not be summarily dismissed because of outmoded assumptions about who needs care, what that care should entail, and what individuals may or may not be willing to do to help them recover from trauma and reduce the risk of lifelong complications. Resources, planning, and training can overcome many obstacles.

REFERENCES

Bryant, R.A., Harvey, A.G., Dang, S., Sackville, T. & Basten, C. (1998). Treatment of acute stress disorder: a comparison of cognitive–behavioral therapy and supportive counseling. *Journal of Consulting and Clinical Psychology*, **66**, 862–866.

Gray, M. & Litz, B.T. (2003). Methodological issues in early intervention research. In *Early Intervention for Trauma and Traumatic Loss*, ed. B. Litz. New York: Guilford Publications, pp. 179–200.

Kessler, R.C., Sonnega, A., Bromet, E., Hughes, M. & Nelson, C.B. (1995). Posttraumatic stress disorder in the National Comorbidity Survey. *Archives of General Psychiatry*, **52**, 1048–1060.

King, D., Vogt, D.S. & King, L. (2003). Risk and resilience factors in the etiology of chronic PTSD. In *Early Intervention for Trauma and Traumatic Loss*, ed. B. Litz. New York: Guilford Publications, pp. 34–64.

Litz, B.T. & Gibson, L. (in press). Conducting research on early interventions. In *Mental Health Intervention Following Disasters or Mass Violence*, eds. M. Friedman & C. Ritchie. New York: Guilford Publications.

Litz, B.T. & Gray, M. (2002). Early intervention for mass violence: what is the evidence, what should be done? *Cognitive and Behavioral Practice*, **9**, 266–272.

Litz, B.T. & Gray, M. (2003). Early intervention for trauma in adults. In *Early Intervention for Trauma and Traumatic Loss,* ed. B. Litz. New York: Guilford Publications, pp. 87–111.

Litz, B.T., Gray, M.J., Bryant, R.A. & Adler, A.B. (2002). Early intervention for trauma: current status and future directions. *Clinical Psychology: Science & Practice*, **9**, 112–134.

Raphael, B. (1977). The Granville train disaster: psychological needs and their management. *Medical Journal Australia*, **1**, 303–305.

Prolonged-exposure treatment as a core resource for clinicians in the community: dissemination of trauma knowledge post-disaster

26

Psychological treatments for PTSD: an overview

Edna B. Foa and Shawn P. Cahill

Among the consequences of the horrific events of September 11, 2001, are increased awareness of and interest in the psychological effects of trauma and their treatment. In this chapter, we provide an overview of the psychosocial treatments for chronic posttraumatic stress disorder (PTSD) and interventions designed to prevent the development of the disorder that have been found to be effective in randomized controlled studies. To date, no controlled studies investigating treatments for PTSD following terrorist attacks have been published. Until then, we must extrapolate from the extensive research on effective treatments for chronic PTSD and acute stress disorder (ASD) following other types of trauma. Such extrapolation can be justified on at least two grounds. First, epidemiological studies conducted within the year following 9/11 (e.g., Galea *et al.*, 2002; Schlenger *et al.*, 2002) indicate that PTSD is a common reaction to terrorist attack and that the various risk factors for the development of PTSD following such attacks are similar to those identified following other kinds of traumatic events (e.g., gender, degree of exposure to the trauma, history of prior stressors, level of social support).

Second, the cognitive behavioral treatments that have been demonstrated to be effective in alleviating PTSD symptoms and associated anxiety and depression have been tested across a wide range of trauma populations including, but not limited to, male combat veterans; female victims of sexual assault; male and female victims of physical assault, survivors of serious accidents (motor vehicle, industrial), and political refugees some of whom were victims of torture. Thus far, there is no evidence that the type of civilian traumas affect differentially the outcome of evidence-based treatments. Moreover, there is one published uncontrolled study of a cognitive therapy program administered to PTSD sufferers after the 1998 terrorist attack in Omagh, Northern Ireland (Gillespie *et al.*, 2002) demonstrating that effect sizes were comparable to those obtained in a randomized controlled trial of the same treatment program administered to a sample of motor vehicle accident survivors (Ehlers *et al.*, 2003).

At the same time, however, it is important to remain mindful of the different environment in which treatment for posttraumatic stress reactions following an act of mass terrorism takes place, compared to the treatment of chronic PTSD following more typical civilian traumas. The most obvious difference is the sheer magnitude of people who are affected by the event who may need psychological interventions at the same time. In a short period of time, the families of nearly 3000 individuals lost a loved one to the ruthless attack of terrorists in New York on 9/11, with many of them repeatedly witnessing the collapse of the two towers via the intense media coverage. In addition, there are the many survivors who were able to escape the buildings before they collapsed, other first hand witnesses of the attacks on the Twin Towers, and the emergency services personnel who worked tirelessly in the days and weeks after 9/11 to rescue lives and recover bodies of the victims. Clearly, many thousands of people experienced severe distress related to the World Trade Center. Providing psychological help to those in need would require mental health infrastructure that does not exist at present.

Historical background of treatments for PTSD

Customarily, overviews of treatments for PTSD focus on knowledge that has accumulated since 1980, when PTSD was introduced into Diagnostic and Statistical Manual of Mental Disorders (DSM-III) (American Psychiatric Association, 1980). While this convention may have a formal justification, it leaves the reader with the erroneous impression that before 1980 we did not have knowledge about post-trauma psychological disturbances and how to treat them, thus obscuring the continuity between current and past conceptualizations and treatments of these disturbances. One body of knowledge that has influenced current views on PTSD and its treatments derives from articles and books, published throughout the 20th century, reflecting particular theoretical perspectives, such as psychoanalysis, describing in detail how treatments were applied to individuals who had experienced trauma-related symptoms with special attention to combat-related experiences (e.g., Hurst, 1919; Grinker & Speigel, 1944). This literature reflects the wide recognition that chronic psychological disturbances following traumatic experiences are a common occurrence, that these disturbances frequently require therapeutic intervention, and that various interventions were observed to alleviate post-trauma symptoms.

Another rich body of knowledge that influenced current cognitive behavior therapy conceptualizations and treatments of post-trauma reactions comes from the learning theory conceptualization of pathological anxiety and the treatments that had been developed to reduce such anxiety. In this tradition, chronic post-trauma symptoms were recognized as severe anxiety or fear reactions acquired through Pavlovian conditioning. Indeed, that post-trauma reactions were perceived as the prototype of pathological fear is exemplified in the work of Dollard and Miller (1950). In a chapter describing how symptoms (phobias) are learned, the authors noted that the simplest and most convincing illustrations of how phobias are acquired through conditioning come from symptoms following traumatic events, describing in detail a case of a pilot who developed intense fear and avoidance of airplanes and related objects and situations after being exposed to intensely fear-provoking stimuli during one of his missions. Rachman's work (1978) on fear and courage, which began in the 1970s, also exemplified the conception of traumatic reactions as rooted in fear and anxiety. Indeed, to study basic mechanisms of fear and courage, he chose military personnel as subjects for his experiments. In the same vein, in his article on emotional processing, Ranchman (1980) conceptualized natural processes of recovery from a traumatic event in terms of anxiety reactions.

The official placement of PTSD among the anxiety disorders in the DSM-III reflected the wide recognition that anxiety is a predominant chronic reaction to trauma. Indeed, the symptoms of PTSD overlap considerably with those of other anxiety disorders. For example, the arousal symptoms such as hypervigilance sleep disturbances, irritability, and difficulty concentrating are common to both PTSD and generalized anxiety disorder (GAD). Fear and avoidance are common to PTSD, specific phobia, social phobia, and agoraphobia. Furthermore, escape/avoidance behaviors in PTSD sufferers, like many avoidance behaviors in individuals with other anxiety disorders, are driven by the strong desire of anxious individuals to avoid or escape states of high anxiety as well as by their bias toward exaggerating the probability of threat (Foa & Kozak, 1986; Foa et al., 1989; Foa et al., 1996). Hence, with the codification of PTSD, cognitive behavioral theories of PTSD have essentially conceptualized the disorder as a phobia with especially extensive generalization (Keane et al., 1985; Foa et al., 1989).

The conceptualization of the acquisition and extinction of pathological fear within learning theory has prompted extensive research on the measurement of fear and anxiety and their treatment with cognitive behavioral therapies (CBT) beginning in the 1960s. The first CBT techniques to be successfully applied to morbid anxiety were variants of exposure therapy (Foa et al., 1989). Specifically, techniques involving imaginal and *in vivo* exposure to feared objects, situations, and memories had already been shown to be effective in the reduction of anxiety in the treatment of specific phobias (Wolpe, 1958; Bandura et al., 1969), agoraphobia (Emmelkamp, 1974; Emmelkamp & Wessels, 1975; Mathews et al., 1976), public speaking phobia (Paul, 1966), and obsessive–compulsive disorder (Meyer, 1966, Meyer et al., 1974; Marks et al., 1975; Foa & Goldstien, 1978).

Interestingly, the knowledge that people who suffer trauma-related disturbances can be helped by exposure to trauma reminders, including traumatic memories, comes not only from the development of exposure treatment of anxiety disorders and from the wide recognition that post-trauma reactions are predominately anxiety related. The "exposure principle" is also clearly imbedded in the much earlier literature on treatment of trauma-related disturbances. For example, as early as 1893 Freud and Breuer noted (Freud, 1973) in a article on the phenomenology and treatment of hysteria (a condition that would be called PTSD in current diagnostic systems) that individual hysterical symptoms disappeared when the therapist succeeded in bringing clearly to light the memory of the event by which it was provoked and in arousing the accompanying affect, and when the patient had described the event in the greatest possible detail and put the affect into words. A similar formulation was offered by emotional processing theory (Foa & Kozak, 1986) and the treatment of PTSD that has ensued from the theory which is focused on systematic, repeated recounting (i.e., imaginal exposure) of the traumatic memory.

The 1970s witnessed another quite separate development in the treatment for anxiety disorders that parallels, and interacts with, the development of exposure therapy described above. This approach is called "anxiety management training" (AMT) (Suinn, 1971) and "stress inoculation training" (SIT) (Meichenbaum & Cameron, 1972). The basic tenet of this treatment is that anxiety symptoms can be ameliorated by educating patients about anxiety symptoms, teaching them how to manage the symptoms, and providing skills to cope with future stresses and anxiety evoking situations. SIT has been successfully applied to phobic patients (Meichenbaum, 1974).

To understand the continuity between treatment of anxiety disorders developed prior to 1980 and treatments developed specifically for PTSD after 1980, it is important to recognize that researchers studying these CBT interventions did not view themselves as developing specific treatments for specific disorders, *per se*. Rather, they viewed themselves as studying processes related to fear reduction generally, with the assumption that knowledge gained from investigating methods of fear reduction with one group of individuals (e.g., agoraphobics) would be relevant to the understanding of fear reduction among other groups (e.g., those with obsessive–compulsive disorder).

These two factors, recognition that the basis of PTSD lies in pathological anxiety and recognition that cognitive behavioral treatment is effective for anxiety disorders, led to the application of the these procedures in the treatment of trauma victims. Initial reports took the form of case studies of treatment for combat veterans (Saul *et al.*, 1946; Kipper, 1977; Schindler, 1980; Black & Keane, 1982; Fairbank & Keane, 1982; Keane & Kaloupek, 1982; Fairbank *et al.*, 1983), rape victims (Wolff, 1977; Veronen *et al.*, 1978; Olasov-Rothbaum & Foa, 1983; Veronen & Kilpatrick, 1983) and motor vehicle accident victims (Kushner, 1965; Kraft & Al-Issa, 1965). Only later were these procedures formally tested in randomized controlled trials (Resick *et al.*, 1988, 2002; Brom *et al.*, 1989; Cooper & Clum, 1989; Keane *et al.*, 1989; Foa *et al.*, 1991, 1999; Marks *et al.*, 1998). But the early case reports demonstrate that trauma experts readily recognized that the treatment for anxiety could naturally apply to trauma-related psychological difficulties.

In summary: (a) there was from early on a wide recognition that trauma-related psychological problems were rooted in fear and anxiety; (b) there was already in the 1960s and 1970s a great deal of knowledge concerning the effectiveness of CBT, in particular exposure therapy, in reducing anxiety symptoms in a variety of anxiety disorders; (c) the traditional descriptions of successful treatments for post-trauma disturbances converge with modern developments in the area of anxiety disorders, both advocating therapeutic exposure to trauma reminders; and (d) there has been knowledge about the effectiveness of stress inoculation programs for anxiety and stress disorders. Thus, in anxiety clinics where behavior and cognitive therapies were conducted, trauma victims were viewed as suffering from pathological anxiety and were treated in the same manner as other anxiety patients.

Current status of psychosocial treatments for chronic PTSD

While numerous case reports, books, and books chapters have described a variety of treatments for post-trauma reactions (Foa *et al.*, 2000), evidence for the efficacy and effectiveness in reducing PTSD and other trauma-related symptoms such as general anxiety and depression comes mostly from programs that utilized cognitive behavioral techniques (Foa & Meadows, 1997; Foa & Rothbaum, 1998; Foa *et al.*, 2003). These programs include variants of exposure therapy, anxiety management, and cognitive therapy. Combinations of these interventions have also been investigated (Marks *et al.*, 1998; Foa *et al.*, 1999). More recently, the efficacy of several programs for PTSD that include non-conventional exposure and cognitive therapy techniques have also been submitted to scientific examination. The most studied of such program is eye movement desensitization and reprocessing (EMDR) (Shapiro, 2001).

Most of the early studies of treatment for PTSD were conducted with two groups of trauma survivors: male Vietnam veterans and female sexual and non-sexual assault victims. In these studies, exposure therapy programs were generally employed with veterans (Brom *et al.*, 1989; Cooper & Clum, 1989; Keane *et al.*, 1989; Foa *et al.*, 1991), and anxiety management programs such as SIT were generally employed with female assault victims (Veronen *et al.*, 1978; Veronen & Kilpatrick, 1983; Foa *et al.*, 1991). More recent CBT studies have examined the efficacy of cognitive therapy and combinations of exposure and cognitive therapy and include patients with traumatic experiences other than combat and assault, such as motor vehicle accidents (Blanchard *et al.*, 2003), childhood sexual abuse (Cloitre *et al.*, 2002), refugees (Paunovic & Ost, 2001), and mixed trauma samples (Marks *et al.*, 1998).

"Conventional" CBT programs

Exposure therapy

As noted earlier, the idea that therapy for trauma-related disturbances should include some form of exposure to memories or reminders of traumatic event has a long history in psychology and psychiatry (Rivers, 1920). In its modern form, this idea is reflected in exposure therapy for PTSD. With PTSD, the core components of exposure programs are imaginal exposure, or repeated recounting of the traumatic memory, and *in vivo* exposure, the repeated confrontation with trauma-related situations and objects that evoke excessive anxiety. For example, a person who directly witnessed the collapse of one of the Twin Towers would be asked to provide a detailed description of the events he or she experienced starting at the moment the person realized that something was wrong and continuing until the point the person recognized that he or she was safely out of the situation. The person would tell this story out loud in first person narrative, using the present tense, and including details about the thoughts and feelings he or she had at the time of the trauma. While telling this story, the person would be instructed to develop a vivid image of the events being described. The goal of this treatment is to promote habituation and processing of the trauma memory (Foa & Kozak, 1986). In between sessions, the person would listen to a recording of the imaginal exposure and would begin to confront safe but feared situations – such as visiting tall buildings (Empire State Building), crowded places, "Ground Zero" and nearby locations – that the person has been avoiding. People whose trauma involved the loss of a loved one in the attack may be encouraged to reminisce with others about the deceased, look at pictures or confront other reminders (clothing). Alternatively, they may be encouraged to begin engaging in normal activities of daily life or pleasant activities they stopped doing, perhaps out of a misplaced sense that it is "too early" to be returning to such activities.

Beyond the core components of imaginal and *in vivo* exposure, programs may vary in the specifics. For example, the program developed by Keane and colleagues for veterans with PTSD included relaxation training (Keane *et al.*, 1989), and the program developed by Foa and colleagues called prolonged exposure (PE), includes breathing training and psychoeducation, as well as discussion and processing following the imaginal exposure to the traumatic memory (Foa *et al.*, 1991; Foa *et al.*, 1999). Moreover, the manner in which imaginal and *in vivo* exposure is implemented varies across programs. In Foa and colleagues' work PE program imaginal and *in vivo* exposure are introduced simultaneously whereas Marks' and colleagues' exposure therapy program introduced imaginal exposure for five sessions followed by *in vivo* exposure for the remaining five sessions (Marks *et al.*, 1998) Furthermore, some exposure programs include imaginal exposure only (Tarrier *et al.*, 1999).

Stress inoculation training (SIT)

Anxiety management approaches were commonly utilized in research on female crime victims. The most researched program for PTSD is SIT (Meichenbaum, 1974), which was adopted for post-rape PTSD by Veronen and Kilpatrick (Veronen & Kilpatrick, 1983). SIT for PTSD includes education about trauma-related symptoms as well as techniques for managing anxiety such as breathing and relaxation training, cognitive restructuring, guided (task-enhancing) self-dialogue, assertiveness training, role-playing, covert modeling, and thought-stopping. Accordingly, a therapist may assist a survivor of the 9/11 attack in New York in the development of a range of anxiety management skills (e.g., breathing and relaxation training) and the use of these techniques to manage anxiety in challenging situations, such as returning to work in a tall building located in lower Manhattan. As with exposure therapy, SIT programs vary from one another. Some include exposure component (Veronen & Kilpatrick, 1983) and others do not (Foa et al., 1991). Number of session also varies, as does the format in which SIT is conducted (group vs. individual). Notably, the interest in studying SIT for PTSD has diminished in the past few years.

Cognitive therapy

Cognitive therapy for PTSD is derived from Beck's model of treatment of depression and anxiety (Beck et al., 1985). With PTSD, the goal of cognitive therapy is to teach the patient to identify trauma-related or symptom-related irrational or dysfunctional beliefs that may influence his/her response to a situation and lead to intense negative emotion (Marks et al., 1998; Tarrier et al., 1999). The patient is taught to challenge these thoughts or beliefs in a logical, evidence based manner. Relevant facts that support/do not support the belief are examined and alternative ways of interpreting the eliciting situation are considered. The therapist assists the patient to weigh the alternative interpretations and consequently decide whether the belief is helpful and accurately reflects reality, and if not, to replace or modify it. For example, fears of being a victim in a future terrorist attack and attendant avoidance of perceived "high risk" situations would be addressed by examining the realistic probabilities for that particular individual being at the future target site at the time of the future attack. Here too, the program varies with respect to length and number of sessions. Moreover, some cognitive therapy programs include an exposure component – Cognitive Processing Therapy (e.g., Resick et al., 2002), Ehlers and clark's cognitive therapy (e.g., Ehlers et al., 2003) – whereas others do not (e.g., Marks et al., 1998).

"Unconventional" exposure and cognitive therapy programs

In addition to the above three categories of CBT programs that include components of conventional cognitive behavioral therapy, the field of treatment of PTSD has witnessed a proliferation of programs that include components of "unconventional" exposure and/or cognitive therapy. By unconventional, we mean that the methods used to implement exposure and cognitive therapy and/or the rationales given to the patient for the efficacy of the technique may differ in significant ways from how these techniques have traditionally been implemented. In addition, these unconventional programs may include distinct features, such as eye movements in the case of EMDR, which are thought to make the treatment unique.

The most studied of these programs is EMDR (Shapiro, 1989, 2001). In EMDR, the therapist asks the patient to generate images, thoughts, and feelings about the trauma (exposure?), to evaluate their aversive qualities, and to make alternative cognitive appraisals of the trauma or their behavior during it (cognitive therapy?). As the patient at first focuses on the distressing images and thoughts, and later focuses on the alternative cognition, the therapist elicits rapid, laterally alternating eye movements by instructing the patient to visually track a finger rapidly waved back and forth in front of his face. Originally, Shapiro regarded these eye movements as essential to the processing of the traumatic memory (Shapiro, 1991). The assertion about the cardinal role of the rapid eye movements component of the treatment has not been supported by studies (Lohr *et al.*, 1998; Cahill *et al.*, 1999). Recently, EMDR programs have replaced the eye movement components with other procedures – patient alternating finger tapping for right to left hand – claiming equivalent mechanisms underlying these various procedures (Shapiro, 2001).

Other programs also seem to include unconventional exposure and cognitive therapy. One such program is Imagery Rehearsal Therapy for nightmares (Krakow *et al.*, 2001), where patients describe their nightmares in writing (exposure?), modify the content of the nightmares (cognitive restructuring?), and then imagine the original and modified dreams (exposure?). In another program, called Emotional-Focused Therapy (Paivio & Nieuwenhuis, 2001), patients are involved in gestalt-driven imaginal confrontation with abusive others (exposure?), access maladaptive cognitions, and change their meaning (cognitive therapy?). A third program, called Interapy (Lange *et al.*, 2001), is conducted via the internet. Patients are instructed to describe the traumatic event in writing (exposure?), to identify and challenge cognitive appraisals about the trauma (cognitive therapy?), and to instruct a hypothetical friend how to process a traumatic event (cognitive therapy?). In contrast to programs that used conventional CBT and EMDR, each of these therapies has been submitted to one controlled study with waitlist as the control condition.

In a comprehensive literature search of recent (1995–2003) outcome studies on PTSD, Foa and colleagues (Foa *et al.*, 2003) identified 21 well-controlled randomized studies that reported on the efficacy of 14 different protocols. We have not included the SIT alone program because of lack of current interest in this program. These studies seem to illustrate that with few exceptions, each researcher invented a new program. Some modifications were minor (e.g., number of sessions) while others were extensive (e.g., writing vs. imagining the traumatic event). Confusing matters even more, similar programs have been given different names – Foa's and colleagues' "PE" program (Foa *et al.*, 1999) vs. Marks' "exposure therapy" program (Marks *et al.*, 1998) and different programs have been given similar names – Ehlers' and colleagues' "cognitive therapy" program, which includes imaginal and *in vivo* exposure (Ehlers *et al.*, 2003) vs. Tarrier's and colleagues' "cognitive therapy" program which includes identifying, challenging, and modifying distorted cognitions, but explicitly avoided exposure procedures (Tarrier *et al.*, 1999).

How can we create order out of the present chaos?

Foa (2003) noted that all 14 identified protocols included at least some variation of exposure or cognitive restructuring, and that most programs combined exposure and cognitive restructuring. They divided the exposure therapy programs into: (1) programs that include both *in vivo* and imaginal exposure, which they labeled Extensive Exposure; and (2) programs they labeled Limited Exposure, which involve either imaginal or *in vivo* exposure, or limited duration of exposure. Foa (2003) further noted that there were two types of programs that combined exposure and cognitive therapy: (1) programs that combined Extensive Exposure with Cognitive Therapy (e.g., Marks *et al.*, 1998; Foa *et al.*, 2005); and (2) programs that combined Cognitive Therapy with Limited Exposure (e.g., Resick *et al.*, 2002; Ehlers *et al.*, 2003). In this way, the existing programs were organized into five categories of conventional CBT and one category of programs involving unconventional exposure combined with cognitive restructuring. These groups are summarized in Figure 26.1.

Table 26.1 summarizes the number of studies that included each of the treatment conditions (*N* Conditions) and the total number of subjects that completed

---

> - All active treatment programs have at least one of the following two ingredients:
>   - ❑ Extensive or limited exposure
>   - ❑ Cognitive restructuring
>
> - Active treatment programs can be organized into six types:
>   - ❑ Extensive exposure (imaginal PLUS *in vivo* exposure)
>   - ❑ Limited exposure (imaginal or *in vivo* exposure; use of brief exposures)
>   - ❑ Cognitive therapy
>   - ❑ Extensive exposure + cognitive therapy
>   - ❑ Cognitive therapy + limited exposure
>   - ❑ Unconventional combined exposure and cognitive therapy

Figure 26.1 Elements present in various treatments for PTSD and categorization of treatment programs.

Table 26.1. Average percent change in PTSD symptoms for different treatments for PTSD

Condition	N conditions	N subjects	Average % change	Group average % change
Cognitive therapy + limited exposure	3	70	67.74	
Extensive exposure	6	170	63.18	63.21
Extensive exposure + cognitive therapy	8	172	61.39	
UCEC	7	158	54.89	
In vivo or imaginal exposure	4	78	41.94	48.88
Cognitive therapy	2	51	40.89	
Relaxation	3	45	33.17	
Supportive counseling	3	59	29.92	28.53
Affect management	2	38	20.86	
Wait list/minimal attention	15	326	9.37	9.37

treatment in each of the conditions (*N* Subjects). Because studies have used different instruments to assess PTSD symptoms, we selected from each study the primary outcome measure, computed the percent change score for each treatment condition, averaged these scores across the number of treatment conditions (average % change), and then computed the average percent change for each of the six types treatment conditions (group average % change). For example, three studies included a condition that combined cognitive therapy with limited exposure, in which a total of 70 patients completed treatment. On average, this treatment resulted in a 67.74% reduction on the severity of PTSD symptoms. Table 26.1 presents the same data for several active control conditions and for waitlist/minimal attention control conditions. Some of the more frequently used outcome measures were the PTSD Symptoms Scale Interview (PSS-I) (Foa *et al.*, 1993), Clinician Administered PTSD Scale (CAPS) (Blake *et al.*, 1990), and the Impact of Event Scale (IES) (Horowitz *et al.*, 1979). For each of these measures, either the patient or an independent evaluator rated the frequency and/or severity of the patient's PTSD symptoms to compute a total symptom severity score.

Inspection of the average percent change for the six active treatment categories and the various control conditions suggests four clusters. The most efficacious cluster consisted of three treatments: cognitive therapy with limited exposure, extensive exposure alone (imaginal and *in vivo* exposure), and extensive exposure therapy combined with cognitive restructuring. Across all the studies that included one or more of these treatment conditions, there was an average reduction of PTSD severity of approximately 63%. The second cluster averaged 49% symptom reduction and included the unconventional combined programs, just imaginal or just *in vivo* exposure programs, and cognitive therapy programs that excluded exposure. The least efficacious clusters included active control conditions such as relaxation or supportive counseling (29% symptom reduction) and waitlist or minimal attention controls (9% symptoms reduction). Interestingly, it seems that the efficacy of cognitive therapy alone (40.89% symptom reduction) was improved by the addition of either limited exposure (67.74% symptom reduction) or extensive exposure (61.39% symptom reduction). In contrast, the efficacy of extensive exposure alone (63.18%) was not enhanced by the addition of cognitive therapy (61.39%). It seems then that the inclusion of exposure to trauma-related material may be necessary for maximizing treatment efficacy. While strong conclusions cannot be drawn from comparisons across studies, there is ample evidence to suggest that the addition of various techniques to Extensive Exposure programs does not enhance and perhaps impedes its efficacy (Foa *et al.*, 2003).

Current status of psychosocial treatments for the prevention of chronic PTSD

Although the majority of trauma survivors recover without intervention, a significant minority develops chronic PTSD (Rothbaum *et al.*, 1992). It is widely believed that a brief intervention administered in the acute aftermath of a traumatic event can speed recovery and prevent the development of chronic PTSD. Two approaches to facilitating recovery following a traumatic event that have been subjected to the most research: psychological debriefing and abbreviated cognitive behavioral packages.

Psychological debriefing

Following the recently published Practice Guidelines from the International Society for Traumatic Stress Studies (Bisson *et al.*, 2000), the term psychological debriefing is used in a general way to refer to very brief (one or a few sessions) interventions that are typically applied shortly after a traumatic event (frequently within 48–72 hours, but not necessarily) and which share a number of features, such as discussing the facts of the traumatic event and the trauma-survivors' perceptions of what happened; expressing thoughts, impressions, and emotional reactions; normalizing the trauma-survivors' reactions; and developing coping strategies for dealing with the trauma and its sequelae. These interventions have been administered in groups and in individual therapy settings. Although psychological debriefing is often offered as a stand alone intervention, proponents of critical incident stress management (CISM) (Everly *et al.*, 2001), one particular type of brief intervention for acute trauma reactions, have recently argued that group psychological debriefing should be offered as part of larger set of services that include follow-up individual counseling sessions.

Results of randomized controlled studies of the effects of debriefing have repeatedly shown high levels of consumer satisfaction with the intervention. However, the effects of debriefing on reducing specific trauma-related symptoms has not been encouraging, with most studies finding either no differences between conditions (Conlon *et al.*, 1999; Rose *et al.*, 1999) or finding less improvement for debriefing than control conditions (Hobbs *et al*, 1996), particularly at long-term follow-up (Bisson *et al.*, 1997; Mayou *et al.*, 2000). The strongest support for debriefing is a study in which emergency medical service workers completed a PTSD symptom questionnaire 3 months after responding to the 1992 Los Angeles civil disturbance, some of whom had received a debriefing session shortly after the riot, others of whom did had not. Debriefed participants endorsed significantly fewer PTSD symptoms than did non-debriefed participants. However, the absence of random assignment and pre-intervention assessment of symptoms preclude any strong conclusions regarding the efficacy of debriefing. Other studies cited as supportive of debriefing also suffer from significant methodological limitations (McNally *et al.*, 2003).

Brief CBT

Brief (i.e., four to five sessions) CBT beginning approximately 2 weeks after the trauma has been shown to speed the rate of recovery in women victims of sexual and non-sexual assault who met symptom criteria for PTSD (Foa *et al.*, 1995) and prevent the development of chronic PTSD in male and female accident survivors and assault victims with ASD (Bryant *et al.*, 1998, 1999, 2003). For the most part, CBT in these studies consisted of a combination of PE plus elements of SIT. In Foa's and colleagues' study, at 2 months after the assault only 10% of women receiving CBT met criteria for PTSD vs. 70% of those in the assessment control group (Foa *et al.*, 1995). However at follow-up, natural recovery in the assessment control group erased the superiority of CBT on PTSD outcome. Thus, CBT sped the rate of recovery but did not reduce the incidence of chronic PTSD.

Across a series of three studies by Bryant and colleagues, between 8% and 20% of participants receiving CBT met criteria for PTSD at the end of treatment and between 17% and 23% at 6-month follow-up, compared to between 56% and 83% immediately following supportive counseling and 58–67% at 6-month follow-up. In addition, Bryant and colleagues compared the full CBT program with five sessions of just the PE elements of the treatment and found no differences between them (Bryant *et al.*, 1999). Thus, as with studies of chronic PTSD (reviewed in the previous section), exposure therapy, either alone or in combination with anxiety management, is an effective treatment. In addition, there is no apparent benefit of a combined treatment program compared to exposure therapy alone.

Discussion

The study of reactions to trauma and their treatments has occupied a central place in psychiatry and psychology since the beginning of the 20th century and continues to draw the interest of clinicians and researchers to date. This work has led to a rich and solid body of knowledge of how to treat PTSD and related disturbances efficiently and effectively. Despite this remarkable achievement, it is important to note that a minority of patients does not improve and many remain somewhat symptomatic. Thus, the search for enhancing treatment effectiveness should continue. We suggest that this endeavor is best served by replicating the best existing programs with various trauma populations and different cultures/ethnic populations as well as by improving these programs rather than by inventing "new" programs.

The need to further improve outcome notwithstanding, our main challenge is to disseminate the excellent programs we have developed to mental health professionals. Recent findings from a survey of clinicians who treat trauma survivors underscore the need for dissemination of effective treatments for PTSD. With respect to PE, the most widely studied program in the most effective cluster, only 20% of the respondents noted that they felt somewhat or very comfortable using imaginal exposure for PTSD, only 17% reported ever using this treatment, and only 4% reported using it most of the time with PTSD. The main three reasons for not using PE were: (1) limited training, (2) a preference for individualized, non-manualized therapy, and (3) the fear that patients will decompensate (Becker et al., 2004).

Based on our review of the literature above and on the few studies that compared several active treatments, we conclude that exposure therapy, SIT, cognitive processing therapy (which includes writing the trauma and cognitive therapy), and various programs that combined exposure with cognitive therapy or SIT procedures produce comparable and excellent outcome. Given limited availability of training resources, what factors should influence the decision of which treatments should be disseminated? The first factor is the strength of the evidence for the efficacy of the program. The excellent outcome of exposure therapy alone and in combination with SIT and cognitive therapy has been evidenced in many studies across a wide range of trauma populations. On the other hand, cognitive processing therapy and SIT alone have fewer replications and their efficacy was proven in women assault victims only. The second factor to consider for selecting treatments for wide dissemination is the simplicity of the program. Presumably, a simpler program will require less time to learn and will be more robust in the hands of non-experts. Given that combined treatments have not yielded superior outcome to exposure therapy alone, this treatment seems a better candidate for dissemination than more complex programs. A third consideration is acceptability of the treatment to patients and its safety. As discussed in detail in Cahill et al. (this volume), there is an erroneous impression that exposure therapy alone is less acceptable and less safe than other treatments (Pitman *et al.*, 1996; Tarrier *et al.*, 1999; Cloitre *et al.*, 2002). However, a full review of the available data does not support this belief (Cahill *et al.*, this volume). Thus, at present it seems that dissemination efforts should focus on exposure therapy. As described in detail in Chapter 27, we are extensively involved in disseminating PE Program in several clinics that treat trauma survivors and examine the success of its dissemination.

REFERENCES

American Psychiatric Association (1980). *Diagnostic and Statistical Manual of Mental Disorders* (3rd ed.). Washington, D.C.: American Psychiatric Press.

Bandura, A., Blanchard, E.B. & Ritter, B. (1969). The relative efficacy of desensitization and modeling approaches for inducing behavioral, affective, and cognitive changes. *Journal of Personality and Social Psychology*, **13**, 173–199.

Beck, A.T., Emery, G. & Greenberg, R.L. (1985). *Anxiety Disorders and Phobias: A Cognitive Perspective*. New York: Basic Books.

Becker, C.B., Zayfert, C. & Anderson, E. (2004). A survey of psychologists' attitudes towards and utilization of exposure therapy for PTSD. *Behaviour Research and Therapy*, **42**, 277–292.

Bisson, J.I., Jenkins, P.L., Alexander, J. & Bannister, C. (1997). Randomized controlled trial of psychological debriefing for victims of acute burn trauma. *British Journal of Psychiatry*, **171**, 78–81.

Bisson, J.I., McFarlane, A.C. & Rose, S. (2000). Psychological debriefing. In *Effective Treatment for PTSD*, ed. E.B. Foa, T.M. Keane & M.J. Friedman, New York, NY: Guilford Press, pp. 39–59.

Black, J.L. & Keane, T.M. (1982). Implosive therapy in the treatment of combat related fears in a World War II veteran. *Journal of Behavior therapy and Experimental Psychiatry*, **13**, 163–165.

Blake, D.D., Weathers, F.W., Nagy, L.N., Kaloupek, D.G., Klauminser, G., Charney, D.S. & Keane, T.M. (1990). A clinician rating scale for assessing current and lifetime PTSD: The CAPS-1. *Behavior Therapist*, **18**, 187–188.

Blanchard, E.B., Hickling, E.J., Devineni, T., Veazey, C.H., Galovski, T.E., Mundy, E., Malta, L.S. & Buckley, T.C. (2003). A controlled evaluation of cognitive behavioral therapy for post-traumatic stress in motor vehicle accident survivors. *Behavior Research and Therapy*, **41**, 79–96.

Brom, D., Kleber, R.J. & Defares, P.B. (1989). Brief psychotherapy for post-traumatic stress disorder. *Journal of Consulting and Clinical Psychology*, **57**, 607–612.

Cahill, S.P., Hembree, E.A. & Foa, E.B. (this volume), Dissemination of prolonged exposure therapy for posttraumatic stress disorder: successes and challenges. In *9/11: Mental Health in The Wake of A Terrorist Attacks*. ed. Y. Neria, R. Gross & R. Marshall. Cambridge, UK: Cambridge University Press, 475–495.

Cahill, S.P., Carrigan, M.H. & Frueh, B.C. (1999). Does EMDR work? And if so, why? A critical review of controlled outcome and dismantling research. *Journal of Anxiety Disorders*, **13**, 5–33.

Cloitre, M., Koenen, K.C., Cohen, L.R. & Han, H. (2002). Skills training in affective and interpersonal regulation followed by exposure: A phase-based treatment for PTSD related to childhood abuse. *Journal of Consulting and Clinical Psychology*, **70**, 1067–1074.

Conlon, L., Fahy, T.J. & Conroy, R. (1999). PTSD in ambulant RTA victims: A randomized controlled trial of debriefing. *Journal of Psychosomatic Research*, **46**, 37–44.

Cooper, N.A. & Clum, G.A. (1989). Imaginal flooding as a supplementary treatment for PTSD in combat veterans: A controlled study. *Behavior Therapy*, **20**, 381–391.

Dollard, J. & Miller, N.E. (1950). *Personality and Psychotherapy; An Analysis in Terms of Learning, Thinking, and Culture*. New York: McGraw-Hill.

Ehlers A., Clark DM., Hackmann A., *et al.* (2003). A randomized controlled trial of cognitive therapy, a self-help booklet, and repeated assessments as early interventions for posttraumatic stress disorder. *Archives of General Psychiatry*; **60**, 1024–1032.

Emmelkamp, P.M.G. (1974). Self-observation versus flooding in the treatment of agoraphobia. *Behaviour Research and Therapy*, **12**, 229–237.

Emmelkamp, P.M.G. & Wessels, H. (1975). Flooding in imagination vs. flooding *in vivo*: A comparison with agoraphobics. *Behaviour Research and Therapy*, **13**, 7–16.

Everly, G.S., Flannery, R.B., Eyler, V. & Mitchell, J.T. (2001). Sufficiency analysis of an integrated multicomponent approach to crisis intervention: Critical incident stress management. *Advances in Mind Body Medicine*, **17**, 174–183.

Fairbank, J.A. & Keane, T.M. (1982). Flooding for combat-related stress disorders: Assessment of anxiety reduction across traumatic memories. *Behavior Therapy*, **13**, 499–510.

Fairbank, J.A., Gross, R.T. & Keane, T.M. (1983). Treatment of posttraumatic stress disorder: Evaluating outcome with a behavioral code. *Behavioral Modification*, **7**, 557–568.

Foa, E.B., (2003, May). *Treatment for PTSD: what do we know and what next?* Invited presentation at the 8th European Conference on Traumatic Stress, Berlin, Germany.

Foa, E.B. & Goldstein, A. (1978). Continuous exposure and complete response prevention in the treatment of obsessive-compulsive neurosis. *Behavior Therapy*, **9**, 821–829.

Foa, E.B. & Kozak, M.J. (1986). Emotional processing of fear: exposure to corrective information. *Psychological Bulletin*, **99**, 20–35.

Foa, E.B. & Meadows, E.A. (1997). Psychosocial treatments for post-traumatic stress disorder: a critical review. In *Annual Review of Psychology*, Vol. 48, Palo Alto, CA: Annual Reviews Inc. pp. 449–480.

Foa, E.B. & Rothbaum, B.O. (1998). *Treating the Trauma of Rape*. New York: Guilford.

Foa, E.B., Rothbaum, B. & Kozak, M.J. (1989). Behavioral treatments of anxiety and depression. In *Anxiety and Depression: Distinctive and Overlapping Features*, ed. P. Kendall & D. Watson, New York: Academic Press. pp. 413–454.

Foa, E.B., Steketee, G. & Rothbaum, B. (1989). Behavioral/cognitive conceptualizations of post-traumatic stress disorder. *Behavior Therapy*, **20**, 155–176.

Foa, E.B., Keane, T.M. & Friedman, M.J. (2000). *Effective Treatments for PTSD: Practice Guidelines from the International Society for Traumatic Stress Studies*. New York: Guilford.

Foa, E.B., Rothbaum, B.O. & Furr, J.M. (2003). Augmenting exposure therapy with other BT procedures. *Psychiatric Annals*, **33**, 47–53.

Foa, E.B., Rothbaum, B.O., Riggs, D.S. & Murdock, T. (1991). Treatment of post-traumatic stress disorder in rape victims: A comparison between cognitive-behavioral procedures and counseling. *Journal of Consulting and Clinical Psychology*, **59**, 715–723.

Foa, E.B., Franklin, M.E., Perry, K.J. & Herbert, J.D. (1996). Cognitive biases in generalized social phobia. *Journal of Abnormal Psychology*, **105**, 433–439.

Foa, E.B., Dancu, C.V., Hembree, E.A., Jaycox, L.H., Meadows, E.A. & Street, G. (1999). The efficacy of exposure therapy, stress inoculation training and their combination in ameliorating PTSD for female victims of assault. *Journal of Consulting and Clinical Psychology*, **67**, 194–200.

Freud, S. (1973). *The New Introductory Lectures in Psychoanalysis*. New York: Penguin.

Galea, S., Ahern, J., Resnick, H., Kilpatrick, D., Bucuvalas, M., Gold, J. & Vlahov, D. (2002). Psychological sequelae of the September 11 terrorist attacks in New York City. *New England Journal of Medicine*, **346**, 982–987.

Gillespie, K., Duffy, M., Hackmann, A. & Clark, D. M. (2002). Community based cognitive therapy in the treatment of posttraumatic stress disorder following the Omagh bomb. *Behaviour Research and Therapy*, **40**, 345–357.

Grinker, R.R. & Spiegel, J.P. (1944). Brief psychotherapy in war neuroses. *Psychosomatic Medicine*, **6**, 123–131.

Hobbs, M., Mayou, R., Harrison, B. & Worlock, P. (1996). A randomized controlled trial of psychological debriefing for victims of road traffic accidents. *British Medical Journal*, **313**, 1438–1439.

Horowitz, M.J., Wilner, N. & Alvarez, W. (1979). Impact of event scale: a measure of subjective stress. *Psychosomatic Medicine*, **41**, 209–218.

Hurst, A.F. (1919). Hysteria in the light of the experience of war. *Journal of Educational Research*, **20**, 771–774.

Keane, T.M. & Kaloupek, D.G. (1982). Imaginal flooding in the treatment of post-traumatic stress disorder. *Journal of Consulting and Clinical Psychology*, **50**, 138–140.

Keane, T.M., Zimering, R.T. & Caddell, J.M. (1985). A behavioral formulation of PTSD in Vietnam veterans. *Behavior Therapist*, **8**, 9–12.

Keane, T.M., Fairbank, J.A., Caddell, J.M. & Zimering, R.T. (1989). Implosive (flooding) therapy reduces symptoms of PTSD in Vietnam combat veterans. *Behavior Therapy*, **20**, 245–260.

Kipper, D.A. (1977). Behavior therapy for fears brought on by war experiences. *Journal of Consulting and Clinical Psychology*, **45**, 216–221.

Kraft, T. & Al-Issa, I. (1965). The application of learning theory to the treatment of traffic phobia. *British Journal of Psychiatry*, **111**, 277–279.

Krakow, B., Hollifield, M., Johnston, L., Koss, M., Schrader, R., Warner, T. D., Tandberg, D., Lauriello, J., McBride, L., Cutchen, L., Cheng, D., Emmons, S., Germain, A., Melendrez, D., Sandoval, D. & Prince, H. (2001). Imagery rehearsal therapy for chronic nightmares in sexual assault survivors with posttraumatic stress disorder: A randomized controlled trial. *Journal American Medical Association*, **286**, 537–545.

Kushner, M. (1965). Desensitization of a posttraumatic phobia. In *Case Studies in Behavior Modification*, ed. L.P. Ullmann & L. Krasner, New York: Holt, Rinehart & Winston. pp. 193–196.

Lange, A., van de Ven, J., Schrieken, B. & Emmelkamp, P.M. (2001). Treatment of posttraumatic stress through the Internet: A controlled trial. *Journal of Behavior Therapy and Experimental Psychiatry*, **32**, 73–90.

Lohr, J.M., Tolin, D.F. & Lilienfeld, S.O. (1998). Efficacy of eye movement desensitization and reprocessing: implications for behavior therapy. *Behavior Therapy*, **29**, 123–156.

Marks, I.M., Hodgson, R. & Rachman, S. (1975). Treatment of chronic obsessive-compulsive neurosis *in vivo* exposure, a 2 year follow-up and issues in treatment. *British Journal of Psychiatry*, **127**, 349–364.

Marks, I., Lovell, K., Noshirvani, H., Livanou, M. & Thrasher, S. (1998). Treatment of post-traumatic stress disorder by exposure and/or cognitive restructuring. *Archives of General Psychiatry*, **55**, 317–325.

Mathews, A.M., Johnston, D.W., Lancashire, M., Munby, M., Shaw, P.M. & Gelder, M.G. (1976). Imaginal flooding and exposure to real phobic situations: treatment outcome with agoraphobic patients. *British Journal of Psychiatry*, **129**, 362–371.

Mayou, R.A., Ehlers, A. & Hobbs, M. (2000). Psychological debriefing for road traffic accident victims: three year follow-up of a randomised controlled trial. *British Journal of Psychiatry*, **176**, 589–593.

McNally, R.J., Bryant, R.A. & Ehlers, A. (2003). Does early psychological intervention promote recovery from posttraumatic stress? *Psychological Science in the Public Interest*, **4**, 45–79.

Meichenbaum, D. (1974). *Cognitive Behavior Modification.* Morristown, NJ: General Learning Press.

Meichenbaum, D. & Cameron, R. (1972). Stress inoculation: a skills training approach to anxiety management (unpublished manuscript), University of Waterloo.

Meyer, V. (1966). Modification of expectations in cases with obsessional rituals. *Behaviour Research and Therapy*, **4**, 273–280.

Meyer, V., Levy, R. & Schnurer, A. (1974). A behavioral treatment of obsessive-compulsive disorders. In *Obsessional States,* ed. H.R. Beech, London: Methuen. pp. 223–258.

Olasov-Rothbaum, B. & Foa, E.B. (1983). Exposure treatment of PTSD concomitant with conversion mutism: A case study. *Behavior Therapy*, **22**, 449–456.

Paivio, S.C. & Nieuwenhuis, J.A. (2001). Efficacy of emotion focused therapy for adult survivors of child abuse: A preliminary study. *Journal of Traumatic Stress*, **14**, 115–133.

Paul, G.L. (1966). *Insight vs. Desensitization in Psychotherapy.* Stanford, CA: Stanford University Press.

Paunovic, N. & Ost, L.G. (2001). Cognitive-behavior therapy vs. exposure therapy in the treatment of PTSD in refugees. *Behaviour Research and Therapy*, **39**, 1183–1197.

Pitman, R.K., Orr, S.P., Altman, B., Longpre, R.E., Poire, R.E., Macklin, M.L., Michaels, M.J. & Steketee, G.S. (1996). Emotional processing and outcome of imaginal flooding therapy in Vietnam veterans with chronic posttraumatic stress disorder. *Comprehensive Psychiatry*, **37**, 409–418.

Rachman, S.J. (1978). *Fear and Courage.* W.H. Freeman, San Francisco, California.

Ranchman, S. (1980). Emotional processing. *Behaviour Research & Therapy*, **18**, 51–60.

Resick, P.A., Jordan, C.G., Girelli, S.A., Hutter, C.K. & Marhoefer-Dvorak, S. (1988). A comparative outcome study of group behavioral therapy for sexual assault victims. *Behavior Therapy*, **19**, 385–401.

Resick, P.A., Nishith, P., Weaver, T.L., Astin, M.C. & Feurer, C.A. (2002). A comparison of cognitive processing therapy with prolonged exposure and a waiting condition for the treatment of chronic posttraumatic stress disorder in female rape victims. *Journal of Consulting and Clinical Psychology*, **70**, 867–879.

Rivers, W.H.R. (1920). Repression and suppression. In *Functional Nerve Disease: An Epitome of War Experience for the Practitioner,* ed. H.C. Miller, London: Henry Frowde (and) Hodder & Stoughton, pp. 88–98.

Rose, S., Brewin, C.R., Andrews, B. & Kirk, M. (1999). A randomized controlled trial of individual psychological debriefing for victims of violent crime. *Psychological Medicine*, **29**, 793–799.

Rothbaum, B.O., Foa, E.B., Riggs, D.S., Murdock, T. & Walsh, W. (1992). A prospective examination of post-traumatic stress disorder in rape victims. *Journal of Traumatic Stress*, **5**, 455–475.

Saul, L.J., Rome, H. & Leuser, E. (1946). Desensitization of combat fatigue patients. *American Journal of Psychiatry*, **102**, 476–478.

Schlenger, W.E., Caddell, J.M., Ebert, L., Jordan, B.K., Rourke, K.M., Wilson, D., Thalji, L., Dennis, J.M., Fairbank, J.A. & Kulka, R.A. (2002). Psychological reactions to terrorist attacks: Findings from the National Study of Americans' Reactions to September 11. *Journal American Medical Association*, **288**, 581–588.

Schindler, F.E. (1980). Treatment by systematic desensitization of a recurring nightmare of a real life trauma. *Journal of Behavior Therapy & Experimental Psychiatry*, **11**, 53–54.

Shapiro, F. (1989). Efficacy of eye movement desensitization procedure in the treatment of traumatic memories. *Journal of Traumatic Stress*, **2**, 199–223.

Shapiro, F. (1991). Eye movement desensitization and reprocessing procedure: From EMD to EMDR: A new treatment model for anxiety and related traumata. *The Behavior Therapist*, **14**, 133–135.

Shapiro, F. (2001) *Eye Movement Desensitization and Reprocessing: Basic Principles, Protocols, and Procedures*, (2nd edn.). New York: The Guilford Press.

Suinn, R.M. & Richardson, F. (1971). Anxiety management training: A nonspecific behavior therapy program for anxiety control. *Behavior Therapy*, **2**, 498–510.

Tarrier, N., Pilgrim, H., Sommertield, C., *et al.* (1999). A randomized trial of cognitive therapy and imaginal exposure in the treatment of chronic posttraumatic stress disorder. *Journal of Consulting and Clinical Psychology*, **67**, 13–18.

Veronen, L.J. & Kilpatrick, D.G. (1983). Stress management for rape victims. In *Stress Reduction and Prevention*, ed. D. Meichenbaum & M.E. Jaremko, New York: Plenum Press, pp. 341–374.

Veronen, L.J., Kilpatrick, D.G. & Resick, P.A. (1978). Stress inoculation training for victims of rape. Paper presented at the *Association for Advancement of Behavior Therapy*, Chicago, November.

Wolff, R. (1977). Systematic desensitization and negative practice to alter the aftereffects of a rape attempt. *Journal of Behavior Therapy and Experimental Psychiatry*, **8**, 423–425.

Wolpe, J. (1958). *Psychotherapy by Reciprocal Inhibition.* Stanford, CA: Stanford University Press.

27

Dissemination of prolonged exposure therapy for posttraumatic stress disorder: successes and challenges

Shawn P. Cahill, Elizabeth A. Hembree and Edna B. Foa

The catastrophic events of September 11, 2001, significantly raised this country's interest in and concern about the psychological consequences of mass trauma and for good reason. Epidemiological studies conducted 1 to 2 months after 9/11 reported prevalence rates of posttraumatic stress disorder (PTSD) in Lower Manhattan of between 7–11% (Galea et al., 2002; Schlenger et al., 2002), a much higher figure than the 4% or less in the rest of the country (Schlenger et al., 2002). Other studies documented an increase in stress-related symptoms across the entire country in the immediate days and weeks after 9/11, although the prevalence of PTSD decreased substantially with distance from ground zero (Silver et al., 2002; Blanchard et al., 2004). In addition, there was a small, but statistically significant increase in the use of psychiatric medications among people living in Manhattan in the month following the attacks on the World Trade Center (Boscarino et al., 2003) and a substantial proportion (29%) of Manhattanites increased their use of alcohol, cigarettes, and marijuana 5–8 weeks later (Vlahov et al., 2002). Individuals who increased their substance use were more likely to experience PTSD and depression (Vlahov et al., 2002). These studies serve to illustrate the significant psychological impact even a single incident of terrorism can have and the need to have appropriate resources available to assist those who develop significant psychological difficulties in the aftermath of such an event.

There has been substantial progress over the last 15 years in the development and validation of effective psychological treatments for PTSD. Yet, as we will discuss later, the majority of mental health providers who treat trauma survivors are not trained in or do not use these empirically supported treatments for PTSD. The catastrophic events 9/11 therefore also serve to highlight the importance of wide dissemination of effective treatments in order to minimize the negative mental health consequences of such incidents. In the remainder of this chapter, we will provide a detailed description of one particular treatment program for PTSD, namely prolonged exposure (PE), summarize the research documenting its efficacy, and then discuss the results of our ongoing attempts to disseminate PE to community therapists and the obstacles we encountered in these efforts.

Description of prolonged exposure

The term *exposure therapy* is used here to refer to a general treatment strategy for reducing anxiety that involves confronting thoughts, situations, activities, and people that are feared and avoided although they are not inherently harmful. Exposure therapy can be conducted in imagination, where the patient is instructed to visualize the feared stimuli, or *in vivo*, where the patient actually confronts the feared stimuli in real life. Exposure therapy is an effective component of treatment for all of the anxiety disorders. The term PE is used here to refer to a specific treatment protocol that has been developed and evaluated as a treatment for PTSD (Foa *et al.*, 1991, 1999; Foa & Rothbaum, 1998). PE is typically administered in nine to twelve 90-minute sessions delivered once or twice weekly.

The first two sessions consist of patient education about the nature of trauma, common reactions to trauma, and factors that maintain posttrauma reactions; assessment of the patient's trauma history; providing a rationale for treatment by exposure; formalizing details about the treatment plan (e.g., creating a hierarchy of feared objects and situations); and training in controlled breathing. *In vivo* exposure is discussed in depth in Session 2 and the first *in vivo* homework assignment is conducted between Sessions 2 and 3. To monitor progress, the patient is instructed to indicate his/her level of anxiety at the beginning and end of each *in vivo* exposure exercise on a scale of subjective units of distress (SUDs) ranging from 0 to 100. Imaginal exposure (IE) is introduced in Session 3. During Sessions 3–5, IE is conducted in a manner that involves the patient describing the entire trauma memory from beginning to end. Patients are instructed to close their eyes, vividly imagine the traumatic event, and recount it in detail, including a description of what had happened as well as the thoughts and emotions they experienced during trauma. The IE is conducted in session for 30–60 minutes and is tape recorded each time for the patient to listen to their story as part of daily homework. The therapist asks the patients to indicate his/hers SUDs levels approximately every 5 minutes throughout IE. Beginning in Session 5 or 6, IE is altered to focus on one or more specific "hotspots" within the overall trauma narrative. By this point in therapy, most patients have experienced some reduction in their anxiety while telling the story, but there usually remain one or a couple of specific points during the trauma narrative that are more distressing than the rest, which we refer to as hotspots. IE is focused repetitively on these hotspots, one at a time, until anxiety to the hotspot is substantially reduced. In the last session, IE involves putting the trauma story back together again and telling the narrative from beginning to end.

At the end of each IE session, the therapist spends 15–20 minutes discussing with the patient his or her experiences during the imaginal reliving of the trauma, including new information or insights that emerged from this experience. This part of the session, called processing, aims at helping the patient to integrate the new information and insights into their memory, thus attaining a more constructive perspective about the trauma. A detailed description of the treatment is found in Foa and Rothbaum (1998).

Efficacy of prolonged exposure and related programs for chronic PTSD

We at the Center for the Treatment and Study of Anxiety (CTSA) have been studying PE for PTSD since the mid-1980s and have completed three outcome studies of this treatment among women assault victims with chronic PTSD (Foa *et al.*, 1991, 1999, 2005). In addition, we have developed and tested a brief treatment, consisting of only four sessions of cognitive behavior therapy (CBT), to be administered starting within 2–4 weeks of a trauma as a method to speed natural recovery (Foa *et al.*, 1995, in Press).

In our first treatment outcome study, we found PE and another form of CBT, stress inoculation training (SIT; Meichenbaum, 1974; Veronen & Kilpatrick, 1983), to be more effective in treating PTSD than waitlist, while supportive counseling (SC) was not more effective than waitlist (Foa *et al.*, 1991). In addition, there was some evidence that SIT was superior to PE immediately after treatment, while the opposite appeared to be case at 3-month follow-up. Foa *et al.* (1991) interpreted this pattern of differential outcome to suggest that the two treatments may operate through distinct mechanisms and that combining the two treatments would optimize outcome. This hypothesis was tested in our second study by comparing the outcome of patients randomized to PE alone, SIT alone, the combination of PE and SIT, and waitlist control (WL) (Foa *et al.*, 1999). On the whole, all three active treatments were very effective whereas the waitlist condition was not. Contrary to expectations, we did not replicate the differential effects of PE and SIT at post-treatment or follow-up. Instead, regardless of whether assessments were at post-treatment or follow-up, PE was found superior to SIT on some measures while on other measures the two treatments did not differ from one another. Also contrary to expectation, there was no evidence that combining PE and SIT improved outcome. However, equating treatments on variables such as treatment length and time with therapist made PE/SIT a fairly demanding treatment for both patient and therapist: patients engaged in IE for the same amount of time as did the patients in PE alone, followed by instruction and practice of each coping skill of SIT. Thus the PE/SIT sessions were jam-packed with tasks and therapists reported that they sometimes sensed "information overload" in patients. It is possible that this format decreased efficacy of the combined treatment. But not all patients that received PE do well and augmentation strategies are still relevant.

Therefore, in our third study, we compared PE alone to a program that included PE and cognitive restructuring (CR), which we thought to be the most vital or important ingredient of SIT, thus reducing the complexity of the combined treatment. To test the hypothesis that the simplified combined treatment would augment the efficacy of PE alone, we randomly assigned women with PTSD to PE alone, PE combined with CR, or WL. Results showed that PE and PE/CR were highly and equally effective at reducing PTSD and depression, and anxiety compared to waitlist. As in the earlier study, combined treatment was not superior to PE alone (Foa *et al.*, 2002a, b). Similar results were reported by Paunovic and Ost (2001) who also compared PE with PE plus CR and found that both treatments produced significant improvement, but PE/CR was not superior to PE alone.

Resick *et al.* (2002) compared PE with cognitive processing therapy (CPT), a form of cognitive therapy originally developed for rape survivors (Resick & Schnicke, 1992) that focuses on the themes of safety, trust, power, esteem, and intimacy. Because Resick and Schnicke considered it important that rape survivors feel the emotions associated with the assault, CPT also includes an exposure component of repeated writing and reading the trauma narrative. This exercise was designed to encourage expression of affect and to ensure that all the important trauma-related feelings and associated beliefs would be elicited. Resick *et al.* (2002) found that, compared to waitlist, both PE and CPT produced large improvement in PTSD severity and depression, and there were no significant differences between groups on these measures.

Rothbaum (2005) compared PE with eye movement desensitization and reprocessing (EMDR). Results revealed that, compared to waitlist, both treatments produced significant improvement in PTSD, depression, and anxiety. Although the treatments did not differ at the posttreatment assessment, PE was superior to EMDR on a composite measure of good and state functioning at 6-month follow-up.

Marks *et al.* (1998) also developed and tested an exposure therapy protocol that combined imaginal and *in vivo* exposure. However, in contrast to PE where the two modalities were administered simultaneously, they were administered sequentially in the Marks *et al.* protocol. The first five sessions were confined to in-session IE and corresponding homework, followed by five sessions of in-session, therapist assisted *in vivo* exposure, and corresponding homework. Patients in this study, whose PTSD resulted from a variety of traumas, were randomized to exposure alone, CR alone, combined exposure and CR, or relaxation training. They found that exposure, CR, and the combination of exposure and CR were highly and equally effective and were superior to relaxation. Follow-up evaluations conducted 3 and 6 months after treatment indicated that patients treated with exposure, either alone or in combination with CR, continued to show decline in PTSD symptoms over time at a greater rate than those treated with CR alone. Taylor *et al.* (2003) utilized an eight-session variation of the Marks *et al.* (1998) exposure therapy protocol (four sessions devoted to each to imaginal and *in vivo* exposure) and compared it with EMDR and relaxation. Significant improvement was obtained in all three groups. Exposure therapy was found to be significantly superior to relaxation, whereas EMDR did not differ from either relaxation or exposure therapy.

Prevention of chronic PTSD/treatment of acute stress disorder

Brief (i.e., four to five sessions) CBT beginning approximately 2 weeks after the trauma has been shown in several studies to either speed the rate of recovery (Foa *et al.*, 1995, in press) and prevent the development of chronic PTSD (Bryant *et al.*, 1998, 1999, 2003). For the most part, CBT in these studies consisted of a combination of PE plus elements of SIT. In the first study, Foa *et al.* (1995) administered four 90-minute sessions of CBT to a group of female sexual and non-sexual assault victims meeting symptom criteria for PTSD. Results indicated that treatment accelerated participants' speed of recovery. Specifically, 2 months after the assault, only one of the ten (10%) participants in the treatment group met criteria for PTSD, which was significantly less than the seven out of ten (70%) women in a matched comparison group who simply underwent repeated assessments. Three months later, however, one of the nine CBT participants who completed the follow-up met criteria for PTSD (11%), which was not different from two of the nine control participants (22%) who were also reached for follow-up. In a replication and extension of this study, Foa *et al.* (in press), found that female survivors of sexual assault who received brief CBT had a greater decrease in self-reported PTSD severity and a trend toward lower anxiety immediately after treatment than participants who received SC. At 3-month follow-up, participants in the CBT condition evidenced lower general anxiety than those in the SC condition and a trend toward lower self-reported PTSD severity. However, at the last available follow-up, no differences were detected between brief CBT and SC, and neither condition was different from an assessment only comparison group.

Using a modified version of the Foa *et al.* (1995) CBT program, Bryant *et al.* (1998, 1999, 2003) conducted three studies investigating the efficacy of five 90-minute sessions of CBT compared to SC among individuals meeting criteria for acute stress disorder (ASD) subsequent to motor vehicle and industrial accidents and non-sexual assault. Harvey and Bryant (1998) had previously found that 78% of motor vehicle accident victims who met full diagnostic criteria for ASD immediately after the trauma met criteria for PTSD 6 months later, as did 60% of participants who were classified as "sub-clinical" ASD, which contrasted with only 4.3% of participants who did not meet the criteria for either classification. Across the three treatments studies by Bryant and colleagues, between 8–20% of participants receiving CBT met criteria for PTSD at end of treatment and between 17–23% at 6-month follow-up, compared to between 56–83% immediately following SC and 58–67% at 6-month follow-up. In addition, Bryant *et al.* (1999) compared the full CBT program with five sessions of just the PE elements of the treatment and found no differences between them. Thus, as with studies of chronic PTSD, both exposure therapy alone and in combination with anxiety management is an effective treatment, and there is no apparent benefit of a combined treatment program compared to exposure therapy alone.

Availability of exposure therapy: the need for and barriers to dissemination

The existence of effective treatments for PTSD such as PE and other forms of CBT is of little benefit to consumers of mental health services unless mental health care providers are trained in and use these treatments. Becker *et al.* (2004) surveyed a large sample of psychologists regarding whether they have treated patients with PTSD, whether they were trained in and used IE with their PTSD patients and, if not, their reasons for not using IE. The most common theoretical orientations of respondents were eclectic (37%), psychodynamic/analytic (28%), behavioral/cognitive-behavioral (21%), and cognitive (9%). Sixty-three percent of the sample reported having treated more than 11 patients with PTSD, yet only 27% of the sample had been trained in the use of IE for PTSD. Given that the efficacy of exposure therapy in treating other anxiety conditions has been known since the end of the 1960s, (phobias, social anxiety, obsessive-compulsive disorder), it is important to note that even fewer respondents (12%) had been trained in the use of IE in the treatment of other anxiety disorders. Only 9% of respondents reported using IE with the majority of their patients with PTSD. Thus, not only are the majority of therapists who see patients with PTSD not trained in the use of exposure therapy, even fewer regularly use exposure therapy to treat PTSD. Why is that?

The three most frequently endorsed reasons for not using exposure therapy to treat PTSD were lack of training (60%), resistance to using manualized treatments (25%), and fears that patients would decompensate from the treatment (22%). Although we are not aware of similar surveys with regard to other specific empirically supported treatments for PTSD, such as CPT and SIT, it is likely that their use is equally limited by lack of training and clinicians negative attitude towards manualized treatment. The third factor, safety, is of course an extremely important issue for any treatment, although this concern seems to get raised more frequently regarding exposure therapy than for other treatments for PTSD. Thus, the question is not simply whether there are risks associated with the use of exposure therapy for PTSD, but how those risks compare to other treatments for PTSD as well as how those risks compare to withholding treatment.

Evaluating the safety of exposure therapy for PTSD

Until recently, the primary evidence offered in support of concerns about the safety of exposure therapy has been a widely cited case series in which Pitman *et al.* (1991) described six cases in which symptom exacerbation were noted taken from an ongoing treatment trial of IE therapy for PTSD among veterans (see Pitman *et al.*, 1996). However, the study from which the case series was obtained did not include a control condition. Therefore, it is unknown how many veterans would have experienced an acute exacerbation of their symptoms during the study period had they not received treatment. Moreover, each of the patients received some additional treatment (e.g., medication, additional psychotherapy) after their treatment with exposure therapy and showed improvement. Because all of the patients were in the Veterans Administration (VA) system before receiving PE, and presumably had been treated with routine treatments without much improvement, it is possible that PE actually enhanced the responsiveness to the subsequent treatment.

More recently, Tarrier *et al.* (1999) conducted a randomized-controlled trial comparing IE with cognitive therapy and reported that, despite overall comparable outcome on measures of PTSD prevalence and severity, anxiety, and depression, significantly more patients treated with IE (31%) showed "symptom worsening" over the course of the study compared to cognitive therapy (9%). Taken on face value, these data would seem to support concerns about the safety of exposure therapy in the treatment of PTSD. However, several considerations caution such a conclusion. First, the operational definition of symptom worsening was a post-treatment PTSD severity score greater than the corresponding pretreatment score by one or more points and Tarrier *et al.* did not report the mean increase in PTSD severity scores. Given that an increase of just one point is easily within the measurement error of the instrument (the Clinician Administered PTSD Scale), it is not clear whether this index reflects actual symptom worsening or is better thought of as a measure failure to improve (see Devilly & Foa, 2001 for an extended discussion). Second, Tarrier *et al.* did not include a waitlist condition, therefore it is not possible to determine whether the observed rates of symptom worsening/failure to improve observed in the IE condition represents an increase, decrease, or no change from what would have been observed had treatment been withheld. Third, the question must be raised as to whether the Tarrier *et al.* (1999) results can be generalized to other samples and other measures of psychopathology that are correlated with PTSD (i.e., depression, general anxiety).

Subsequent research has failed to support the potential concerns about the safety of exposure therapy raised by the Tarrier *et al.* study. Cloitre *et al.* (2002) investigated the efficacy of a treatment that sequentially combines skills training in affect and interpersonal regulation (STAIR), based on principles of Dialectical Behavior Therapy (Linehan, 1993), with IE to treat PTSD in women victims of childhood abuse. Applying the Tarrier *et al.* definition of symptom worsening, Cloitre and colleagues reported that 4.5% of patients receiving STAIR/IE had some increase in PTSD severity following treatment compared to 25% in the waitlist comparison group. While limitations on the design of this study preclude conclusions about whether or not the low rate of symptom worsening can be attributed to treatment with STAIR prior to administering exposure, the results do illustrate that treatment with exposure therapy does not necessarily result high rates of symptom worsening. Taylor *et al.* (2003) also investigated symptom worsening following treatment in their study comparing imaginal plus *in vivo* exposure with EMDR and relaxation. Rates of symptoms worsening were uniformly low across conditions (0%, 7%, and 7% respectively).

We (Cahill *et al.*, 2003) recently analyzed data from the Foa *et al.* (1999) study of PE vs. SIT vs. PE/SIT vs. waitlist and our recently completed comparing PE alone vs. PE with CR (PE/CR) vs. waitlist (Foa *et al.*, 2005). Across 162 participants who completed one of active treatments, only one person (0.6%) showed symptom worsening defined as an increase in PTSD severity by one or more points on the PTSD Symptom Scale – Interview (PSSI), our primary outcome measure. Interestingly, that one person had received the PE/SIT combination, not PE alone. In the waitlist conditions, three out of 39 participants (7.7%) showed symptom worsening. Cahill and colleagues also investigated symptom worsening across self-report measures of depression and general anxiety. Only 6 out of 159[1] participants receiving active treatment (3.8%) showed an increase on depression, compared to 11 out of 36 waitlist participants (30.6%). For general anxiety, the corresponding numbers were 12 out of 159 active treatment participants (7.5%) and 13 out of 34 waitlist participants (38.2%). Combining across measures, there were a total of 16 out of 159 active treatment participants (10.1%) who showed worsening on one or more measures, compared to 20 out of 35 waitlist participants (57.1%). Across the active treatments, rates of symptom worsening on at least one of the three measures were 6.8% for PE alone, 10.5% for PE/CR, and 27.3 for PE/SIT.

The results from the studies by Cloitre and colleagues and Taylor and colleagues, along with the analyses from two of our studies all found low rates of symptom

---

[1] Three participants completed PSSI but did not complete self-report measures of anxiety and depression, thus accounting for the discrepancy between the sample sizes for the PSSI ($N = 162$) and the sample size for the measures of depression and anxiety ($N = 159$).

worsening associated with treatment, regardless of the type of treatment and failed to support the hypothesis that exposure therapy was associated with a greater risk of symptom worsening than other treatments (Cloitre *et al.*, 2002; Taylor *et al.*, 2003). Indeed, the studies that included WLs would suggest that, if anything, it is withholding treatment that is associated with symptom worsening. None of these analyses takes into consideration that an increase of just a single point or even a few points could reflect measurement error, rather than actual worsening of symptoms. Therefore, Cahill *et al.* also investigated instances of "reliable" symptom worsening, defined as an increase from pre to posttreatment that was as large or larger than the standard error of the difference between two measurements (*cf.* Devilly & Foa, 2001). Across all measures, there were 19 instances of symptoms worsening, defined as at least a one-point increase, among participants receiving an active treatment. Six of those instances (32%) met the criteria for reliable symptom worsening, one person in each of the PE, PE/CR, and SIT conditions and three in PE/SIT. In the waitlist conditions, there were 27 instances of worsening by at least one point, 9 of which (33.3%) met criteria for reliable worsening.

In summary, the primary evidence used to support concerns about the safety of exposure therapy for PTSD have been cases studied from Pitman *et al.* (1991) and the Tarrier *et al.* (1999) results, neither of which included an appropriate comparison condition to determine how frequently symptom worsening occurred when treatment was withheld. Other investigations have failed to replicate the high rate of symptom worsening observed in the Tarrier *et al.* exposure therapy condition and have not found exposure therapy to be associated with higher rates of symptom worsening than other forms of treatment. In addition, studies that included waitlist conditions found that, if anything, withholding treatment was associated with increased risk for symptom worsening. Finally, the analysis by Cahill *et al.* found that even when "symptom worsening" was observed, the increase was generally small and easily within the margin of measurement error. The frequency of a significant exacerbation in symptoms was in fact relatively rare, even in the waitlist conditions.

Evaluating efforts to disseminate CBT for PTSD

Clinicians commonly report that although they are attracted by the efficacy and efficiency of exposure therapy, and are interested in using it with their PTSD patients, they are also concerned about being able to implement it independently. We have trained many professionals of various disciplines in workshops. With few exceptions, training time in these workshops vary from 2 hours to 2 days. We are fairly certain that a sizable number of these clinicians do not end up using PE in their practices. Many clinicians commented that although the workshops were quite informative, their confidence at implementing PE would be increased by extending the workshops.

Even many of those who received an extended workshop (3–5 days) expressed a desire for ongoing consultation or supervision by knowledgeable clinicians.

In many cases, we concur. An intensive workshop is often adequate training for clinicians who are already trained in CBT strategies and who have been using it for other disorders in general and for anxiety disorders such as phobias and panic disorder in particular. These clinicians are often already grounded conceptually and experientially in the exposure model of treatment and can readily apply the principles and the procedures to PTSD patients. But for those who have been trained in very different models of therapy – psychodynamic, systems, SC – learning to apply PE in their practices frequently involves thinking and working with patients in a whole new way.

This can be challenging even for seasoned therapists, and many clinicians would be more comfortable learning to use PE with their first few cases while under expert supervision. This is because PE, like other CBT treatment programs, differs from traditional therapies in several important ways. First, CBT programs focus on reducing specific symptoms whereas the focus of other types of therapies may be on processes such as therapist–patients relationship, or on providing support to the patient in order to increase immediate comfort level. Second, the agenda of CBT sessions is largely defined by therapists, whereas in traditional therapies the treatment agenda is often dictated by the patient. Third, many CBT programs, including PE, follow detailed protocols that specify the content and the techniques that are utilized in each session, whereas traditional therapies do not follow specific protocols. Thus, non-CBT therapists need to learn not only how to conduct imaginal and *in vivo* exposure, but also how to take an active role in implementing the protocol and preventing the patients from setting their own agenda, how to instruct patients in doing home exercises, etc.

As reviewed above, the efficacy and efficiency of PE has been demonstrated in numerous studies both in the USA and abroad. Therefore, the next crucial task is to develop and test models of training and dissemination of PE to clinicians working in community settings. Based on our own work and a review of the literature, two dissemination models have emerged. In the first model, experts provide intensive training and direct, ongoing supervision of the therapists that will be administering the treatment. In the second model, experts provide the intensive initial training of the therapists but ongoing supervision of the therapists and initial training of new therapists is provided by local supervisors, who with time become experts themselves.

Model I: Intensive initial training of therapists followed by ongoing expert supervision

We recently completed a study (Foa *et al.*, 2005) that utilized this model to disseminate PE with and without CR to two community-based clinics in Philadelphia: women organized against rape (WOAR), a clinic whose mission includes support and treatment of sexual assault victims, and the sexual assault counseling and education (SACE) division of Temple University's Counseling Center. Prior to our involvement with WOAR and SACE, their treatments consisted of individual and group SC, which was present-focused and aimed at helping sexual assault victims cope with their reactions to the trauma and their daily-life stressors. Group therapy, in which 5–8 women were seen in closed groups that ran for 10 weeks, utilized social support, normalization of reactions to assault, and exercises designed to heal and empower the group members.

The community therapists who participated in this first dissemination study were women with Master's degrees in counseling or social work. They had all been working with survivors of sexual assault for several years, and were extremely committed and active advocates for women rape victims. None were previously trained in cognitive behavioral interventions and none had prior research skills or experience in delivering manualized treatment protocols. In fact, some of them were outspoken about their reservations regarding the ethics of doing research with rape victims and were initially reluctant to use manualized treatments with their clients. Interestingly, they were not opposed to the concept of using exposure therapy with rape survivors: they accepted the notion that confronting painful memories, images, and feelings promotes healing.

In the first step of our dissemination of PE to WOAR and SACE, CTSA experts provided the community therapists with a 5-day intensive workshop. In the first day, participants were provided with background into the theory and efficacy data supporting the use of PE in the treatment of PTSD. In the remaining days, they were provided with instruction in the administration of PE interventions. The second and third days were devoted to teaching and practicing how to deliver the overall rationale for the treatment, rationales for imaginal and *in vivo* exposure, and how to implement the two forms of exposure. This was done via detailed instructions of "how to do it", watching excerpts from videotapes of expert therapists demonstrating each aspect of PE, and role plays in small groups. Therapists were also trained in how to treat patients who present with under-engagement or over-engagement with the traumatic memory (i.e., portraying too little or too much distress during reliving of the traumatic memory), how to address motivational problems such as non-compliance with homework instructions, and how to address therapists' distress and fatigue. A second week of intensive training was devoted to CR and was conducted by Dr. David M. Clark of London, England, and the CTSA experts. This training in how to implement CR was tailored to working with trauma survivors and began with a detailed theoretical presentation of the profound impact trauma has on the survivor's thoughts and beliefs about the self, others, and the world. It is important to note that an integral part of our training has been to familiarize the clinicians with assessment tools to measure PTSD and related symptoms before and after treatment in order to evaluate the results of the treatment and to emphasize the importance of such assessment.

Each therapist then completed at least two training cases under intense supervision by a CTSA supervisor. Supervision was conducted weekly for 3 hours by CTSA experts on the premises of the community sites. All therapists working in the study attended the supervision sessions, in which each ongoing case was discussed, and videotapes of that week's therapy sessions were viewed. After completion of the training cases, female sexual assault victims seeking services through the usual referral networks were invited to participate in a study that involved random assignment to treatment with nine to twelve sessions of PE alone, PE combined with CR, or to waitlist followed by active treatment with PE or PE/CR. For the first 2 years of the study, the CTSA experts conducted 2-day booster workshop every 6 months in which all therapists from both community clinics presented cases and videotapes of therapy sessions. Throughout the course of the 6-year study, a CTSA supervisor continued to provide weekly supervision to the WOAR and SACE therapists as described above.

In parallel fashion, participants were also recruited through the CTSA and randomly assigned to PE, PE/CR, or WL provided by CTSA therapists with expertise in CBT for PTSD. The CTSA therapists also participated in weekly supervision that included discussing ongoing cases and viewing the videotapes of therapy sessions. Indeed, the supervision established at WOAR and SACE was modeled after our standard supervision practices at the CTSA. As noted above in the section on the efficacy of PE, the results from this study revealed that, compared to WL, both treatments were very effective in reducing symptoms of PTSD and depression. Also, contrary to expectations, PE/CR was not superior to PE alone. Of greatest relevance to evaluating our success at disseminating PE, comparisons between participants seen at the CTSA with those seen in the community settings indicated that both samples were similar in their pretreatment levels of PTSD and depression and, most importantly, there were no differences in treatment outcome between the two sites. On average, participants treated by community therapists under CTSA supervision showed the same reduction in symptoms as participants treated by CTSA expert therapists.

We are currently conducting two additional dissemination studies in Philadelphia. The first study is a continuation of the work with WOAR therapists in which the weekly supervision by CTSA experts has been replaced with supervision by one of WOAR's senior clinical staff members who was a therapist in the previous study and thus was supervised by the CTSA experts. The aim of this research is to determine whether therapists at WOAR can maintain adherence to the treatment protocol without intensive involvement of experts and to compare the outcome they achieve with internal supervision to that achieved with intensive expert supervision in the previous dissemination stage. In the second study, the basic training and intensive supervision procedures that were given to WOAR are being replicated with another community mental health agency, the Joseph J. Peters Institute. If the initial dissemination to this new clinic is successful, we will withdraw expert supervision in order to examine the ability of the agency to maintain their level of treatment adherence and outcome with internal supervision.

In another application of this model, several members of the CTSA were involved with training a group of New York City therapists in the use of PE for individuals suffering significant symptoms of PTSD after the attacks on the World Trade Center. This training was part of a larger program sponsored by the New York Times Foundation to bring in a variety of experts in trauma and PTSD to provide therapists in New York City familiarity with a variety of treatment modalities for PTSD and other psychological difficulties (e.g., complicated bereavement). In addition, we conducted a collaborative research project with the Mount Sinai School of Medicine designed to compare the efficacy of a brief course of PE (four sessions) to that of SC. The study lasted approximately 1 year, with data collection beginning in January of 2002. The therapy sessions were video or audiotaped and supervisors from the CTSA reviewed each tape and provided therapists with weekly supervision conducted through weekly telephone calls and frequent trips (approximately every 2 to 3 weeks) to New York for direct group supervision where videotapes of therapy sessions were viewed and discussed. Assessments were conducted before and after treatment and at follow-up. While data analyses have not been completed, the clinical impression of the CTSA supervisors is that both brief interventions seemed to be quite effective in alleviating PTSD symptoms and associated depression.

An ongoing multi-site study that compares PE to present centered SC. PCT is being conducted within the Cooperative Studies Program of the VA by Paula P. Schnurr, Ph.D., Matthew J. Friedman, M.D., Ph.D., and Charles C. Engel, M.D., M.P.H. The purpose of this study is to evaluate the efficacy of these treatments in ameliorating PTSD and associated problems in female veterans and active duty military personnel. Our role in this study is to train and supervise the therapists who provide PE. Here again, the model for training was an intensive 5-day training workshop for a group of 25 therapists who were designated to administer the PE treatment, followed by ongoing supervision of training and study cases by PE experts. Supervisors watch session videotapes and provide the therapists regular feedback and supervision via telephone. No data are yet available on the outcome of this study.

A similar model for training therapists to provide cognitive therapy based on Ehlers's and Clark's (2000) model of PTSD was utilized by Gillespie *et al.* (2002) for survivors of the 1998 car bombing of Omagh in Northern Ireland. Shortly after the bombing, community therapists were given intensive training in this form of cognitive therapy, which includes exposure therapy and behavioral experiments in addition to more traditional cognitive therapy techniques. The five study therapists came from varying backgrounds (psychiatry, nursing, and social work) and none had previously specialized in psychological trauma. Initial training consisted of three steps. First, there were several phone consultations with David M. Clark to identify key therapeutic procedures and discuss how they were to be applied to the current circumstances. Second, there was a lecture on PTSD and cognitive models of PTSD. Third, Dr. Clark and his colleagues conducted a 2-day workshop in Omagh. In addition regular ongoing supervision was provided locally by a CBT expert (Gillespie) and by Clark and colleagues via teleconferencing technology once every 4–6 weeks. Although the treatment permitted flexibility in the total number of sessions, the median number of sessions was eight and 76% of participants completed treatment within 15 sessions. On average, participants displayed a 64% reduction in PTSD severity, ranging between 20–100% reduction. These results are comparable to those obtained in a randomized-controlled trial completed by Ehlers *et al.* (2003).

In summary, the existing evidence suggests a dissemination model that includes an intensive several day workshop and ongoing supervision by experts on CBT for PTSD can be quite effective. Indeed, it has been heartening to witness the natural ripple effect that our work at WOAR has had in the Philadelphia rape-treatment community. PE has been adopted as one of the primary treatment interventions for survivors of rape and childhood sexual abuse at WOAR and the therapists and administrators who were originally trained for the dissemination study have continued training community clinicians in the use of PE. The WOAR clinicians have become staunch PE advocates and educators. In fact, when experts in the CTSA developed a PE protocol for children, WOAR clinicians immediately began to use it with their sexually abused clients and are currently collecting data on the efficacy of this treatment. In an initial group of seven children (ages 7–15 years) treated with the pediatric PE manual, five showed clinically meaningful improvement, with an overall average of 58% reduction in PTSD symptom severity. However, formal evaluation of the protocol in the context of a randomized-controlled study has yet to be conducted. Therapists at WOAR also took the initiative to have the PE manual translated into Spanish, and used the translated manual to train local Latino community therapists so that Spanish-speaking clients can also benefit from this treatment. They have even developed and begun using a PE intervention program for incarcerated women with PTSD.

While it has been very gratifying to see this outgrowth, our experience is that the method of disseminating PE we used in community settings in Philadelphia is labor intensive and requires the proximity of the expert site in order to provide the training for an extended period of time. This requirement combined with the high cost of such intense and long expert supervision may limit the practicality of this training model.

Model II: Intensive initial training of therapists and a local supervisor

A second model of treatment dissemination aims at reducing experts' involvement in the dissemination process, thus not only limiting costs, but also enabling dissemination to places that do not have access to local experts. In this model, community clinicians come to train in expert clinics for various length of time, with the expectation that they will go back to their communities where they will train and supervise local clinicians in the delivery of CBT treatments, but no efforts were made to systematically follow-up and evaluate the success of this dissemination method. At the same time, experts provide workshops outside their city on CBT treatments of anxiety disorders. To our knowledge, no systematic evaluation has been conducted about the impact of the training and the workshops on treatment delivery.

A more systematic dissemination program has been instituted in Israel in the past 2 years. As in other countries, over the years one of us (EBF) has delivered numerous workshops on PE in Israel, varying from 3 hours to 2 days, with no efforts to evaluate the impact of these workshops. After the onset of the *Aktza Intifada* at the end of September 2000, and with the increased number of victims exposed to terrorists attacks or combat, the interest in training therapists to deliver effective short-term treatment for PTSD has increased significantly, and this interest has taken two forms. First, clinicians working in treatment centers for recent victims of terrorist attacks and/or patients with combat-related PTSD have applied for training at the CTSA, lasting between 2 to 5 weeks. Second, organizations (e.g., hospitals, universities, the Joint Distribution Committee) and government institutions (e.g., the Ministry of Defense) sponsored 3–5 day workshops for clinicians whose work focuses on trauma related psychological disturbance, with an emphasis on PTSD.

In the remainder of this section, we describe these dissemination efforts by discussing in detail the program that has been sponsored by the Joint Distribution Committee under the direction of Dr. Ruth Ragulant-Levy. The Joint Distribution Committee is an American Jewish charitable organization that funds a number of aid programs. The program to disseminate PE was built in part on our accumulation of experiences described previously with the training of therapists at WOAR, the New York therapists following 9/11, and the ongoing VA study. The training sponsored by the Joint Distribution Committee began in July, 2002, with a 5-day workshop for 35 therapists who work in clinical centers for trauma victims (e.g, the PTSD unit in the Israel Defense Forces (IDF), social security clinics, hospitals). Five trainers participated in the workshops, two faculty of the CTSA, and three clinicians who had been trained at the CTSA in PE for various lengths of time prior to the workshop. The content and form of the workshops were based on those used in training therapists at WOAR, New York, and the VA.

After the workshops, three supervision groups were formed, one in Hadassah hospital in Jerusalem; one in Tel Hashomer, a hospital near Tel Aviv; and one in the Kiriat Shmona Trauma Center, situated near the northern borders with Lebanon. The Hadassah and Tel Hashomer groups were supervised by a clinician who previously trained at the CTSA. Dr. Yadin from the CTSA supervised the Kiriat Shmona group via weekly teleconferences. Six months after the 5-day workshop, there was a 2-day meeting with the original participants, where videotapes and audiotapes from PE sessions were presented and discussed by a CTSA expert (EBF). The supervision groups meet regularly to date, viewing tapes and discussing the patients' treatment plans and progress. Although we remain available for consultation to the supervisors on an as-needed basis, our involvement as consultants at this point has been very limited. In July 2003, again under the auspices of the Joint Distribution Committee, two experts from the CTSA, with the help of two Israeli psychologists who had been trained in the CTSA, replicated the 5-day workshop with 35 additional therapists who work in Afula Hospital, which serves many victims of terrorists attacks. Two clinicians, a psychologist and a psychiatrist from the army who participated in the first 5-day and have treated a number of PTSD patients with PE, recently received 3-weeks training at the CTSA with the goal of becoming the supervisors of the Afula group.

Results from the first 10 patients treated by the Tel Hashomer group were presented in the Annual Meeting of the Israeli Psychiatric Association (Nacasch *et al.*, 2003). Patients were all men, most had chronic PTSD related to combat, some had suffered from PTSD symptoms for 30 years and were in psychiatric treatment for many years with no or little improvement. After 10–12 sessions of PE, the mean reduction of symptoms was 58%. The outcome was quite impressive and is comparable to that of our clinic and at WOAR with women victims of sexual and nonsexual assault. Thus, although our experience with this second dissemination method is more limited at this point, preliminary results attests to its success. We hope that this model will provide a solution to the limitations noted of the first model, particularly with regard to creating a local culture of expertise, training, and supervision that will be able to be sustained without extensive involvement with outside experts.

Summary and conclusions

While the catastrophic events of September 11, 2001, may have heightened general awareness about the consequences of mass trauma, it has specifically heightened our awareness of the need for effective dissemination of empirically supported treatments for PTSD. Our research group together with other research groups in the USA, Canada, the UK, the Netherlands, and Australia have built a solid data base demonstrating the efficacy of cognitive behavior therapies across a wide range of trauma populations (e.g., veterans, crime victims, accident survivors; see also Foa & Cahill, this volume). However, these treatments are not yet widely available to consumers of mental health services. Three factors that contribute to the unavailability of empirically supported treatments for PTSD. First and foremost is lack of training. Although, as noted above, members of the CTSA faculty regularly offer 1- and 2-day workshops in the use of PE for PTSD, our strong impression is that such trainings serve to heighten many therapists interest in PE, but neither they nor we feel such training is generally adequate to learn how to effectively implement PE. Indeed, in our dissemination research where we have obtained positive results, the level of initial training and ongoing supervision has been far more extensive than a 2-day workshop. We are actively studying methods to disseminate PE to a variety of different agencies in order to develop a model that is both effective and efficient. The method of intensively training therapists and providing ongoing supervision over an extended period of time has proven effective, but is very time consuming. As we have demonstrated, an alternative model is to intensively train the first generation of therapists via a 4- to 5-day workshop and to provide even more intense training (2–5 weeks) and extended consultation to clinicians who will serve as local supervisors. While we have less formal experience with this model, it seems to be promising as both an effective and a more efficient method of creating local, self-sustaining expertise.

The other two factors impeding dissemination of empirically supported treatments for PTSD involve negative attitudes by therapists toward manualized therapies and concerns about the safety of PE. In our own approach to utilizing and teaching manualized PE, we emphasize the need for therapists to learn not only the specific skills and techniques of the treatment, but also to understand the underlying principles on which treatment is based. As noted earlier, a good portion of our intensive 4- or 5-day training is devoted to discussing modifications to the standard protocol to deal with problems of patient such as under-engagement and over-engagement. We have begun to disseminate the need for balance between adhering to treatment protocols that received empirical support and modifying certain procedures for a minority of patients when such modifications are needed (e.g., Jaycox & Foa, 1996; Hembree *et al.*, 2001, 2003; Feeny *et al.*, 2003).

We have also dispelled the myth that PE is harmful in publications that empirically examined this myth. As discussed in this chapter, the primary empirical basis for these concerns emanate from a series of uncontrolled case studies (Pitman *et al.*, 1991) and one recently published randomized-controlled trial of IE vs. cognitive therapy (Tarrier *et al.*, 1999). Although both of these sources suggested significant symptom worsening with the use of exposure therapy, neither of them provides a comparison with untreated participants to determine the effects of withholding treatment the likelihood of on exacerbation in PTSD and associated psychopathology. A more comprehensive review of the available data from randomized-controlled trials has failed to find any replications of the high rates of symptom worsening reported by Tarrier and colleagues. In addition, exposure therapy has been found to have similar or lower rates of symptom worsening than other ostensibly less anxiety provoking treatments such as SIT (Cahill *et al.*, 2003) and relaxation (Taylor *et al.*, 2003).

In conclusion, advances in treatments for PTSD have resulted in several empirically supported treatments that are not only effective but also safe, with PE being the most thoroughly studied of these treatment programs. However, they are generally unavailable to consumers of mental health services. Accordingly, if we are to heed one of the many lessons taught to us by the events of 9/11, our field needs to set among the highest of its priorities the widespread dissemination of effective treatments, the development and evaluation of different dissemination models to insure the use of these treatments, and the assessment of their efficacy in the field compared to outcomes obtained in randomized-controlled trials.

REFERENCES

Becker, C.B., Zayfert, C. & Anderson, E. (2004). A survey of psychologists' attitudes towards and utilization of exposure therapy for PTSD. *Behaviour Research and Therapy*, **42**, 277–292.

Blanchard, E.B., Kuhn, E., Rowell, D.L., Hickling, E.J., Wittrock, D., Rogers, R.L., Johnson, M.R. & Steckler, D.C. (2004). Studies of the vicarious traumatization of college students by the September 11th attacks: effects of proximity, exposure, and connectedness. *Behaviour Research and Therapy*, **42**, 191–205.

Boscarino, J.A., Galea, S., Ahern, J., Resnick, H. & Vlahov, D. (2003). Psychiatric medication use among Manhattan residents following the World Trade Center disaster. *Journal of Traumatic Stress*, **16**, 301–306.

Bryant, R.A., Harvey, A.G., Basten, C., Dang, S.T. & Sackville, T. (1998). Treatment of acute stress disorder: a comparison of cognitive-behavior therapy and supportive counseling. *Journal of Consulting and Clinical Psychology*, **66**, 862–866.

Bryant, R.A., Sackville, T., Dangh, S.T., Moulds, M. & Guthrie, R. (1999). Treating acute stress disorder: an evaluation of cognitive behavior therapy and supportive counseling techniques. *American Journal of Psychiatry*, **156**, 1780–1786.

Bryant, R.A., Moulds, M., Guthrie, R. & Nixon, R.D.V. (2003). Treating acute stress disorder following mild traumatic brain injury. *American Journal of Psychiatry*, **160**, 585–587.

Cahill, S.P., Riggs, D.S., Rauch, S.A.M. & Foa, E.B. (2003). *Does Prolonged Exposure Therapy for PTSD Make People Worse?* Poster presented at the *Annual Convention of the Anxiety Disorders*, Association of America, Toronto, Ontario, Canada, March 2003.

Cloitre, M., Koenen, K.C., Cohen, L.R. & Han, H. (2002). Skills training in affective and interpersonal regulation followed by exposure: a phase-based treatment for PTSD related to childhood abuse. *Journal of Consulting and Clinical Psychology*, **70**, 1067–1074.

Devilly, G.J. & Foa, E.B. (2001). The investigation of exposure and cognitive therapy: comment on Tarrier *et al.* (1999). *Journal of Consulting and Clinical Psychology*, **69**, 114–116.

Ehlers, A. & Clark, D.M. (2000). A cognitive model of posttraumatic stress disorder. *Behaviour Research and Therapy*, **38**, 319–345.

Ehlers, A., Clark, D.M., Hackmann, A., McManus, F., Fennell, M., Herbert, C. & Mayou, R. (2003). A randomized controlled trial of cognitive therapy, self-help booklet, and repeated assessment as early interventions for PTSD. *Archives of General Psychiatry*, **60**, 2024–1032.

Feeny, N.C., Hembree, E.A. & Zoellner, L.A. (2003). Myths regarding exposure therapy for PTSD. *Cognitive and Behavioral Practice*, **10**, 85 90.

Foa, E.B. & Cohill, S.P. (present volume). Psychological treatments for PTSD: An overview. In *Mental Health in the wake of Terrorists Attacks*, ed. Y Neria, R. Gross. & R. Marshall. Cambridge, UK: Cambridge University Press, pp. 457–474.

Foa, E.B. & Rothbaum, B.O. (1998). *Treating the Trauma of Rape: Cognitive-Behavioral Therapy for PTSD*. New York: Guilford.

Foa, E.B., Rothbaum, B.O., Riggs, D.S. & Murdock, T.B. (1991). Treatment of posttraumatic stress disorder in rape victims: a comparison between cognitive-behavioral procedures and counseling. *Journal of Consulting and Clinical Psychology*, **59**, 715–723.

Foa, E.B., Hearst-Ikeda, D. & Perry, K.J. (1995). Evaluation of a brief cognitive-behavior program for the prevention of chronic PTSD in recent assault victims. *Journal of Consulting and Clinical Psychology*, **63**, 948–955.

Foa, E.B., Dancu, C.V., Hembree, E.A., Jaycox, L.H., Meadows, E.A. & Street, G.P. (1999). A comparison of exposure therapy, stress inoculation training, and their combination for reducing posttraumatic stress disorder in female assault victims. *Journal of Consulting and Clinical Psychology*, **67**, 194–200.

Foa, E.B., Hembree, E.A., Cohil, S.P., Pauch, S.A., Riggs, D.S., Feeny, N.C. & Yodin, E. (2005). Randomized trial of prolonged exposure for PTSD with and without cognitive restructuring: Outcome at academic and community clinics. *Journal of Consulting and Clinical Psychology*, **73**, 953–964.

Foa, E.B., Zoellner, L.A. & Feeny, N.C. (in press). An evaluation of three brief programs for facilitating recovery after trauma. *Journal of Traumatic Stress*.

Galea, S., Ahern, J., Resnick, H., Kilpatrick, D., Bucuvalas, M., Gold, J. & Vlahov, D. (2002). Psychological sequelae of the September 11 terrorist attacks in New York City. *New England Journal of Medicine*, **346**, 982–987.

Gillespie, K., Duffy, M., Hackmann, A. & Clark, D.M. (2002). Community based cognitive therapy in the treatment of posttraumatic stress disorder following the Omagh bomb. *Behaviour Research and Therapy*, **40**, 345–357.

Harvey, A.G. & Bryant, R.A. (1998). The relationship between acute stress disorder and posttraumatic stress disorder: a prospective evaluation of motor vehicle accident survivors. *Journal of Consulting and Clinical Psychology*, **66**, 507–512.

Hembree, E.A., Marshall, R., Fitzgibbons, L. & Foa, E.B. (2001). The difficult to treat PTSD patient. In *The Difficult to Treat Psychiatric Patient*, eds. M. Dewan & R. Pies. Washington, DC: American Psychiatric Press.

Hembree, E.A., Rauch, S.A.M. & Foa, E.B. (2003). Beyond the manual: the insider's guide to prolonged exposure for PTSD. *Cognitive and Behavioral Practice*, **10**, 22–30.

Jaycox, L.H. & Foa, E.B. (1996). Obstacles to implementing exposure therapy for PTSD: case discussions and practical solutions. *Clinical Psychology and Psychotherapy*, **3**, 176–184.

Linehan, M.M. (1993). *Cognitive-Behavioral Treatment of Borderline Personality Disorder*. New York: Guilford.

Marks, I., Lovell, K., Noshirvani, H., Livanou, M. & Thrasher, S. (1998). Treatment of post-traumatic stress disorder by exposure and/or cognitive restructuring. *Archives of General Psychiatry*, **55**, 317–325.

Meichenbaum, D. (1974). *Cognitive Behavior Modification*. Morristown, NJ: General Learning Press.

Nacasch, N., Cohen-Rapperot, G., Polliack, M., Knobler, H.Y., Zohar, J. & Foa, E.B. (2003). Prolonged exposure therapy for PTSD: the dissemination and the preliminary results of the implementation of the treatment protocol in Israel. Abstract in the *Proceedings of the 11th Conference of the Israel Psychiatric Association*, Haifa, Israel, April, 2003.

Paunovic, N. & Ost, L.G. (2001). Cognitive-behavior therapy vs. exposure therapy in the treatment of PTSD in refugees. *Behaviour Research and Therapy*, **39**, 1183–1197.

Pitman, R.K., Altman, B., Greenwald, E., Longpre, R.E., Macklin, M.L., Poire, R.E. & Steketee, G.S. (1991). Psychiatric complications during flooding therapy for posttraumatic stress disorder. *Journal of Clinical Psychiatry*, **52**, 17–20.

Pitman, R.K., Orr, S.P., Altman, B., Longpre, R.E., Poire, R.E., Macklin, M.L., Michaels, M.J. & Steketee, G.S. (1996). Emotional processing and outcome of imaginal flooding therapy in Vietnam veterans with chronic posttraumatic stress disorder. *Comprehensive Psychiatry*, **37**, 409–418.

Resick, P.A. & Schnicke, M.K. (1992). Cognitive processing therapy for sexual assault victims. *Journal of Consulting and Clinical Psychology*, **60**, 748–756.

Resick, P.A., Nishith, P., Weaver, T.L., Astin, M.C. & Feurer, C.A. (2002). A comparison of cognitive processing therapy with prolonged exposure and a waiting condition for the treatment of chronic posttraumatic stress disorder in female rape victims. *Journal of Consulting and Clinical Psychology*, **70**, 867–879.

Rothbaum, B.O., Astin, M.C. & Marsteller, F. (2005). Prolonged exposure versus eye movement desensitization and reprocessing (EMDR) for PTSD rape victims. *Journal of Traumatic Stress*, 18, 617–629.

Schlenger, W.E., Caddell, J.M., Ebert, L., Jordan, B.K., Rourke, K.M., Wilson, D., Thalji, L., Dennis, J.M., Fairbank, J.A. & Kulka, R.A. (2002). Psychological reactions to terrorist attacks: findings from the National Study of Americans' Reactions to September 11. *Journal of the American Medical Association*, **288**, 581–588.

Silver, R.C., Holman, E.A., McIntosh, D.N., Poulin, M. & Gil-Rivas, V. (2002). Nationwide longitudinal study of psychological responses to September 11. *Journal of the American Medical Association*, **288**, 1235–1244.

Tarrier, N., Pilgrim, H., Sommerfield, C., Faragher, B., Reynolds, M., Graham, E. & Barrowclough, C. (1999). A randomized trial of cognitive therapy and imaginal exposure in the treatment of chronic posttraumatic stress disorder. *Journal of Consulting and Clinical Psychology*, **67**, 13–18.

Taylor, S., Thordarson, D.S., Maxfield, L., Fedoroff, I.C., Lovell, K. & Ogrodniczuk, J. (2003). Comparative efficacy, speed, and adverse effects of three PTSD treatments: exposure therapy, EMDR, and relaxation training. *Journal of Consulting and Clinical Psychology*, **71**, 330–338.

Veronen, L.J. & Kilpatrick, D.G. (1983). Stress management for rape victims. In *Stress Reduction and Prevention*, eds. D. Meichenbaum & M.E. Jaremko. New York: Plenum Press, pp. 341–374.

Vlahov, D., Galea, S., Resnick, H., Ahern, J., Boscarino, J.A., Bucuvalas, M., Gold, J. & Kilpatrick, D. (2002). Increased use of cigarettes, alcohol, and marijuana among Manhattan, New York, residents after the September 11th terrorist attacks. *American Journal of Epidemiology*, **155**, 988–996.

28

Mental health community response to 9/11: training therapists to practice evidence-based psychotherapy

Lawrence V. Amsel, Yuval Neria, Eun Jung Suh and Randall D. Marshall

Introduction

The events of 9/11 continue to have profound consequences for the sense of physical safety and psychological well-being of Americans. In particular, as epidemiological research revealed the full magnitude of the mental health consequences of the 9/11 attacks (Galea *et al.*, 2002), there was an unprecedented level of outreach aimed at insuring that those in need of mental health services are identified and treated (Felton, 2002). As part of this campaign, members of the general public were encouraged to examine their own distress levels and, if needed, to seek assessment and treatment.

These campaigns, and the public response to them, represent a sea change in attitudes toward mental health in our culture. The public discussion of the mental health consequences of 9/11 has been relatively free of stigmatizing and shaming attitudes that are often associated with mental health disorders. As noted by Jack Rosenthal, the Pulitzer Prize winning president of the New York Times Foundation, in the wake of 9/11, the word "victim" no longer held its pejorative connotation (J. Rosenthal, personal communication, 2001).

Of course, even with this reduction in stigma, many needing psychological help as a result of the events of 9/11 will still feel resistant to seek help. A survey by DeLisi and colleagues reported that only 27% of those with severe post-9/11 psychological symptoms were obtaining treatment (DeLisi *et al.*, 2003). Nevertheless, even conservative estimates predict that over 100,000 persons could be expected to seek help for 9/11-related psychological trauma in the New York area alone (Herman *et al.*, 2002). Moreover, the public health outreach effort, with its focus on reducing stigma and increasing acceptance of psychological treatment, can be expected to further increase the demand for quality mental health services, and will hopefully reduce the number of untreated sufferers.

These laudable gains in public understanding and acceptance, however, raise questions about the availability of services. Is there an adequately trained mental health workforce with the expertise to treat the psychological sequelae of terrorism including post-traumatic stress disorder (PTSD) and traumatic grief? While effective treatments for PTSD have been developed and tested in the last decade, it is unclear how many mental health practitioners have received the appropriate training in how to carry out these new treatments.

There is unfortunately little empirical information available on mental health workforce preparedness for mass trauma, as indicated by the following open questions. What treatment modalities are being practiced by those community clinicians who are treating post-traumatic psychological sequelae? What kinds of treatment results are being achieved? Among those community clinicians who treat post-traumatic psychological sequelae, including PTSD and traumatic grief, how many are aware of the current evidence-based assessment and treatment guidelines for these problems? For those clinicians who are not experienced with trauma, how many would be willing and logistically able to obtain special training? How many clinicians do we need to train in order to adequately meet the current need? If there are further attacks, how will that impact on the need for appropriately trained therapists?

While hard evidence on these questions is not readily available, it was clear that prior to 9/11 most mental health clinicians had little specialized training in treating the psychological sequelae of mass trauma. By raising awareness of treatable mental health disorder and reducing stigma, the public health response to 9/11 may have in fact exposed a fault line in the preparedness of the mental health community. At the same time, recent research has raised serious questions about the effectiveness of traditional continuing professional education (CPE).

Traditional CPE has been shown to be ineffective at enhancing clinicians' skill at delivering new therapeutic interventions or at changing their clinical behavior (Poses, 1999). Traditional CPE treats dissemination of clinical innovation as if it were a well-defined commodity that accumulates at research centers and that can be easily distributed. In the current interactive informational economy this model of knowledge transmission has been abandoned. Instead of delivering a self-contained commodity to a passive recipient, what is needed is an efficient, active and interactive process that enhances the skills of recipients, enables changes in clinical behaviors, and encourages adoption of innovative treatments.

Thus, the challenge facing the academic mental health community in greater New York was to develop effective training programs that would augment the existing capacity of mental health practitioners to deal with the psychological sequelae of trauma. What follows is a description of the dissemination efforts of the Trauma Studies and Services Group at the New York State Psychiatric Institute.

We will describe our initial attempts at creating a dissemination model to deal with these issues. This consisted of developing training programs which simultaneously disseminated an evidence-based psychotherapy for PTSD to a large number of community clinicians; collected information on the clinicians' attitudes, beliefs, experience, and previous training regarding trauma and its cognitive–behavioral treatment (CBT); and lastly, gathered information from participants about which training techniques were most effective at promoting adoption of these clinical techniques. While this is very much a work in progress, we believe it may serve as a useful prototype for trainings in public mental health preparedness.

In this chapter we will first describe how we applied an evidence-based paradigm to selecting the material for training clinicians to respond to mass trauma. This paradigm led us to choose a form of cognitive–behavior assessment and therapy for our dissemination trainings. Next we will discuss the process of creating a manageable set of component recommendations that could be rapidly learned, and effectively applied in clinical practice. We then explored trainees' attitudes toward these recommendations, as well as their perceived skill levels at implementing them. This gave us a set of training goals organized into the following categories: imparting information, addressing negative attitudes, enhancing practice skills, anticipating application barriers, and supplying requisite motivation for these recommendations to actually be adopted into clinical practice. With this set of educational and behavior change goals in hand, we designed a workshop consisting of lectures, clinical demonstrations and role-play exercise based on basic science theories of effective behavior change methodology. Finally, we collected trainees' perceptions of how the training affected their beliefs, skills, attitudes, and behavioral intentions (BI) with regard to incorporating these therapeutic modalities into their practices.

The evidence-based mental health paradigm

The theoretical foundations of this project began with a commitment to promulgating treatments that had a proven record of effectiveness; that is, an evidence-based practice paradigm. Historically the numerous disciplines and schools of thought involved in mental health have held very divergent views on the nosology, etiology, and best-practice approaches to mental illness. In the last few decades, however, consensus and standards have emerged for a number of disorders. Moreover, the emergence of the evidence-based paradigm, first in medicine and later in mental health, has introduced some empirical benchmarks against which the therapeutic debates can be evaluated (Drake *et al.*, 2001). The pillars of evidence-based interventions are standardization, measurability, and replication.

Because mental health has always been focused on the uniqueness of the individual, the attitude of evidence-based practice toward the standardization of psychotherapy techniques has often met with an understandable skepticism (Marshall *et al.*, 1997; Grimshaw *et al.*, 2002). Nevertheless, as more empirical evidence on psychotherapy becomes available, practitioners can be expected to integrate these scientific findings into their everyday practice (for a review, see Beutler *et al.*, 2002).

Complicating these issues is the fact that much of the evidence that exists for psychotherapy speaks to the question of treatment *efficacy*, that is the evidence shows that the treatment works well in a highly structured, well-controlled research setting. This leaves open the question of *effectiveness*: that is will the treatment also work well in community settings? Fortunately, in the last few years a number of researchers have begun to conduct these effectiveness studies (Drake *et al.*, 2001). Of particular relevance to our work is the study by Gillespie *et al.* (2002) conducted in the wake of a terrorist bombing in the small town of Omagh in Northern Ireland, which killed 29 people and injured 370. As part of a community recovery project, five clinicians, who were not researchers and had only modest prior PTSD experience, were given a brief training in an evidence-based cognitive treatment for PTSD, and then treated patients referred for bombing-related psychological symptoms under expert supervision from David Clark's group at University of London. A total of 91 consecutive patients were treated, and then assessed for rates and degree of recovery from PTSD. These patients as a whole showed highly significant improvement, comparable to that seen in efficacy research. This study suggests that it may be possible to train community-based clinicians to deliver a specific, high-quality therapy to address the psychological sequelae of terrorism, at least on this relatively small scale. Unfortunately the challenges in the greater New York area, in terms of lives lost and population affected, was orders of magnitude larger and thus required a much more ambitious training program.

To better understand the clinical application of the evidence-based approach, it is useful to follow a five-step procedure described by Sackett *et al.* (1996). The first step is to clarify a clinical problem by reframing it in the form of an empirically answerable question. In our case we begin with the clinical problem of how to best help people who have PTSD symptoms as a result of having been exposed to a trauma. While much attention has been focused on acute interventions for the peri-traumatic period, the evidence indicates that it is chronic reactions and symptoms that are the greatest source of public health concern (Shalev, 2002). Moreover, while there is evidence that certain medications can ameliorate PTSD symptoms, we were interested in promulgating a treatment program that could be practiced by a broad set of mental health clinicians. Thus, our clinical challenge was refined to identifying a well-established, efficacious, time-limited psychosocial intervention for chronic PTSD in the wake of a terrorist attack.

This seemingly simple step is fundamental to the subsequent success of the dissemination effort. It forces a clear focus on well-defined diagnostic or clinical problems, and a single, or at most a few comparable, treatment approaches. More-over, in order to be empirically answerable, the relevant clinical situation must be amenable to standardized assessment tools, treatment protocols, and outcome measurements. This methodology moves our clinical technique away from a general psychotherapeutic approach and toward highly specific treatments for well-defined disorders, such as chronic PTSD. As we shall see below, for many community-based therapists, this process of standardization, which is an irreducible core concept of evidence-based treatments, represents a radical break from usual practice patterns.

The second step in the evidence-based approach is to track down relevant clinical trials. The third step is to critically evaluate this literature for its validity (was it a high-quality study that avoided biased conclusions), its impact (the effect size or clinical significance of a positive finding), and its applicability (how close were the study subjects and their clinical problems to our current situation). It is beyond the scope of this chapter to review all the evidence supporting various cognitive–behavioral psychotherapies for PTSD. However, a key finding is that all empirically validated psychotherapies for PTSD incorporate some form of exposure to the traumatic memory: that is, a clinician-guided remembering and retelling of the traumatic events. Moreover, these exposure techniques currently have the strongest clinical evidence to support their efficacy as a treatment for PTSD (Taylor *et al.*, 2003). Thus, we selected the treatment manual developed by Edna Foa and colleagues for conducting CBT including prolonged exposure (PE) therapy in adults with chronic PTSD (Foa *et al.*, 1999).

It is important to note, however, that much of the research on CBT for PTSD had been done with victims of rape and other individual traumas, which raises the question of its applicability to mass trauma, such as in a terrorist attack. However, these different trauma types all produce PTSD symptoms, presumably through similar psycho-physiologic mechanisms. This would tend to support the idea that treatments proven helpful for one type of trauma would also be applicable to PTSD symptoms resulting from other types of trauma. This is further supported by the results obtained by Gillespie in the study cited above involving PTSD resulting from terrorism (Gillespie *et al.*, 2002).

The fourth step in the evidence-based approach is using clinical expertise to integrate the existing evidence with an individual patient's values, circumstances, and physiology. The final step is to evaluate the outcome of this whole process and make ongoing adjustments. These last steps are perhaps the most controversial. Some researchers have insisted that a proven treatment must be applied with a high degree of adherence to its original formulation in order to be useful (Waltz *et al.*, 1993). In direct contradiction, others have focused on the need to adapt the proven treatment to a variety of situations, and explicitly recognize the need to modify the techniques accordingly (Schulte, 1996). We refer to this debate as the Adopt vs. Adapt controversy, and will return to it below.

Evidence-based psychotherapy is also controversial because it touches on questions of professional autonomy and the role of the professional's individuality as a therapeutic tool, as explicated by Jerome Frank in his book, *Persuasion and Healing* (Frank, 1973). Thus, as our research confirmed, the very notion of standardization in psychotherapy may be the most difficult adjustment for psychotherapists without prior CBT training to make. These therapists often find the standardization of CBT techniques at odds with their usual psychotherapy practices. Therefore, the dissemination of evidence-based treatments involves more than mere communication of information, as presumed by traditional CPE programs, and this may account for their limited effect on clinician behavior. Instead, dissemination requires a fundamental attitudinal shift as well as significant behavior change on the part of the clinician-trainees, and the training model must address these issues. Our goal was to begin to develop such a training model within the given set of constraints on training programs. We will return to this point after further discussing the detailed structure of the CBT for PTSD that we chose to disseminate.

CBT for PTSD: what it is and what clinicians think of it

As discussed above, applying the evidence-based paradigm to PTSD led us to adopt an exposure-based CBT as the treatment of choice. Our first challenge then was to identify the active components of this treatment and to frame them in a way that could be easily applied by individual practitioners. In this regard we identified aspects of the treatment that were both central to the therapy, and that distinguished it from traditional psychotherapy as practiced in the community. As we developed our training workshops it became clear that therapists with different theoretical orientations might view these recommendations quite differently. Thus, the educational experience might be very different for a psychodynamic-oriented therapist and a CBT-oriented therapist, even if both had no PTSD experience. It was therefore instructive to consider the findings of Blagys & Hilsenroth (2002) on the distinctive activities of CBT as a therapeutic modality.

Blagys and colleagues conducted an exhaustive review of the psychotherapy-process literature, in particular focusing on differences between psychotherapy processes in psychodynamic treatments and those in CBT treatments. The studies they reviewed involved clinicians rating different types of therapy sessions for the presence or absence of particular therapeutic activities. They identified six activities that were consistently rated as present in CBT sessions but not in the psychodynamic sessions, and thus could be reasonably shown to be distinctive elements of CBT.

The six distinct activities were: (1) use of homework and outside-of-session activities; (2) direction of session activity by manualized guidelines; (3) teaching of skills to be used by patients to cope with symptoms; (4) emphasis on patients' future experiences rather than past experiences; (5) providing patients with information about their treatment, disorder, or symptoms; and (6) an intrapersonal cognitive focus, that is cognitive restructuring.

While this represents an important starting point, there are some clear difficulties with this list. First, exposure techniques are missing from Blagys' list of distinctive activities of CBT. Blagys explains that the research has tended to focus on studies of psychotherapy for depression, in which exposure does not play a role. While acknowledging that exposure techniques are of central importance in the CBT treatment of PTSD, obsessive–compulsive disorder (OCD), social anxiety disorder, and simple phobias, Blagys concludes that, thus far, there is not enough therapy-process research in these diagnostic areas to conclude that exposure is a practice unique to CBT.

Second, while there is some general appeal to the idea that psychodynamic sessions tend to look backward while CBT sessions tend to look forward, the idea that CBT uniquely emphasizes a patient's future experience is problematic. Granted, Blagys did find that in six out of seven studies independent raters confirmed this past/future distinction, nevertheless, if one includes exposure techniques (including exposure to detailed memories as in PE for PTSD), these time frame orientations would change.

Third, Blagys does not list the use of structured instruments for initial evaluation and for assessing therapeutic progress. Yet, in practice CBT therapists tend to use them more often than psychodynamic therapists. From an evidence-based practice perspective of course, these are not distinctive to CBT but rather should be part of the systematic assessment of any psychotherapy treatment.

Lastly, despite the older stereotype of the silent psychodynamic therapist, the idea that providing clinical information to patients is a distinctively CBT activity is questionable. Blagys acknowledges this, and even found that in more experienced clinicians this difference disappeared. Moreover, as we shall discuss below, supplying adequate psycho-education was the most universally accepted of all our recommendations.

Keeping this research in mind we developed a set of ten distinguishable component recommendations which together constituted the core of the CBT treatment program for PTSD. These are listed in Table 28.1 and will be briefly described below:

(1) The initial *diagnostic evaluation* must distinguish patients who can benefit from PE from patients who are not appropriate for this treatment, and who will require a different treatment approach. As part of this evaluation we also recommend using structured clinical instruments to increase reliability and to establish a baseline against which to measure improvement.

Table 28.1. PE therapy for chronic PTSD

Component recommendations

(1) It is important to conduct an initial *diagnostic evaluation* in order to distinguish patients with who can tolerate and benefit from PE from patients who cannot tolerate this procedure, and who will require a different treatment approach.

(2) It is helpful for patients to participate in *prolonged exposure*, even if this causes the patient significant distress.

(3) Incorporate *breathing retraining* exercises early in the therapy.

(4) Incorporate *psycho-education* as an integral part of the therapy.

(5) It is helpful for patients to participate in *in vivo exposures* to situations that they have been avoiding due to their association with the trauma, even if doing so causes distress.

(6) It is important for the therapist to conduct the treatment according to the principles *outlined in the manual* for each session, though this may leave little time for exploratory interpersonal discourse.

(7) Assess salient factors using a *structured instruments* or forms.

(8) It is important for patients to actively carry out structured weekly *homework* assignments and to document these experiences on structured patient report forms, which are then reviewed by the therapist.

(9) *Restructure cognitions* or change patients' distorted belief structures, or schema, by eliciting patients' belief structures and directly challenging them.

(10) Train the patient to be able to identify their *subjective units of distress*, as an integral part of the exposure experience.

(2) In treating patients with PTSD in a CBT modality, it is helpful for them to participate in *prolonged exposure*, even if this causes the patient distress. This technique is one of the key elements of this psychotherapy. Although there are different CBT models, as mentioned above recent work by Taylor *et al.* (2003) confirms that including exposure-based approaches makes for the most effective of the currently available treatments. The technique involves a detailed recounting of the traumatic event done repeatedly. This leads to a reduction in anxiety and fear associated with the traumatic memories and reduces PTSD symptoms, over which patients initially have no control. Like other exposure techniques this can be a temporarily uncomfortable experience for patients.

(3) Incorporate *breathing retraining* exercises. Breathing exercises have been shown to reduce anxiety and autonomic responses to stress. This also serves an important cognitive function by concretely demonstrating to patients that they can have more control over their emotional responses than they had initially believed.

(4) Incorporate *psycho-education* as an integral part of the therapy. We do not view this as unique to CBT; rather it is a standard part of any good therapy.

Nevertheless, for patients suffering with PTSD in particular, accurate information on the illness, its precipitants, common symptoms, common responses to symptoms, and treatment rationale are extremely important and are very helpful in establishing an alliance, and in fostering the belief that the therapist understands the symptoms and has expertise in their treatment.

(5) It is helpful for patients to experience *in vivo exposures* to situations that they have been avoiding due to their association with the trauma, even if doing so causes distress. In conjunction with imaginal exposures, these exposures to places, objects, or situations are done by the patients as an out-of-session exercise. The experience of successfully reducing one's own anxiety response in a feared situation can be quite empowering and can serve as a motivating factor for the rest of the therapy.

(6) In treating patients with PTSD, it is important for the therapist to conduct the treatment according to the principles *outlined in the manual* for each session, though this may leave little time for exploratory interpersonal discussion. (This is one of the most controversial recommendations, as will be discussed below.)

(7) In treating patients with PTSD, it is important for the therapist to assess initial symptoms and treatment progress using *structured instruments* or forms. Within this therapy modality the objective feedback of symptomatic improvements is extremely important in keeping patients motivated for the difficult therapeutic work, as well as being needed for the planning of ongoing interventions and therapeutic exercises. Patients with severe anxiety often cannot appreciate real symptomatic improvements at a subjective level; however, if they see objective evidence of improvement they may gain a sense of mastery and confidence, so helpful to this therapeutic work.

(8) In treating patients with PTSD, it is important for patients to actively carry out structured weekly *homework* assignments, and to document these experiences on structured patient report forms, which are then reviewed by the therapist and patient together. As mastery over anxiety and avoidance are central goals of this therapy, each experience of mastery that a patient has can help remove behavioral restrictions and undermine false, fear-driven beliefs. The word "homework" has some negative connotations, and patients often respond more positively to the phrase "between-session exercises."

(9) *Restructure cognitions* (i.e., change patients' distorted beliefs or schema) by eliciting them and then gently but directly challenging them. Traumatic experiences by their very nature tend to produce intense beliefs about ongoing risks, the safety of the world, personal powerlessness, and related themes that are often over-generalized in ways that create an unnecessarily grim and frightening view of the world. Therapists should use a cognitive framework to challenging these trauma-related distortions and automatic thoughts.

(10) Train the patient to be able to identify their *subjective units of distress* as an integral part of the exposure experience. Identifying one's level of distress on a scale from 1 to 100, while experiencing the distress, is an integral part of the exposure technique for several reasons. It lets the therapist and patient know how intense a particular memory or exposure is; it highlights the variability of distress; it demonstrates the therapeutic function of exposure as the distress diminishes as the exposure proceeds; finally, it gives the patient an ability to simultaneously experience and observe distress.

Having identified these ten component recommendations, our next task was to assess our clinician-trainees attitudes toward these recommendations. At the start of each workshop, therefore we asked our trainees to rate each recommendation on a scale ranging from -5 (very unfavorable attitude) to $+5$ (very favorable attitude). We also asked them to rate their ability, or self-efficacy, to carry out the recommendation, again rated on a scale from -5 (very hard to implement) to $+5$ (very easy to implement). In addition, participants were asked to describe in a qualitative fashion their perception of benefits and barriers related each component recommendation. These qualitative written comments were then coded and analyzed.

The results of the questionnaires reported here are based on an analysis of an initial group of 104 clinicians who participated in the training workshops and completed the questionnaires. The group was 81% female, with a mean age of 49, and was 81% white, 10% Hispanic, 6% Asian, and 2% African American. The participants had a mean of 17 years in practice, and were in a variety of disciplines, with 57% in social work, 18% in psychology, 8% in psychiatry, 2% in nursing, and the rest in miscellaneous helping professions. An additional group of 23 participants completed the qualitative written comments only.

As mentioned, our prediction was that the use of psycho-education would be seen differently than the other recommendations, in that it was familiar to most therapists who have positive expectations regarding its usefulness, and who generally perceive themselves as skillful in its implementation. This prediction was borne out. Psycho-education scored higher than all other recommendations, receiving a mean favorability rating of 4.6 (SD = 0.7) out of a possible 5, and a self-efficacy score of 3.8 (SD = 1.8) out of a possible 5. Thus, the trainees' ratings on psycho-education can be used as a benchmark of familiarity, as it were, against which we could measure clinicians' attitudes and self-efficacy for the other, less familiar, components of CBT for PTSD.

Indeed, by using psycho-education as a benchmark we found that clinicians had serious attitudinal reservations about a number of the other recommendations, as well as rating their self-efficacy for carrying out those recommendations significantly lower than it was for psycho-education. The only exception was breathing retraining, which clinicians rated highly on both favorability 4.1 (SD = 1.3) and self-efficacy 3.2 (SD = 2.2).

Second, there was a large difference between the attitude score and self-efficacy score for many of the recommendations. This indicates that, even for recommendations that were seen as quite favorable, the clinicians had low confidence in their own ability to successfully apply them. We created a variable designated as the *implementation gap*, which represents this difference between favorability and self-efficacy score for a component recommendation. When it is large there is a dissonance between what a trainee believes to be good practice and what the trainee has confidence in doing. Therapists are obviously less likely to apply a recommendation, when they have little confidence in their ability to carry it out successfully.

In theory we would expect to see four patterns here. In the first, clinicians both have positive attitude toward a recommendation and are confident in their ability to implement it. For this pattern there is no implementation gap and there is a high likelihood of the recommendation being implemented. This is exactly the pattern seen in psycho-education and breathing retraining which proved to have the smallest gaps of 0.8 and 0.9, respectively, which is then used as the standard for further comparisons. In the second pattern clinicians give the recommendation a low favorability rating and have low confidence in their ability to implement it. We expect recommendations with this pattern to be un-ambivalently rejected.

The third pattern involves a high (or moderate) favorability rating but a low self-efficacy rating. Recommendations with this pattern should be the major targets of any skill-based training, as this pattern implies an implementation gap in which clinicians have a favorable attitude toward a recommendation, but believe they lack the ability to implement it. Thus, if participants gain the skills and confidence to implement these recommendations they are likely to adopt them.

Moreover, these recommendations would be expected to show the greatest change in a skills-oriented training. The final pattern of low favorability but high self-efficacy did not show up in our ratings. Presumable, this rating is for techniques with which a trainee is quite familiar but dissatisfied, these are not areas for which clinicians would seek instruction.

Keeping these patterns in mind, the most dramatic finding was that use of a manual to conduct psychotherapy received the lowest favorability rating, with a score 1.5 (SD = 2.6). In addition to having the lowest favorability score, manualization had the second lowest rating on self-efficacy at 0.3 (SD = 2.9). This was also reflected in the qualitative comments, where manualization was seen as: restricting the therapeutic process (45 comments), harmful to the therapeutic alliance (40 comments), and a source of resistance by both the patient and by clinical institutions (46 comments). Attitudes toward standardization were clearly mixed as indicated by the fact that manualization was also seen as helpful in structuring the therapy (61 comments), but not necessarily in improving a patient's condition (only ten comments suggested such improvement).

In our experience with training research staff, manuals are often seen as a very helpful tool in learning a new therapy procedure. They serve as a road map, sometimes even minute-to-minute guide on what to do in a therapy session, and our research trainees find this very reassuring. Thus, one might expect that using a manual would help clinicians overcome concerns about their own clinical skills when adopting a new technique, and, in fact, this is a major motivation for the creation of these manuals in the first place. Those who promulgate manualized therapies see the manuals as part of the solution to low self-efficacy; not, as our trainees did, as another self-efficacy problem. This suggests that there needs to be a more intense, in-depth discussion about the advantages and disadvantages of using manuals at all future trainings.

Interestingly, the mixed attitude of our trainees toward manualized psychotherapy is reflected among psychotherapy researchers themselves. Garfield (1998) argued that, under certain circumstances, strict adherence to a manual might be detrimental to the efficacy of psychotherapy, as therapists would not be able to deviate constructively and respond to patients' individual and unique needs. Similarly, Castonguay *et al.* (1996) found that, in treatment for depression, an overly rigid adherence to CBT manual correlated negatively with treatment outcome. Gibbons *et al.* (2002) takes an intermediate position. While she argues for the usefulness of manuals, she believes they need to be applied with flexibility. Her study demonstrated that highly trained therapists actually applied manuals with considerable flexibility and sensitivity to patients' needs. What is certain is that manualization remains a key controversial issues in disseminating evidence-based psychotherapies and is in need of more research.

As noted above, PE is a core intervention for CBT treatment of PTSD. It rated moderately well on favorability at 2.5 (SD = 2.2), but very low on self-efficacy at 0.3 (SD = 2.8), indicating that trainees see themselves as lacking the skills to effectively implement this psychotherapy intervention. The *in vivo* exposure recommendation showed a similar response pattern. In our qualitative data, participants strongly endorsed the idea that PE could lead to clinical improvement (72 comments), however, they also expressed strong concern that PE could harm patients (49 comments). Thus, there were ambivalent clinical attitudes within the group of trainees, and even within individual trainees, regarding the emotional cost–benefit of PE.

Trainees might be fearful that a poor implementation of exposure techniques would not only be ineffective, but may actually be harmful to their patients. Concerns about potentially harming the patient, or making the condition worse, were, for the most part, restricted to these two recommendations, and may be based on concerns about "re-traumatizing" the patient. In fact there have been some published reports claiming that exposure techniques can cause harm (Tarrier *et al.*, 1999), while more recent work has not found this to be the case (Foa *et al.*, 2002). Any training involving exposure techniques should incorporate a full discussion of this issue as it is reflected in the current literature. In addition, the high implementation gap here indicates that clinicians need an effective skill-building training to feel comfortable adopting this technique.

The scores for recommendations regarding cognitive restructuring, assigning therapeutic homework, and use of structured assessment instruments were close to each other and higher than PE on favorability, thus falling somewhere in the middle of all recommendations. They were probably seen as the workhorse components of the treatment – not well known, but not particularly controversial. Again, skill-building training could be expected to have an important effect on the adoption of this group of recommendations.

Trainees clearly appreciated that the first step to effective treatment is correctly identifying those who could benefit, those in need, and excluding inappropriate candidates. Thus, the high favorability rating of 3.8 (SD = 1.9) for the assessment recommendation, though expected, is encouraging. Moreover, assessment is a core skill for all therapists, and so we would expect its self-efficacy score to be relatively higher than for more unfamiliar techniques, and at 1.9 (SD = 2.8) this is borne out. On the other hand, there still was a high gap between favorability and self-efficacy, reflecting concerns about getting the assessment right, and not enrolling inappropriate patients.

Finally, the breathing retraining recommendation received very high scores, with a favorability score of 4.1 (SD = 1.3) and self-efficacy score of 3.2 (SD = 2.2). This was the only component statistically indistinguishable from psycho-education. In the qualitative remarks this had the strongest endorsement of all the recommendations for contributing to clinical improvement (80 comments). Together, these ratings indicate that therapists were already incorporating breathing techniques into their therapies, even if they used no other CBT techniques. Breathing techniques are not part of psychodynamic therapy training or practice, and so, from our many discussions with our trainees we have learned that their knowledge of breathing techniques seems to be originated in the general cultural popularity of complementary and alternative therapies and from the general popularity of yoga exercise (Wolsko *et al.*, 2004). To our knowledge this may constitute the first empirical documentation of how widespread the use of breathing retraining has become for psychotherapists.

In summary, at entry into our training, clinicians' attitudes divided the ten recommendations into five subgroups. (1) Manualization, representing the structured approach to psychotherapy, is in a class by itself both for the opposition it raises and the low self-efficacy most clinicians feel toward this approach to the interpersonal work of psychotherapy. (2) Exposure work, both in-session imaginal exposure and at-home *in vivo* exposure, raise concerns about harming the patient, and many clinicians feared that they lacked the skills to execute these techniques properly. At the same time their potential benefit was acknowledged. (3) Cognitive restructuring, homework assignments, teaching patients to quantify their subjective units of distress, and using structured instruments, are seen as useful but unfamiliar techniques, without significant risks, but requiring more skills and practice. (4) Thorough initial assessment is seen as an essential skill important to proper delivery of therapy, and a skill that clinicians are mostly comfortable with, though it is acknowledged to be difficult. (5) Psycho-education and use of breathing retraining are already adopted parts of everyday clinical practice, though how this happened remains unclear.

The process of developing and conducting our trainings also illustrates the vital importance of incorporating research methods into post-disaster efforts. By assessing trainees' baseline attitudes and self-perceived self-efficacy for the basic components of CBT, we were able to further clarify what areas of training were most needed. As these results became available, we were able to modify our trainings to address trainees' needs.

Dissemination to achieve clinician behavior change: teaching psychotherapy in a 2-day workshop

When considering the methodology of psychotherapy training, one must differentiate between initial professional education and CPE. The traditional model for initial psychotherapy training arose from psychoanalysis and consisted of three parts: a didactic training that tended to be highly theoretical meta-psychology, closely supervised case work based on process notes and resembling an apprenticeship, and finally a personal therapy. The latter two experiences served to foster close personal observation of a master psychotherapist and were conducted with an implicit master-disciple structure that incorporated as much of a personal-transformation model as an educational model (Strupp *et al.*, 1988). Cognitive and behaviorally oriented trainings held very different meta-psychology and de-emphasized the personal therapy or personal-transformation model. They have tended to focus on technical proficiency and adherence to established protocol through repeated practice, but they also rely on close supervision, reminiscent of an apprenticeship (Milne *et al.*, 1999).

On the other hand, traditional CPE has tended to focus on knowledge transmission, usually with lectures dominating the contact time, and with knowledge acquisition as its intended endpoint. While adequate for imparting new information within an existing treatment paradigm, this training model has been repeatedly shown to be inadequate to achieving the kind of clinical behavior change required for clinicians to adopt a new practice (Davis *et al.*, 1999).

To enhance behavior change by clinicians a number of different theoretical models have been explored, ranging from adult education theories to stages of change models (Prochaska & Velicer, 1997), each with highly variable success (Poses, 1999). Instead, we sought an easily applied but scientifically sound motivational model based on the basic sciences of decision-making and motivation, that links specific educational interventions to measurable aspects of attitudes, cognitions, and behaviors. The relevant theories include the Theory of Reasoned Action, TRA (Fishbein & Ajzen, 1975) as well as the Theory of Planned Behavior, TPB (Ajzen, 1988). These theories build upon the simple proposition that intentions precede and direct actions. As a first approximation, people do what they intend to do, and do not do what they do not intend to do. Such intentions are called BI and, in the present context, refer to a clinician's intention to adopt CBT techniques in the treatment of post-traumatic patients. Jaccard (1975) and others have identified and described the three key factors that together predict the strength of such BI. The stronger a BI is the greater the likelihood that a person will perform the given behavior (Figure 28.1).

The first factor is the *expected value of the outcome*, that is the positive consequences that are expected to result from the behavior. In the clinical situation this would involve a clinician's expectation and beliefs about the efficacy of a given

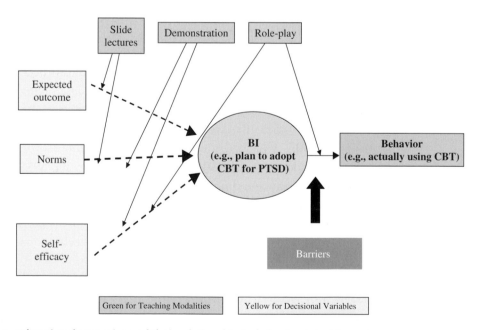

Figure 28.1 Educational strategies and their relationship to behavioral decision science.

treatment modality. This expectation may be based on prior training or experience, on published literature, or on convincing information presented in a training program. This factor is what we are trying to measure with the favorable attitude ratings introduced above. In traditional economic theory this expected value is the only factor incorporated in decision analysis, but empirical work has shown that human behavior is more complex than that of *homoeconomicus* (Fishbein & Ajzen, 1975).

The second factor is one's *belief about existing norms*. Even when we believe that some action would benefit us, we are unlikely to adopt the behavior if it is not supported by the norms of behavior in our environment. Similarly, even when a clinician has strong belief in the helpfulness of an intervention, a contrary opinion by peers, supervisors, or respected experts, creates powerful peer-pressure disincentives that limit the likelihood that a clinician will perform the intervention. Thus, a clinician's belief about the attitudes of her peers and/or the attitudes of thought-leaders in her professional circles may affect practice more than the available evidence in the given clinical field (Poses, 1999).

The third key factor is *self-efficacy*, the belief that one can successfully and effectively perform the behavior. This is what we measured when asking clinicians about the relative ease or difficulty of adopting a recommendation into their practice. Even when these conditions are met, however, a wide range of factors, especially unanticipated barriers, may prevent a BI from effectively becoming an actual behavior. The near universal failure of New Year's resolutions makes the point.

These theoretical considerations influenced the design and implementation of the various educational modalities that made up the training workshops we developed. An important caveat, however, is that we were working within the limitations implied by a 2-day training program. Trainings were, therefore, structured to maximize their impact on each of the relevant factors contributing to BI (see Figure 28.1). We believed that lectures followed by discussion periods would have most of their impact on clinicians' beliefs regarding expected outcomes of recommended interventions. Lectures, therefore, needed to contain a convincing rationale for the treatment design, as well as convincing evidence for treatment efficacy. Lectures may also affect perceived norms, and should include information about the current use of CBT for PTSD in a variety of treatment centers.

Clinical demonstrations consist of a clinical expert modeling a specific technique, for example an intake assessment. This is done either with a patient, or an actor who has been given vignettes and dialog from actual patient sessions. These demonstrations are expected to have their greatest impact on the perception of norms. They may also be expected to influence skill acquisition, contributing to improved self-efficacy. Videotapes of these clinical interactions may also be substituted for live demonstrations in this modality, though the difference in educational effectiveness between live interview and tape needs further study.

Both lectures and clinical demonstration are passive teaching modalities for the participants, while research has shown that active practice is required to actually alter skill levels (Smith, 2000). We, therefore, included role-play sessions in which all participants paired off and alternated playing the role of therapist or client. By allowing the practice of unfamiliar techniques in a supportive setting, this training modality was expected to have the strongest impact on skill acquisition. Moreover, by encouraging participants to experience a clinical situation, albeit an artificial one, role-play can also be expected to help clinicians anticipate and overcome barriers via an experiential process.

In summary, by building on previous empirical findings and introducing theory from the basic behavioral sciences, we developed an initial workshop design that was aimed at having maximum impact on those factors that influence behavior change. To test these assumptions, we asked participants to complete the questionnaires mentioned above as well others on the training experience, and on changes in attitudes resulting from the training.

In the Teaching Modality Questionnaire, participants were asked to rate (on a scale from -5 to $+5$) how effective each of the three modalities (lectures, demonstrations, and role-play) was at influencing each of seven educational factors, namely: (1) Conveying Theoretical Principles, (2) Conveying Methodological Details of the Therapy, (3) Changing Beliefs, (4) Changing Initial Reservations or Objections, (5) Helped to Overcoming Barriers to Implementation, (6) Helping with Skill Acquisition, and (7) Motivating Practice Change.

While confirming some of our training assumptions, the results were both surprising and illuminating. First, Demonstrations rated highest on every dimension, even where our theoretical assumptions would have predicted otherwise. Thus, Demonstration was rated superior to lectures in changing beliefs (2.8 vs. 1.5, $p < 0.005$), reversing reservations (3.0 vs. 1.4, $p < 0.005$), and most surprisingly, even in conveying the theoretical model (3.8 vs. 3.3, $p < 0.05$). These are functions that usually attributed to lectures as they are the information-laden part of a training. Equally surprising, Demonstration rated higher than role-play on skill acquisition (2.9 vs. 2.2, $p < 0.05$), even though role-play was designed specifically for that function. An important caveat here is that watching clinical demonstration of a PTSD treatment can be a highly dramatic and emotionally salient experience, and may thereby bias participants assessment of how each training modality affected their learning process.

It is therefore helpful to examine each modality by itself, to determine its relative effect on each of the educational factors. For example, focusing on role-play alone, it had its greatest impact on Skill Acquisition (2.9), followed by Methodological Details (2.8), and Motivation (2.7). Lectures had their greatest impact on Conveying Theoretical Principles (3.3), and Conveying Methodological Details (3.0), and do poorly on Skill Acquisition (2.2), and Overcoming Barriers (1.3), as expected. Contrary to expectation, lectures have little effect on Changing Beliefs (1.5) or Changing Initial Reservations (1.4). We also expected that the experience of role-play would have more impact on Overcoming Barriers, yet this was rated quite poorly (2.3).

This discussion represents only a preliminary analysis of our training data, and more definitive conclusions will need to await further analysis. Yet there seem to be some trends that may be used in improving training and education programs for evidence-based psychotherapy techniques:

(1) Lectures, the usual mainstay of training conferences, rated quite poorly. Perhaps lectures should not be abandoned but reconfigured to serve different goals than what we have always presumed. It might be worth testing if changing lectures significantly can make them more effective at changing beliefs and behaviors. Instead of merely conveying scientific information, lectures might need to make a motivational case for behavior change, while avoiding frank manipulation. For example, incorporating more explicit argument as to why the existing evidence should motivate behavior change by clinicians, or directly addressing expected resistance to the recommendations, or encouraging more open debate during the lecture, or incorporating a discussion of the level of acceptance of a practice within the profession.

(2) When it comes to imparting information, the goal of lectures should not be to teach all the details but to motivate trainees to further educate themselves. Lectures should continue to carry the burden of conveying the overall theoretical foundations, which they do well, but be less focused on therapeutic details, which are best conveyed in other ways. Lectures can do this by introducing the key theoretical and empirical reasons that motivate the adoption of a given treatment, and by allowing sufficient time for interactive questioning and debate.

(3) Role-play may not be the place to change belief systems or convey theory, but should be used for the purpose of promoting skill acquisition, and enhancing motivation. Given the highly positive results for demonstrations, perhaps the role-play should be modified to a hybrid model somewhere between the passive observation of an expert and the active try-out of role-play. For example, experts might participate in role-play with participants, making role-play more like supervision. Further interactivity could be explicitly introduced by asking dyads to role-play administrative meetings, such as that of the therapeutics committee deciding which interventions to introduce into the clinic or mental health system. This may allow clinicians to take on the role of advocating for or against the given therapy and may increase appreciation for the evidence base.

(4) There may also be a role for documentary-style videotapes involving a number of patients and therapists discussing their experiences with the treatment.

By incorporating patient experience with expert therapist commentary, these videotapes can serve a powerful motivating function that lectures cannot achieve. We have begun to test the effect of such videos on training efficacy.

(5) Finally, it should be noticed that all three modalities were relatively ineffective on overcoming potential barriers to implementation. As we shall see in the next section, barriers play a much larger role in preventing adoption of new therapies than was previously believed, and overcoming them may require an entirely new and dedicated training modality. Alternatively, some form of supervision after trainings may be essential to the process. Supervision involves trial and error learning and allows for highly individualized instruction, focused exactly where the trainee is having difficulty. Unfortunately it is also very expensive and time consuming, and therefore, in the post-9/11 setting, and given the scale of this training project, it was not feasible to implement as part of these workshops. Thinking into the future, for a subgroup of dedicated clinicians, expert-led group supervision or peer group supervision in addition to the workshop may prove to be a reasonable and cost-effective preparedness strategy.

Attitudes, skills, and motivation: what changes with training

At the end of the 2-day training, trainees were asked to rate, again on a scale from -5 to $+5$, how the training changed each of five domains for each of the ten recommendations. Scores on skill and motivation changes were statistically significantly higher than those for beliefs, barriers, and reservations. Because the range was narrow, we are careful not to over-interpret these results. Nevertheless, it is interesting that the traditional goal of CPE, namely to impart information and change minds, scored lower than skill acquisition and motivation changes. If, however, the goal of training is to change behavior rather than minds, this is an overall positive finding.

At the same time the fact that perceived barrier to implementation scored the lowest of any of these dimensions, raises serious concerns. As indicated by the behavioral models above, barriers can easily thwart BI. In order for clinicians to actually carry out these recommendations, further work is needed to directly address ways to help trainees overcome the barriers to implementation that will inevitably arise.

Returning to trainees' rating of the workshop effects, another way to examine the change scores is by looking at how the workshop affected attitudes toward individual recommendations. The recommendations that were predicted to show the greatest changes were those with correctable skill-deficits or implementation gaps. Most importantly, imaginal exposure and *in vivo* exposure were rated low on perceived self-efficacy at the start of the trainings, giving them large implementation gap scores. As predicted these recommendations showed the highest change scores. If confirmed with additional research, these findings are important on two levels.

First, given the low initial self-efficacy scores it is encouraging to see that the training was able to overcome perceptions of skill-deficits and impact trainees' attitudes toward adopting these techniques. Second in terms of dissemination research in general, these findings suggest that we may be able to design more effective trainings by systematically identifying, and specifically addressing, perceived skill-deficits.

Recent work in the area of human motivation has identified two self-regulatory strategies that can improve motivation and help subjects overcome or circumvent barriers standing in the way of their adopting recommended behaviors. The first involves the exercise of mental contrasting (MC), in which a subject anticipates the positive outcomes of a behavior as well as anticipating probable barriers to actually carrying out this behavior. Empirical research (Oettingen, 2000) has demonstrated that MC increases motivation to carry out a behavior. It is important to recognize, however, that this is only true for behaviors that one agrees with, but has been unable to accomplish due to barriers or lack of self-efficacy. Perhaps MC can be used to augment motivation in a non-coercive fashion and enhance clinicians' ability to translate their own intentions into clinical behaviors.

The second exercise is implementation intentions (II) in which subjects anticipate barriers, then strategize about solutions to these barriers, and finally commit to specific courses of action long before the barriers are encountered. Gollwitzer (1999) distinguishes between goal intentions such as, "I intend to improve my golf score," and II, which are detailed plans to overcome particular obstacles that facilitate the actual implementation. One is more likely to attain a goal when it is supported by II, because (a) the barriers become more readily attended to, more easily detected, and more easily recalled, and (b) the intended behavior to overcome the barrier is initiated immediately, without the necessity of inventing a plan *de novo*. Empirical research (summarized in Gollwitzer, 1999) has found strong support for the effectiveness of coordinating the exercises of II and MC as a combined self-regulatory strategy that helps people achieve their goals. We have begun research to test if these strategies can be incorporated as part of training workshops and if they enhance adoption of new techniques.

Future directions and research agendas

The events of 9/11 leave little doubt as to the need for us to be prepared for the psychological consequences of terrorism and other mass traumas. This preparation involves at least two components. One is a public mental health strategy that informs the community about the nature of psychological consequences of trauma and encourages help-seeking where needed. The second is ensuring that there is an adequate, well-trained, self-confident, and highly motivated mental health workforce to treat those in need and support the general public education effort.

Clearly the current mental health workforce does not have enough practitioners with adequate skills to meet our public mental health requirements in regards to psychological trauma. There is therefore an urgent and ongoing need for training and skill enhancement. Moreover, we cannot afford to simply run traditional training courses, which have focused on knowledge dissemination with little impact on important factors such as skill building, anticipating and overcoming barriers, and active motivational interventions to promote adoption of the training recommendations. Instead, we need trainings that will be highly effective at getting clinicians to adopt evidence-based treatments and to upgrade their skills at evaluating and treating psychological consequences of trauma.

Finally, in this effort we cannot afford to just hope that trainings are working, we need to be sure that the therapeutic knowledge and skills will be available when needed. Research into effective dissemination is thus an integral part of this effort. Research into effective dissemination is still in its infancy, yet the imperative of public mental health preparedness requires dissemination techniques that have been proven effective, as much as it needs effective treatments and public health outreach.

In closing we might ask, if the products of mental health research are not getting delivered to our patients, what is the point of research? If clinicians are not delivering the best available treatment what is the point of clinical practice? While evidence-based mental health has been accepted as an ideal for nearly a decade, actually getting clinicians to practice by its tenets has proven more challenging than anticipated. This represents a serious public mental health challenge to both clinicians and researchers, and raises serious questions about the relationship of the research and clinical enterprises in mental health. We hope this work contributes to answering these pressing problems.

REFERENCES

Ajzen, I. (1988). *Attitudes, Personality and Behavior*. Chicago: Dorsey Press.

Blagys, M.D. & Hilsenroth, M.J. (2002). Distinctive activities of cognitive–behavioral therapy. A review of the comparative psychotherapy process literature. *Clinical Psychology Review*, **22**, 671–706.

Beutler, L.E., Moleiro, C. & Talebi, H. (2002). How practitioners can systematically use empirical evidence in treatment selection. *Journal of Clinical Psychology*, **58**, 1199–1212.

Castonguay, L.G., Goldfried, M.R., Wiser, S., Raue, P.J. & Hayes, A.M. (1996). Predicting the effect of cognitive therapy for depression: a study of unique and common factors. *Journal of Consulting and Clinical Psychology*, **64**, 497–504.

Davis, D., O'Brien, M.A., Freemantle, N., Wolf, F.M., Mazmanian, P. & Taylor-Vaisey, A. (1999). Impact of formal continuing medical education: do conferences, workshops, rounds, and other traditional continuing education activities change physician behavior or health care outcomes? *Journal of the American Medical Association*, **282**, 867–874.

DeLisi, L.E., Maurizio, A., Yost, M., Papparozzi, C.F., Fulchino, C., Katz, C.L., Altesman, J., Biel, M., Lee, J. & Stevens, P. (2003). A survey of New Yorkers after the September 11, 2001, terrorist attacks. *American Journal of Psychiatry*, **160**, 780–783.

Drake, R.E., Goldman, H.H., Leff, H.S., Lehman, A.F., Dixon, L., Mueser, K.T. & Torrey, W.C. (2001). Implementing evidence-based practices in routine mental health service settings. *Psychiatric Services*, **52**, 179–182.

Felton, C.J. (2002). Project Liberty: a public health response to New Yorkers' mental health needs arising from the World Trade Center terrorist attacks. *Journal of Urban Health*, **79**, 429–433.

Fishbein, M. & Ajzen, I. (1975). *Belief, Attitude, Intention and Behavior: An Introduction to Theory and Research.* Reading, MA: Addison-Wesley.

Foa, E.B., Dancu, C.V., Hembree, E.A., Jaycox, L.H., Meadows, E.A. & Street, G.P. (1999). A comparison of exposure therapy, stress inoculation training, and their combination for reducing posttraumatic stress disorder in female assault victims. *Journal of Consulting and Clinical Psychology*, **67**, 194–200.

Foa, E.B., Zoellner, L.A., Feeny, N.C., Hembree, E.A. & Alvarez-Conrad, J. (2002). Does imaginal exposure exacerbate PTSD symptoms? *Journal of Counsulting and Clinical Psychology*, **70**, 1022–1028.

Frank, J.D. (1973). *Persuasion and Healing* (revised edition). Baltimore: John Hopkins University Press.

Galea, S., Resnick, H., Ahern, J., Gold, J., Bucuvalas, M., Kilpatrick, D., Stuber, J. & Vlahov, D. (2002). Posttraumatic stress disorder in Manhattan, New York City, after the September 11th terrorist attacks. *Journal of Urban Health*, **79**, 340–353.

Garfield, S.L. (1998). Some comments on empirically supported treatments. *Journal of Consulting and Clinical Psychology*, **66**, 121–125.

Gibbons, M.B., Crits-Christoph, P., Levinson, J., Gladis, M., Siqueland, L., Barber, J.P. & Elkin, I. (2002). Therapist interventions in the interpersonal and cognitive therapy sessions of the Treatment of Depression Collaborative Research Program. *American Journal of Psychotherapy*, **56**, 3–26.

Gillespie, K., Duffy, M., Hackmann, A. & Clark, D.M. (2002). Community based cognitive therapy in the treatment of posttraumatic stress disorder following the Omagh bomb. *Behavior Research Therapy*, **40**, 345–357.

Gollwitzer, P.M. (1999). Implementation intentions: strong effects of simple plans. *American Psychologist*, **54**, 493–503.

Grimshaw, J.M., Eccles, M.P., Walker, A.E. & Thomas, R.E. (2002). Changing physicians' behavior: what works and thoughts on getting more things to work. *Journal of Continuing Education Health Professionals*, **22**, 237–243.

Herman, D., Felton, C. & Susser, E. (2002). Mental health needs in New York State following the September 11th attacks. *Journal of Urban Health*, **79**, 322–331.

Jaccard, J. (1975). A theoretical analysis of selected factors important to health education strategies. *Health Education Monograms*, **3**, 152–167.

Marshall, R.D., Vaughan, S.C., Mackinnon, R.A., Mellman, L. & Roose, S.P. (1997). Assessing outcome in psychoanalysis and long-term psychodynamic psychotherapy. *Journal of the American Academy of Psychoanalysis*, **24**, 575–604.

Milne, D.L., Baker, C., Blackburn, I.M., James, I. & Reichelt, K. (1999). Effectiveness of cognitive therapy training. *Journal of Behavior Therapy Experimental Psychiatry*, **30**, 81–92.

Oettingen, G. (2000). Expectancy effects on behavior depend on self-regulatory thought. *Social Cognition*, **18**, 101–129.

Poses, R.M. (1999). One size does not fit all: questions to answer before intervening to change physician behavior. *Joint Commission Journal on Quality Improvement*, **25**, 486–495.

Prochaska, J.O. & Velicer, W.F. (1997). The transtheoretical model of health behavior change. *American Journal of Health Promotion*, **12**, 38–48.

Sackett, D.L., Rosenberg, W.M., Gray, J.A., Haynes, R.B. & Richardson, W.S. (1996). Evidence based medicine: what it is and what it isn't. *British Medical Journal*, **312**, 71–72.

Schulte, D. (1996). Tailor-made and standardized therapy: complementary tasks in behavior therapy. A contrarian view. *Journal of Behavior Therapy Experimental Psychiatry*, **27**, 119–126.

Shalev, A.Y. (2002). Acute stress reactions in adults. *Biological Psychiatry*, **51**, 532–543.

Smith, W.R. (2000). Evidence for the effectiveness of techniques to change physician behavior. *Chest*, **118**(Suppl. 2), 8S–17S.

Strupp, H.H., Butler, S.F. & Rosser, C.L. (1988). Training in psychodynamic therapy. *Journal of Consulting and Clinical Psychology*, **56**, 689–695.

Tarrier, N., Pilgrim, H., Sommerfield, C., Faragher, B., Reynolds, M., Graham, E. & Barrowclough, C. (1999). A randomized trial of cognitive therapy and imaginal exposure in the treatment of chronic posttraumatic stress disorder. *Journal of Consulting and Clinical Psychology*, **67**, 13–18.

Waltz, J., Addis, M.E., Koerner, K. & Jacobson, N.S. (1993). Testing the integrity of a psychotherapy protocol: assessment of adherence and competence. *Journal of Consulting and Clinical Psychology*, **61**, 620–630.

Wolsko, P.M., Eisenberg, D.M., Davis, R.B. & Phillips, R.S. (2004). Use of mind–body medical therapies. *Journal of General Internal Medicine*, **19**, 43–50.

Part V

Disasters and mental health: perspectives on response and preparedness

29

The epidemiology of 9/11: technological advances and conceptual conundrums

Naomi Breslau and Richard J. McNally

The terrorist attacks of September 11, 2001 prompted a wave of epidemiologic research, as the chapters in this edited volume illustrate. The three investigators, who have summarized their field work and selected findings in the first section of this volume, deserve much praise for their initiative in launching and completing their studies in the midst of local and national upheaval (Galea *et al.*, this volume; Hoven *et al.*, this volume; Silver *et al.*, this volume). The three epidemiologic studies implemented field procedures, designed to produce data on the psychological responses to the 9/11 attacks that are representative of the targeted populations. These include New York City (NYC) public schoolchildren, adult residents of the NYC metropolitan area and all American adults. These investigators applied well-tested state-of-the-art survey technologies to assure timeliness and efficiency. Data produced in these studies have been presented in multiple publications in leading medical journals and more publications are sure to follow. The chapters included herein focus primarily on the conduct of the research, organizational support, design options that were considered and the rationale for the choices that were made. In giving these accounts, the chapters contribute an interesting and instructive perspective that is often hidden from view. The more difficult goal of outlining lessons that could influence policy remains elusive. Recommendations for prevention programs that are not based on rigorous evaluation would be unwarranted.

Perhaps because of the enormity of the terrorist attacks or because of the upsurge in patriotic sentiment occurring in their wake, critical discussion of the conceptual underpinnings and implications, or even the methodological aspects of this work, has been largely absent. For example, no questions have been raised about the meaning of children's replies to questions about their relatives' direct exposure to the attacks or about the validity of children's endorsement of symptoms, such as sleep or concentration problems, given social expectations at that time. In this brief commentary, we omit appraisal of methodology and techniques in favor of addressing selected important issues that have largely been ignored.

September 11, 2001: the mental health crisis that wasn't

In the days following the attacks, many mental health experts predicted that an epidemic of stress-induced psychiatric disease, chiefly posttraumatic stress disorder (PTSD), would sweep through NYC and possibly throughout the rest of America as well (for documentation of these ominous predictions, see Sommers & Satel, 2005, pp. 177–214). Government responded quickly, authorizing funds for treating the 2.5 million New Yorkers believed to require psychotherapy as a result of the attacks. But as of the Spring of 2003, only about 25% of the predicted number of New Yorkers sought help from clinicians operating under the auspices of Project Liberty (Gittrich, 2003). And many of these individuals sought help for preexisting problems unrelated to the attacks.

As the studies summarized in this volume make clear, the epidemic of mental illness never materialized. Established definitions of *epidemic*, such as that of the Centers for Disease Control, specify that an epidemic is characterized by increase in the incidence of disease beyond expected rates that occurs within a specific geographic location during a specific time period. On the one hand, the increase in reported PTSD symptoms in NYC following the terrorist attacks might be interpretable in these terms. On the other hand, the uptick in apparent PTSD in NYC quickly subsided (Galea *et al.*, this volume), suggesting that survey interviewers had mainly detected reactions of expectable emotional distress rather than symptoms of disease. Indeed, there was no convincing evidence that these emotional responses produced any genuine functional impairment for those reporting them. Ergo, because there was no increase in *disease*, there was no *epidemic*. Finally, the reports of the empirical findings explicitly avoided any reference to formal psychiatric diagnoses, and used qualifiers, such as "probable" PTSD or symptom counts. As Sommers and Satel (2005) aptly remarked, September 11th was "the mental health crisis that wasn't" (p. 177).[1]

What counts as "exposure" to trauma?

Contemporary research on the psychological consequences of terrorist attacks relies on the *Diagnostic and Statistical Manual for Mental Disorders-IV* (DSM-IV) definition of PTSD (American Psychiatric Association (APA), 1994). The DSM-IV PTSD criteria differ in two important ways from its predecessors. The inclusion of Criterion

---

[1] The 9/11 terrorism attacks also focused attention on the limitations of psychological debriefing, a popular crisis intervention method designed to prevent subsequent posttraumatic psychopathology (For a review, see McNally *et al.*, 2003). Despite its popularity among many clinicians specializing in traumatic stress, research has shown that it may impede natural recovery from the effects of trauma (Bisson *et al.*, 1997; Mayou *et al.*, 2000).

F in DSM-IV specified that the disturbance arising in the aftermath of a trauma must produce significant distress or functional impairment for the person to receive the diagnosis. This criterion reflects the acknowledgment that people may experience intrusive thoughts, distressing dreams, startle and so forth, and yet be capable of functioning at their usual level in everyday life. The inclusion of the clinical significance requirement renders the diagnostic criteria for PTSD more stringent.

The second major change was the expansion of Criterion A, which defines the etiologic stressor, to include a far wider range of stressors than were envisioned under DSM-III (APA, 1980). The original concept of trauma was confined to extraordinary events falling outside the boundary of everyday stressful experiences. Thus, the authors of DSM-III distinguished traumatic stressors from non-traumatic stressors by furnishing examples of the former, such as confinement to a concentration camp, combat or rape.

To ensure that individuals deemed by clinicians to be suffering from the PTSD syndrome following non-catastrophic stressful experiences would not be ruled out from the diagnosis, subsequent DSM PTSD committees expanded the range of stressors, to bring the definition in line with clinical practice. This conceptual bracket creep in the definition of trauma (McNally, 2003a) now enables a very wide range of people to qualify as having been exposed to PTSD-level trauma. For example, according to one epidemiologic estimate, nearly 90% of adults residing in Southeastern Michigan qualify as having been exposed to at least one traumatic stressor yet only 9.2% of those exposed ever-developed PTSD (Breslau & Kessler, 2001). That is, approximately 90% of American adults are "trauma survivors."[2] Bracket creep in the definition of trauma now means that "the population's total life experiences that can be used to diagnose PTSD has increased materially by 59.2%" (Breslau & Kessler, 2001, p. 703).

From one perspective, bracket creep in the definition of trauma is a non-problem. Some clinical scholars may believe that regardless of whether the range of qualifying traumatic stressors is broad or narrow, the number of people meeting symptomatic criteria for PTSD should not change. According to this view, one cannot legislate phenomenology by fiat: a person either does or does not exhibit the signs and symptoms of the disorder, regardless of the apparent seriousness or triviality of the etiologic event. The problem with this view, however, is that it presupposes a cultural vacuum in which trauma occurs. On the contrary, a broadened concept of trauma and its close link to psychological disease has leaked into the discourse of everyday life, encouraging people to interpret the vicissitudes of life through the

---

[2] In addition to the bracket creep in the definition of what counts as a traumatic stressor, the concept of *survivor* has also broadened. Although Lifton (2005) has written, "A survivor is one who has been exposed to the possibility of dying or has witnessed the death of others yet remained alive" (p. 2263), the concept now applies to those exposed to stressful, but not potentially fatal, events (e.g., survivor of sexual abuse; someone viewing media coverage of the 9/11 terrorist attacks).

lens of trauma. Emotional responses to life's misfortunes are increasingly experienced as symptoms of disease. For example, PTSD allegedly triggered by exposure to obscene jokes in the workplace has been reported (McDonald, 2003). And as one eminent historian of military psychiatry asked:

"Will psychiatrists have the sense to realize that by medicalizing the human response to stressful situations, they have created a culture of trauma and thus undermined the general capacity to resist trauma? They could make a start by dismantling the unitary concept of trauma, an idea that has long outlived its purpose. Any unit of classification that simultaneously encompasses the experience of surviving Auschwitz and that of being told rude jokes at work must, by any reasonable lay standard, be a nonsense, a patent absurdity."
(Shephard, 2004, p. 57).

Shephard, however, is not sanguine about the prospects for the field now that "trauma has been vectored into the wider society by the law and the media" (Shephard, 2004, p. 58).

The expansion of the meaning of traumatic stressor in DSM-IV has influenced epidemiologic work on the response to the 9/11 terrorist attacks. If, for example, one can qualify for having been exposed to trauma if one reacts with "horror" when "confronted with an event" that poses "a threat to the physical integrity" of "others" (APA, 1994, pp. 427–428), then anyone who watched television coverage of the carnage of 9/11 counts as a trauma survivor. The upshot is to group together in a single category the countlessly diverse, unspecified experiences of New Yorkers on September 11, and the following weeks and months.

Questions on surveys designed to measure PTSD are supposed to link symptoms to a specific, identifiable traumatic event. Unfortunately, epidemiologic research related to the terrorist attacks has not followed this practice. For example, many symptoms of PTSD are nonspecific (e.g., difficulty falling or staying asleep, feeling of detachment or estrangement from others), and it is not at all clear that such symptoms were caused by a specific trauma that occurred on that date in history. Survey questions on symptoms that are related in their content to a specified event were asked in reference to " the attacks on the World Trade Center." Indeed, "being exposed to 9/11" does not reference any identifiable trauma.

The assumption in the epidemiologic projects is that all residents of the NYC metropolitan area (or even the USA) were exposed to the attacks and could "plausibly develop PTSD." What actually happened to most of them remains obscure.

There are two problems here: one is expansion of the concept of traumatic stressor and the other is the ambiguity surrounding the concept of exposure. Behaviorally oriented clinical psychologists have appealed to animal fear conditioning models in their attempts to come to grips with PTSD (Keane *et al.*, 1985; Foa *et al.*, 1992). Whatever the limitations of these models, they did have the virtue of relative clarity regarding the concept of exposure. Traumatic exposure was likened to contact with the unconditioned stimuli (USs; e.g., electric shocks) of Pavlovian fear conditioning preparations, whereas the cues evocative of re-experiencing symptoms were likened to the conditioned stimuli (CSs; e.g., tones, lights) that predicted the onset of USs. But when a person is not the direct recipient of life threat, the meaning of the concept of traumatic exposure becomes increasingly amorphous. And this poses problems for epidemiologists. How do we determine who counts as "exposed" among those in NYC? "Exposure to 9/11" is not like being exposed to a Pavlovian US despite the continuing invocation of fear conditioning models as relevant to the etiology of PTSD.

Resilience?

The concept of resilience is gaining currency within the field of traumatic stress studies. In many ways, this is a welcome development. Several years ago, anyone emphasizing resilience would have run the risk of being either condemned for "silencing the voices of survivors" or of "being in denial" regarding the consequences of trauma. Indeed, only a half dozen years ago, certain leaders of the trauma field joined forces with politically conservative members of the House of Representatives to engineer a formal congressional condemnation of a meta-analytic review article (Rind *et al.*, 1998) that concluded that adults who were sexually abused children are more resilient than most clinicians had hitherto suspected (See McNally, 2003b, pp. 22–26). Evidently, many clinicians specializing in trauma managed to misread the message of resilience as somehow authorizing the sexual abuse of children.

The failure of epidemiologists to detect a marked upsurge in trauma-induced mental disease following 9/11 was interpreted by trauma researchers and commentators as evidence of resilience. The non-epidemic of PTSD has not prompted a critique of traumatology's basic assumption: the expectation of breakdown. Rather, the non-epidemic has been interpreted as confirming that assumption by invoking a complementary aspect of trauma and victimization, that of resilience, an unexpected capacity to go on with life with minimal psychological damage.

However, one cannot infer mechanisms of resilience from the mere absence of psychopathology following exposure to trauma. Indeed, such an inference poses problems akin to inferring inhibitory mechanisms in Pavlovian fear conditioning. That is, confirming a stimulus as a conditioned inhibitor requires the failure of fear responding in the presence of a cue otherwise known to evoke the fear response (McNally & Reiss, 1984). For example, to confirm that a stimulus does possess inhibitory properties, one must expose the subject (human being or animal) to this stimulus in compound with another stimulus known to elicit fear. If the joint presentation of these two stimuli results in less fear than does the joint presentation of the known fear stimulus and a novel, neutral stimulus, then one can infer inhibitory capacity to the alleged inhibitory stimulus.

Invoking resilience when PTSD fails to emerge implies adherence to a trauma paradigm that presupposes that pathology is the normative response, but for operation of these inferred inhibitory mechanisms.

Conclusions

With the passage of time since the terrorist attacks of September 11, 2001, there is likely to be less reluctance to examine critically the growing literature on psychological trauma, and, specifically, studies of the aftermath of these events (McNally, 2004; Shephard, 2004; Young, 2004). In this commentary, we addressed two issues – exposure and resilience – that warrant conceptual precision. The epidemiologic projects summarized in this volume provide an opportunity to raise questions about general assumptions in research on trauma, including the assumption of expectable breakdown.

As Malcolm Gladwell's recent essay illustrates, the expectation that severe stressors cause psychic damage is not a timeless one (Gladwell, 2004). Gladwell contrasts two novels about combat veterans, one concerning a World War II veteran, published in 1955 (Wilson's *The Man in the Grey Flannel Suit*) and one concerning a Vietnam War veteran, published in 1994 (O'Brien's *In the Lake of the Woods*). In both novels, the combat veteran suffered extreme traumas. In the first novel, the veteran-protagonist "put the war behind him," but in the second, his traumatic memories dominate his life for many years and finally destroy him. As Gladwell observed, "Somehow in the intervening decades our understanding of what it means to experience a traumatic event has changed." And, as he suggests – "it's worth wondering whether we've got it right" (p. 76).

REFERENCES

American Psychiatric Association (1980). *Diagnostic and Statistical Manual of Mental Disorders* (3rd ed.). Washington, DC: American Psychiatric Press.

American Psychiatric Association (1994). *Diagnostic and Statistical Manual of Mental Disorders* (4th ed.). Washington, DC: American Psychiatric Press.

Bisson, J.I., Jenkins, P.L., Alexander, J. & Bannister, C. (1997). Randomised controlled trial of psychological debriefing for victims of acute burn trauma. *British Journal of Psychiatry*, **171**, 78–81.

Breslau, N. & Kessler, R.C. (2001). The stressor criterion in DSM-IV posttraumatic stress disorder: an empirical investigation. *Biological Psychiatry*, **50**, 699–704.

Foa, E.B., Zinbarg, R. & Rothbaum, B.O. (1992). Uncontrollability and unpredictability in posttraumatic stress disorder: an animal model. *Psychological Bulletin*, **112**, 218–238.

Galea, S., Ahern, J., Resnick, H. & Vlahov, D. (this volume). Post-traumatic stress symptoms in the general population after a disaster: implications for public health: evidence from a study of the NYC metropolitan area in the aftermath of September 11. In *9/11/2001: Treatment, Research and Public Mental Health in the Wake of a Terrorist Attack*, eds. Y. Neria, R. Gross & R. Marshall. Cambridge, UK: Cambridge University Press.

Gittrich, G. (2003). $90 million in Project Liberty mental health funds remains unspent. *New York Daily News*. Available at http://www.nydailynews.com/05-27-2003/front/story/87199p-79357 c.html

Gladwell, M. (2004). Getting over it. *The NewYorker*, **80**, 75–79.

Hoven, C.W., Mandell, D.J., Duarte, C.S., Wu, P. & Giordano, V. (this volume). An epidemiological response to disaster: the New York City Board of Education's Post 9/11needs assessment. In *9/11/2001: Treatment, Research and Public Mental Health in the Wake of a Terrorist Attack*, eds. Y. Neria, R. Gross & R. Marshall. Cambridge, UK: Cambridge University Press.

Keane, T.M., Zimering, R.T. & Caddell, J.T. (1985). A behavioral formulation of posttraumatic stress disorder in Vietnam veterans. *Behavior Therapist*, **8**, 9–12.

Lifton, R.J. (2005). Americans as survivors. *New England Journal of Medicine*, **352**, 2263–2265.

Mayou, R.A., Ehlers, A. & Hobbs, A. (2000). Psychological debriefing for road traffic accidents: three-year follow-up of a randomised controlled trial. *British Journal of Psychiatry*, **176**, 589–593.

McDonald Jr., J.J. (2003). Posttraumatic stress dishonesty. *Employee Relations Law Journal*, **28**, 93–111.

McNally, R.J. (2003a). Progress and controversy in the study of posttraumatic stress disorder. *Annual Review of Psychology*, **54**, 229–252.

McNally, R.J. (2003b). *Remembering Trauma*. Cambridge, MA: Belknap Press/Harvard University Press.

McNally, R.J. (2004). Conceptual problems with the DSM-IV criteria for posttraumatic stress disorder. In *Posttraumatic Stress Disorder: Issues and Controversies*, ed. G.M. Rosen, Chichester, UK: Wiley, pp. 1–14.

McNally, R.J. & Reiss, S. (1984). The preparedness theory of phobias: the effects of initial fear level on safety-signal conditioning to fear-relevant stimuli. *Psychophysiology*, **21**, 647–652.

McNally, R.J., Bryant, R.A. & Ehlers, A. (2003). Does early psychological intervention promote recovery from posttraumatic stress? *Psychological Science in the Public Interest*, **4**, 45–79.

Rind, B., Tromovitch, P. & Bauserman, R. (1998). A meta-analytic examination of assumed properties of child sexual abuse using college samples. *Psychological Bulletin*, **124**, 22–53.

Shephard, B. (2004). Risk factors and PTSD: a historian's perspective. In *Posttraumatic Stress Disorder: Issues and Controversies*, ed. G.M. Rosen, Chichester, UK: Wiley, pp. 39–61.

Silver, R.C., Holman, E.A., McIntosh, D.N., Poulin, M., Gil-Rivas, V. & Pizarro, J. (this volume). Coping with a national trauma: a nationwide longitudinal study of responses to the terrorist attacks of September 11th. In *9/11/2001: Treatment, Research and Public Mental Health in the*

Wake of a Terrorist Attack, eds. Y. Neria, R. Gross & R. Marshall. Cambridge, UK: Cambridge University Press.

Sommers, C.H. & Satel, S. (2005). *One Nation Under Therapy: How the Helping Culture is Eroding Self-reliance*. New York: St. Martin's Press.

Young, A. (2004). When traumatic memory was a problem: on the historical antecedents of PTSD. In *Posttraumatic Stress Disorder: Issues and Controversies*, ed. G.M. Rosen, Chichester, UK: Wiley, pp. 127–146.

30

Searching for points of convergence: a commentary on prior research on disasters and some community programs initiated in response to September 11, 2001

Krzysztof Kaniasty

Close to 100 years ago, after his visit to San Francisco, severely devastated by the 1906 earthquake, William James noted that "In California every one, to some degree, was suffering and one's private miseries were merged in the vast general sum of privation and in the all-absorbing practical problem of general recuperation" (James, 1912, p. 225). These insightful words illuminate two paramount characteristics of community-wide tragedies. Most importantly, whether they are caused by the forces of nature, technological mishaps or errors, or result from premeditated acts of violence and terrorism, they are more than individual-level events. They are "a basic disruption of the social context within which individuals and groups function" (Fritz, 1961, p. 651). Even if they strike geographically bounded environments such as tornados coiling one side of a street, floods submerging a neighborhood along the river banks or explosions shattering the heart of a city, their impact "ripples outward" inflicting harm and damages, and over time creating a greater sense of loss to larger and larger numbers of people. Consequently, the coping efforts aimed at recovery from the oppressive forces of these events become a shared responsibility and collective activity. The chapters presented in this volume all underscored this dynamic interplay of individual and community experiences that emerged in the hours, days, weeks and months in the aftermath of the terrorist attacks of September 11, 2001.

What were the recurring themes in this diverse set of reports describing a variety of outreach efforts to hundreds of thousands of Americans brutally awakened to the unprecedented levels of terror and grief? Undoubtedly the scope of these acts of terror and the devastation they brought about have no match in the history of the USA, if not in the history of the modern world. Of course, the world has experienced a plethora of tragedies and many of them were extensively studied by scientists in the past few decades. Hence it might prove useful to explore the extent to which the difficulties and complexities observed and experienced by the authors of this volume can be traced back to the difficulties and complexities of coping with large-scale trauma uncovered by prior research on disastrous events. Can the themes exposed in the context of intervention efforts following the destruction of the World Trade Center (WTC) in New York City and part of the Pentagon complex in Washington, DC be placed within a larger empirical milieu of studies describing psychological and societal reactions to natural and human-induced disasters and catastrophes?

Undoubtedly, the first hours following the attacks were overwhelmed by fright and chaos but, overall, even the immediate exodus from the areas of the fallen Towers and burning Pentagon was directed and enacted in a remarkably composed way. The instantaneous heroic actions of emergency professionals and volunteers selflessly bursting into rescuing and protecting others from ensuing harm were extraordinary. These first hours following the attacks showed again that when faced with an unambiguous crisis situation, people quickly regain a collective sense of determination and even the most calamitous pains and fears do not render them inept. In that way, the overall public response to the events of September 11 resembled reactions to many other disasters. "Terrorist attack offers a clear threat with a clear need to respond" (Hobfoll, this volume). In spite of the great dose of uncertainty about the actual nature of the events, there was neither need nor time to question the brutal force of the stressor and thus appraisals of it were rapid and undebatable. Mass panic and chaotic disorganization are not frequently reported following natural disasters and other horrifying events with clearly visible impacts (Wenger et al., 1985; Fischer, 1998). "Disaster victims do not exhibit irrational and self-destructive behavior nor do they become helpless and dependent. While some are killed or injured, most victims are not. They become resources" (Dynes & Drabek, 1994, p. 12).

What happened in the days to follow in New York City and at the Pentagon, and in fact in the entire country, again resembled often documented social dynamics emerging in the aftermath of many other disasters, especially those caused by forces of nature. Nothing better exemplifies the initial surge of coping frenzy than the instantaneous post-disaster mobilization of help and support. Disasters elicit an outpouring of immense mutual helping. In essence, this is exactly what people expect in times of crisis: when help is needed, supporters provide it. James (1912) observed on the day an earthquake struck San Francisco that the level "of helpfulness [have gone] beyond the counting" (p. 225). This immediate phase has been referred as a "democracy of distress" (Kutak, 1938), "post-disaster utopia" (Wolfenstein, 1957) and most often as "altruistic community" (Barton, 1969). Decidedly distinguishing features of this collective entity are heightened internal solidarity, disappearance of community conflicts, utopian mood and an overall sense of altruism. Some researchers have also suggested that the experience of the same fate can cause previous race, ethnic and social class barriers to fade away, at least temporarily (Drabek, 1986; Bolin, 1989; Eranen & Liebkind, 1993).

For the moment we were as one, and I was the brother of the toothless Filipino crone who sat besides me and smoked a big black cigar. Near me was a charming Southern woman, the widow of an old friend of mine. She accepted a cigarette from a Negro piano player. A millionaire tourist from Chicago sat on a pile of luggage with one of Shanghai's well-known beach-combers, and the two found a great deal to talk about. Ours was the democracy and brotherhood of common disaster …

Carl Crow's account of the bombing of Shanghai, *Harper's Magazine*, December 1937, cited in Kutak, 1938.

Undoubtedly, one of the paramount aims of terrorism is to bring on a sense of horror, helplessness and chaos extending well beyond the target of the attack. As we have seen, unfortunately so many times, this is exactly what happens. However, as the early spirals of terror spin far and past "Ground Zero", more and more people amalgamate against it. Thus the most strategically potent force of organized terrorism is also its greatest point of weakness. Often times, and as it happened following the mayhem of September 11, the initial shock and pain is followed by a passionate collective resolve and determination. Just as the victims of natural disasters have their "altruistic and heroic" stage, the victims of terrorism may have their "altruistic and patriotic" stage (Kaniasty & Norris, 2004). In the history of the world the acts of murderous terror are prevalent, yet not more common than illustrations of how communities endured various perils bounded together in a sense of common outrage, collective purpose and fearless drive to survive. Indeed a few empirical studies have documented the resilience of communities and nations experiencing violent social turbulences (e.g., Mira, 1939; Fogelson, 1970; Greenley *et al.*, 1975; Milgram, 1986; Curran, 1988). Efforts of the authorities, professionals and countless citizens described in the chapters presented here add to this list.

The authors of featured interventions quite explicitly mentioned an extraordinarily high desire of many professionals to offer their services in aiding the victims. Such instantaneous influx of volunteers and helping professionals have been often observed (Kaniasty & Norris, 1999), yet it appears that in the context of this tragedy it reached unprecedented heights. Interestingly, a consistent finding in disaster literature is that victims are quite reticent in utilizing assistance from sources outside their immediate network, even if such formalized aid offered by governmental and relief agencies is readily available, and rely mainly on their families, relatives, friends and neighbors. The pattern of help utilization following disasters resembles a pyramid with its broad foundation being family and other members of the immediate networks and its narrow top being aid provided by professionals and formal agencies (Barton, 1969; Drabek & Key, 1984; Carr *et al.*, 1992; Kaniasty & Norris, 2000). It is reasonable to assume that again on 9/11 the family, relatives and friends enacted their routine roles of leading social support providers but the professional response to attacks in New York City, at the Pentagon and in Shanksville, Pennsylvania, was exceptional. Exceptional also was the level of help-seeking among thousands of affected individuals. Hence possibly in years to come, help-utilization literature will refer to this aspect of the aftermath of 9/11 as a "trapezoid of post-disaster aid." Notwithstanding the incredible magnitude and the scope of these horrific acts, a large share of the reason for why so many people turned to professionals for help could be the great care with which these programs presented themselves to individuals and communities in need. It radiates in all the narratives that these "mass drives" of "psychological first aid" (see Litz, this volume), whether in the corridors of the Pentagon, in the screening rooms of the Mount Sinai Medical Center, during community forums in Lower Manhattan, on the phone lines of LIFENET, or in various media and educational appeals of Project Liberty, were conducted with the utmost dose of respect and sensitivity. It appears that these attempts effectively minimized eternal traps for potential stigmatization, marginalization and medicalization of help-seekers (Gist *et al.*, 1998).

Great attention has been also paid to cultural and ethnic diversity represented in targeted populations. Projects such as LIFENET (Draper *et al.*, this volume) and Project Liberty (Felton *et al.*, this volume), as well the WTC Worker/Volunteer Mental Health Screening Program (Katz *et al.*, this volume) and the Primary Care Survey in Northern Manhattan (Neria *et al.*, this volume), have adopted multicultural and multilingual approaches. This may seem an obvious thing to do given the "melting pot" distinction of New York City, yet studies document with some regularity that victims representing minorities and lower socioeconomic resource echelons do not always fully participate in post-disaster altruistic communities (Bolin & Bolton, 1986; Kaniasty & Norris, 1995; Webster *et al.*, 1995; Beggs & Haines, 1996; Oliver-Smith, 1996; Kaniasty, 2003). Factors such as race/ethnicity, age and education attainment (proxy for socio-economic status indicators, SES) are key variables affecting distribution of resources in recovery. It is important to remember that post-crisis exchanges of support, distribution of aid, and formalized intervention efforts take place in a context of pre-existing socio-political and cultural structures, with established rules and norms of resource distribution that regulates the quality and quantity of supportive relations (Kaniasty & Norris, 1999). Although the most obvious and familiar *rule of relative needs* may dominate, other ways of distribution may surface as well. In a fervor of benevolence, frequently accompanied with organizational confusion ("post-disaster culture of chaos," see Norris, this volume), it is easy to leave out some subgroups of victims just because of their historically and culturally sanctioned separation from the mainstream of the society. This might result in a *pattern of neglect* such that some of the victims could receive less help and support than other people comparably affected (Kilijanek & Drabek, 1979; Kaniasty & Norris, 1995).

The intervention and outreach programs described in this volume were very much tuned to these juxtapositions of the rule of relative needs and the potential of patterns of omission: "The thesis of community recovery and mutuality is to give the greatest aid to those in greatest need, without creating deficits for other vulnerable groups" (Fullilove & Saul, this volume). Nevertheless, both LIFENET and Liberty Projects reported relative underutilization of their services by Asian and, to a lesser extent, Latino populations. The importance of psychological and cultural factors affecting reluctance to seek help from formal and informal sources of support must be recognized and dealt with (Griffith & Villavicencio, 1985; Barrera & Reese, 1993; Norris & Alegria, 2006). Minorities and people from lower socioeconomic strata often incur greater losses in disasters (Bolin, 1982; Perilla *et al.*, 2002) but their elevated needs do not necessarily translate into a greater propensity to communicate them. Our studies with culturally diverse samples of disasters victims from the USA (Kaniasty & Norris, 2000) and Central Europe (Kaniasty, 2003) clearly documented that people in need receive help but they may receive altogether less help than they might have because of their reticence in asking for support. "People do not get what they do not ask for" and thus help-seeking discomfort or its opposite help-seeking comfort, as an important psychological asset affecting the efficacy of coping processes, could render some individuals to be more vulnerable to additional resource loss in crisis situations (see Hobfoll, this volume). Culturally savvy intervention efforts are always essential (Norris, this volume).

Within the ecology of collective stress, every asset has its liabilities, every benefit has its costs. The critical role of support providers in the first moments following the impact of the catastrophe is obvious. However, once past the initial havoc, the coordination and modes of providing professional and volunteer assistance require more than just good will. "The desire to assist is without question laudable, but not all forms of help, of course, prove equally helpful" (Gist *et al.*, 1998). Ironically, but not surprisingly, the surge of "the wonderful helpers" created logistic as well as philo-sophical dilemmas for the people in charge of post-September 11 outreach efforts. "For weeks, it seemed that we received more calls from well-intentioned individuals seeking to give assistance than from persons actually seeking help. Sorting through qualifications from many hundreds of volunteers to determine fitness for deployment was often a precarious endeavor" (Draper *et al.*, this volume). Helpers' working models of how to help, of what help is needed, or of what is appropriate and when are direct reflections of their own cultural and societal worldviews and professional preferences. Many of these beliefs are based on very vivid individualized professional experiences of past successes but are infrequently systematically evaluated for their efficacy. Stereotypes about the so-called "appropriate ways of coping" that in turn determine "appropriate ways of helping" may compromise the potential for various intervention activities to be supportive (Jerusalem *et al.*, 1995; McFarlane, 1995; Wortman & Silver, 2001). "In general, both command and soldiers were receptive to the briefings. However, long 'debriefings' provided at the end of a long shift were not always welcomed. Invitations for smoking cessation classes were definitely anathema"

(Ritchie *et al.*, this volume). Sincere concerns of mental health providers with predictions of looming rates of post-traumatic stress disorder (PTSD) and other major disorders in the aftermath of major traumatic events (McNally *et al.*, 2003) may focus their conceptualizations of a disaster as an individual, not social or community experience, and enhance their convictions that they are chiefly responsible for providing resolutions. Overreliance on the medical model of helping (Brickman *et al.*, 1982) and *overhelping* could, in the long run, undermine autonomy of those affected and beget dependence and a sense of helplessness. Even in the context of colossal trauma, professionals cannot act as "surrogate frontal lobes" for people in crisis, thereby slowing down the process of marshaling communal healing resources by the victimized communities on their own (Oliver-Smith, 1996; Kaniasty & Norris, 1999). The initiatives described in this volume were very aware of these potential pitfalls, as eloquently stated by Fullilove and Saul (this volume): "In many societies post-calamity, affected people have to struggle to articulate to their would-be helpers that recovery lay in group interactions, not in individual therapy."

With that many resources available in the aftermath of the 9/11 tragedy, it became crucial to determine how to funnel these assets into efforts extending beyond the immediate areas of destruction and for the time to come. "Numerous chaplains and mental health personnel went to the crash site, instead of planning for the ripple effect on the community" (Ritchie *et al.*, this volume). The psychological distress for many victims may surface later than the duration of some of the crisis interventions. Although often calamities occur suddenly, the stress they inflict is not just acute. Disasters evoke an array of secondary stressors that continuously challenge affected communities and strain their coping resources at a rate faster than the progress of recovery. As time passes following the event "the more difficult it is for emotionally affected persons to identify 9/11 as a significant factor related to their current concern" (Draper *et al.*, this volume). A number of studies have found that subsequent life events and losses are good predictors of disaster victims' symptom levels and recovery (Norris *et al.*, 2002). The role of forthcoming secondary stressors as mediators of the impact of the focal event (Norris & Uhl, 1993) has to be recognized from the very outset such that the initial overabundance of helping resources is preserved for the future. In other words, mental health workers and volunteers should also direct their efforts toward planning, advertising and implementing later services to resource-depleted communities. At the time of this writing, two and half years after 9/11 many activities of the projects described here have not yet ceased.

Such a longer-term approach is always imperative simply because the post-crisis instantaneous heroic and altruistic struggle to fulfill immediate needs represent only one side of the disaster experience. As "a rise and fall of utopia" (Giel, 1990), disasters are vivid portrayals of how communal upheavals move from an initial profusion of coping activities and helping to an often inadvertent and slowly unfolding depletion of supportive resources. Resource loss is difficult to prevent and more powerful than resource gain (Hobfoll, 1988, 2001, this volume). More often than not, the *mobilization* phase may not be sufficient to block subsequent progression of *deterioration* of victims' quality of life and interpersonal relations in their communities (Kaniasty & Norris, 1997, 1999, 2004). Deterioration may be particularly potent in the context of human-caused disasters and oppression. It has been generally accepted in the literature that the stress associated with many human-induced catastrophes is more persistent than that of natural disasters (Baum, 1987; Norris *et al.*, 2002). It appears that these events, whether they are just unfortunate mishaps or deliberate acts of organized violence, exert their destructive powers that go beyond their ability to destroy, injure or kill. Such events are mediums or weapons of terror and their strength should be measured by their capability to petrify. Not surprisingly then, the words used by victims of technological disasters and victims of terror to describe their experiences are frighteningly similar. A victim of an underground gasoline spill interviewed by Kai Erikson for his essays on human-provoked traumas said: "Of the words up here – 'hostage,' 'prisoner,' 'besieged,' and 'trapped' – I think I personally like 'trapped,' because trapped is definitely how I feel. Going on day to day with existence, with work and carrying on a routine, but trapped in it." (Erikson, 1994, p. 112).

The victims of human-induced disasters and oppression are hostages because they are trapped in often fuzzy, chaotic, secretive, nonlinear, convoluted and drawn-out features that are most characteristic for these events. Not denying the potential of natural disasters to create chronic stress, their victims are "afforded the luxury" of a finite conclusion declaring the end to destructive powers of natural forces that commences the process of relief and recovery. After the clear low point (Baum *et al.*, 1992), recovery activities begin and the improvements of life conditions are in sight. On the other hand, people are psychologically besieged by human-caused catastrophes and terror because of repeatedly voiced concerns and worries: *who did it and why?, will it happen again?, when will we be safe?* These questions, frequently not easily answerable, prevent the identification of the psychological "rebound point" keeping all affected unclear whether the incident is really over (Erikson, 1994; Kaniasty & Norris, 2004).

There are a multitude of ways through which disasters and catastrophes exert their deleterious influence on community life. From the very moment of the 9/11 assaults the public reactions were augmented by a "belief that 'anything was possible' in the hours, days and weeks following the attack" (see Hobfoll, this volume). Directly affected victims, and the entire citizenry for that matter, entered a "psychological minefield" where individuals' fears and ways to cope with them potentially collided and may have amplified the experience of shock and stress. Hobfoll (this volume) noted that victims of stressful events that impact larger groups often subject themselves to "pressure cooker" (Hobfoll & London, 1986) or "stress contagion" (Riley & Eckenrode, 1986) phenomena, whereby, paradoxically, social interactions and sharing of feelings and worries may exacerbate their perceptions of distress. Undoubtedly, the events that followed the attacks – the anthrax scare, the Washington, DC sniper attacks, the plane crash in Rockaway (Queens, New York City), the war in Afghanistan and later the uncertainty and actual war in Iraq – fueled concerns and heated debates among many, quite possibly straining their social relationships.

Of course, many catastrophes remove significant supporters from victims' networks through death, injury and relocation. The extent of bereavement and injuries resulting from the attacks was horrifying. Furthermore, just a look at what stands now at "Ground Zero" is more than enough to help us understand why on the top of the long list of "victims' categories eligible for services" presented by Draper *et al.* (this volume) were the people who lost their residences, and quite possibly, their employment. Not discounting the global impact of these undeniable personal dramas, social network losses such as these also force people to make downward adjustments in their expectations of social support availability (Kaniasty *et al.*, 1990; Solomon *et al.*, 1993; Warheit *et al.*, 1996). Residents of places ruined by disasters often report decreased participation in social activities with relatives, friends, neighbors and community organizations (Hutchins & Norris, 1989; Bolin, 1993; Kaniasty, 2003). People in affected areas must prioritize and expend prudently their energies, often putting their "social life" on hold (Golec, 1983). "I have friends but I do not call" said one of the respondents in Katz *et al.* (this volume) case examples. Overexposure to emotional disclosures about trauma can be psychologically threatening and emotionally draining. "All these media, these reminders … it's killing me" (Draper *et al.*, this volume; Neria *et al.*, this volume). People may become weary of unending exposures to news and testimonials of others about their experiences (Pennebaker & Harber, 1993; Mehl & Pennebaker, 2003). Those who need to talk and seek help in validating their subjective realities of trauma risk social disapproval. Empirical work has clearly documented that sharing traumatic experiences with respectful and supportive others helps people in discovering the mean-ing of the experience, gaining control over their emotional reactions and rebuilding shattered assumptions about the world (Pennebaker, 1990; Janoff-Bulman, 1992; Lepore & Smyth, 2002).

Ironically, the progress of recovery activities can also bring about feelings of apprehensiveness, isolation or even divisiveness (Golec, 1983; Steinglass & Gerrity, 1990). Some individuals, some communities, may recover at a faster rate than others and these victims may want to move on with their lives and leave behind those still immersed in the experience. "Some people were more ready than others to have their children return to the school, and the differences between peoples' feelings about the safety of the environment and the visibility of the destruction were topics that caused tension in the community" (Fullilove & Saul, this volume). Such communal tensions and animosities may add to an already diminished sense of social connectedness and victims' beliefs in goodness of the world and its people (Kaniasty, 2003). Lack of personal resolution, continuous fatigue and disagreements about the meaning and consequences about the event could incite interpersonal conflicts including family distress and disharmony (Erikson, 1976, 1994; Adams & Adams, 1984; McFarlane, 1987; Picou et al., 1992; Bowler et al., 1994; Harvey et al., 1995). Victims depicted in Katz's and colleagues' case examples mentioned a separation from a spouse and difficulties relating to close ones, "I know I love my family, but it is still hard to be around them. This is the biggest problem." (Katz et al., this volume).

The miasma of disasters' influence on personal and communal relationships grows in scope and virulence. Fullilove and Saul talked about the destruction of the WTC as a loss reaching beyond its immediate surroundings. "All people in the metropolitan area had lost a neighborhood that was important to them and had a right to consider themselves injured" (Fullilove & Saul, this volume). Loss of attachments to places is psychologically hurtful because physical structures with their familiar symbolic, social and cultural dimensions are foundations of self- and collective identities. How many New Yorkers, how many Americans, actually appreciated beforehand the psychological magnitude of these symbols? Significance of many places is usually only fully recognized when they have been disrupted or removed and when that happens, they could be grieved in a way analogous to mourning loved ones (Erikson, 1976; Brown & Perkins, 1992; deVries, 1995; Oliver-Smith, 1996). When the search for the causal factor moves away from the *nature* toward the *human* agent, more systemic community animosities and divisions become likely to surface (Drabek, 1986). Following September 11, shared experience of the lethal assault on American liberties and values and ensuing common threats undoubtedly amplified the sense of patriotism and national identity but this increased sense of togetherness was also responsible for some occurrences of escalation of political, societal and cultural divides. "The defensive posture accentuates in group-out group differences as a knee jerk reaction" (Hobfoll, this volume; see also Pyszczynski et al., 2003). All in all, the aftermath of disasters, those with clear fault lines of human culpability in particular, is a dynamic stage for many accelerating cycles of losses exerting their toll on very different planes: psychological, social, individual, community, political, cultural and economic.

I understood my task of this commentary as an attempt to identify the points of convergence between empirical literature on social reactions to natural and technological disasters and the dynamics described in this volume summarizing major community outreach efforts that followed the 9/11 terrorists attacks. Just like all of us, I have been humbled by the enormity of these events, the extent of human suffering and heroism, and the professionalism and foresight of people responsible for and involved in the continuous activities aimed at alleviating psychological and social consequences of these atrocities. Although unique and unprecedented, the suffering of the victims of September 11 echoes many similarities to the suffering of countless victims and communities traumatized by other disasters and catastrophes. Traumatic events are often very different from one another, and each may beget inimitable demands and create very specific needs. Yet the differences and a general sense of distinctiveness behind these events pale if we shift our attention to the backgrounds against which they unveil. Reactions and struggles of individuals are interwoven with reactions and struggles of their communities. The reality of individual victimization cannot be understood without consideration of the collective reality. Hence helping the victims also means deterring the erosion of sense of belonging to a community that "provides a channel for intimate communication and expression, and a major source of physical and emotional support and reassurance" (Fritz, 1961, p. 689). The heart of Charles Fritz's "therapeutic community" notion is a belief that post-disaster deterioration of social support and community relations is not inevitable (see also, *the social support deterioration model*, in Norris, this volume). The same conviction was present in all of the intervention efforts described here. "Such actions are not only essential to rebuilding the society, but also are curative for the symptoms of trauma-related illnesses. Overcoming aloneness, feeling the support of the larger group, having a manifestation of the higher power that lies in collective action are the best antidotes to lingering feelings related to terror" (Fullilove & Saul, this volume).

REFERENCES

Adams, P. & Adams, G. (1984). Mount St. Helen ashfall: evidence for a disaster stress reaction. *American Psychologist*, **39**, 252–260.

Barrera, M. & Reese, F. (1993). Natural social support systems and Hispanic substance abuse. In *Hispanic Substance Abuse*, eds. R. Sanchez Mayers, B. Kail & T. Watts. Springfield, IL: Charles C. Thomas, pp. 115–130.

Barton, A.M. (1969). *Communities in Disaster*. Garden City, NJ: Doubleday.

Baum, A. (1987). Toxins, technology, and natural disasters. In *Cataclysms, Crises, and Catastrophes: Psychology in Action*, eds. G. VandenBos & B. Bryant. Washington, DC: American Psychological Association, pp. 9–51.

Baum, A., Fleming, I., Israel, A. & O'Keeffe, M.K. (1992). Symptoms of chronic stress following a natural disaster and discovery of a human-made hazard. *Environment and Behavior*, **28**, 347–365.

Beggs, J.J. & Haines, V.A. (1996). Situational contingencies surrounding the receipt of informal support. *Social Forces*, **75**, 201–223.

Bolin, R. (1982). *Long-Term Family Recovery from Disaster*. Boulder, CO: University of Colorado.

Bolin, R. (1989). Natural disasters. In *Psychological Aspects of Disaster*, eds. R. Gist & B. Lubin. New York: Wiley, pp. 61–85.

Bolin, R. (1993). Natural and technological disasters: evidence of psychopathology. In *Environment and Psychopathology*, eds. A.-M. Ghadirian & H.E. Lehmann. New York: Springer, pp. 121–140.

Bolin, R. & Bolton, P. (1986). *Race, Religion, and Ethnicity in Disaster Recovery*. Boulder, CO: University of Colorado.

Bowler, R.M., Mergler, D., Huel, G. & Cone, J.E. (1994). Psychological, psychosocial and psychophysiological sequelae in a community affected by a railroad chemical disaster. *Journal of Traumatic Stress*, **7**, 601–624.

Brickman, P., Rabinowitz, V., Karuza, J., Coates, D., Cohn, E. & Kidder, L. (1982). Models of helping and coping. *American Psychologist*, **37**, 368–384.

Brown, B.B. & Perkins, D.D. (1992). Disruptions in place attachment. In *Place Attachment*, eds. I. Altman & S. Low. New York: Plenum Press, pp. 279–304.

Carr, V.J., Lewin, T.J., Carter, G. & Webster, R. (1992). Patterns of service utilization following the 1989 Newcastle earthquake: findings from phase 1 of the Quake Impact Study. *Australian Journal of Public Health*, **16**, 360–369.

Curran, P.S. (1988). Psychiatric aspects of terrorist violence: Northern Ireland 1969–1987. *British Journal of Psychiatry*, **153**, 470–475.

deVries, M.W. (1995). Culture, community and catastrophe: issues in understanding communities under difficult conditions. In *Extreme Stress and Communities: Impact and Intervention*, eds. S.E. Hobfoll & M.W. deVries. Dordrecht, the Netherlands: Kluwer, pp. 375–393.

Drabek, T.E. (1986). *Human System Responses to Disaster*. New York: Springer-Verlag.

Drabek, T.E. & Key, W.M. (1984). *Conquering Disaster: Family Recovery and Long-Term Consequences*. New York: Irvington Publishers.

Draper, J., McCleery, G. & Schaedle, R. (this volume). Mental health services support in response to September 11th: the central role of the Mental Health Association of New York City. In *9/11: Mental Health in the Wake of Terrorist Attacks*, eds. Y. Neria, R. Gross & R.D. Marshall. Cambridge, UK: Cambridge University Press.

Dynes, R.R. & Drabek, T.E. (1994). The structure of disaster research: its policy and disciplinary implications. *International Journal of Mass Emergencies and Disasters*, **12**, 5–23.

Eranen, L. & Liebkind, K. (1993). Coping with disaster: the helping behavior of communities and individuals. In *International Handbook of Traumatic Stress Syndromes*, eds. J.P. Wilson & B. Raphael. New York: Plenum Press, pp. 957–964.

Erikson, K. (1976). *Everything in Its Path*. New York: Simon & Schuster.

Erikson, K. (1994). *A New Species of Trouble: The Human Experience of Modern Disasters*. New York: W.W. Norton & Company.

Felton, C.J., Donahue, S., Lanzara, C.B., Pease, E.A. & Marshall, R.D. (this volume). Project Liberty: responding to mental health needs after the World Trade Center terrorist attacks. In *9/11: Mental Health in the Wake of a Terrorist Attacks*, eds. Y. Neria, R. Gross & R. Marshall. Cambridge, UK: Cambridge University Press.

Fischer III, H.W. (1998). *Response to Disaster: Facts versus Fiction and Its Perpetuation* (2nd ed.). Lanham, MD: University Press of America.

Fogelson, R.M. (1970). Violence and grievances: reflections on the 1960s riots. *Journal of Social Issues*, **26**, 141–163.

Fritz, C.E. (1961). Disasters. In *Contemporary Social Problems*, eds. R.K. Merton & R.A. Nisbet. New York: Harcourt, pp. 651–694.

Fullilove, M.T. & Saul, J. (this volume). Rebuilding communities postdisaster in New York. In *9/11: Mental Health in the Wake of Terrorist Attacks*, eds. Y. Neria, R. Gross & R.D. Marshall. Cambridge, UK: Cambridge University Press.

Giel, R. (1990). Psychosocial process in disasters. *International Journal of Mental Health*, **19**, 7–20.

Gist, R., Lubin, B. & Redburn, B.G. (1998). Psychological, ecological, and community perspective on disaster response. *Journal of Personal and Interpersonal Loss*, **3**, 25–51.

Golec, J.A. (1983). A contextual approach to the social psychological study of disaster recovery. *International Journal of Mass Emergencies and Disaster*, **1**, 255–276.

Greenley, J.R., Gillespie, D.P. & Lindenthal, J.J. (1975). A race riot's effects on psychological symptoms. *Archives of General Psychiatry*, **32**, 1189–1195.

Griffith, J. & Villavicencio, S. (1985). Relationships among acculturation, sociodemographic characteristics and social support in Mexican American adults. *Hispanic Journal of Behavioral Sciences*, **7**, 75–92.

Harvey, J., Stein, S., Olsen, N., Roberts, R., Lutgendorf, S. & Ho, J. (1995). Narratives of loss and recovery from a natural disaster. *Journal of Social Behavior and Personality*, **10**, 313–330.

Hobfoll, S.E. (1988). *The Ecology of Stress.* New York: Hemisphere.

Hobfoll, S.E. (2001). The influence of culture, community, and the nested-self in the stress process: advancing conservation of resources theory. *Applied Psychology*, **50**, 337–370.

Hobfoll, S.E. (this volume). Guiding community intervention following terrorist attack. In *9/11: Mental Health in the Wake of Terrorist Attacks*, eds. Y. Neria, R. Gross & R.D. Marshall. Cambridge, UK: Cambridge University Press.

Hobfoll, S.E. & London, P. (1986). The relationship of self-concept and social support to emotional distress among women during war. *Journal of Social and Clinical Psychology*, **12**, 87–100.

Hutchins, G. & Norris, F.H. (1989). Life change in the disaster recovery period. *Environment and Behavior*, **21**, 33–56.

James, W. (1912). *Memories and Studies (On Some Mental Effects of the Earthquake)*. New York: Longmans, Green, & Co.

Janoff-Bulman, R. (1992). *Shattered Assumptions: Towards a New Psychology of Trauma.* New York: Free Press.

Jerusalem, M., Kaniasty, K., Lehman, D., Ritter, C. & Turnbull, G. (1995). Individual and community stress: integration of approaches at different levels. In *Extreme Stress and Communities: Impact and Intervention*, eds. S.E. Hobfoll & M.W. deVries. Dordrecht, the Netherlands: Kluwer, pp. 105–129.

Kaniasty, K. (2003). *Kleska zywiolowa czy katastrofa spoleczna? Psychospoleczne konsekwencje polskiej powodzi 1997 roku.* [*Natural Disaster or Social Catastrophe? Psychosocial Consequences of the 1997 Polish Flood.*] Gdansk, Poland: Gdanskie Wydawnictwo Psychologiczne.

Kaniasty, K. & Norris, F. (1995). In search of altruistic community: patterns of social support mobilization following Hurricane Hugo. *American Journal of Community Psychology*, **23**, 447–477.

Kaniasty, K. & Norris, F. (1997). Social support dynamics in adjustment to disasters. In *Handbook of Personal Relationships* (2nd ed.), ed. S. Duck. London, UK: Wiley, pp. 595–619.

Kaniasty, K. & Norris, F.H. (1999). The experience of disaster: individuals and communities sharing trauma. In *Response to Disaster: Psychosocial, Community, and Ecological Approaches*, eds. R. Gist & B. Lubin. Philadelphia, PA: Brunner/Maze, pp. 25–61.

Kaniasty, K. & Norris, F.H. (2000). Help-seeking comfort and receiving social support: the role of ethnicity and context of need. *American Journal of Community Psychology*, **28**, 545–581.

Kaniasty, K. & Norris, F. (2004). Social support in the aftermath of disasters, catastrophes, and acts of terrorism: altruistic, overwhelmed, uncertain, antagonistic, and patriotic communities. In *Bioterrorism: Psychological and Public Health Interventions*, eds. R. Ursano, A. Norwood & C. Fullerton. Cambridge, UK: Cambridge University Press, pp. 200–229.

Kaniasty, K., Norris, F. & Murrell, S.A. (1990). Received and perceived social support following natural disaster. *Journal of Applied Social Psychology*, **20**, 85–114.

Katz, C.L., Smith, R., Herbert, R., Levin, S. & Gross, R. (this volume). The World Trade Center Worker/Volunteer Mental Health Screening Program. In *9/11: Mental Health in the Wake of Terrorist Attacks*, eds. Y. Neria, R. Gross & R.D. Marshall. Cambridge, UK: Cambridge University Press.

Kilijanek, T. & Drabek, T.E. (1979). Assessing long-term impacts of a natural disaster: a focus on the elderly. *The Gerontologist*, **19**, 555–566.

Kutak, R.I. (1938). The sociology of crises: the Louisville flood of 1937. *Social Forces*, **16**, 66–72.

Lepore, S.J. & Smyth, J. (eds.) (2002). *The Writing Cure: How Expressive Writing Promotes Health and Emotional Well-being*. Washington, DC: APA.

Litz, B.T. (this volume). Learning lessons from the early intervention response to the Pentagon. In *9/11: Mental Health in the Wake of a Terrorist Attacks*, eds. Y. Neria, R. Gross & R. Marshall. Cambridge, UK: Cambridge University Press

McFarlane, A.C. (1987). Family functioning and overprotection following a natural disaster: the longitudinal effects of post-traumatic morbidity. *Australian and New Zealand Journal of Psychiatry*, **21**, 210–218.

McFarlane, A.C. (1995). Stress and disaster. In *Extreme Stress and Communities: Impact and Intervention*, eds. S.E. Hobfoll & M.W. deVries. Dordrecht, the Netherlands: Kluwer, pp. 247–266.

McNally, R., Bryant, R. & Ehlers, A. (2003). Does early psychological interventions promote recovery from posttraumatic stress? *Psychological Science in the Public Interest*, **2**, 45–79.

Mehl, M. & Pennebaker, J. (2003). The social dynamics of a cultural upheaval: social interactions surrounding September 11, 2001. *Psychological Science*, **6**, 578–579.

Milgram, N. (1986). *Stress and Coping in War: Generalizations from the Israeli Experience*. New York: Brunner/Mazel.

Mira, E. (1939). Psychiatric experience in the Spanish war. *British Medical Journal*, **1**, 1217–1220.

Neria, Y., Gross, R., Olfson, M., Gamerrof, M.J., Das, A., Feder, A., Lantigua, R., Shea, S. & Weissman, M.M. (this volume). Screening for PTSD in low income predominantly Hispanic primary care patients in NYC one year after 9/11 attacks. In *9/11: Mental Health in the Wake of Terrorist Attacks*, eds. Y. Neria, R.Gross & R.D. Marshall. Cambridge, UK: Cambridge University Press.

Norris, F. (this volume). Community and ecological approaches to understanding and alleviating post disaster distress. In *9/11: Mental Health in the Wake of Terrorist Attacks*, eds. Y. Neria, R.Gross & R.D. Marshall. Cambridge, UK: Cambridge University Press.

Norris, F. & Alegria, M. (2006). Promoting disaster recovery in ethnic minority individuals and communities. In *Intervention following mass violence and disorders: strategies of mental health practice,* eds. C. Ritchie, P. Watson & M. Friedman. New York: Guildford Press, pp. 319–342.

Norris, F. & Uhl, G. (1993). Chronic stress as a mediator of acute stress: the case of Hurricane Hugo. *Journal of Applied Social Psychology,* **23**, 1263–1284.

Norris, F., Friedman, M., Watson, P., Byrne, C., Diaz, E. & Kaniasty, K. (2002). 60,000 disaster victims speak. Part I: An empirical review of the empirical literature, 1981–2001. *Psychiatry,* **65**, 207–239.

Oliver-Smith, A. (1996). Anthropological research on hazards and disasters. *Annual Reviews of Anthropology,* **25**, 303–328.

Picou, J.S., Gill, D., Dyer, C. & Curry, E.W. (1992). Disruption and stress in an Alaskan fishing community: initial and continuing impacts of the Exxon Valdez oil spill. *Industrial Crisis Quarterly,* **6**, 235–257.

Pennebaker, J.W. (1990). *Opening Up: The Healing Power of Confiding in Others.* New York: Morrow.

Pennebaker, J.W. & Harber, K. (1993). A social stage model of collective coping: the Loma Prieta earthquake and the Persian Gulf War. *Journal of Social Issues,* **49**, 125–145.

Perilla, J., Norris, F. & Lavizzo, E. (2002). Ethnicity, culture, and disaster response: identifying and explaining ethnic differences in PTSD six months after Hurricane Andrew. *Journal of Social and Clinical Psychology,* **21**, 28–45.

Pyszczynski, T., Solomon, S. & Greenberg, J. (2003). *In the Wake of 9/11: The Psychology of Terror.* Washington, DC: APA.

Riley, D. & Eckenrode, J. (1986). Social ties: subgroup differences in costs and benefits. *Journal of Personality and Social Psychology,* **51**, 770–778.

Ritchie, C.E., Leavitt, D.T. & Hanish, S. (this volume). The mental health response to the 9/11 attacks on the Pentagon. In *9/11: Mental Health in the Wake of Terrorist Attacks*, eds. Y. Neria, R. Gross & R.D. Marshall. Cambridge, UK: Cambridge University Press.

Solomon, S.D., Bravo, M., Rubio-Stipec, M. & Canino, G. (1993). Effect of family role on response to disaster. *Journal of Traumatic Stress,* **6**, 255–270.

Steinglass, P. & Gerrity, E. (1990). Natural disasters and post-traumatic stress disorder: short-term versus long-term recovery in two disaster-affected communities. *Journal of Applied Social Psychology,* **20**, 1746–1765.

Warheit, G.J., Zimmerman, R.S., Khoury, E.L., Vega, W.A. & Gil, A.G. (1996). Disaster related stresses, depressive signs and symptoms, and suicidal ideation among a multi-racial/ethnic sample of adolescents: a longitudinal analysis. *Journal of Child Psychology and Psychiatry,* **37**, 435–444.

Webster, R., McDonald, R., Lewin, T. & Carr, V. (1995). Effects of a natural disaster on immigrants and host population. *Journal of Nervous and Mental Disease,* **183**, 390–397.

Wenger, D.E., James, T.F. & Faupel, C.E. (1985). *Disaster Belief and Emergency Planning.* New York: Irvington.

Wolfenstein, M. (1957). *Disaster: A Psychological Essay.* Glencoe, IL: Free Press.

Wortman, C.B. & Silver, R.C. (2001). The myths of coping with loss revisited. In *Handbook of Bereavement research: Consequences, Coping and Care,* eds. M.S. Stroebe, R.O. Hansson, W. Stroebe & H. Schut. Washington, DC: APA, pp. 405–429.

31

What mental health professionals should and should not do

Simon Wessely

Introduction

I don't live in America, let alone in New York. I live in Central London under the Heathrow flight path. It was not long ago that my house was shaken by the final flights of the last three Concordes. On September 11, 2001, we experienced the opposite, a strange week of silence, when all flights were banned for a week. And when they resumed for a while I looked out of my window as each plane came past and experienced a frisson of anxiety. Like virtually everyone I know, it took sometime to shake off those hypnotic images imprinted in my memory from those hours glued to our TV screens throughout the horrors of that first day.

But not for a moment did I consider that I had a problem, let alone seek help for it. And after a few weeks these emotions disappeared. Yes, my view of the world had changed, as had my appraisal of the society we live in and the threats we face. The world seemed, and probably was, a riskier place (Halpern-Felsher & Millstein, 2002; Roberts & Em, 2003). But emotionally and physically I felt the same as I had been before, for better or worse.

When I visited America only a few weeks later, to take part, ironically, in a pre-arranged conference on psychological responses to mass violence (National Institute of Mental Health, 2002), I observed something else. September 11th had also brought about positive changes in the society that I have visited so many times. Was it my imagination, or were people genuinely more talkative, more likely to engage with me in the bars, waiting rooms and queues that are the staple of travel these days? No, on everyone's lips was the observation that adversity had brought us together, and indeed that upsurge in communitarian feelings for once even involved myself as a Britisher, finally forgiven for George III. It was confirmation of the "democracy and brotherhood of common disaster" (Kutak quoted in Kaniasty, this volume).

Should we be surprised by this? It was Durkheim himself who suggested that during periods of external threat group cohesion increases, and suicide rates decrease (Durkheim, 1897). Indeed, tentative evidence of a lowering of the suicide rate in the UK after 9/11 has been presented (Salib, 2003), and it would be interesting to know if the same will be observed in the USA. We are robust nations and our citizens repeatedly surprise us by their resilience in the face of adversity in the past (Jones *et al.*, in press) and of course during the terrible events of 9/11, when panic was noticeable by its absence (Glass & Schoch-Spana, 2002).

September 11th did bring about changes in most of us. These were a complex mixture of both negative and positive changes. But were these abnormal? Did I need treatment for my compulsive checking of the sky over my house, or the dreams I experienced? Did I need to consult with a mental health professional?

It is a general principle, and one to which I shall return, that professionals should refrain from treating ailments that are going to get better fairly quickly anyway, since to do so wastes resources and exposes patients to the risks of side effects of unnecessary treatment. What do we know about the emotional responses that were indeed so common after 9/11?

The contributions in this book tell us much. The Rand team reported that 44% of Americans had "substantial stress" in the wake of 9/11 (Schuster *et al.*, 2001). One does wonder if "having trouble falling or staying asleep", or "having difficulty concentrating", scoring on either item at the "quite a bit" level being sufficient to qualify for "substantial stress" was really compatible with the word "substantial", but never mind. This figure had halved at Wave 2, taken during November 2001, only a few weeks later. And we can compare this with the contribution from Sandro Galea and colleagues, who conducted an equally elegant follow-up study carried out solely in New York City at 1, 4 and 6 months after the attacks (Galea *et al.*, 2003). Probable post-traumatic stress disorder (PTSD) declined from 7.5% to 0.6% at 6 months, the latter figure comfortably within expected population norms. Thus, we can expect that the Rand study, if it had been repeated at 6 months after the attacks would show further decline, and I suspect would likewise return to the baseline level of psychological distress in the community. According to the National Comorbidity Survey, taken prior to 9/11, the lifetime prevalence of PTSD in the USA is less than 8%. We should not make the error of assuming that all PTSD in New York City is due to the events of 9/11.

Likewise, it is intriguing to note that according to the contribution by Katz and colleagues, 60% of rescue workers screened positive, a figure not changing over time, whilst 40% were cases on the General Health Questionnaire (GHQ) (Katz *et al.*, this volume). The former statistic makes one wonder what the pre-9/11 rate of "caseness" would have been, not least because there is a vast literature attesting to high symptom scores in many emergency workers anyway, and the latter statistic is comfortably within population norms. Katz and colleagues note the strangely reduced rates of major depression in this sample – one wonders if there has simply been a diagnostic shift rather than a true increase in morbidity. Either way, when analysing any uncontrolled post-9/11 mental health data, we should beware of assuming that America pre-9/11 was free of mental health problems.

And just how serious or abnormal were these manifestations anyway? We all know that there are no clear cutoffs between the normal and abnormal in psychiatry. In general, we strive to treat the abnormal clinical depression, for example, and not the normal sadness after the death of a loved one. After exposure to traumatic events we often expend considerable efforts to remind people that it is normal to feel upset, shaken, or to have difficulty sleeping, and this is not a psychiatric disorder nor the inevitable precursor to one. Indeed, the inherent ambiguity of many post-disaster interventions, which simultaneously proclaim that it is normal to feel upset when bad things happen, and then suggest a variety of therapeutic interventions, points to the importance of non-therapeutic factors underlying many institutional and professional responses to trauma. Deciding on the boundaries between the normal and abnormal will always be a matter of discretion. And as a sociologist Frank Furedi has recently argued, there is a danger that we are now getting these boundaries wrong (Furedi, 2003), and actively professionalizing or pathologizing normal feelings with consequences that can be unforeseen and undesirable.

Symptoms are not disorders

One increasingly recognized boundary is the one existing between symptoms and disorder. In our work on members of the United Kingdom Armed Forces after the 1991 Gulf War we found elevated rates of every symptom that we inquired after, including those indicative of possible PTSD (Unwin et al., 1999). Yet when we interviewed these service personnel using standardized psychiatric instruments the rate of PTSD was elevated, but only from 1% in the well veterans to 3% in the sick (Ismail et al., 2002). Many veterans had symptoms, fewer had discrete disorders mandating treatment.

Symptoms alone are a poor guide to disorder, and what we should be concerned about is disorder and its implications on functioning. The focus should be on people unable to earn their living or look after their families, not on those who felt transiently alarmed or anxious in a world growing increasingly alarming. Symptoms might indicate disorder, but then again, as Carol North notes in this volume, they might not.

So how do we interpret what happened after 9/11? We have vast numbers of people like myself – people who felt both emotional distress and greater social involvement in the days after 9/11. People who did indeed experience emotional change, and sometimes visible distress, but emotions that were understandable, not abnormal, did not indicate a lifetime of psychiatric illness, and indeed had begun to disappear in a matter of weeks. And we have people, in New York City, who rose to the challenge of 9/11 in a variety of community and adaptive actions, as described by Fullilove and Saul (this volume).

There are certainly exceptions to the above – those in whom psychiatric disorder might be expected to either develop or persist. These "high risk" groups (those with low socio-economic status (SES), pre-existing disorder and/or acute stress disorders, and those with direct intense exposure to the traumatic event – not simply hearing about, reading or watching it) will be considered later. Ever since the development of a recognizable professional psychiatry early in the twentieth century these people have been considered to be the appropriate concern of the mental health services. However, in the last decade or so, attention has shifted from this minority to the majority – people who have been exposed to adversity, but who are not suffering from any psychiatric disorder as yet, and who have not been considered to need, require or demand mental health interventions. And it is this potentially vast group, and the attempts to engage, educate and even treat this group, that forms the principal focus and interest of this book.

Two approaches have been particularly advocated for this majority group, were tried in an *ad hoc* fashion after 9/11, and are likely to be tried again should circumstances repeat themselves. These involve, first of all, some form of screening, and second, some form of immediate psychological intervention such as psychological debriefing. Neither, however, is without problems and pitfalls.

The seductions of screening and the disappointment of debriefing

PTSD, like all psychiatric disorders, is bad news if you develop it. And because it seems so obvious that prevention is better than cure, who can argue with a plea for better prevention? So how might post-traumatic psychiatric disorders be prevented? Historically two principal strategies have been tried. The first of these involves screening for vulnerability to breakdown either before exposure (as for example in the military or the emergency services to determine who should or should not be put in harm's way, or screening after exposure, to determine those who should receive support and/or treatment). The second involves a direct psychological intervention aimed at all those exposed to trauma, with the purpose of preventing subsequent psychiatric disorder. Both are problematic. I shall consider the pitfalls of screening for vulnerability to psychiatric disorder first.

The rules of screening

Screening is never an end in itself, it is a means to an end, and that end is the delivery of treatment that might make a difference. If we consider for a moment why certain screening programmes are indeed successful, we can see what are the hurdles that need to be overcome before we can recommend a mental health screening programme after trauma, and how unlikely it is that we will ever be able to do this in practice.

These principles are straight forward, well understood, and crucial to understanding the general record of failure in screening for mental health vulnerability or disorder. They are described in any textbook of screening, public health or epidemiology (Hennekens & Buring, 1987; Muir Gray, 1997; National Screening Committee, 1998).

The first principle concerns the method used to detect those one wishes to identify, which in this situation is most likely to be a questionnaire. These must have certain properties. Technically these are known as sensitivity, specificity, positive predictive value and negative predictive value. The instrument must detect a substantial proportion of those we aim to detect (those who either have, or will get, the disorder in question) – this is sensitivity. Likewise, it must not detect very many of those who do not have, or will not get, the disorder – this is specificity. Finally, when we are talking about detecting those who have not yet developed the disorder in question, the key statistic here is the positive predictive value – of those who are detected by our screening programme, how many will go on to develop the disorder itself (Rose, 1992).

The second principle is that screening is worthwhile. There must be a benefit to the individual, and to society, from detecting people by this method. Several requirements must therefore be satisfied. First, one only screens for disorders for which proven effective interventions exist and are available. There is no point in screening for disorders that cannot be treated effectively. Likewise, there is little point in screening for disorders that will improve spontaneously. A knowledge of the natural history of the disorder is thus a prerequisite. Screening for conditions in which the natural tendency is towards recovery is hard to justify on ethical, clinical and economic grounds. Second, screening must be cost effective. There is little point in mounting a complex and costly screening programme if there is evidence that most people with the disorder are going to be detected by existing methods or services anyway.

All screening carries a risk of harm. As Muir Gray puts it "all screening programmes do harm, some can do good as well" (Muir Gray, 1997). Those detected may be exposed to investigations or treatments with side effects. Screening itself has hazards – side effects of the instrument, or increased anxiety about the condition. Those who are identified by the programme may not realize, and indeed probably don't realize, they are "at risk". Once they learn that they are now at increased risk of an adverse outcome, their behaviour may change in many unforeseen ways. They may become more careful or solicitous about their health, or conversely adopt a wide range of risky behaviours – "because it is going to happen to me anyway".

Their view of themselves as a healthy person has been altered, and their mood and psychological well-being may be adversely effected. There is a wide, extensive and compelling literature on the adverse psychological consequences of screening (Shaw *et al.*, 1999). For those who are identified as at risk, but actually are not going to develop the disorder (false positives) it will be clear that screening can only be a source of harm – the question is how much. Exactly the same applies to those correctly identified as having a disorder, but one which will spontaneously remit without treatment.

Screening: a lesson from history

That is the theory, but how has screening for mental health problems fared in reality? There is one very good example that should give pause for thought. It is the story of mental health screening as practiced by the military authorities over the last hundred years (Jones *et al.*, 2003). One can understand why this is appealing to the military mind. If we could know beforehand who was going to breakdown in battle, we could screen them out beforehand. This would give us a stronger military, and would be better for the men themselves, their families, and the national budget.

The historical record is indeed full of pleas made by those having to command men in battle to those responsible for selection imploring them to do a better job (Jones *et al.*, 2003). My favourite is quoted in Ben Shephard's classic account of psychiatrists at war (Shephard, 2000), and is a signal sent by a senior officer in the eighth Army in Egypt in 1942 back to the War Office begging them not to send him men who "can't stand the brothels of Cairo, let alone the Afrika Corp".

One answer seemed to be mass psychological screening. Back in World War II, the Americans believed that they could identify those who were going to make bad soldiers and become future psychiatric cases. They enlisted the enthusiastic help of the best psychiatrists in the land, led by no less a figure than Harry Stack Sullivan. The psychiatrists gave their all for the war effort, removing over two million men from the draft on the basis of personality testing that predicted who would and who would not break down (Jones *et al.*, 2003).

But patriotism and good intentions were not enough. Indeed, the consequences of the mass psychological screening programme was that the Americans nearly lost the war. By 1944, when no less a person that George C. Marshall called a halt to the screening programmes, they were running out of men (Ginzberg, 1959). What then happened was that many of those rejected on psychiatric grounds were re-enlisted – a vast natural experiment. To everyone's surprise studies showed that most made perfectly good, and sometimes very good, soldiers. Some broke down, more than those who had not been screened out – the psychiatrists were not totally wrong, but up to 85% actually made perfectly adequate soldiers (Aita, 1949).

There were many reasons why the screening programme failed, some of them relevant to the debate on the consequences of terrorist trauma, some of them less so. A major risk factor for breakdown is experiencing a traumatic event – but that hasn't happened yet, and may not, so predeployment screening is deprived of the best single predictive factor. And what remains are a collection of risk factors, which while statistically significant, are all relatively weak individual predictors of future breakdown (Brewin *et al.*, 2000). Of course, after an incident such as 9/11 the event has happened, and while we can say in general terms that the greater the exposure to the traumatic event, the greater the risk of PTSD, the various predictive factors remain too weak to allow the level of individual prediction necessary to say who will, and who will not, develop later disorder.

Less relevant to the post-trauma situation, but nevertheless still necessary when considering any screening programme, are the adverse effects of the procedure. For example, if screening is used to exclude individuals from military service, or perhaps the emergency services, further problems can be anticipated. Excluding people who have risk factors for developing disorder after trauma – coming from a single parent family, having a family history of psychiatric disorder, a poor school record and so on, would have many untoward consequences. Denying military service to people with these risky backgrounds, for example, would clearly have a serious effect on recruitment, since both the British and American militaries traditionally recruit from areas of social disadvantage. Furthermore, it would also deny some of the social goals and benefits of military service – giving people from disadvantaged backgrounds a chance to learn a skill and gain self-respect.

Definitely relevant to the trauma situation is that labelling people as potentially psychologically unstable, liable to breakdown if something is not done to prevent this, is also not without risks. It changes peoples' views of themselves in unpredictable ways, and exposes them to stigma. The American World War II experience showed that many of those denied the opportunity to serve their country because of concerns for their psychological stability returned to their home communities and were exposed to shame and ridicule.

Questions that must be answered before we can recommend screening for psychological vulnerability or disorder

Armed with that historical example, what questions should be answered before we can advise the implementation of a psychological screening programme in the aftermath of a disaster? First, do services exist to deal with the disorder that is going to be detected? If so, do we know that those people who require treatment are not already accessing it? If those who are the target of that screening would have presented to medical services anyway, then there is clearly no case for launching an expensive and elaborate screening system. The answer will differ from country to country, depending on the characteristics of different health care systems. There is less of a case for screening in countries such as the UK, in which there is a comprehensive primary health care system, which is very permeable indeed (most people see their family doctor between three and four times a year). Likewise, many military health systems are exceptionally easy to access. Even if it is found that those who should be detected are being overlooked, this may be a case for better recognition, or better education and training of the physician, but not screening *per se*.

However, even if an efficient and effective system for managing psychological disorder existed (and regrettably despite the above examples of efficient and effective systems for managing psychological disorder, they are conspicuous by their absence in all the health care systems I have knowledge of), there is still a possible case for a screening programme if it can be shown that those who would benefit from treatment fail to access the services available.

There are various reasons why people might not access services when they should do so, and hence may be potential beneficiaries of screening. One reason may be that they have not yet actually developed the disorder in question – in this context the question of delayed PTSD. Such people will not gain from screening in the aftermath of trauma for obvious reasons.

What about people who have the disorder, but have not sought help? There are numerous studies describing the characteristics of those who seek treatment, since such studies are easy to perform, but what is required are studies in which those who do not seek treatment but are also suffering from psychological distress are compared to those with similar conditions who have sought assistance. This kind of data is harder to find. However, studies that are able to compare treatment seeking and non-treatment seeking populations generally show that those who present to services are more symptomatic than those who do not, which is encouraging (Solomon *et al.*, 1989; Kulka *et al.*, 1990; Bramsen & Ploeg, 1999) but weakens the case for screening.

Why do many people not present? Some do not wish to, as indeed is their basic human right. Some are aware of the stigma of psychiatric disorder, and either feel ashamed of their symptoms or are concerned that others might see them as weak. Like the author, the readership of this book almost certainly do not share this attitude, but there can be no doubt that many others do. Perhaps it is as Amsel and colleagues state, 9/11 has led to a sea change in our acceptance of mental distress and disorder (Amsel *et al.*, this volume), but this process had begun before 9/11 anyway (Furedi, 2003).

We have as a society become more sensitive to the plight of "victims", but nevertheless, stigma remains a powerful issue, and many people will continue to be very uncomfortable with a psychiatric label. As no one is advocating compulsory treatment for post-traumatic stress and its variants, these wishes must be respected. Mental health professionals all too easily forget the low esteem in which we and our patients are held by the general public. And because I am not in favour of compulsory psychiatric treatment except under the provisions of the existing mental health legislation, I regret I cannot share the call made by Difede and colleagues in their otherwise excellent contribution for mandatory psychological screening either. If it is to be done, it must be on the basis of consent, not compulsion. Already many of us have heard of disquiet and resentment among emergency workers forced to attend compulsory debriefing after 9/11.

Others do not present because of the nature of the disorder. For some, avoidance of reminders of the source of their distress is a powerful force. The disorder itself plays a role in preventing them from seeking help. These people may be persuaded to access services if correctly identified and sensitively managed, and are perhaps the group that stand most to benefit from screening, if only they can be identified.

Finally, comes the issue of prognosis. One screens for cervical or breast cancer because neither spontaneously improves or disappears. This is far from the case for the disorders we are concerned with. The evidence presented in this book makes it clear that most distress after 9/11 improved anyway. Likewise, Solomon's prospective studies of Israeli combat veterans show PTSD can and does improve over time (Solomon, 1989). This is a major obstacle to implementing any screening programme – it will detect a great deal of symptomatic distress that is going to clear up anyway. These people will then be exposed to the risks and costs of treatment for no reason.

Choices of measures

The next question is that if screening is desirable, is there an effective instrument? As already stated, the key statistics in assessing the performance of any screening instrument are its sensitivity, specificity and positive predictive value.

There are currently many instruments that have been used to detect PTSD. Several of the newer ones have shown acceptable psychometric properties in specific populations. For example, the scale devised by Davidson, reported in 1997, has at its best cut off a sensitivity of 0.69, a specificity of 0.95, and a positive predictive value of 92%, which is very respectable (Davidson *et al.*, 1997). However, that data comes from the validation study in which the prevalence of PTSD was very high – 67 out of 129 subjects had the disorder. In a sample with far lower prevalences of PTSD, which is the case in any population or public health setting, the scale will perform far worse.

A more relevant comparison was provided by Shalev and colleagues (Shalev *et al.*, 1997). They compared the ability of four different questionnaires to predict

PTSD in those attending an Accident and Emergency Department. This is more relevant to the current discussion, because the overall prevalence of PTSD was lower than in previous studies (30% at 1 month and 17% at 4 months), albeit still higher than the population. The results showed that whereas all the questionnaires did predict PTSD better than chance alone, none had the properties required for a screening programme – in particular the positive predictive values were all low, and would be unacceptable as a basis for any screening programme (Shalev *et al.*, 1997).

Screening and treatment

It is a requirement of all screening programmes that there be a benefit to the person who is identified as a result of the screening – in other words that treatments of proven efficacy exist and are available. In certain conditions such as cervical cancer, where early intervention is virtually curative of what would otherwise be a fatal condition, treatment clearly passes the risk benefit equation with flying colours, and hence the case for screening is strengthened. Edna Foa and colleagues have addressed issues of treatment for PTSD, and concluded that the long-term effects of treating trauma related psychiatric disorder are reasonable, but not outstanding (Foa *et al.*, 2000). This relatively modest, albeit worthwhile, success means that the case for screening for PTSD in low prevalence populations is always going to be problematic.

The more recent optimistic reports on the use of new treatment modalities in some populations of patients with acute stress disorders (Andre *et al.*, 1997; Bryant *et al.*, 1998, 1999) are an important step forward, but may not necessarily relate to screened populations. Randomized controlled trials of treatment are almost invariably based on those who come forward spontaneously for assistance. In contrast, it seems likely that those identified by a screening programme are less motivated to change, and hence less likely to gain benefits from treatment than those who form the subject of the cited statistics on treatment success and failure.

Is it effective?

We now reach the final requirement, that there be evidence that the screening programme is effective – that at the end of the day, there has been a demonstrable difference in health outcomes for the population that has been screened, taking into account both the positive and negative aspects of the programme. Throughout this book most contributors have been meticulous in only promoting "evidence-based treatments" for very cogent reasons. The arguments for only promoting evidence-based screening are as compelling.

The only way in which one can assess the success or failure of such a strategy is via the randomized controlled trial, since there is no other safe way of knowing what would have happened without the screening, and no way of assessing the size and scale of any adverse effects. I have been unable to locate any such studies relevant to PTSD, but there is evidence concerning general psychiatric disorders that is relevant.

A recent high quality systematic review found nine randomized controlled trials of the results of screening for mental health problems linked with some method of feeding back the results of the tests to doctors – which would be one simple way in which post-trauma screening would be carried out in countries with reasonable primary care services (Gilbody *et al.*, 2001).

First, routine administration and feedback did not increase the overall recognition of mental disorders. Second, if only those with high scores were fed back to the doctors (removing the noise and concentrating on the signal, as it were) then there was evidence that the recognition of disorders did increase. However, even if recognition increased, it did not lead to any differences in intervention nor could any effect on patient outcome, which is the point of the exercise, be demonstrated. The conclusions do not support the policy of routine screening for psychiatric disorders (Gilbody *et al.*, 2001).

Likewise, another recent review detected seven studies which examined the actual results of screening for mental health problems in routine practice – "none of these studies found an advantage for detecting patients" (Coyne *et al.*, 2000). While the authors still do not discount the possibility that there may still be as yet undemonstrated benefits to such systems, "the lack of contrary evidence is disconcerting" (Coyne *et al.*, 2000).

The answer seems to be that with the best intentions in the world, mental health programmes based on screening for existing disorders have not been a success.

In conclusion, it is hard to see how a psychological screening programme instituted to prevent psychiatric disorder after trauma could ever fulfil the criteria that the National Health Service insists upon before introducing any new screening programme (Muir Gray, 1997). It remains the case that screening without evidence of efficacy cannot be justified, and that "screening of unproven value should not be advocated" (Law, 2004). Perhaps this may change, but at present the evidence does not exist.

The disappointments of debriefing

Just as with screening, the idea that immediate psychological interventions could prevent later breakdown sounds intuitively appealing, and has had numerous supporters over the years. However, just as the negative experiences of psychological screening during the Second World War should give us pause for thought, we have the example of psychological debriefing to provide us with another cautionary tale.

Most people will be familiar with the concept of single session psychological debriefing. There are many different forms of debriefing, but in essence all are variations on a similar theme. It is a fairly structured procedure in which a mental health professional carries out an intervention with people, either individually or in groups, very shortly after they have been exposed to some form of adversity. The procedure involves some element of telling the story of the event, asking how people felt emotionally during the event and now, and teaching about likely further emotional reactions over time. Its purpose, enthusiastically proclaimed by its protagonists, is to prevent later psychiatric disorder such as PTSD.

In our contemporary culture, the arrival of what the media inevitably call "trained counsellors", has become as much a part of the theatre of disaster as that of the emergency services. It has become part of the social recognition of disaster, and our collective desire that "something must be done" (Gist, 2002).

But the problem is that single session psychological debriefing clearly does not work, and indeed there is more than a suggestion that it may actually increase the risk of subsequent psychological disorder (Wessely *et al.*, 2000; Emmerik *et al.*, 2002). Since the publication of these systematic reviews there are at least four more randomized controlled trials currently under review, all of which give similar results and add to the robustness of the conclusions of the reviews. Let there be no doubt – single session psychological debriefing, no matter what it is called or what label it carries, if it is based on the concept of "better out than in" and promoting emotional disclosure immediately after trauma, does not work and probably makes some people worse.

There are many reasons for the ineffectiveness and possible adverse effects of debriefing. I favour the view that it impedes the normal ways in which we deal with adversity – talking to our friends, family, general practitioner, clergy, etc. and instead professionalizes distress. As Kaniasty puts it in this volume – "victims are quite reticent in utilizing assistance from sources outside their immediate network, even if such formalized aid offered by governmental and relief agencies is readily available, and rely mainly on their families, relatives, friends, and neighbours".

I also feel that immediate formal psychological interventions such as debriefing may actively disempower people from "doing what comes naturally". I am aware of increasing instances of counselors being sent to local schools when a tragic event strikes a child in a school. We had an incident near us in which a child was killed during a school outing. The school authorities that night requested immediate help from our local mental health services so that counselors could be on hand in the morning to help the children comes to terms with the tragedy. I know one of teachers in the school, and asked her afterwards why she did not feel able to talk to the children in her class about the death of the child in another class. Her answer was that although she felt instinctively it was part of her role as a classroom teacher, perhaps there were special "professional" skills needed that she did not possess. Meanwhile, the Headmaster who had made the request later told me that he did so "in order to make clear how seriously we took this tragedy". What this shows is first, the teacher felt that in some ill defined way she was not qualified to talk to the children in her class about the loss, even though common sense suggests the classroom teacher may be the person best placed to do this. Second, how the institution itself reached for the counselors as a signal or symbol of how seriously they were taking the tragedy, rather than because of any particular reason, need or evidence that such an intervention was necessary. I rarely resort to anecdote, but I do so now, confident in the knowledge that what I am describing has become commonplace.

I also detect similar concerns in Fullilove's account in this volume of how providing counselling services to New York City schools left parents and teachers feeling disenfranchised. This must be a cause for concern. Schecter and Coates remind us of Anna Freud's observations of children during the London blitz (Schecter & Coates, this volume). We should take to heart her and others' conclusions that children were relatively unaffected by exposure to danger and adversity, providing family ties were maintained (it was the evacuation more than the blitz itself, that created problems). Instead, children's responses were and continue to be primarily determined by the actions of parents and guardians (Freud & Burlingham, 1943; Carey Trefzer, 1949).

Likewise, in the contribution from Draper and colleagues, describing the demands made on Lifenet after 9/11, comes the phrase that requests came "from shaken schools, community centers and workplaces around the city seeking an outreach worker to conduct group crisis counselling". It is legitimate to ask if the people themselves made that request, or if they perceived a need, or whether this was again an institutional response designed to show that the employer "cares". Of course, there is no reason why an employer should not demonstrate they "care" about their staff, employees or children, but one is also entitled to question if this now reflex response is the best or only way of demonstrating that.

I suspect that the adverse effects of crisis debriefing are sociological, relating to inculcating the belief that people have a mental health problem, and that either they themselves, or their teachers/leaders, are not competent to cope with these feelings without professional help. But there are other possibilities. Perhaps it is too early. Perhaps it exposes people to distressing memories without allowing habituation – a form of re-traumatization or exposure without the gradual exposure and habituation of formal exposure based treatments over many sessions (Devilly *et al.*, 2006). Perhaps by describing emotional reactions that have not yet occurred but might occur it encourages suggestibility.

Perhaps there is no right or wrong answer as to how we should manage our emotions. Emotional responses like everything else are subject to fashion. And fashions can change. So during the 1960s and beyond stiff upper lip was satirized by Beyond the Fringe and Monty Python, while emotional expression was encouraged and rewarded, until we reach the *reductio ab absurdam* of Jerry Springer and the talk show culture. Emotional expression is now very much in fashion (Furedi, 2003), but it is not the only way of handling adversity.

Anyway, it matters less precisely why debriefing does not work, but more that we finally acknowledge this fact. The debriefing saga is a warning against well-intentioned efforts that we can prevent, and I emphasize the word, prevent, the psychological consequences of trauma (Wessely, 2005: in press). It also reminds us that people are different, and handle and process emotions differently. Given that fairly obvious statement, it should come as no surprise that a single type of intervention, the psychological debriefing, should not be suitable or acceptable for all. One size certainly does not fit all.

And there is a profounder meaning as well. When bad things happen normal people feel distressed. And when very bad things happen, such as the loss of a loved one, the pain and suffering can continue for many weeks, months or years. It is a natural human instinct to want to alleviate such suffering, but short of bringing back the deceased, perhaps it cannot be done, at least not for sometime. Immediate psychological interventions to reduce distress may make us, the bystanders or observers, feel better and reassured that something has "been done". It may indeed be a social validation of the scale and impact of disaster, and recognition by the rest of us of the tragedy, but that does not mean it does any good for those in grief. Sometimes we must acknowledge that there are "no simple solutions for complex problems" (Gist & Woodhall, 1999).

That's all very well, but …

I am aware that I have been rather negative about two proposed methods of reducing distress after disaster – implementing screening programmes and using short psychological interventions aimed at normal people. I am also aware that such advice is hard to implement when the need to do something is overwhelming, as Cam Ritchie's contribution on the aftermath of the Pentagon crash demonstrates so eloquently (Ritchie *et al.*, this volume). The answer is that yes, there are things that the authorities, the emergency services and others can and should do that will have a mental health impact.

First, for the majority of people emotional support when needed can and should come from people's own social networks, such as family, friends, colleagues, general practitioners, clergy, etc. It is therefore the task of the authorities to facilitate this support and not impede it. Special efforts may need to be directed at certain groups, such as those with low incomes, the elderly, ethnic minorities and so on, but even then the default position is to assist people to link with their own social networks rather than replacing them with professional assistance.

Second, immediate mental health support in the acute situation comes indirectly from practical support. The task of the authorities is to ensure security, provide timely and accurate information, provide food and drink, ensure communications with family and friends and provide all practical support necessary regarding accommodation, transport and so on. That is a mental health intervention par excellence.

The importance of rapid, accurate communication can hardly be overestimated. This can and should take two forms. First, communication between those affected by a disaster and their families. We know that after 9/11 there was a dramatic upsurge in mobile phone communications within minutes, and indeed this brought the systems in New York City to a halt. Emergency services frequently view this immediate response, which happens after every terrorist incident in Israel, as at best an irritation, and at worst a threat to their own communications. But it is in fact a vital coping mechanism. The Israeli experience shows that provided people receive fast and accurate information from the mass media, and can at the same time make rapid contact with their families, then they can continue with their activities, and/or make rational choices about what they should do in the situation. Shalev has shown in the current Israeli situation of continuous terror that anxiety about families is more powerful than anxiety about personal safety (Shalev & Freedman, 2004). The Japanese experience after the Sarin attack on the Tokyo subway shows that the absence of mobile phone network coverage was one reason for an increase in anxiety in those trapped in the subway system but not actually exposed to the attack. Our technologies improve from month to month, and ensuring that mobile phone systems can be maintained after a terrorist attack is not just a matter of allowing the emergency services to communicate with each other, but of allowing people to do the same. Communication increases control, and reduces the chance of panic.

Third, the provision of information is vitally important. It is unnecessary to labour the point that after any terrorist event people need information quickly. This will need to be delivered speedily, so much so that information for various eventualities will need to be prepared well in advance. The speed of modern news delivery means that the so called "media window" for the responsible authorities to get their message across before others do that for them is measured in minutes, perhaps an hour, and no more. All of that is well understood, even though in many emergency simulations and rehearsals that I have attended, there is still a tendency for some of those commanders on the ground to instinctively feel that information needs to be restricted to "prevent panic". Nothing could be further from the case. The provision of timely, accurate information (including the admission of uncertainty when that is the real situation) is not just an end in itself, it is also a mental health intervention, one whose impact probably outweighs anything that mental health professionals can do. It is instructive to note from this volume that the calls to the Lifenet hotline in the immediate aftermath of 9/11 were indeed related to basic needs and information.

It is also important not to neglect psychological factors relevant to the emergency services. Again, there is no evidence for the effectiveness of, or need for, formal psychological interventions for all. However, simple measures must not be neglected, such as insisting on adequate rest, and demonstrating leadership, support and appreciation that should be part of all high quality management systems. Boyatzis and colleagues show how some possess such leadership skills, while others do not. Likewise, it is clear that some organizations are better equipped to demonstrate support and appreciation of their employees than others.

Fourth, financial and administrative support is very valuable. It would be tedious to reference all the post-disaster literature that emphasizes that what survivors and the bereaved most appreciate in the immediate aftermath is practical help. Cam Ritchie's account of the response to the Pentagon attack describes how each bereaved family was assigned a "casualty assistance care officer (CACO)", who stayed with the family to help them negotiate all of the financial and other issues related to sudden death (Ritchie *et al.*, this volume). It is this type of "nuts and bolts" help that is the immediate and most pressing priority, and is itself a mental health intervention in all but name.

Finally, it is a leitmotif of this contribution that our role as professionals is to step back and "play the long game". We will be needed when the emergency services have gone home, and normal life has resumed for most. Later it may be important to know just who was affected in the event – to establish a denominator of those at risk. Many of the problems that continue to echo around the aftermath of the 1992 El Al plane crash in Amsterdam could have been better addressed if someone had kept a record of precisely who was involved at the start, since establishing this years later as a baseline for health impact studies, not to mention financial recompense, proved both difficult and also an additional point of contention (Yzermans J, 2002). For that reason one of the tasks of our mental health team in our acute disaster planning is the mundane one of trying to keep a register of who has been involved, and the name of their family doctor. We do this partly so we can later communicate with the individual's general practitioner if necessary, and partly as a first step towards carrying out research should that become necessary.

It's all over ... now what?

I continue to have some scepticism about the immediate role of the mental health professional in the acute drama, other than his or her role as a good citizen, believing that immediate mental health support is best delivered indirectly by non-mental health professionals (although they in turn may need support and encouragement). Instead, I continue to be surprised by the capacity of people to show courage and resilience in adversity, and by the capacity of their systems to recover and adapt.

But this is not my view about our role in the longer term, which I will arbitrarily define as being after 3 months. Experience tells us that in the acute situation altruism, solidarity and even resources are not hard to find. If psychological support is to be offered, there is no shortage of volunteers – after the shootings at the Columbine High School the authorities received thousands of offers of help from people offering their services as counselors or debriefers – "trauma tourists" as Richard Gist has labelled them.

In my own hospital here in London when there was a bomb outrage in our vicinity some 4 years ago we too were overwhelmed with offers of help from mental health professionals, all of them doing so out of a sense of altruism and the desire to help. It was therefore predictable that this happened on a vast scale after 9/11, and posed many problems of its own. Simply offering to help does not mean that help is needed, nor that a particular individual is qualified to give that help (Gist & Redburn, 1998). Our own disaster plan now includes a section on how to deal with the expected surge of helpers who will converge on our emergency facilities.

But in the long term memories fade, priorities change, and enthusiasm declines. The majority of those affected have now recovered and resumed their own lives. But now there will be a small number of people who remain not just distressed, but also disabled. And it is then that accessing services becomes much as it was before the incident – difficult! As Felton and colleagues (this volume) point out, mental health services remain preoccupied with the care of the psychoses, and although evidence-based treatments exist for the non-psychotic disorders such as depression, panic disorder and PTSD, obtaining them remains difficult. What is required now is not simple support and counselling, but evidence-based directive psychotherapies, which require both time and skilled trained professionals, not enthusiastic amateurs.

So the first challenge in post-disaster mental health management is to ensure that once the dust has settled, literally or figuratively, those with defined psychiatric disorders can now access decent quality treatments. Our work with UK veterans after they have left the Armed Forces shows that to be the exception and not the rule, and the contributors to this book affirm that the situation was not radically different in the USA prior to, and indeed after, 9/11.

Knowing what to do for the small numbers of people with prolonged post-traumatic psychiatric disorders is not difficult conceptually, even if it is often difficult to organize in practice. But there is a second scenario that causes far more problems, and has a far greater impact not just on the individuals concerned, but with the entire community and political system, and can potentially significantly add to the impact of a terrorist event.

Consider the following scenario. There has been a terrorist event, involving a chemical, biological or radiation weapon. After a brief initial chaos, the emergency services coped heroically in difficult circumstances. People pulled together. Politicians united in displays of solidarity. Soon the experts declared the surrounding area, if perhaps not the site itself, to be clean. Transport runs again and the economic life of the affected city resumes. Behind the scenes the emergency planners began the usual "lessons learned" exercises, but were privately relieved – things could have been a lot worse.

And then 6 months later someone in the affected area, or perhaps one of the rescue workers, develops a cancer. Another develops strange physical symptoms such as fatigue, headache, malaise or myalgia, of no known cause. Physicians suggest the problems might be psychological, but this is vehemently rejected. Or perhaps a third gives birth to or fathers a child with obvious congenital handicaps.

And now the rumours start. Were the experts right? Was the surrounding area really safe? Perhaps another agent was used in the attack. Do the authorities know more than they are saying? A scientist who has worked in the field before the incident, albeit from a very maverick perspective, appears in the media claiming that the official lower limit of substance X is actually still hazardous. People remember other mishandled episodes in the past – Gulf War Syndrome, Agent Orange, or, if they are British, the "Mad Cow" crisis. It seems that science is fallible, and governments cannot be trusted. And now more and more cases start to appear. No matter that the public health officials claim that people have always developed cancer, that chronic fatigue is extremely common, and some pregnancies end tragically anyway. For the individuals concerned this is all irrelevant – before the incident they did not have cancer, felt well and had given birth to normal children. What else could be responsible but the single most dramatic and dangerous event in their lives? And why do the doctors and politicians seem to deny this, or suggest the problems are psychosomatic, which is almost as bad?

The reader will recognize this scenario. It has been played out many times. And its consequences can be profound. Communities divide. Trust is eroded. Confidence drops. Suspicion rises. And unless we are careful, the objectives of terrorism – in which the physical destruction of people and property is but a means to an end, are achieved.

And it is at this stage that wise heads are needed. In every contribution to this book is the assumption that there is an implicit, and indeed explicit, assumption that the main problems that arise after mass terrorism in general, and 9/11 in particular, relate to emotional responses, and that people will share those assumptions. But history tells us this is not always the case. Fear and anxiety takes many forms, as does depression. Not all, indeed not even the majority, of mental health problems present with clear-cut emotional problems. Many people do not acknowledge, even to themselves, that their symptoms may have an emotional basis, and react angrily to such a suggestion. And there are many people who experience symptomatic ill-health in the absence of formal mental health problems such as PTSD or depression – the under-researched problem of medically unexplained symptoms.

It is from these symptomatic templates that new syndromes arise. Unexplained respiratory complaints that are not substantiated by pulmonary investigations are reported. Cases of strange allergies or chemical sensitivities that are not associated with immunological mechanisms arise, and so on. It is the management of these syndromes that can prove the most problematic, and have the potential for the most rapid loss of trust between the population and the political and public health authorities (Engel et al., 2002; Hyams et al., 2002).

It would be tempting at this stage to now discuss how these scenarios can be managed. However, the truth is that we do not really know, and are better able to point to what not to do, rather than what to do (Havenaar & Bromet, 2002; Fischoff & Wessely, 2003). However, it is at this stage that sound epidemiological research comes into its own – not simply for its own sake, but as part of the risk management process and to address legitimate health concerns, a point well made in the contribution from Bromet and Havenaar (Havenaar & Bromet, this volume).

Conclusions

I began this chapter by admitting that I am not American, let alone a resident of New York City or Washington DC. I am actually a graduate of an American (Texan) high school, and have long since lost count of the number of visits I have made to American shores. But, nevertheless, I am conscious that the meaning of the events of 9/11 must inevitably differ from my transatlantic perspective. I was not there.

But perhaps I am also in a position to take one step back, and observe from afar. Like any thinking human being I cannot claim to be immune from personal emotional reactions to the events of that day, but perhaps these were reduced because of the protection of distance and passport. Finally, I have also attempted to derive some more general observations and conclusions on the subject of how we should respond to terrorist attacks, rather than specific comments on the events around 9/11.

So how should we respond to the next major terrorist attack? The answer is still unclear. At the conference on early psychological interventions after trauma that was held coincidentally soon after 9/11 it would be fair to say that a consensus was not reached. The weight of opinion was against giving blanket interventions to normal people, most of whom were either not distressed or if so, were going to get better anyway, although the corridor conversations indicated that this was precisely what was happening on the ground even as we debated. Some, this author included, worried about the possibility of causing more harm than good, and remain troubled by the proliferation of interventions, high in enthusiasm and charisma, but low in evidence of effectiveness. Our past should leave us in no doubt that as mental health professionals we do have the power to create disorder as well as treat it (Dineen, 1996; McHugh, 1999). We have a rather better record in treatment than prevention.

It is also unclear to me how large scale mobilization of mental health professionals fits with the universally agreed need to promote resilience. Historical examples of population resilience – London during the Blitz, German cities during the Strategic Air Offensive, Leningrad during the siege – achieved this without the aid of mental health services. Instead, resilience and resistance to adversity comes not from counselling, but from having a shared sense of purpose – of knowing why one is under threat, and even more importantly, being able to do something about it. By 1944 up to 80% of the British population had some active participation in the war effort (Jones et al., in press). We are still struggling to find some equivalent way of popular participation in the so called "war on terror" – but if we do, we may find that such a shared sense of purpose and participation conveys more strength and resilience than our mental health programmes do.

Other speakers at the Mass Violence Conference preferred to target scarce resources on the immediate minority who really needed help, rather than the majority who didn't. This is not the conclusion of Sandro Galea and his colleagues (this volume) but is echoed by a recent review authored by three noted authorities on psychological interventions (McNally et al., 2003), highlighting a rapidly developing literature which is starting to suggest that the strategy with the most promise is to target only the minority with acute stress reactions. And we must bear in mind that successful intervention involves not a single session stress debriefing, but a more focussed and lengthy cognitive behavioural intervention, which not everyone is qualified to deliver (McNally et al., 2003). This is not an intervention to be implemented on a population level, and is not meant to be.

So what do we do for the rest? Here's the hard bit. Why do we, speaking now as a mental health professional, need to do anything at all? Yes, psychological management is vital from the start of any event, if we are to minimize its impact and disruption, but I have outlined that I do not consider this is the task of a mental health professional. Instead it is imperative that crisis managers and leaders remain alert and attuned to the psychological impact of their actions and messages. It is also imperative that they do everything they can to enable people to connect to their own sources of social support and not provide ersatz sources instead.

For the rest of us there is a desire to "do something". None of us like to see people in distress. The desire to help our fellow human beings is one of the more attractive aspects of human nature. In times of crisis we should strive to be good neighbours, loving parents, loyal colleagues, and sensitive employers. This is what Raphael has labelled "psychological first aid", and just as physical first aid does not need a medical degree, psychological first aid does not need a mental health qualification.

But beyond this good citizenship, is there an immediate role for us as psychiatrists, psychologists or other mental health professionals? I remain to be convinced. The balance between getting people to talk to people, and getting people to talk to professionals, has not been established (Wessely, 2002). Instead I am persuaded that the descriptions of the assistance provided at the Pentagon crash site by Ritchie and colleagues – in which the general policy, in so much as there was a policy, was to be non-intrusive and supportive, to use accepted community figures (namely military padres) at the forefront, and to concentrate on information-based interventions, seems to be generally sensible (Ritchie *et al.*, this volume). We do not know, as Litz correctly says, whether or not it did any good (Litz, this volume), but one can also say that it probably had the lowest chances of doing harm, and that is no bad thing. We also do not know if the extraordinary effort and expense represented by Project Liberty likewise "worked". If by "work" we mean demonstrate our concerns and the importance we give to mental health issues, then yes it did. Likewise, if we judged efficacy solely by satisfaction, then again I am sure it did "work". After all, debriefing almost invariably is associated with high satisfaction from the debriefed and the debriefers, but does not reduce mental distress. But the fundamental question, did Project Liberty achieve any further reduction of mental distress over and above natural recovery remains unanswered and unanswerable.

But when the acute incident has been managed, then we should remind those who provide and resource services that we now have evidence-based treatments to help the minority of citizens who do go on to develop serious psychiatric disorders, including, but not restricted to, PTSD after trauma. I do not need to reference all the contributions to this volume who repeat that it takes time, months certainly, years occasionally, for those most seriously affected by trauma to eventually suffer its consequences. This is rarely due to true delayed onset of disorder, but delayed presentation, but the effects are much the same. Those most in need of mental health care will not become visible for some time.

We also know that many, perhaps most, of these people do not receive the best available treatments. For this reviewer, our policy should not be to throw resources at those who probably don't need our help, but instead concentrate our resources on those who would benefit from our modern interventions, but are most likely not receiving it.

Finally, we must remember the fundamental goal of terrorism – to demoralize and render people fearful, and to disrupt society. We can be thankful that this is far from easily achieved. People respond to adversity in general, and terrorism in particular, in many varied and sometimes contradictory ways. These responses will differ according to the political and cultural setting of the terrorism. But there are also considerable differences in responses to even a single event of terror, as exemplified by the variety of responses to 9/11. Americans became more fearful, but also more unified (Roberts & Em, 2003). Continuous terror in Israel has had many adverse psychological effects, but has also unified communities and families (Bleich *et al.*, 2003; Shalev, 2004). Deliberate area bombing of civilian targets in Britain and later Germany during the Second World War not only did not destroy civilian morale, it arguably achieved the opposite (Jones *et al.*, in press). This may well occur if people can see and share a wider purpose to enduring risk, deprivation and danger.

Assuming that we do not share the goals of terrorism, we will all agree that our goal as professionals must be to promote such resilience. But what is not so clear is how we can achieve this. To promote resilience, independence and coping and to oppose victimhood while continuing to support victims, is a delicate balance, but one that must be achieved. As mental health professionals we are traditionally and compassionately concerned with the plight of victims – people who are defined by what has been done to them. But societies that successfully resist terror also require heroes – people who are known for what they do.

What 9/11 has forced us to do, and this book is a vital part of this process, is to undertake an open and honest assessment not of our intentions or motives, but of our results. We need a judicious assessment of not just the benefits, but also the risks of our interventions. It is the latter that is harder, more challenging and perhaps more important than the former.

Suggested policy framework for planners/crisis managers/local authorities concerning the mental health/psychological management of terrorist incidents

Beforehand
- Prepare communication messages for likely scenarios.
- Identify and train spokespersons.
- Prepare crisis cards to be held in major centres/hospitals.

During

- Concentrate on providing basic needs – security, accommodation, information and communication.
- Ensure people access their own social networks and support as quickly as possible.
- Avoid formal psychological interventions/debriefing.
- Trust your population – they are more resilient than you expect.
- Try and keep a register of those in the affected area.
- Have a plan for managing volunteerism in a constructive way.
- Make sure your emergency services get adequate support, sleep and rest.

After

- Facilitate community driven collective and commemorative responses.
- Liaise with mental health provider units to ensure adequate resources for the minority who remain symptomatic and disabled.
- Make sure that your professionals are able to deliver evidence-based treatments.
- Be alert for the emergence of rumours, myths and legends, and have a communication strategy to deal with this.
- Think about a research strategy as part of the risk management process if concerns about physical health outcomes start to emerge.

REFERENCES

Aita, J. (1949). Efficacy of brief clinical interview method in predicting adjustment: 5 year follow up study of 304 Army inductees. *Archives of Neurology and Psychiatry*, **61**, 170–178.

Amsel, L.V., Neria, Y., Suh, E.J. & Marshall, R.D. (this volume). Mental health community response to 9/11: training therapists to practice evidence-based psychotherapy. In *9/11: Mental Health in the Wake of a Terrorist Attacks*. eds. Y. Neria, R. Gross & R. Marshall. Cambridge, UK: Cambridge University Press.

Andre, C., Lelord, F., Legeron, P., Reignier, A. & Delattre, A. (1997). Etude controlee sur l'efficacite a 6 mois d'une prise en charge precoce de 132 conducteurs d'autobus victimes d'agression. *L'encephale*, **23**, 65–71.

Bleich, A.G.M., Solomon, Z. & Gelkopf, M. (2003). Exposure to terrorist attacks, stress-related mental health symptoms, and coping behaviors among a nationally representative sample in Israel. *Journal of the American Medical Association*, **290**, 612–620.

Bramsen, I. & Ploeg, H. (1999). Use of medical and mental health care by World War II survivors in the Netherlands. *Journal of Traumatic Stress*, **12**, 243–261.

Brewin, C., Andrews, B. & Valentine, J. (2000). Meta-analysis of risk factors for posttraumatic stress disorder in trauma exposed adults. *Journal of Consulting and Clinical Psychology*, **68**, 748–766.

Bryant, R., Harvey, A., Dang, S. & Sackville, T. (1998). Treatment of acute stress disorder: a comparison of cognitive-behavioral therapy and supportive counselling. *Journal of Consulting and Clinical Psychology*, **66**, 862–866.

Bryant, R., Sackville, T., Dang, S., Moulds, M. & Guthrie, R. (1999). Treating acute stress disorder: an evaluation of cognitive behavior therapy and supportive counselling techniques. *American Journal of Psychiatry*, **156**, 1780–1786.

Carey-Trefzer, C. (1949). The results of a clinical study of war-damaged children who attended the Child Guidance Clinic, The Hospital for Sick Children, Great Ormond Street, London. *Journal of Mental Science*, **95**, 535–539.

Coyne, J. C., Thompson, R., Palmer, S. C., Kagee, A. & Maunsell, E. (2000). Should we screen for depression? Caveats and potential pitfalls. *Applied & Preventive Psychology*, **9**, 101–121.

Davidson, J.R.T., Book, S., Colket, J., Tupler, L., Roth, S., Dav, D., Hertzberg, M., Mellman, T., Beckham, J., Smith, R., Davison, R., Katz, R. & Feldman, M. (1997). Assessment of a new self-rating scale for post-traumatic stress disorder. *Psychological Medicine*, **27**, 153–160.

Devilly, G., Gist, P. & Cotton, P. (2006). Ready! Fire! Aim! The status of psychological debriefing and therapeutic interventions – in the workplace and after disasters. *Review of General Psychology in press.*

Dineen, T. (1996). *Manufacturing Victims.* Montreal: Robert Davis.

Durkheim, E. (1897). *Suicide: a study in sociology.* NY: The Free Press of Glenco.

Emmerik, A., Kamphuls, J., Hulsbosch, A. & Emmelkamp, P. (2002). Single session debriefing after psychological trauma: a meta-analysis. *Lancet*, **360**, 736–741.

Engel, C., Adkins, J. & Cowan, D. (2002). Caring for medically unexplained symptoms after toxic environmental exposure: the effect of contested causation. *Environmental Health Perspectives*, **110** (Suppl. 4), 641–647.

Felton, C.J., Donahue, S., Lanzara, C.B., Pease, E.A. & Marshall, R.D. (this volume). Project Liberty: responding to mental health needs after the World Trade Center terrorist attacks. In *9/11: Mental Health in the Wake of a Terrorist Attacks.* eds. Y. Neria, R. Gross & R. Marshall. Cambridge, UK: Cambridge University Press.

Fischoff, B. & Wessely, S. (2003). Predictable care for inexplicable health problems. *British Medical Journal*, **326**, 595–597.

Foa, E., Keane, T. & Friedman, M. (2000). Guidelines for Treatment of PTSD. *Journal of Traumatic Stress*, **13**, 539–588.

Freud, A. & Burlingham, D. (1943). *War and Children.* New York City: Medical War Books.

Fullilove, M. & Saul, J. (this volume). Rebuilding communities post-disaster in New York. In *9/11: Mental Health in the Wake of a Terrorist Attacks.* eds. Y. Neria, R. Gross & R. Marshall. Cambridge, UK: Cambridge University Press.

Furedi, F. (2003). *Therapy Culture: Cultivating Vulnerability in an Anxious Age.* London: Routledge.

Galea, S., Vlahov, D., Resnick, H., Ahern J., Susser, M., Gold, J., Bucuvias, M. & Kilpatrick, D. (2003). Trends of probable post-traumatic stress disorder in New York City after the September 11th terrorist attacks. *American Journal of Epidemiology*, **158**, 514–524.

Galea, S., Ahern, J., Resnick, H. & Vlahov, D. (this volume). Post-traumatic stress symptoms in the general population after a disaster: implications for public health. In *9/11: Mental Health in the Wake of a Terrorist Attacks.* eds. Y. Neria, R. Gross & R. Marshall. Cambridge, UK: Cambridge University Press.

Gilbody, S., House, A. & Sheldon, T. (2001). Routinely administered questionnaires for depression and anxiety: systematic review. *British Medical Journal*, **322**, 406–409.

Ginzberg, E. (1959). *The Lost Divisions*. NY: Columbia University Press.

Gist, R. (2002). What have they done to my song? Social science, social movements and the debriefing debates. *Cognitive and Behavioral Practice*, **9**, 273–279.

Gist, R. & Woodhall, S. (1999). There are no simple solutions to complex problems. The rise and fall of critical incident stress debriefing as a response to occupational stress in the fire services. In *Response to Disaster: Psychological, Community and Ecological Approaches*, eds. R. Gist & B. Lubin, Philadelphia: Brunner/Mazel, pp. 211–235.

Gist, R.L.B. & Redburn, B.G. (1998). Psychological, ecological, and community perspective on disaster response. *Journal of Personal and Interpersonal Loss*, **3**, 25–51.

Glass, T. & Schoch Spana, M. (2002). Bioterrorism and the people: how to vaccinate a city against panic. *Clinical Infectious Diseases*, **34**, 217–223.

Halpern-Felsher, B. & Millstein, S. (2002). The effects of terrorism on teens' perceptions of dying: the new world in riskier than ever. *Journal of Adolescent Health*, **30**, 308–311.

Havenaar, J.M. & Bromet, E.J. (2002). *Toxic Turmoil: Psychological and Societal Consequences of Ecological Disasters*. NY: Plenum.

Havenaar, J.M. & Bromet, E.J. (this volume). Capturing the impact of large scale events through epidemiological research. In *9/11: Mental Health in the Wake of a Terrorist Attacks*. eds. Y. Neria, R. Gross & R. Marshall. Cambridge, UK: Cambridge University Press.

Hennekens, C. & Buring, J. (1987). *Epidemiology in Medicine*. Boston: Little, Brown and Company.

Hyams, K., Murphy, F. & Wessely, S. (2002). Combatting terrorism: recommendations for dealing with the long term health consequences of a chemical, biological or nuclear attack. *Journal of Health Politics, Policy and Law*, **27**, 273–291.

Ismail, K., Kent, K., Brugha, T., Hotopf, M., Hull, L., Seed, P., Palmer, I., Reid, S., Unwin, C., David, A., Wessely, S. (2002). The mental health of UK Gulf war veterans: phase 2 of a two-phase cohort study. *British Medical Journal*, **325**, 576–579.

Jones, E., Hyams, K. & Wessely, S. (2003). Screening for vulnerability to psychological disorders in the military: an historical inquiry. *Journal of Medical Screening*, **10**, 40–46.

Jones, E., Woolven, R., Durodie, W. & Wessely, S. (2004). Public panic and morale: a reassessment of civilian reactions during the Blitz and World War 2. *Journal of Social History*, **17**, 463–479.

Kaniasty, K. (this volume). Searching for points of convergence: A commentary on prior research on disasters and some community programs initiated in response to September 11, 2001. In *9/11: Mental Health in the Wake of a Terrorist Attacks*. eds. Y. Neria, R. Gross & R. Marshall. Cambridge, UK: Cambridge University Press.

Katz, C.L., Smith, R., Herbert, R., Levin, S. & Gross, R. (this volume). The World Trade Center worker/volunteer mental health screening program. In *9/11: Mental Health in the Wake of a Terrorist Attacks*. eds. Y. Neria, R. Gross & R. Marshall. Cambridge, UK: Cambridge University Press.

Kulka, R., Schlenger, W., Fairbank, J., Hough, R., Jordan, B., Marmar, C. & Weiss, D. (1990). *Trauma and the Vietnam War Generation: Report of Findings from the National Vietnam Veterans Readjustment Study*. NY: Brunner/Mazel.

Law, M. (2004). Screening without evidence of efficacy: screening of unproven value should not be advocated. *British Medical Journal*, **328**, 301–302.

Litz, B.T. (this volume). Learning lessons from the early intervention response to the Pentagon. In *9/11: Mental Health in the Wake of a Terrorist Attacks*. eds. Y. Neria, R. Gross & R. Marshall. Cambridge, UK: Cambridge University Press.

McHugh, P. (1999). How psychiatry lost its way. *Commentary*, 32–38.

McNally, R., Bryant, R. & Ehlers, A. (2003). Does early psychological intervention promote recovery from traumatic stress? *Psychological Science in the Public Interest*, **4**, 45–79.

Muir Gray, J. (1997). *Evidence-Based Healthcare: How to Make Health Policy and Management Decisions*. Edinburgh, London: Churchill Livingstone.

National Institute of Mental Health (2002). *Mental Health and Mass Violence: Evidence Based Early Psychological Intervention for Victims/Survivors of Mass Violence*: US Government printing office.

National Screening Committee (1998). First report of the National Screening Committee. London: Health Departments of the United Kingdom.

North, C., Pfefferbaum, B. & Hong, B. (this volume). Historical perspective and future directions in research on psychiatric consequences of terrorism and other disasters. In *9/11: Mental Health in the Wake of a Terrorist Attacks*. eds. Y. Neria, R. Gross & R. Marshall. Cambridge, UK: Cambridge University Press.

Ritchie, E.C., Leavitt, W.T. & Hanish, S. (this volume). The mental health response to the 9/11 attack on the Pentagon. In *9/11: Mental Health in the Wake of a Terrorist Attacks*. eds. Y. Neria, R. Gross & R. Marshall. Cambridge, UK: Cambridge University Press.

Roberts, J. & Em, M. (2003). Fear at work, fear at home: surveying the new geography of dread in America Post-9-11. *International Journal of Mass Emergencies and Disasters*, **21**, 41–55.

Rose, G. (1992). *The Strategy of Preventive Medicine*. NY: Oxford University Press.

Salib, E. (2003). Effect of 11 September 2001 on suicide and homicide in England and Wales. *British Journal of Psychiatry*, **183**, 207–213.

Schecter, D.S. & Coates, W.S. (this volume). Relationally and developmentally focused interventions with young children and their caregives in the wake of terrorism and other violent experiences. In *9/11: Mental Health in the Wake of a Terrorist Attacks*. eds. Y. Neria, R. Gross & R. Marshall. Cambridge, UK: Cambridge University Press.

Schuster, M., Stein, B., Jaycox, L., Collins, R., Marshall, G., Elliott, M., Zhou, A., Kanouse, D., Morrison, J. & Berry, S. (2001). A national survey of stress reactions after the September 11, 2001 terrorist attacks. *New England Journal of Medicine*, **345**, 1507–1512.

Shalev, A. (2004). The Israeli experience of continuous terrorism: 2000–2004. In *Disasters and Mental Health*, eds. J.J. Lopez-Ibor, M. Maj, N. Sartorius & A. Okasha. London: John Wiley.

Shalev, A. & Freedman, S. (2005). PTSD following terrorist attacks: a prospective evaluation. *American Journal of Psychiatry*, **162**, 1188–1191.

Shalev, A., Freedman, S., Peri, T., Brandes, D., Sahar, T. (1997). Predicting PTSD in trauma survivors: prospective evaluation of self-report and clinician-administered instruments. *British Journal of Psychiatry*, **170**, 558–564.

Shaw, C., Abrams, K. & Marteau, T. (1999). Psychological impact of predicting individuals' risks of illness: a systematic review. *Social Science and Medicine*, **49**, 1571–1598.

Shephard, B. (2000). *A War of Nerves, Soldiers and Psychiatrists 1914–1994*. London: Jonathan Cape.

Solomon, Z. (1989). A three-year prospective study of PTSD in Israeli combat veterans. *Journal of Traumatic Stress*, **2**, 59–73.

Solomon, Z., Kotler, M., Shalev, A. & Lin, R. (1989). Delayed onset of PTSD among Israeli veterans of the 1982 Lebanon War. *Psychiatry Interpersonal and Biological Processes*, **52**, 428–437.

Unwin, C., Blatchley, N., Coker, W., Ferry, S., Hotopf, M., Hull, L., Ismail, K., Palmer, I., David, A. & Wessely, S. (1999). The health of United Kingdom Servicemen who served in the Persian Gulf War. *Lancet*, **353**, 169–178.

Wessely, S. (2002). Proceedings of a NATO Workshop on the Social and Psychological Consequences of Chemical, Biological and Radiological Terrorism. NATO Headquarters.

Wessely, S. (2005). Risk, Psychiatry and the Military, the 15th Liddell Hart Lecture. *British Journal of Psychiatry*, and http://www.kcl.ac.uk/kcmhr/information/lecture_notes/liddell_hart_lecture_by_ Professor_Wessely.pdf **186**, 459–466.

Wessely, S., Bisson, J. & Rose, S. (2000). A systematic review of brief psychological interventions ("debriefing") for the treatment of immediate trauma related symptoms and the prevention of post traumatic stress disorder. In *Depression, Anxiety and Neurosis Module of the Cochrane Database of Systematic Reviews*, eds. M. Oakley-Browne, R.Churchill, D. Gill & S.Wessely. Oxford: Update Software.

Yzermans, J.G.B. (2002). The chaotic aftermath of an airplane crash in Amsterdam: a second disaster. In *Toxic Turmoil: Psychological and Societal Consequences of Ecological Disasters*. eds. J.M. Havenaar & E.J. Bromet. NY: Plenum, pp. 85–99.

32

Coping with the threat of terrorism

Shira Maguen and Brett Litz

The terrorist attacks on September 11, 2001 created fear, dread, and uncertainty among most Americans. Although many Americans have been aware of terrorism in the world, it is unprecedented for Americans to feel unsafe at home and abroad. Indeed, terrorist groups have launched a total of 3300 attacks on US targets since 1968. However, on 9/11, more than three times the number of Americans were killed than those that died in terrorist attacks over the last 33 years (Hoffman, 2002).

Since September 11, 2001, the threat of another terrorist attack has been a chronic stressor for many. For example, about two-thirds of Americans report fears of future terrorism (Silver *et al.*, 2002) and 44% think that terrorism will increase over the next few years (Schuster *et al.*, 2001). Fears of future terrorism are not limited to adults. Following the attacks on 9/11, 47% of children were worried about their own safety or the safety of a loved one, and there was a significant association between child and adult stress (Schuster *et al.*, 2001). The terrorist events on 9/11 and their aftermath, including wars in Afghanistan and Iraq and the uncertainty of future attacks on the US, have led to increased feelings of insecurity, fearfulness, and anxiety among many Americans.

How can Americans cope with this ongoing threat of terrorism? Is having some anxiety and vigilance normative? Are there forms of adaptation to the threat of terrorism that do not result in optimal mental health or functioning? Can we learn any lessons from how citizens in other countries cope with the chronic threat of terrorism? In this chapter we address these questions by describing the psychological impact of the threat of terrorism, reviewing studies of coping with terror, both nationally and internationally, highlighting implications of existing research and outlining a framework that can serve as a guide for future research.

What is terrorism?

According to the Institute of Medicine (IOM), "Terrorism involves the illegal use or threatened use of violence, is intended to coerce societies or governments by inducing fear in their populations, and typically involves ideological or political motives (Butler *et al.*, 2003). Terrorism is "psychological warfare," in which terrorists "invoke a pervasive fear in the civilian population by personalizing the threat so that everyone feels vulnerable" (Tucker, 2003). Terrorists propagate their message by promulgating fear among the masses and inducing the belief that the probability of a future terrorist act is much higher than statistically indicated. Fear affects far more individuals than the terrorist act itself, often leading to behavioral changes (e.g., decreasing or eliminating air travel). These changes are caused by the expectation that another terrorist attack is possible or imminent, despite the low probability of any one individual being directly involved in a terrorist attack. Behavioral changes and avoidance fulfill the terrorists' goals by drastically affecting the economy and acting to reinforce feelings of fear, helplessness, and insecurity.

While most Americans proved to be resilient in the face of the threat of future terrorism, our knowledge of the psychological sequelae that lead some to demonstrate impairment and others psychological adaptation and hardiness in the face of terrorism is limited. In a recent report, the IOM concluded that research on the psychological sequelae of terrorist attacks is extremely limited. According to the IOM, while there is good cross-sectional evidence about the mental health problems resulting from exposure to terrorism, there is little knowledge about the trajectory of coping with the lingering threat of terror and the manner in which terror affects functioning (Butler *et al.*, 2003). We concur and as a result, in our view, exclusively relying on existing models of direct exposure to trauma when examining the psychosocial impact of *the threat of future terrorism* is misguided and limits our understanding of long-term coping in a chronically threatening environment. Indeed, exposure to terrorist events and any resulting mental health problem is one of multiple variables that affect coping with threats of future terror and the degree to which functioning is altered.

The psychological burden of terrorism

In the months that followed the tragedies of 9/11, Americans were told to return to "business as usual," yet many had a difficult time doing so, and rates of depression and posttraumatic stress disorder (PTSD) increased following the terrorist attacks (Schuster *et al.*, 2001; Galea *et al.*, 2002). Two months after the attacks, 12% of Americans were experiencing clinically significant distress (Schlenger *et al.*, 2002), 30% were reporting symptoms of stress and anxiety, and 27% reported avoiding situations that reminded them of 9/11 (Silver *et al.*, 2002).

However, the initial high level of anxiety decreased over time, and only about 11% of Americans reported symptoms of stress, anxiety, and avoidance half a year after the attacks (Silver *et al.*, 2002). As would be expected, the majority of Americans proved resilient and did not develop a formal psychiatric condition following the national trauma. One of the challenges following tragedies such as 9/11 is to distinguish between psychopathology and the range of normative reactions that are expected following national trauma (Litz *et al.*, 2002; North & Pfefferbaum, 2002). Although crucial from a public health standpoint, there is very little research that helps distinguish those who need immediate psychological assistance from those who will recover alone over time.

We also know little about the degree to which the average individual's life has changed with respect to perceived safety, anxiety, and the functional impact of lingering concerns about future terrorism (e.g., behavioral decisions about travel). We argue that mental health problems (e.g., PTSD) resulting from exposure to terrorism events are one of many factors that affect how people function over time in the face of the threat of future terrorism.

Coping with uncertain future threats

There has been very little research examining coping with terrorism, yet there is a great deal of research concerning how individuals cope with stress generally. Individual responses to stressors have been categorized as *emotion-focused* coping, consisting of strategies to decrease emotional distress, or *problem-focused* coping, consisting of methods that deal directly with the stressor (Folkman & Lazarus, 1991). Moos employs the parsimonious concepts of *avoidance-* and *approach-based* coping (Roth & Cohen, 1986; Moos, 1990; Skinner *et al.*, 2003). Individuals who use problem-focused coping strategies generally fare better on a number of mental health outcomes in comparison to those who employ more emotion-focused coping strategies (Florian *et al.*, 1995). However, following a traumatic event, the efficacy of problem- and emotion-focused coping may vary, depending on the type of stressor (Sharkansky *et al.*, 2000; Suvak *et al.*, 2002). We know little about coping with the chronic threat of *potential* trauma.

Under unpredictable and chronically stressful conditions, emotion-focused coping and denial may be more beneficial than problem-focused coping (Lazarus & Folkman, 1984). Although this seems relevant to coping with the threat of future terrorist attacks, which are unpredictable and chronically stressing, the categorical distinction between emotion- and problem-focused coping seems limited when applied to coping with impending threat. First, emotion-focused coping seems overly inclusive. For example, making efforts to acquire social support may produce different results than "venting" about fears in an unproductive fashion. Incorporating such different responses into a single category causes any association of emotion-focused coping with adjustment to become difficult to interpret (Stanton *et al.*, 2000). Second, conceptualizing coping in a bipolar fashion disregards the dimensional variation inherent in these categories. It also assumes that emotion- and problem-focused coping categories are mutually exclusive and orthogonal (Skinner *et al.*,

2003). Third, with respect to coping with the threat of terrorism, existing coping categories do not account for the moderating influences of personality, past history, and the influence of culture.

Employing *The Brief Cope* (Carver, 1997), Silver and colleagues measured coping with the uncertainty of future US terrorist attacks in a national sample (Silver *et al.*, 2002). They reported that active coping (e.g., "I've been taking action to try and make the situation better") was inversely associated with general anxiety and distress 6 months after the 9/11 attacks, whereas behavioral disengagement (i.e., "giving up"), denial, and self-blame predicted higher levels of distress. Acceptance (e.g., "I've been learning to live with it"), behavioral disengagement, denial, seeking social support (e.g., "I've been getting emotional support from others"), self-blame, and self-distraction (e.g., "I've been turning to work or other activities to take my mind off of things") all independently predicted PTSD symptom severity 6 months after 9/11 (Silver *et al.*, 2002). Although differing from the findings reported in other countries exposed to the threat of terrorism, active coping led to the best adaptation.

Following 9/11, there is also some evidence that emotional coping was associated with better mental health outcome. For example, there was an association between satisfaction with emotional support from friends and family, and the number of individuals providing instrumental support and lower rates of distress (Butler *et al.*, 2002). Additionally, 90% of Americans reported engaging in prayer or turning to religion or spirituality in order to cope (Schuster *et al.*, 2001).

Studying the conditions that create resilience is particularly important given that most Americans will cope effectively with the threat of terrorism. According to Masten, resilience arises from the normative functions of human adaptation and, as a result, is quite common (Masten, 2001). Illuminating these resilient processes of adaptation in the context of coping with terror becomes important since it will likely lead to more robust functioning. For example, Fredrickson and colleagues found that individuals that were more resilient, defined as the capacity to "modulate effectively and monitor an ever-changing complex of desires and reality constraints" (Block & Kremen, 1996), were more likely to find positive meaning with daily hassles and stressors (Fredrickson *et al.*, 2003). More positive emotions and fewer negative emotions were reported by more resilient individuals following the attacks in New York, and resilience was negatively correlated with symptoms of depression. Positive emotions mediated the relationship between resilience and growth in psychological resources and between resilience and development of depressive symptoms. Despite the prospective nature of this study, the study is limited because of the small sample size and because the participants were not directly impacted by an actual terrorism event (e.g., did not know anyone who was killed). Limitations aside, Fredrickson and colleagues suggest a mode of coping that promotes resilience in the face of the threat of terror (Fredrickson *et al.*, 2003). There is also some evidence that humor is a coping mechanism that serves to reduce threat-induced anxiety (Yovetich *et al.*, 1990). When faced with a threatening situation, individuals who used humor consistently rated themselves as less anxious and reported less increase in stress.

Coping with the threat of terrorism internationally

Research on coping with the ongoing threat of terrorism in other nations that are terror-prone could shed light on current American challenges. For example, individuals who were at risk for SCUD attacks (Weisenberg *et al.*, 1993) and individuals who were at risk of transportation explosions (Gidron *et al.*, 1999) were surveyed in two studies in Israel. Results indicated that both adults and children who employed problem-focused coping fared worse (Weisenberg *et al.*, 1993; Gidron *et al.*, 1999). Furthermore, concurrent with developmental changes, children's coping styles become more effective as they mature (Weisenberg *et al.*, 1993). For instance, as compared to older children, younger children may not be able to distort or deny external threats. Older children are more likely to use emotion-focused coping in the face of terror-related threat, which Weisenberg and colleagues hypothesize is a more effective way of coping.

According to some researchers, employing problem-focused coping emphasizes the uncontrollable nature of terror, thereby increasing distress and symptomatology in those that use this coping strategy (Forsythe & Compas, 1987). This "goodness of fit" hypothesis (Masel *et al.*, 1996; Park *et al.*, 2001) emphasizes the need for a fit between coping (e.g., self-soothing and emotion-focused coping) and individual appraisal (e.g., uncontrollable nature of terror). However, problem-focused coping can be helpful in some terrorist-related situations (e.g., looking out for and identifying suspicious individuals), and may provide individuals with a sense of mastery over their environment. Gidron and colleagues argue that the use of problem-focused coping in and of itself is not associated with poorer outcome, but rather that a higher ratio of problem to emotion-focused coping may be associated with increased levels of anxiety among individuals (Gidron *et al.*, 1999).

There are problems with measurement that should be underscored in both of the Israeli studies. A six-item coping measure was used by Gidron and colleagues with two items for emotion-, problem-focused, and denial (Gidron *et al.*, 1999). The emotion-focused coping strategies included: (1) During the bus ride, I calm myself down by reading a newspaper or by looking at the view and (2) During the bus ride I think about pleasant things, or people whom I like. A questionnaire containing 25 items, and rated on a 3-point scale was created by Weisenberg and colleagues, with the final scale reduced to 13 items (Weisenberg *et al.*, 1993).

Emotion-focused coping was defined as avoidance and distraction strategies, and a reliability measure for the final scale was not reported. Given these measurement limitations, these findings should be interpreted with caution.

Both of these studies were also based around a specific terrorist event, and individuals were surveyed shortly thereafter. Gidron and colleagues surveyed bus commuters 4–5 days after a bus explosion, and Weisenberg and colleagues surveyed children 3 weeks following the SCUD missile launching (Weisenberg *et al.*, 1993; Gidron *et al.*, 1999). Consequently, it is unclear whether measured coping strategies are beneficial in chronically threatening situations as opposed to immediately following a terror event. It is also unclear whether general ways of coping were surveyed vs. methods specific to the terrorist events that preceded the survey. Additionally, results from the Israeli studies and Silver's and colleagues' study (Silver *et al.*, 2002) may differ in part because of the time frame of the surveys (i.e., Americans were surveyed 6 months post-terrorism). For example, active coping may be more helpful after a few months. The ways of conceptualizing coping and measurements employed differed in the Israeli studies, which surveyed individuals within the framework of Folkman's and Lazarus' "Ways of Coping" and the Silver's and colleagues' study, which used Carver's Brief Cope measure (Folkman & Lazarus, 1991; Silver *et al.*, 2002).

Cairns and Wilson investigated two forms of coping in Northern Ireland: distancing, which they used as a proxy for denial, and social support (Cairns & Wilson, 1989). They also surveyed individuals' appraisals of violence in their communities. Results indicated that those living in more violent areas used more distancing, and those who appraised the violence as more severe, regardless of their actual neighborhood violence, engaged in more social support seeking and less distancing coping. In this study, it was appraisals of violence, rather than actual levels of violence, that determined coping strategies. Furthermore, women were more likely to cope by using social support as compared to men. Cairns and Wilson concluded that denial might be a strong source of coping in terrorism-prone areas of Northern Ireland (Cairns & Wilson, 1989). This study only examined two types of coping and did not include measures of problem-focused coping; as a result, comparison with other studies is impossible. Appraisals of violence play a large part in this study; however, the authors do not examine "appraisal-focused coping," in which appraisals are used to define the changing meaning of a situation (Moos & Billings, 1982). The relationship between coping and ratings of mental health outcome measures was not included in the study.

The authors suggest that those living in more dangerous areas are more likely to cope with uncontrollable future threats by employing distancing, a combination which is reminiscent of the "goodness of fit" hypothesis. The Cairns and Wilson study is unable to shed light on which type of coping is most utilized due to the few types of coping surveyed (Cairns & Wilson, 1989). Regardless, other studies did not find that denial is more frequent in terror-prone areas. For example, Israelis used emotion-, problem-focused, and denial coping fairly equally (Gidron *et al.*, 1999). We hypothesize that existing ways of conceptualizing coping may not be the best fit when the threat of terrorism is elevated, and assumptions about "healthy coping" may differ under these conditions.

Children and coping with terrorism

The process by which children comprehend and react to the threat of terror may differ significantly from that of adults. Depending on age, children may have varying abilities to understand, process, and cope with acts of terror and the ongoing threat of terror. In helping children cope with terror, the American Psychological Association's (APA) Task Force on Resilience in Response to Terrorism recommended that parents talk to children about terrorism in developmentally appropriate ways and additionally, exert control of media exposure of terrorism (APA, 2003). It appears that following terrorist events, such as the events of 9/11, 85% of Americans with children reported that they or another adult in the household had spoken to their child about the terrorist attacks for an hour or more (Schuster *et al.*, 2001). However, what parents are telling children is unclear, as is the extent to which developmentally appropriate material is being conveyed and children's follow-up questions are being addressed in the aftermath. Arguably, communication about terrorism should be ongoing, especially as threat levels rise and public warnings ensue. For young children, ongoing warnings may be confusing, and children may create their own meaning behind what these warnings mean if they are not clearly explained and discussed. There is also evidence that exposure to terror-related media is not necessarily helpful, and may even be harmful for children in large doses. In children who are not directly exposed to terrorism, there seems to be a correlation between television viewing (i.e., indirect exposure) and stress symptoms (Pfefferbaum *et al.*, 1999, 2001; Schuster *et al.*, 2001). Although some families may use television viewing or media exposure to cope with the ongoing threat of terrorism by staying informed (Bleich *et al.*, 2003), studies indicate that this might increase stress symptoms in children.

The association between media exposure and stress symptoms has also been demonstrated internationally in children at high risk of exposure to terror events. Thabet and colleagues found that in a high terror-prone area in the Gaza strip, children exposed to terror events indirectly, through media and adults, reported greater *anticipatory anxiety* than children who had their houses bombarded and demolished (Thabet *et al.*, 2002). Those who were directly exposed, in turn, exhibited greater PTSD symptoms. One possibility for this finding is that children who were not directly exposed might have anticipated that they would be next, especially given high rates of exposure among their neighbors, and were consumed with thoughts, worries, and ruminations about the threat of destruction.

Finally, in children directly exposed to terrorism, fears related to future terrorism may persist and worries may be slow to subside. In children present at the 1993 World Trade Center bombing, fear of another bombing was endorsed at both 3 and 9 months post-attack, and fear ratings did not significantly decrease during the 6-month interval ($M = 3.86$ on a 5-point scale at 3 months, $M = 3.81$ at 9 months; Koplewicz et al., 2002). Ways of coping were not assessed during this study.

Appraisal-tendency theory

According to appraisal-tendency theory, cognitive appraisals, which are elicited by emotions, affect cognitions, physiology, and action (Lerner & Keltner, 2001). Emotions may differ on multiple appraisal dimensions (e.g., control and certainty) and a schema is activated by each emotion causing individuals to appraise future events in a schema-consistent and automatic fashion. Consequently, emotions initiate perceptions, judgments, and behavioral choices, which may or may not be appropriate. For example, exaggerated risk estimates result in response to fear in multiple situations, completely independent of the intrinsic level of risk.

Appraisal-tendency theory was applied in a study following the terrorist attacks on 9/11 (Lerner et al., 2003). On two separate occasions a probability sample of Americans was assessed through Knowledge Networks, an organization that provides WebTV and free interactive Internet access to 75,000 households that closely match the US census. In exchange, these families complete occasional surveys. The first survey, consisting of an anxiety questionnaire and a desire for vengeance scale, was completed by 1786 individuals on September 20, 2001. The second survey was completed by 973 of the same individuals 2 months later, and each participant was assigned to one of three emotion conditions: anger, sadness, or fear. Participant's current mood was assessed, followed by a two-part emotional induction. For the first part, depending on the emotional condition to which they were assigned, individuals described in detail what made them angry, sad, or afraid concerning the terrorist attacks on 9/11. For the second part, a picture was presented with accompanying audio material evoking the target emotion (e.g., celebrations of the attacks by people in Arab countries in the anger condition). Questions about resulting emotional states were surveyed, as were policy preferences and risk perceptions for the self and for the average American.

Lerner and colleagues concluded that both naturally occurring and induced negative emotions result in related appraisals and decisions (Lerner et al., 2003). More specifically, reports of fear were associated with more precautionary plans (e.g., "you will screen your mail carefully for suspicious items") and higher-risk estimates (e.g., "I feel that future terrorist attacks can happen anytime anywhere and there is no way of predicting when or where"), and fewer beliefs that punitive public policy was warranted (e.g., "deport foreigners in the US who lack valid visas"). Reports of anger were associated with fewer precautionary measures, lower-risk estimates, and more frequent beliefs that punitive public policy was warranted. These findings suggest that emotional responses to a terrorist episode may impact judgments about coping with terrorism-related threat.

Situational determinants of threat appraisal

Patterson and Neufeld offer a heuristic of the determinants of threat appraisal (Patterson & Neufeld, 1987). They highlight the importance of original event severity, imminence, and probability of reoccurrence. They argue that anticipatory anxiety results when threat cues signal the future occurrence of a stressful event (e.g., terrorist attack), and that there is a correlation between the severity of the threatened event and the resulting anticipatory anxiety. In the case of 9/11, the level of destruction and loss was unprecedented, and as a result, cues signaling a future attack (e.g., bomb threats, raising the level of security alert, etc.) might be associated with the tragedies of 9/11, resulting in increased anticipatory anxiety.

The level of anticipatory anxiety is also directly influenced by imminence of the stressor (Patterson & Neufeld, 1987). It is unclear to what extent this proposition generalizes to the future threat of terrorism. For example, there have been multiple instances following 9/11 where the federal government issued warnings about imminent attacks that they postulated would occur at specific times. Because no attack on American soil has occurred thus far since 9/11, is the level of anticipatory anxiety still high when the government informs us that the attack is imminent or have we become habituated to these warnings?

According to the theory, which is based mostly on laboratory studies, when the event is imminent, the longer the "incubation" period (i.e., the anticipation), the greater the anticipatory stress will be. However, in one reported study, anticipatory anxiety was not increased with a prolonged delay, which may be due to participants performing some arousal-reducing coping activity during the interval, rather than a distraction task, as was done in most other studies (Folkins, 1970). In the case of 9/11, the incubation period has been extended over a period of several years without a subsequent attack; however, Americans are constantly reminded that another attack is a certainty. Although some individuals will undoubtedly continue to have high levels of anticipatory anxiety, one possibility is that the delay has allowed Americans to learn to cope effectively with the ongoing threat. There is evidence that in other countries, such as Israel, where the threat of attack is chronic, on the whole individuals cope effectively with the threat and may even habituate to a chronic level of threat (Thabet *et al.*, 2002; Bleich *et al.*, 2003). As further evidence of coping well, the majority of Israelis indicate high self-efficacy concerning their ability to function in a terrorist attack (Bleich *et al.*, 2003).

Patterson and Neufeld also postulate that anticipatory stress is reduced when the probability of an event's occurrence is decreased (Patterson & Neufeld, 1987). This could be empirically tested by surveying whether anticipatory stress of the average individual in the US decreases when the color-coded warnings are lowered and federal warnings from the government cease to be issued. Additionally, it is unclear whether there is a point at which this postulation no longer holds true due to habituation. In other words, what is the threshold at which this tenet no longer holds true? Patterson and Neufeld suggest that in some cases individuals will inflate the probability of danger as an unconscious strategy in order to "prepare for the worst" (Patterson & Neufeld, 1987). With terrorism warnings, probabilities are difficult to gage, and governments tend to err on the side of informing the public, producing many "false alarms," as we have witnessed in the last few years. How do the numerous false alarms influence subjective assessments of probability? One study suggests that anticipatory anxiety will decrease with false alarms (Breznitz, 1967); however, it is unclear whether this is due to changes in subjective probability of threat, habituation, or better coping. For example, with each false alarm of a terrorism threat, individuals may realize that the probability of harm is much lower than originally assumed; alternatively, reduced anxiety may be a product of habituating to warnings of threat or learning to more effectively cope with these warnings.

To complicate the picture, there are certain dispositionally anxious individuals who may overestimate the probability of aversive outcomes each time there is a warning of threat, and in this case, anxiety is associated with an expectancy bias (Chan & Lovibond, 1996). Indeed, previous studies have found that anxiety is associated with an attentional bias toward threatening stimuli (Mathews & MacLeod, 1994), especially in ambiguous situations. The terrorism threat fits perfectly into the paradigm of an ambiguous situation whose occurrence could produce magnanimous outcomes.

Implications and suggestions for future research

Are there conclusions that can be drawn regarding coping with the threat of terrorism? In reviewing existing studies it becomes apparent that there are many unresolved issues. As a result of the paucity of studies that address coping with the threat of future terrorism, coupled with limitations of consistency and timing of measurement, little can be gleaned about how to cope with the threat of terrorism most effectively. Emotion-focused coping was found to produce better mental health outcomes in two Israeli studies; however, these studies assessed coping directly following a terrorist event, and as a result may not necessarily generalize to coping daily with the threat of terrorism. Israelis also live in an environment in which attacks are more frequent than in the US and terrorism is a constant threat and as a result, some of the differences in the coping findings may be due to chronicity and/or culture. The long-term efficacy of more "emotion-focused" coping as well as the assumptions of the "goodness of fit" hypothesis were called into question following a nationwide survey of Americans after 9/11, which found that active, problem-focused coping was associated with better mental health for months afterward. Furthermore, appraisal-tendency theory may provide clues concerning interactions between types of coping and emotional/cognitive processes. Situational determinants of threat appraisal may also offer clues as to how threat is processed and appraised, leading to higher anticipatory anxiety as a result.

In order to appreciate the time course of managing the threat of terrorism, future studies should examine coping in a longitudinal fashion. Individual coping strategies may alter over time as a result of ever-changing appraisals of terrorism. "Appraisal-focused coping" (i.e., how people re-appraise a situation in order to define its meaning) is also a process that unfolds over time and as a result is important to gage at several time points (Moos & Billings, 1982).

When examining individual differences in coping with the threat of terrorism, the existing framework for measuring coping might not be a good fit. As discussed, "emotion-focused" coping includes different types of coping, with varying degrees of utility in the context of coping with uncontrollable, high-threat events. More fine-grained analyses of coping strategies should be conducted in the future in order to understand how people cope with terrorism threats (e.g., what specific strategies to people engage in day-to-day cope with the threat of terrorism?).

There are several treatment and policy implications that are important to discuss despite literature limitations. For example, Fredrickson and colleagues suggest that positive emotionality may create resilience in an increasingly dangerous environment (Fredrickson et al., 2003). Given that it reduces depressive symptoms, emphasizing the importance of positive emotionality is important for mental health professionals who work with individuals coping with the threat of terrorism. Specific relaxation techniques have also been suggested as age-appropriate preventive interventions with children in the context of terrorism (Klingman, 1992). We also suggest that individuals who are unduly burdened by the threat of terrorism and have thoughts and beliefs that create significant restrictions and functional impairments may benefit from cognitive–behavioral therapy (CBT). While CBT can be helpful for those suffering from the threat of terrorism, most individuals cope adequately with the threat and will not require professional assistance. Yet, focusing on positive emotionality and challenging occasional maladaptive thoughts may be helpful, even for the average person (Somer et al., 2003).

Despite the fact that terrorism is a low-probability event, most Americans likely consider the personal risk to be higher than statistically indicated. This may be a rational assessment, given that the government prepares us for the possibility of future terrorism events. Some individuals may have a liberal decision-making criterion for deciding to act on their fears, due to assuming the worst case, which increases anxiety and likely impacts decisions about leisure or planning (e.g., sealed rooms). This "personalization of terror" may impact citizens across many spheres of daily life and result in a downward spiral. "Immunizing" citizens against this "personalization of terror," would require beginning in the schools with age-appropriate information aimed at education about terrorism and ultimately involving citizens of all ages (Tucker, 2003). Children in elementary school through college could attend talks given by terrorism experts who would travel around the US. These talks would also consist of teaching about the motivations and strategies of terrorists in a developmentally appropriate fashion. These talks would also be attended by community groups (e.g., churches, social organizations) that would, in turn, help others cope with the threat of terrorism. Ultimately, the terrorists' primary mission will be foiled by reducing the level of anxiety and panic among US citizens as a result of encouraging dialog and demystifying terrorism (Tucker, 2003).

It is also important to provide education and information about potential bio-terrorism, and the behavioral and social impacts of bio-terrorism need to be incorporated as part of any comprehensive planning initiative (Holloway et al., 1997). First, psychological reactions account for a significant portion of the cases reporting to emergency rooms following a terrorism attack (Karsenty et al., 1991; Bleich et al., 1992). As a result, information about risks of bio-terrorism events, coping with bio-terrorism, and specific education about bio-terrorism agents (e.g., the types of different agents, how to recognize symptoms) might help increase adaptation and coping with this threat among citizens (Noy, 2002). Benedek and colleagues argue that clear, consistent, accessible (e.g., on the web through a government agency, through public mailings), reliable and redundant information that is given from trusted sources will help individuals cope by diminishing public uncertainty about a cause of a symptom that might cause seeking unnecessary treatment (Benedek et al., 2002). Therefore, dissemination of information is a public health issue because it arguably reduces anxiety, assists in the process of coping, and reduces the prevalence of somatic and psychological casualties, thus saving medical resources for those who truly need them following a chemical attack. Citizens in Israel were taught about chemical and bio-terrorism agents and how to protect themselves against the adverse risks of these chemicals during a heightened time of risk. More specifically, children in schools and adults were taught how to use gas masks as well as antidote injections in case of an attack. In comparison, the US government provided vague instructions about using duct tape and storing supplies during a time of heightened threat. Ambiguous suggestions provided by the government may increase anxiety because they are neither educative nor prescriptive. However, we appreciate the complexities inherent in the provision of prescriptive protections and government warnings in the face of possible terror. Inadvertently inaccurate information may produce unfounded reassurances of safety or lead citizens to overestimate the possibility of harm, resulting in iatrogenic fear (Hall *et al.*, 2002), which may lead to mistrust of the government during a critical time.

The fashion in which the American government and media deliver the message of terrorism can also be guided by existing research. Given that emotions affect appraisals that are linked to particular emotional states (Lerner & Keltner, 2001), information should be delivered without inducing fear or anger in citizens, and in the most unbiased and informative way possible. Additionally, terrorist threats should be publicized following reliable and specific support from intelligence offices, and only when they appear imminent. Recent terrorism-related warnings have been criticized as "poorly coordinated and overly vague" and the current color-coded terrorism warning system has been called unhelpful due to fear invocation without information dissemination (Tucker, 2003).

The Gilmore Commission, a federally chartered group also known as the Advisory Panel to Assess Domestic Response Capabilities for Terrorism Involving Weapons of Mass Destruction, has also made several policy-related recommendations (Gilmore Commission, 2003). The purpose of the Gilmore Commission was to make recommendations in order to help create "*a new normalcy*," defined as a way of life which acknowledges that the threat of terrorism will not disappear but one that also preserves civil liberties that are central to the American value system. The report argues that to promote better coping in the public, A Terrorist Threat Integration Center, which is separate from the CIA and FBI, should be established and ultimately provide information to federal, state, and local governments so that efforts and information can be centralized and coordinated. The Gilmore Commission also recommends an ongoing, well-coordinated strategy that is aimed at public education on prevention, risk, signs of exposure, resulting symptoms, and treatment for intervention before, during, and after a potential attack. The Gilmore Commission also stresses that individuals need to prepare to cope with a wide range of terrorist scenarios, not only the worst-case situations; they predict that the future will hold an increase in smaller-scale attacks. They argue that a terror event that will cause "mass destruction" is a lower-probability event than a smaller-scale terror event, especially since a smaller-scale event will be easier to carry out and psychologically, will still have the effects that terrorist seek to achieve (i.e., mass terror). Although we have pieces of the puzzle that help inform our understanding of coping with terrorism, overall we know little about how individuals cope with the threat of terrorism. There is a great deal to learn about how coping varies across individuals and cultures, and about normative ways of coping that lead to the lowest levels of anxiety and the least functional impairments. We also need theoretical models that attempt to explain coping in the context of terrorism, and research concerning the most effective ways of portraying threat and other important policy choices. Ideally, we want to better understand ways of promoting the least functional impairment in citizens, coupled with the requisite preparation and vigilance.

A working conceptual framework

We offer a working conceptual framework that depicts an initial set of constructs that may mediate the relationship between a terrorist event and subsequent responses to the threat of future terrorist events as a heuristic guide for future research. Part of our model is reminiscent of Barlow's "triple vulnerability model," which posits that psychological and biological vulnerability interact with existing stressors to influence the development of anxiety (Barlow, 2002). Additionally, we borrow from existing frameworks that illustrate the psychological repercussions of disasters (La Greca *et al.*, 1996, 1998; Vernberg *et al.*, 1996). However, our model differs from others in the sense that we believe that the most important outcome should be the *functional impact of terrorism*, as opposed to psychopathology. Existing models of traumatic stress capture psychological adaptation to direct or indirect exposure to *specific terrorism events*. We are more concerned with generating a model depicting how uncertain future exposure to terrorism impacts functioning. Rather than depicting psychopathology as the outcome of interest, our model portrays functioning as the most important outcome measure because the threat of future terrorism is not a traumatic event and relying on symptom-based outcomes does not sufficiently capture existing resilience and individuals' behavioral and cognitive responses. However, we argue that exposure to terrorism and subsequent post-traumatic responses are among several important factors that are depicted in our model.

The following categories are included in this working conceptual framework: (1) *terrorism impact variables*, (2) *person/history variables*, and (3) *culture/environment variables*. We will describe the model in general terms since details are provided elsewhere (Maguen & Litz, 2003).

The exogenous variable in our model is an *actual terrorism event*, which is the precursor to any concerns and behaviors related to future terror threat. Alerts about future terrorist attacks would be less meaningful if the terrorist attacks on 9/11 had never happened. Individuals can experience acts of terrorism directly or indirectly, via the media (Schuster *et al.*, 2001; Pfefferbaum *et al.*, 2003).

Terrorism impact variables are the first set of variables depicted in our model and include: (1) immediate reaction to the terrorist event, (2) resource loss, and (3) long-term psychological impact of exposure to terror. Although the effects of exposure to terrorism unfold over time, an individual's immediate reaction to an act of terrorism is constituted of: (a) an individual's appraisal of the event and (b) an individual's acute emotional reaction to the event. Multiple situational determinants influence individual appraisal of a terror event (Patterson & Neufeld, 1987). Appraisal-tendency theory suggests a specific link between the initial appraisal, emotional reaction, and long-term adaptation (Lerner & Keltner, 2001). Personal and collective resources are negatively impacted by traumas or severe stressors, creating risk for enduring posttraumatic problems (Hobfoll *et al.*, 1995). This is especially true for mass disasters, and terrorism on 9/11 created resource loss on multiple ecological levels (e.g., family, organization, and community). Finally, exposure to terrorism may result in a number of psychological reactions, including PTSD and depression symptoms (Bleich *et al.*, 2003). For example, some individuals may experience acute symptoms following an act of terror, which may pass with time (e.g., exaggerated startle response), while others may develop PTSD, demonstrating chronic and severe reactions.

Person and history variables are the second set of variables depicted in our model and include: (1) psychiatric history and mental health, (2) personality factors, (3) trauma history, (4) construction of the meaning of terrorism, and (5) social and self-schemas. Person variables may be altered as a result of a terrorist act, although they are partially pre-existing. A terrorist event may interact with a number of diatheses, creating new, renewed, or exacerbated mental health problems. Shariat and colleagues found that 26% of survivors of a terrorism incident reported pre-existing depression that was exacerbated after the bombing (Shariat *et al.*, 1999). Enduring personality characteristics, such as negative affectivity or neuroticism, will influence the acute and long-term experience of an act of terror, as well as aspects of adaptation to the threat of future terrorism. Personality factors can also play a crucial role in the ability to cope with and respond to threatening information (Chan & Lovibond, 1996; Miller & Patrick, 2000). Furthermore, as compared to those without trauma, individuals with a past trauma history have more difficulty recovering from subsequent life stressors, and prior exposure to trauma is a risk factor for PTSD resulting from ensuing trauma (Stretch *et al.*, 1998; King *et al.*, 1999; Dougall *et al.*, 2000).

Additionally, individuals attempt to establish coherence and meaning in the face of confusion, conflict, and other threats to well-being following terrorist attacks such as those that occurred on 9/11. Constructions about the meaning of the original attacks will partially determine how a person copes with the threat of future terrorist acts. Finally, although schemas about terrorism and threat may be greatly impacted by prior history, individuals may over-accommodate new acts of terror, thereby influencing future perceptions of threat.

Culture/environment variables are the third and final set of variables depicted in our model and include: (1) social network and support and (2) information about the threat from the government and the media. These macro system variables form the milieu in which individuals function post-terrorism. They include smaller more personalized networks at the individual level and larger networks, such as the government and media, at the societal level. Close relationships serve as a terror management mechanism (Florian *et al.*, 2002), and well-functioning social support systems post-disaster serve as a protective factor against long-term mental health consequences (Norris *et al.*, 2002). The media, a very powerful tool, induces strong emotions in individuals, which may unintentionally influence threat appraisals and future policy judgments (Lerner *et al.*, 2003). More care and thought should guide construction of messages sent by both the government and via the media, given the power that these tools exert on the general public.

According to our framework, coping repertoires are the final mediator of the functional impact of the threat of terrorism. Coping strategies will differentially influence functional impact related to fears of future terrorist attacks and will vary considerably from person to person. For instance, individuals who have an avoidant coping style may refuse to engage in outdoor activities or use public transportation. On the other hand, individuals who cope well with the threat of terror may be less hindered and restrictive when engaging in daily living activities.

Functional impact of the threat of terrorism is the final outcome variable in our model. Little is known at present about how terrorism impacts functioning well after the tragedy has passed or after multiple successive events. The IOM's report on the psychological outcomes of terror suggests that research efforts should examine the chronic functional impact of terrorism, including divorce, domestic or interpersonal violence and conflict, and school dropout rates (Butler *et al.*, 2003).

In the aftermath of direct exposure, victims' work capacities, social bonds, and self-care routines are severely disrupted. For example, in the days following the terrorist attacks in New York City, 27% of workers missed work (Melnik *et al.*, 2002). On the other hand, individuals may work harder than normal in order to avoid any emotional reactions or memories that resulted from a terror event, which is also important to capture when assessing functioning. Any acute vocational interruption or change is multiply determined, and is typically a rational choice or evidence of self-care, rather than a sign of poor functioning. For instance, individuals may have suffered resource losses that make it difficult to return to a normal routine, they may want to ensure that the family unit is stabilized before returning to routines of functioning, and/or they may choose to spend more time with significant others in order to garner support. School absences occurred following the sniper attacks in the Washington, DC metropolitan area in October 2002, and attendance rates were as low as 10% at several elementary schools (Schulte, 2002). Again, given that one of the victims was a child walking to school, this was a cogent choice for many parents. At least one study indicates that children with high exposure to other traumatic events may not necessarily fare worse in the context of terrorism. Pfefferbaum and colleagues found that Kenyan children exposed to a terror bombing demonstrated high levels of resilience and low levels of functional impairment (e.g., problems at home and at school, problems with interpersonal relationships) (Pfefferbaum *et al.*, 2003). Functional impact of a terror event may be highly influenced by environmental and cultural variables.

On the other hand, one set of findings may provide some clues about the long-term functional impact of terror. According to surveys that were conducted post-9/11, 21% of cigarette smokers reported an increase in smoking after the attacks (Melnik *et al.*, 2002), 25% of individuals reported an increase in alcohol consumption, and 3% of New Yorkers reported increases in marijuana use (Vlahov *et al.*, 2002). Furthermore, drinking to cope was significantly associated with indicators of poorer functioning following the Oklahoma City bombing (North *et al.*, 2002). These findings suggest that individuals may appeal to unhealthy practices in attempt to soothe and temper anxiety related to terror exposure, which could have sustained impact over the life course. Indeed, there is some evidence of an association between fear and use of substances. For example, individuals with lower perceived safety 7 months after September 11, 2001 were more likely to have increased alcohol use (Grieger *et al.*, 2003). Following the Oklahoma City bombing, increased smoking and increased alcohol use were independently associated with worry about safety and functional impairment (Pfefferbaum *et al.*, 2002). These studies all suggest that identifying increased substance use may be a possible way to screen for functional impairment. Overall, existing studies demonstrate that the large majority of individuals cope very well with the threat of future terrorist attacks and do not evidence long-term functional impairments. Yet we are still uncertain about what constitutes the ideal form of adaptation.

Summary

If terrorism creates lingering anxiety and worry about the potential for future malicious mass violence, then terrorism is effective. As a result, the goal becomes to increase effective coping and reduce incapacitating and disabling fears among citizens. We know very little about how people cope with the unique possibility of future terrorist attacks, although we know something about the mental health impact of direct and indirect exposure to terrorism in different contexts (e.g., Oklahoma City, 9/11). With respect to theory and research depicting risk and resilience factors that contribute to the mental health impact of trauma and traumatic loss, the field of traumatic stress has evolved considerably (Gray *et al.*, 2003; King *et al.*, 2003), and research on the threat of terrorism will likely continue in this tradition. In this chapter we argued that long-term adaptation to terror requires a paradigm shift away from psychopathology and toward coping and functional impact in the face of concerns about future terrorism, and we presented a conceptual framework based on this argument. As evidence accumulates in this important research area, we expect our working conceptual framework to be modified considerably. In order to test the validity of various risk and resilience indicators, causal modeling studies are needed. Our hope is that research examining key elements of the model will reveal information that will guide future terror-related educational and clinical intervention efforts.

REFERENCES

American Psychological Association (2003). Fostering resilience in response to terrorism: for psychologists working with children. Retrieved on December 28, 2003 from http://www.APAHelpCenter.org/resilience

Barlow, D.H. (2002). *Anxiety and Its Disorders: The Nature and Treatment of Anxiety and Panic* (2nd ed.). New York: Guilford Press.

Benedek, D.M., Holloway, H.C. & Becker, S.M. (2002). Emergency mental health management in bioterrorism events. *Emergency Medicine Clinics of North America*, **20**, 393–407

Bleich, A., Dycian, A., Koslowsky, M., Solomon, Z. & Wiener, M. (1992). Psychiatric implications of missile attacks on a civilian population. Israeli lessons from the Persian Gulf War. *Journal of the American Medical Association*, **268**, 613–615.

Bleich, A., Gelkopf, M. & Solomon, Z. (2003). Exposure to terrorism, stress-related mental health symptoms, and coping behaviors among a nationally representative sample in Israel. *Journal of the American Medical Association*, **290**, 612–620.

Block, J. & Kremen, A.M. (1996). IQ and ego resiliency: conceptual and empirical connections and separateness. *Journal of Personality and Social Psychology*, **70**, 349–361.

Breznitz, S. (1967). Incubation of threat: duration of anticipation and false alarm as determinants of the fear reaction to an unavoidable frightening event. *Journal of Experimental Research in Personality*, **2**, 173–179.

Butler, L.D., Koopman, C., Azarow, J., Desjardins, J.C., Seagraves, D., McCaslin, S. & Hastings, T.A. (2002). Predictors of distress and resiliency following the tragedy of 9-11-01. Paper presented at the annual meeting of the International Society of Traumatic Stress Studies (ISTSS). Baltimore, MD.

Butler, A.S., Panzer, A.M., Goldfrank, L.R. & Institute of Medicine of the National Academies (2003). *Preparing for the Psychological Consequences of Terrorism: A Public Health Strategy*. Washington, DC: National Academies Press.

Cairns, E. & Wilson, R. (1989). Coping with political violence in Northern Ireland. *Social Science and Medicine*, **28**, 621–624.

Carver, C.S. (1997). You want to measure coping but your protocol's too long: consider the brief COPE. *International Journal of Behavioral Medicine*, **4**, 92–100.

Chan, C.K.Y. & Lovibond, P.F. (1996). Expectancy bias in trait anxiety. *Journal of Abnormal Psychology*, **105**, 637–647.

Dougall, A.L., Herberman, H.B., Delahanty, D.L., Inslicht, S.S. & Baum, A. (2000). Similarity of prior trauma exposure as a determinant of chronic stress responding to an airline disaster. *Journal of Consulting and Clinical Psychology*, **68**, 290–295.

Florian, V., Mikulincer, M. & Taubman, O. (1995). Does hardiness contribute to mental health during a stressful real-life situation? The roles of appraisal and coping. *Journal of Personality and Social Psychology*, **68**, 687–695.

Florian, V., Mikulincer, M. & Hirschberger, G. (2002). The anxiety-buffering function of close relationships: evidence that relationship commitment acts as a terror management mechanism. *Journal of Personality and Social Psychology*, **82**, 527–542.

Folkins, C.H. (1970). Temporal factors and the cognitive mediators of stress reaction. *Journal of Personality and Social Psychology*, **14**, 173–184.

Folkman, S. & Lazarus, R.S. (1991). Coping and emotion. In *Stress and Coping: An Anthology*, eds. A. Monat & R.S. Lazarus (3rd ed.). New York: Columbia University Press, pp. 207–227.

Forsythe, C.J. & Compas, B.E. (1987). Interaction of cognitive appraisals of stressful events and coping: testing the goodness of fit hypothesis. *Cognitive Therapy and Research*, **11**, 473–485.

Fredrickson, B.L., Tugade, M.M., Waugh, C.E. & Larkin, G.R. (2003). What good are positive emotions in crisis? A prospective study of resilience and emotions following the terrorist attacks on the United States on September 11th, 2001. *Journal of Personality and Social Psychology*, **84**, 365–376.

Galea, S., Ahern, J., Resnick, H., Kilpatrick, D., Bucuvalas, M., Gold, J. & Vlahov, D. (2002). Psychological sequelae of the September 11 terrorist attacks in New York City. *New England Journal of Medicine*, **346**, 982–987.

Gidron, Y., Gal, R. & Zahavi, S. (1999). Bus commuters' coping strategies and anxiety from terrorism: an example of the Israeli experience. *Journal of Traumatic Stress*, **12**, 185–192.

Gilmore Commission (2003). *The Fifth Annual Report to the President and the Congress*. Retrieved on January 2, 2004 from http://www.rand.org/nsrd/terrpanel/

Gray, M., Prigerson, H. & Litz, B.T. (2003). Conceptual and definitional issues in traumatic grief. In *Early Intervention for Trauma and Traumatic Loss*, ed. B. Litz. New York: Guilford Publications, pp. 65–84.

Grieger, T.A., Fullerton, C.S., Ursano, R.J. (2003). Posttraumatic stress disorder, alcohol use, and perceived safety after the terrorist attack on the Pentagon. *Psychiatric Services*, **54**, 1380–1382.

Hall, M.J., Norwood, A.E., Ursano, R.J., Fullerton, C.S. & Levinson, C.J. (2002). Psychological and behavioral impacts of bioterrorism. *PTSD Research Quarterly*, **13**, 1–7.

Hobfoll, S.E., Dunahoo, C.A. & Monnier, J. (1995). Conservation of resources and traumatic stress. In *Traumatic Stress: From Theory to Practice*, eds. J.R. Freedy & S.E. Hobfoll. New York: Plenum Press.

Hoffman, B. (2002). Rethinking terrorism and counter-terrorism since 9/11. *Studies in Conflict and Terrorism*, **25**, 303–316.

Holloway, H.C., Norwood, A.E., Fullerton, C.S., Engel, C.C. & Ursano, R.J. (1997). The threat of biological weapons: prophylaxis and mitigation of psychological and social consequences. *Journal of the American Medical Association*, **278**, 425–427.

Karsenty, E., Shemer, J., Alshech, I., Cojocaru, B., Moscovitz, M., Shapiro,Y. & Danon, Y.L. (1991). Medical aspects of the Iraqi missile attacks on Israel. *Israel Journal of Medical Sciences*, **27**, 603–607.

King, D.W., King, L.A., Foy, D.W., Keane, T.M. & Fairbank, J.A. (1999). Posttraumatic stress disorder in a national sample of female and male Vietnam veterans: risk factors, war-zone stressors, and resilience-recovery variables. *Journal of Abnormal Psychology*, **108**, 164–170.

King, D.W., Vogt, D.S. & King, L.A. (2003). Risk and resilience factors in the etiology of chronic PTSD. In *Early Intervention for Trauma and Traumatic Loss*, ed. B. Litz. New York: Guilford Publications, pp. 34–64.

Klingman, A. (1992). Stress reaction of Israeli youth during the Gulf War: a quantitative study. *Professional Psychology: Research and Practice*, **23**, 521–527.

Koplewicz, H.S., Vogel, J.M., Solanto, M.V., Morrissey, R.F., Alonso, C.M., Abikoff, H., *et al.* (2002). Child and parent response to the 1993 World Trade Center bombing. *Journal of Traumatic Stress*, **15**, 77–85.

La Greca, A.M., Silverman, W., Vernberg, E.M. & Prinstein, M.J. (1996). Symptoms of posttraumatic stress in children after Hurricane Andrew: a prospective study. *Journal of Consulting and Clinical Psychology*, **64**, 712–723.

La Greca, A.M., Silverman, W. & Wasserstein, S.B. (1998). Children's predisaster functioning as a predictor of posttraumatic stress following Hurricane Andrew. *Journal of Consulting and Clinical Psychology*, **66**, 883–892.

Lazarus, R.S. & Folkman, S. (1984). *Stress, Appraisal, and Coping*. New York: Springer Publishing Company.

Lerner, J.S. & Keltner, D. (2001). Fear, anger, and risk. *Journal of Personality and Social Psychology*, **81**, 146–159.

Lerner, J.S., Gonzalez, R.M., Small, D.A. & Fischhoff, B. (2003). Effects of fear and anger on perceived risks of terrorism: a national field experiment. *Psychological Science*, **14**, 144–150.

Litz, B.T., Gray, M.J., Bryant, R. & Adler, A.B. (2002). Early intervention for trauma: current status and future directions. *Clinical Psychology: Science and Practice*, **9**, 112–134.

Maguen, S. & Litz, B.T. (2003). Psychological response to the threat of terrorism: what do we know and where do we go from here? (under review).

Masel, C.N., Terry, D.J. & Gribble, M. (1996). The effects of coping on adjustment: re-examining the goodness of fit model of coping effectiveness. *Anxiety, Stress and Coping: An International Journal*, **9**, 279–300.

Masten, A.S. (2001). Ordinary magic: resilience processes in development. *American Psychologist*, **56**, 227–238.

Mathews, A.M. & MacLeod, C. (1994). Cognitive approaches to emotion and emotional disorders. *Annual Review of Psychology*, **45**, 25–50.

Melnik, T.A., Baker, C.T., Adams, M.L., O'Dowd, K., Mokdad, A.H. & Brown, D.W. (2002). Psychological and emotional effects of the September 11 attacks on the World Trade Center Connecticut, New Jersey, and New York, 2001. *Morbidity and Mortality Weekly Report*, **51**, 784–786.

Miller, M.W. & Patrick, C.J. (2000). Trait differences in affective and attentional responding to threat revealed by emotional Strop interference and startle reflex modulation. *Behavior Therapy*, **31**, 757–776.

Moos, R. (1990). *Coping Responses Inventory Manual.* Palo Alto, CA: Stanford University and Department of Veterans Affairs Medical Centers.

Moos, R.H. & Billings, A.G. (1982). Conceptualizing and measuring coping resources and coping processes. In *Handbook of Stress: Theoretical and Clinical Aspects*, eds. L. Goldberger & S. Breznitz. New York: Free Press, pp. 212–230.

Norris, F., Friedman, M.J., Watson, P.J., Byrne, C.M., Diaz, E. & Kaniasty, K. (2002). 60,000 disaster victims speak. Part I: An empirical review of the empirical literature, 1981–2001. *Psychiatry: Interpersonal and Biological Processes*, **65**, 207–239.

North, C.S. & Pfefferbaum, B. (2002). Research on the mental health effects of terrorism. *Journal of the American Medical Association*, **288**, 633–636.

North, C.S., Tivis, L., McMillen, J.C., Pfefferbaum, B., Cox, J., Spiznagel, E.L., *et al.* (2002). Coping, functioning, and adjustment of rescue workers after the Oklahoma City bombing. *Journal of Traumatic Stress*, **15**, 171–175.

Noy, S. (2002). Early dissemination of information: an essential ingredient in the prevention of biological warfare. *Harefuah*, **141**, 119.

Park, C.L., Folkman, S. & Bostrom, A. (2001). Appraisals of controllability and coping in caregivers and HIV+ men: testing the goodness-of-fit hypothesis. *Journal of Consulting and Clinical Psychology*, **69**, 481–488.

Patterson, R.J. & Neufeld, R.W. (1987). Clear danger: situational determinants of the appraisal of threat. *Psychological Bulletin*, **101**, 404–416.

Pfefferbaum, B., Nixon, S., Tucker, P., Tivis, R., Moore, V. & Gurwich, R. (1999). Posttraumatic stress response in bereaved children after the Oklahoma City bombing. *Journal of the American Academy of Child and Adolescent Psychiatry*, **38**, 1372–1379.

Pfefferbaum, B., Nixon, S., Tivis, R., Doughty, D., Pynoos, R., Gurwich, R., *et al.* (2001). Television exposure in children after a terrorist incident. *Psychiatry*, **64**, 202–211.

Pfefferbaum, B., Vinekar, S.S., Trautman, R.P., Lensgraf, S.J., Reddy, C. & Patel, N. (2002). The effect of loss and trauma on substance use behavior in individuals seeking support services after the 1995 Oklahoma City bombing. *Annals of Clinical Psychiatry*, **14**, 89–95.

Pfefferbaum, B., Sconzo, G.M., Flynn, B.W., Kearns, L.J., Doughty, D.E. & Gurwitch, R.H. (2003). Case finding and mental health services for children in the aftermath of the Oklahoma City bombing. *Journal of Behavioral Health Services and Research*, **30**, 215–227.

Roth, S. & Cohen, L. (1986). Approach, avoidance, and coping with stress. *American Psychologist*, **41**, 813–819.

Schlenger, W.E., Caddell, J.M., Ebert, L., Jordan, B.K., Rourke, K.M., Wilson, D., *et al.* (2002). Psychological reactions to terrorist attacks: findings from the National Study of Americans' Reactions to September 11. *Journal of the American Medical Association*, **288**, 581–588.

Schulte, B. (2002). Schools shaken by threat but won't shut down. *Washington Post*, Section A, p. 1.

Schuster, M.A., Stein, B.D., Jaycox, L.H., Collins, R.L., Marshall, G.N., Elliott, M.N., *et al.* (2001). A national survey of stress reactions after the September 11, 2001 terrorist attacks. *New England Journal of Medicine*, **345**, 1507–1512.

Shariat, S., Mallonee, S., Kruger, E., Farmer, K. & North, C. (1999). A prospective study of long-term health outcomes among Oklahoma City bombing survivors. *Journal of the Oklahoma State Medical Association*, **92**, 178–186.

Sharkansky, E.J., King, D.W., King, L.A., Wolfe, J., Erickson, D.J. & Stokes, L.R. (2000). Coping with Gulf War combat stress: mediating and moderating effects. *Journal of Abnormal Psychology*, **109**, 188–197.

Skinner, E.A., Edge, K., Altman, J. & Sherwood, H. (2003). Searching for the structure of coping: a review and critique of category systems for classifying ways of coping. *Psychological Bulletin*, **129**, 216–269.

Silver, R.C., Holman, E.A., McIntosh, D.N., Poulin, M. & Gil-Rivas, V. (2002). Nationwide longitudinal study of psychological responses to September 11. *Journal of the American Medical Association*, **288**, 1235–1244.

Somer, E., Tamir, E., Maguen, S. & Litz, B.T. (2003). Brief cognitive–behavioral phone-based intervention targeting anxiety about the threat of attack: a pilot study. *Behaviour Research and Therapy*, **43**, 679.

Stanton, A.L., Danoff-Burg, S., Cameron, C.L., Bishop, M., Collins, C.A., Kirk, S.B., et al. (2000). Emotionally expressive coping predicts psychological and physical adjustment to breast cancer. *Journal of Consulting and Clinical Psychology*, **68**, 875–882.

Stretch, R.H., Knudson, K.H. & Durand, D. (1998). Effects of premilitary and military trauma on the development of post-traumatic stress disorder symptoms in female and male active duty soldiers. *Military Medicine*, **163**, 466–470.

Suvak, M.K., Vogt, D.S., Savarese, V.W., King, L.A. & King, D.W. (2002). Relationship of war-zone coping strategies to long-term general life adjustment among Vietnam veterans: combat exposure as a moderator variable. *Personality and Social Psychology Bulletin*, **28**, 974–985.

Thabet, A.A.M., Abed, Y. & Vostanis, P. (2002). Emotional problems in Palestinian children living in a war zone: a cross-sectional study. *Lancet*, **359**, 1801–1804.

Tucker, J.B. (2003). Strategies for countering terrorism: lessons from the Israeli experience. *Journal of Homeland Security* [online]. Available at http://www.homelanddefense.org/journal/Articles/tucker-israel.html

Vernberg, E.M., La Greca, A.M., Silverman, W. & Prinstein, M.J. (1996). Prediction of posttraumatic stress symptoms in children after Hurricane Andrew. *Journal of Abnormal Psychology*, **105**, 237–248.

Vlahov, D., Galea, S., Resnick, H., Ahern, J., Boscarino, J.A., Bucuvalas, M., et al. (2002). Increased use of cigarettes, alcohol, and marijuana among Manhattan, New York, residents after the September 11th terrorist attacks. *American Journal of Epidemiology*, **155**, 988–996.

Weisenberg, M., Schwarzwald, J., Waysman, M., Solomon, Z. & Klingman, A. (1993). Coping of school-age children in the sealed room during scud missile bombardment and postwar stress reactions. *Journal of Consulting and Clinical Psychology*, **61**, 462–467.

Yovetich, N.A., Dale, J.A. & Hudak, M.A. (1990). Benefits of humor in reduction of threat-induced anxiety. *Psychological Reports*, **66**, 51–58.

33

Life under the "new normal": notes on the future of preparedness

Irwin Redlener and Stephen S. Morse

Introduction

Being prepared for emergencies is not a new concept. At every level of government there are contingency plans for natural disasters, accidental catastrophes, local events and personal emergencies of every conceivable manner. Organizations from the Red Cross to the Federal Emergency Management Agency to hospital emergency departments are in a constant state of readiness. Often, regionally specific plans are in place based on expectations of particular kinds of disasters: earthquakes in the West, hurricanes on the East Coast, tornados in the Midwest. In fact, long before 9/11, even terrorism had been on the minds of at least a handful of stalwart preparedness experts – mostly in the military and in special governmental agencies (Benjamin & Simon, 2002; Stern, 2003; Clarke, 2004).

Yet the attacks of 9/11 on New York City, Washington, DC, the downing of a hijacked passenger airliner in Pennsylvania and the many events that followed have radically changed our perceptions and expectations of what it means to be prepared for emergencies. The USA can be seen as undergoing a societal and political transformation of major proportions, similar in many ways to the Great Depression or the Japanese attack on Pearl Harbor, as two examples of transformational events of the last century.

And, as if to emphasize this transformation, the terrible events of 9/11 were followed by other tragedies, marking just the beginning of a series of traumatic experiences that have, collectively, affected the nation in a profound, multi-dimensional way. Hard on the heels of the 9/11 attacks, in the fall of and into the Winter of 2001, we confronted the still unexplained anthrax attacks, followed by sniper shootings in the Washington, DC region, and then the prospect of needing to vaccinate the entire country against smallpox. Meanwhile, terrorist attacks continue to occur regularly across the globe, while suicide bombings remain dramatically frequent in the Mideast and have now spread to other areas such as Russia. Adding further to the stress, the USA is engaged in major military incursions in Afghanistan and Iraq, with continuing terrorist actions against troops and civilians.

Future terrorist attacks seem virtually inevitable. Attacks with unconventional weapons, such as biological or chemical agents, have been widely discussed. The prospect of bioterrorism, and other non-conventional means of attack, raises unprecedented levels of anxiety among people who believe such means might well be used indiscriminately against civilians. Clearly, the idea of terror is to create extreme levels of psychological stress (Susser *et al.*, 2002). The prospect of shadowy foreign nationals using deadly violence against civilians, with or without the so-called "weapons of mass destruction", produces precisely the kind of stress that makes individuals and communities vulnerable to the psychological consequences of terrorism, either actual or anticipated.

Through all of this, the nation is attempting to develop a massive new capacity to prevent, fight and respond to terrorism, of any type, on American soil or against US interests abroad. Internationally driven terrorism is now an irrefutable fact of life in the USA and the response to terrorism and the threat of terrorism will require both technical and psychological strategies.

On the technical side, there will be a full range of programs designed to coordinate better protection and prevention under the rubric of "homeland security". Where and how this goes will be discussed later. But the players on this field will be on relatively familiar ground. Members of the intelligence communities, military and academic experts, first responder systems, public sector agencies, and the like will have roles in presumably developing and engaging new technologies, creating better means of communications and ensuring that a properly trained disaster workforce is at the ready.

But, on the psychological and societal fronts we will need to face an entirely different set of challenges. It is in these matters that a new agenda, and perhaps a new lexicon, will emerge over the next few years. This is because the nation is confronting a series of realities that, collectively, represent a truly transformational development for the country at large, for its government and for all of its citizens.

There are actually few events in recent American history that provide lessons or a sociological roadmap with respect to how America responded to 9/11 and where it needs to go in the future. Even though smaller terrorist attacks have occurred in the USA in the past, including the bombing of the same World Trade Center Tower in 1993, and the bombing of the Murrah Federal Building in Oklahoma City in 1995, there is little to compare to the catastrophic impact that rocked the nation in 2001.

There have been other such occurrences in US history where an unanticipated trauma caused a sudden, extraordinary disruption of business as usual, but these have been rare, especially in the last century. In the 19th century, the Civil War was wrenching for the nation, still in its infancy and prior to its first centennial celebration. But in the 20th century, one is drawn to the analogy between the attacks on Pearl Harbor, drawing the USA into World War II, and the terrorism of 9/11, as perhaps the closest parallel. On December 6, 1941, Americans were certainly aware of the German aggression in Europe and a sense of a growing threat in Asia from Japan, a nation clearly preparing for an expanding war. Yet there was little public or political agreement around the possibility of American engagement on either front. Isolationism was a viable and popular perspective in response to substantial turmoil and military confrontation in other parts of the world. But the events of Pearl Harbor virtually stopped the arm-chair deliberation among Americans with respect to the nation's proper role in a world increasingly at war. That surprise attack had extraordinary and epochal consequences for America. In an immediate sense, war was declared by the USA against aggressors in Europe and Japan. The entire country became mobilized both in terms of military response and what amounted to a virtual upending of the national economy. Beyond the obvious, however, was a transformation of the country and its citizens from a heterogeneous, though internationally isolated, nation still recovering from the great economic depression of a decade or so earlier to a suddenly united, invigorated protagonist in one of the great wars in all of history. Clearly American society was fundamentally different, on many levels, in 2001 than it had been 60 years earlier. Yet there are striking similarities between the attack on Pearl Harbor and the terrorist assaults of 9/11. As in 1941, the attacks of 9/11 were a stunning and horrific surprise to Americans. Both were conceived and carried out by foreign nationals without clear provocation, against targets not generally thought to be particularly vulnerable. At the moment of the attacks, the country was, in both instances, in a relatively isolationist geopolitical frame of mind. Both instances disturbed long-standing complacency and galvanized the country. In addition, the elements of surprise and unpredictability were common to both Pearl Harbor and 9/11. Surprise, and the psychological stress it causes, is one of the most potent allies of the terrorist.

The future of preparedness: challenges and strategies

It is no surprise, then, that bioterrorism, and the other non-conventional means of attack, raises unprecedented levels of anxiety among people who believe such means might well be used indiscriminately against civilians. So the question of how prepared are we to respond to a bioterror attack, or to other types of unconventional attack, is a reasonable and urgent issue for the public. After all, in a post-9/11 world, none of this is out of the question as a future scenario of increased aggression against the USA.

Several years after 9/11, although some significant progress has been made, there is still no cohesive national plan for ensuring optimal preparedness in the USA. In the absence of a national domestic security and response plan, it is difficult to understand the goals or establish working benchmarks for accountability at the level of the implementing agencies. The development of such a plan would be a crucial initial step in working towards a better-prepared nation. In order to establish an appropriate national blueprint there needs to be a realistic assessment of risk and vulnerabilities, new ways of organizing and coordinating critical intelligence and interdiction strategies, clear definitions of "functional preparedness", thorough analysis of estimated costs and appropriation of sufficient resources. Virtually none of this has yet happened to a sufficient degree.

We will consider below a number of the elements that we consider essential in developing our preparedness strategies.

Define "prepared" and establish preparedness benchmarks

One of the most difficult challenges will be defining what is meant by "prepared", especially for terrorism. There is no functional definition of "preparedness" that is consistent throughout government or that is universally accepted by departments of public health, first responders or healthcare systems around the nation. Should a community need the ability to respond to an intentionally poisoned water supply that creates 200 or 2000 very sick people in a short period of time? Should the definitive diagnosis and management protocols for such a calamity be developed by the local health department, a state agency or the federal government? Should hospitals in a community have the capacity to quarantine 10 patients or 100, or 10,000? Should the community be able to decontaminate people covered with radioactive dust at the rate of 6 an hour or 60? What equipment is needed and who needs to be trained? Should a major city be planning for terrorist scenarios with 100,000 casualties or 1 million? In addition, there is a need to understand and include the needs of special vulnerable populations, such as children (Redlener & Markenson, 2003).

Since total preparedness is essentially not achievable, a better approach might be to seek a goal of "functionally and appropriately prepared". This is not simply an academic exercise. In the absence of a definition it is virtually impossible to set benchmarks, understand true costs or evaluate outcomes.

A personal analogy is useful. Paraphrasing an oft-stated response to the question of what does "prepared for a terrorist emergency" mean to an individual, the answer might be stated as "somewhere on the continuum between uninformed complacency and overt paranoia". For a larger system or society as a whole, the concept of functionally and appropriately prepared may be applied similarly. Does the nation need to prepare for *simultaneous* attacks with weaponized smallpox, explosions of "dirty" bombs in six metropolitan areas and several attacks on major infrastructure facilities? Does Chicago's health and public health systems need to plan for 500 or 5000 victims of a nerve gas attack? Or 50,000? There are no obviously correct answers for most of these questions. But a set of decisions needs to be made in order to calculate the resources needed to reach whatever level of preparedness is determined to be appropriate.

Beyond the immediate necessity to define preparedness, there is a real need to establish appropriate benchmarks in many aspects of the planning process. Benchmarks establish a means of describing specific needs, developing cost models and enabling proper monitoring of programs and policies established as part of the preparedness agenda.

Hospital planning illustrates these points. Even with the availability of significant resources for emergency planning, institutions need to understand what they are aiming toward. These questions cannot be left up to local facilities or even entire communities to decide on their own, but require analysis and guidance from high-level planners who can synthesize information on threat assessment, availability of emergency resources from outside the community and other key factors. In the absence of large-scale strategic guidance in these matters, local communities, acute care facilities and public health agencies will have no way of establishing appropriate benchmarks, quantifying need demonstrating efficacy of established preparedness programs.

The potential scenarios are virtually limitless. The money and resources needed for planning are entirely dependent on the scenarios selected. Furthermore, it is impossible to test or plan for every possible scenario; therefore, the selection of scenarios must, by definition, represent choices about the most likely threats, or those for which planning would prove the most generally useful.

In the USA, the call for standardization was recently embodied in Homeland Security Presidential Directive (HSPD) 8, of 2003 (White House, 2003). In response to this directive, the Office of Domestic Preparedness in the Department of Homeland Security is planning to develop 15 standardized scenarios for drills and exercises, and to standardize drill evaluation criteria for all responders.

For public health and the healthcare response, there have also been some attempts toward more specific definition and benchmarks. In public health, the National Association of County and City Health Officials (NACCHO, 2004), which represents local health departments, recently began a program (in collaboration with Centers for Disease Control and Prevention (CDC) and academic partners) called "Public Health Ready" to help agencies define minimum standards of emergency preparedness. Criteria are based on having an adequate plan, providing appropriate training on emergency preparedness to staff, and then testing agency preparedness through drills and exercises. At the hospital level, federal bioterrorism funding to hospitals, implemented through the Health Resources and Services Administration (HRSA) has set certain benchmarks for hospitals receiving these funds. The Joint Commission on the Accreditation of Healthcare Organizations (JCAHO), the standard-setting organization for the USA, has also set increasing standards for hospital emergency preparedness, beginning with having emergency plans and regular drills that also include the community. These are good starts, but obviously represent only the beginning. Preparedness is a process as much as it is a specific list of capabilities, and the endpoint still remains to be defined.

Manage the bureaucracy

Most look to the federal government for standards, but first the federal government must get its own house in order. There is no escaping the fact that the prevention of terrorism and the capacity to respond effectively to major disasters, human made or otherwise, in a society as large and complex as the USA is a monumental task, akin to mounting, and maintaining a credible and effective military. However, the current bureaucracies responsible for managing the process of preparedness, on all levels, are enormous and unwieldy. There are serious concerns regarding the lack of coordination, even among agencies of the same department. The principal preparedness and response functions fall to the US Department of Homeland Security, a newly formed entity that consolidates a number of federal agencies. Its workforce includes nearly 180,000 workers in some 23 different agencies. Yet important management and control questions need to be urgently addressed. Both the Congress and the White House will need to collaborate on the establishment of a properly funded, cohesive system for developing and implementing strategies. The system should expect minimization of redundancy and full accountability from all relevant agencies.

The response to any terrorist event requires coordinating many federal agencies. But, at the same time, emergency response is local and therefore requires local agencies to be prepared and to work together with these numerous federal partners. The blueprint for integrating response across agencies at the federal and local levels is the recently announced National Incident Management System (NIMS). While this is an essential first step, NIMS, like all plans, requires continual practice by those who must use it. If past experience is a guide, communications will remain a major challenge. The integration of response sectors is a particular issue, including integration of healthcare, emergency medical services (EMS) and public health, and their relationship to the "standard" regular first responders.

The proper interface between public health and other government agencies in the post-9/11 world is another fundamental, but unanswered, question. In the age of terrorism in America, we urgently need to define and clarify the dynamic relationship between national security and public health. In 2002, when the possibility of vaccinating large numbers of Americans against smallpox was first raised, experts in the health and public health communities were repeatedly asked if this was an appropriate decision. As the eradication of smallpox in the 1970s was truly one of the great public health accomplishments of all time, so the return of small-pox as a viable possible consequence of an act of terrorism was an astonishing and disconcerting idea to contemplate. But the decision to develop a contingency plan to deal with a smallpox outbreak should not have been a matter of the "opinion" of public health experts. No legitimate expert in this field would ever consider such a notion *unless* smallpox was considered to be a clear threat. This was in fact a decision that had to be made based on information from the national security and intelligence communities, not public health. Public health experts would be integral in the *development and implementation* of a plan, but only if a serious threat of smallpox could be convincingly established.

Monitor dual use and trade-offs

Does a massive investment in preparedness, especially in the health and public health systems, simply shift resources and attention from the traditional or core agendas of these systems, or do innovations related to preparedness have secondary beneficial effects with respect to the capacity of the system to function more generally? Or perhaps both factors are operative in different situations and at different times. There is a case to be made, for instance, that enhancing surveillance for diseases induced by biological weapons can improve mechanisms for early identification of any infectious disease, including newly emerging naturally occurring infections like severe acute respiratory syndrome (SARS) and West Nile, or pandemic influenza (Morse, 2002). Indeed, there is an exact historical precedent. In 1950, during an earlier period of concern about bioterrorism, the CDC started the Epidemic Intelligence Service (EIS). The EIS was intended to provide investigative and public health capacity to respond in case of a bioterrorist attack (Langmuir & Andrews, 1952; Henderson, 1993). While it was never needed for this purpose (before the anthrax attacks in 2001), the EIS has provided expertise for responding to many natural disease outbreaks and has served as a major training mechanism for generations of epidemiologists and other public health experts.

On the other hand, there is considerable concern that "terror preparedness" is swallowing up resources that are needed to deal with the long-standing critical issues, which still require enormous attention, by public health officials. Problems like the spread of HIV/AIDS, control of drug-resistant tuberculosis or ensuring access to childhood immunizations for all children, among many other challenges, remain high priorities for the public health community.

There is evidence that resources for core programs have been eroding, especially as state budgets have come under greater economic pressure (Gursky, 2004; Turnock, 2004). This was particularly evident during the push to vaccinate health, first responder and public health workers against smallpox. Several health departments reported the need to shift personnel, originally assigned to traditional pediatric vaccination or tuberculosis control activities, to the smallpox program (Gursky, 2004).

Over the next few years, it is imperative that non-governmental "watchdog" organizations monitor the consequences of identifying and investing preparedness resources. The potential for degrading vital, core public health and safety net programs is real. In addition, the sustainability of these public health funding increases remains a concern.

Address bioethical and legal ramifications of preparedness

As we confront terrorism, protecting the public without eroding civil liberties and our core democratic values remains an important issue in general. Virtually every aspect of large-scale preparedness planning can evoke critical issues of ethical or legal concern. The USA PATRIOT Act of 2002, giving broad, new investigatory powers to domestic law enforcement officials seeking to identify or detain potential terrorists, has become a major source of concern to legal professionals and civil liberties advocates. Serious questions have been raised regarding privacy of citizens, due process and other matters central to American values, and protected by fundamental principles of the US Constitution and Bill of Rights.

For example, in planning for managing bioterrorist attacks, governmental agencies, law enforcement and public health experts are considering responses including forced evacuation and quarantine. There is a need for systematic examination of the legal and civil liberties implications of such measures. In fact, public health law in general, as well as the relationships among public health, police and military jurisdictions in these matters, is extremely unclear. Principles and governing laws and regulations vary widely among states. Clarifying the implications of these matters with respect to large-scale preparedness planning is an essential near-term objective (Gostin *et al.*, 2002). In many states the process of rewriting public health law is already in process.

Ensure future workforce

Competent and well-prepared personnel are key to any agency's successful preparedness efforts. At least one major recent report reviewed the status of the public health workforce and noted the prospect of severe shortages in the workforce as the current pool aged and retired (Institute of Medicine, 2003). It was predicted that half of the current public health workforce would be lost by attrition within the next decade. Grave concerns were raised about the capacity of the pipeline to ensure appropriate workers to fill needed slots for public health, whether for preparedness or traditional public health. Clearly, an important agenda for public health train-ing and educational institutions would be consideration of efforts to expand and diversify existing programs.

In addition, it is likely that new programs will need to be developed. The develop-ment of the EIS over 50 years ago, and of Project Public Health Ready in the last few years, have already been mentioned. In the last 5 years, the CDC also established a net-work of Centers for Public Health Preparedness to involve academe in helping to train the public health workforce as well as to help replenish the pipeline (Morse, 2003).

National deliberation of short-term and alternative solutions would need to include the possibility of training public health workers at the undergraduate level, as well as graduate programs as is currently the case (Institute of Medicine, 2003). In a similar vein, certificate programs and rapid transition of individuals in related professions to fulfill particular public health preparedness functions would have to be considered. Such efforts would require buy-in and support from the federal government in order to ensure sufficient support.

Engage local communities in emergency preparedness planning

In general, we have a long way to go with community preparedness, and in engaging the community as an essential partner in all preparedness efforts. Clearly, commu-nity resilience is an important goal of preparedness. The response to 9/11 and other tragedies shows that, in fact, there is a surprising amount of resilience in most com-munities. However, with the exception of a few, minimally funded efforts, such as the Community Emergency Response Teams (CERT) Program, there have been few efforts to really engage citizens and local communities in the process of emergency readiness. To date the entire process has been essentially "top down". Government issues terror alert warnings. Officials advise citizens to "be vigilant" and make plans to accommodate a need to evacuate an area or "shelter in place". But, general cyni-cism about the government's ability to respond effectively in the event of a bioterror attack and a decreasing level of confidence in the health and public health system's capacity to provide care in the aftermath of such an event has resulted in little actual cooperation or participation in emergency planning on the part of everyday citizens.

The color-coded alert system has been unhelpful in the absence of explanation or direction regarding what people need to do in response to a change in the level of concern. At the same time, journalists and officials have not fully come to grips with what messages ought to be communicated to the public around terrorism and emergency readiness. In large part, this is due to substantial absence of clarity on this subject from government, lack of publicly trusted, consistent communicators and a general sense that the media has not gotten a clear sense of its own mission during this time of continuing crisis in America.

In a 2003 Marist institute survey commissioned by the National Center for Disaster Preparedness of the Columbia University Mailman School of Public Health and the Children's Health Fund, Americans were found to be very concerned about the possibility of new terrorism, yet many lacked confidence in government or the public health system's ability to respond effectively. In a follow-up poll conducted in July 2004, public confidence had declined even further (National Center for Disaster Preparedness and Children's Health Fund, 2004). While 76% of Americans remain concerned about terrorism, only 53% expressed confidence in the government's ability to protect local areas, contrasted with 62% a year earlier. Even more disconcerting was the finding that more than 63% of Americans had not made their own basic emergency plans, and only 21% (in the July 2004 poll) considered themselves familiar with their own community's terrorism response plan. In fact, in the August 2003 survey, 90% of Americans said they would not cooperate with official directives to evacuate an area considered to be under attack. This dramatic level of potential dissent in the time of an emergency was due to frequently expressed concerns about the whereabouts and safety of family members and loved ones. In other words, if parents are unsure about what's happening with their children in a major emergency, they will not leave an area, even if ordered to do so.

All of these suggest that individuals, and their communities, remain disconnected from the planning process. Work needs to begin immediately to ensure that families take appropriate steps to improve their abilities to survive in an emergency. Citizens also need to be more engaged in working on community-based emergency plans. Research with respect to enhancing individual engagement as well as defining appropriate roles for volunteer programs, local institutions such as schools, neighborhood organizations, faith-based communities and the like will all be the near-term goals in national preparedness.

However, there is still no established methodology for developing community resilience or even for measuring it. Risk communications for pre-event messaging remain among the key strategies, but there is little consistency in either the messages or how they are presented. It is likely that different ethnic communities will have different trusted sources and preferred methods of receiving information. One strategy could be identifying community leaders who are perceived as trusted information sources in their communities, and understanding how risk information can be presented to them for maximum clarity and usefulness.

Nonetheless, this is only meaningful if consensus can be developed on what communities should be doing to prepare for major emergencies. Both risk communications and community preparedness activities remain an evolving area. In the USA, there is a long history of preparedness, including intensive efforts during the Cold War. Many Americans of a certain age remember "duck and cover" drills and other activities that, in retrospect, seem naïve and uninformed, an attempt to show that something was being done. It is possible that the experiences of these Cold War activities have hampered our willingness to develop new civil defense measures and to examine more constructive ways to engage the community in laying the foundations for its own psychological defense against terror.

Efforts to engage the public are in nascent stages in the USA. Programs such as "Ready.gov" or, in New York City, "NYC Aware", are encouraging starts, but only first steps. A number of other countries, such as Britain, Israel, Sri Lanka and Colombia, have had to confront terrorist activities for a number of years, and comparisons might be instructive. There is much to be said for demystifying preparedness and providing individuals with tools to increase resiliency. In Israel, for example, basic emergency preparedness lessons are presented as part of the school curriculum beginning as early as age 6, so that children have had some time to become familiar with basic prepared-ness concepts and to practice them. The lessons at school also encourage discussion of these questions at home, making family discussions easier and ensuring that parents are also confronting these questions along with their children (Boaz Tadmor, personal communication, 2003).

Improve understanding of the psychological and behavioral ramifications of terrorism

The chapters in this volume survey the state of our understanding of the psycholog-ical response to terrorism and other exigent events. It is clear that much has been learned. At the same time, many questions remain. What are the best interventions post-event? How do we recognize those in most immediate need, or those who may be most susceptible, other than those with pre-existing psychopathology? (North *et al.*, this volume). What sorts of pre-event messages are the most useful for prepar-ing the community?

One unmet need is a paradigm for integrating mental health intervention into our preparedness and response activities. For example, some hospitals in Israel assign teams of mental health professionals in the emergency department during major disasters. Other teams of mental health professionals are also assigned specif-ically to work with victims' families, and are trained to address their concerns.

There will also be a need to train response professionals to be competent in mental health issues. There are two obvious components of mental health involved in this. First, responders must be sensitive to mental health issues among those they encounter during the response. They must be able to calm fears among mem-bers of the affected community and must be able to triage quickly and refer those who need immediate counseling. Secondly, and just as importantly, they must be trained to recognize when they are showing signs of stress themselves and get appropriate relief. Even today, there is widespread recognition that responders may be particularly vulnerable, but uncertainty remains about the best way to prevent stress in responders (North *et al.*, this volume).

Conclusions

These are some of the key issues needing careful attention as the nation continues the process of preparedness for disasters and terrorism. We are moving at a level of urgency unprecedented in a modern society. But will the resources for preparedness be distributed equitably throughout our communities? Will already underserved populations see disparities in this arena, as is already the case with traditional health and other services? Who will monitor this potential area of concern? And, perhaps most important, can such efforts be made sustainable?

As society ponders how far we can go in efforts to prevent or respond to terrorism, there are difficult challenges to be faced. Can we do what is prudent and appropriate, without infringing on cherished values or legal rights that are the hallmarks of our society? We all hope so, but only time will tell.

REFERENCES

Benjamin, D. & Simon, S. (2002). *The Age of Sacred Terror*. New York: Random House.

Clarke, R.A. (2004). *Against All Enemies*. New York: Free Press.

Gostin, L.O., Sapsin, J.W., Teret, S.P., Burris, S., Mair, J.S., Hodge Jr., J.G. & Vernick, J.S. (2002). The Model State Emergency Health Powers Act: planning for and response to bioterrorism and naturally occurring infectious diseases. *Journal of the American Medical Association*, **288**, 622–628.

Gursky, E. (2003). *Progress and Peril: Bioterrorism Preparedness Dollars and Public Health*. New York: The Century Foundation. (Also available on the Century Foundation web site, at: http://www.tcf.org/Publications/HomelandSecurity/Gursky_Progress_Peril.pdf).

Henderson, D.A. (1993). Surveillance systems and intergovernmental cooperation. In *Emerging Viruses*, ed. S.S. Morse. New York: Oxford University Press.

Institute of Medicine (2003). *Who Will Keep the Public Healthy?* Washington, DC: National Academy Press.

Langmuir, A.D. & Andrews, J.M. (1952). Biological warfare defense. 2: The Epidemic Intelligence Service of the Communicable Disease Center. *American Journal of Public Health*, **42**, 235–238.

Morse, S.S. (2002). The vigilance defense. *Scientific American*, **287**(4), 88–89.

Morse, S.S. (2003). Building academic–practice partnerships: the Center for Public Health Preparedness at the Columbia University Mailman School of Public Health, before and after 9/11. *Journal of Public Health Management and Practice*, **9**, 427–432.

NACCHO (2004). Project Public Health Ready. Available from NACCHO web site at: http://www.naccho.org/topics/emergency/pphr.cfm. Accessed April 2006.

National Center for Disaster Preparedness and Children's Health Fund (2004). How Americans feel about terrorism and security: Three years after September 11. Marist Institute for Public Opinion Poll, July 2004. Available from NCDP web site at http://www.ncdp.mailman.columbia.edu/files/Annual_Survey_2004.pdf. (Additional survey can be accessed at: http://www.ncdp.mailman.columbia.edu/research.htm.) Accessed April, 2004.

North, C.S., Pfefferbaum, B. & Hong, B. (this volume). Historical perspective and future directions in research on psychiatric consequences of terrorism and other disasters. In 9/11: *Mental Health in the Wake of Terrorist Attacks*, eds. Y. Neria, R. Gross & R. Marshall. Cambridge, UK: Cambridge University Press.

Redlener, I. & Markenson, D. (2003). Disaster and terrorism preparedness: what pediatricians need to know. *Advances in Pediatrics*, **50**, 1–37.

Stern, J. (2003). *Terror in the Name of God*. New York: Harper Collins.

Susser, E.S., Herman, D.B. & Aaron, B. (2002). Combating the terror of terrorism. *Scientific American*, **287**(2), 70–77.

Turnock, B.J. (2004). *Public Health Preparedness at a Price: Illinois*. New York: The Century Foundation. (Also available on the Century Foundation web site, at: http://www.tcf.org/Publications/HomelandSecurity/Turnock.pdf).

White House (2003). Homeland Security Presidential Directive 8 (Hspd-8). Available at http://www.whitehouse.gov/news/releases/2003/12/20031217-6.html. Accessed April 2006.

34

Lessons learned from 9/11: the boundaries of a mental health approach to mass casualty event

Arieh Y. Shalev

Introduction

For a foreigner who visits New York City, population heterogeneity is among the most striking features. There is also something futuristic about what one sees: A conglomerate of extreme opposites, somehow "functioning" together, bound by unannounced and apparently complex rules. Throwing a rock into such pond promises extreme reverberation, but also a somewhat better, though forced and transient, synchrony of waves and reactions.

For a time, following 9/11, one is told, hearts and minds in New York City became closer. Furthermore, since then "the City has changed," acknowledge savvy New Yorkers, and cite as a proof the blackout night of August 14, 2003, in which people "were just out of themselves," offering help and "acting like true community." From anecdotes of ice-cream being given away by merchants on the streets, one can also appraise the extent to which charity, in New York, is typically combined with practicality. These will have melted anyhow, by the next morning.

Notwithstanding, in this book, the lessons of September 11, 2001, are mainly ones of "trauma," "disaster" and "decline in mental health." This is surprising, given the sense of common fate that should be hovering over the city since – or has it gone? Arguably, it is not the role of mental health specialists to identify resiliency – but rather to treat the diseased. To ignore it, however, is certainly not a good practice.

Additionally, this book highlights the presence of threat, fear, and post-traumatic symptoms, and one wonders what, indeed, was the relative part of loss, and by extension whether, beyond narrating the story of a "trauma," mental health professionals actually have the vocabulary that properly expresses what has been, and is regularly being observed under duress?

One question that this chapter raises, therefore, concerns the extent to which some change in perception, appraisal and formulation of major negative events should occur as a result of the events of September 11, 2001, and the subsequent experiences of the professional community. Such necessary changes might be difficult to identify. However, to the extent that this volume should offer more than historical documentation, they must be formulated, be it tentatively.

And what a peculiar choice it is to leave this task to a fellow-professional from abroad, who might be close enough to echo the sentiment, yet far enough not to simply resonate.

Clearly unable to do justice to the richness of the observations reported in this volume, I have chosen five dimensions for discussing the material brought here. These include the following: (a) The particularities of the event itself; (b) The approach taken to evaluate its effect on people and construe action to be taken; (c) The conceptual and cultural framework within which the discipline of "mental health," was firstly chosen as prime responder *and interpreter* of reality, and then scrambled, within its inherent constraints, to find "solutions" to dubiously formulated "problems." (d) An attempt to draw a line between "reactions" and "disorders" and similarly between "help," "intervention" and "treatment" and also address the related issue of reluctance, stigma, and avoidance of care. (e) Action taken, observations made, learning curves experienced and their implications for the future.

Uniqueness of the 9/11 experience

The combined attacks on the Twin Towers in New York and the Pentagon were both unprecedented and surprising; hence an understandable hesitancy and delays in mounting organized responses. Notwithstanding, The 9/11 Commission Report (National Commission on Terrorist Attacks Upon the United States, 2004) provides important details about early individual responses to the rolling drama, such as those of airlines – and US security forces, of rescue teams in New York and at the Pentagon, and of ordinary people, caught in the action (e.g., in a staircase at one of the towers) who were already helping, soothing, comforting, trying to make sense, communicating and actually reducing both the death toll – and the psychological burden.

Consequently the most important lesson of 9/11 might be that each of the potential clients for any intended "intervention" or "treatment" already has a record of skillfully and actively helping himself or herself, and often others – and of trying to cope with multiple forms of adversity and with his or her own reaction. Somehow, identifying distressed survivors by a set of symptoms neither requires nor promotes a view of each of them as active participant, which is where we often fall short of paying respect to the strength of humans, and than lament that they avoid us.

Chapters in this volume provide an account of a somewhat hesitant but rapidly developing professional and paraprofessional response to the events. Given the novelty of the events, it is not surprising that they mark the beginning of a learning curve. In the absence of subsequent occurrences, however, all learning is based on a single occurrence, and necessarily reflects the particularities of that experience.

Several unique features of the New York 9/11 experience are worth mentioning. The event was of rather short duration, unprecedented magnitude, extremely visual and of extremely powerful symbolism. It made very few injured survivors – and very few identifiable human remains to be buried and properly mourned. As much as the hole in New York City's skyline, 9/11 created human loss without remains. It also left a hallo of suspended threat, which, like the cloud of smoke over Ground Zero and parts of Manhattan, remained "in the air," never truly disappearing, never giving a concrete target for protective action. Given the vertical collapse of the towers, and their location, structural damage was also contained. Cleaning and reconstruction were, therefore, left to dedicated personnel, whereas most people remained participants by observation – rather than action. Thus, for those not directly affected, that is, for most New Yorkers, the drama of 9/11 was essentially psychological. It also required little concrete response from most people – leaving many in a search for ways to act, and others in a state of passive worry and objectless anticipation.

Additionally, there was little damage to the city's infrastructure and to its institutional stability. Electricity, transportation, communication, food supply, and core social institutions were quickly restored. Thus, in the concrete sense of a disaster exhausting community's core resources, the New York City community was far from being "disastrously" affected. This may again have contributed to the salience of psychological reactions, which, in other disasters can become second in importance to other needs, such as food and shelter needs.

A prototype of modern disasters, the 9/11 death toll affected a wide array of proximal and distant communities, making the disaster's painful impact (and subsequent supportive efforts) both widespread and poorly focused.

In another such "modern" feature, the events of the morning of 9/11 could be observed, and therefore "directly" (or, at least, immediately) experienced by innumerable spectators – from those strolling in the streets of downtown New York – or rushing to balconies or roofs, to those living on the New Jersey bank of the Hudson River – to those glued to TV screens elsewhere across the country. Not only were the flashes of fire and debris visible to eventually everyone – the 9/11 events also had, from the first moments, a distinct ex-temporal quality, since, unlike concrete or somewhat "less photogenic" events, of which we mainly see the aftermath, or which *happen* and then become a memory, in 9/11, emotionally overwhelming images of the airliners' impact kept being broadcasted, time and again in a sort of extended present.

In addition, the relevance of the events' embedded threats gave them extended and poorly defined spatial boundaries. It takes time, for a visitor of New York, to gather how personally relevant the 9/11 were events to many – or most residents. One didn't know where the next blow was going to come from, but many felt, and some are still convinced, that more is coming, and soon, and from another and totally unexpected angle.

Thus, many who would not be in personal peril in other types of disasters, experienced imminent and personal threat following 9/11. Unlike the bloodiest air raids in war, there was no trusted safety signal (e.g., a siren announcing the end of an attack) and no safe places (e.g., the underground). A theft in one's own bedroom whilst one sleeps has similar effects: safety itself isn't safe any more.

Consequently, the boundaries between direct and indirect exposure were blurred – and indeed a matter of *degree*: geographic, to some extent (e.g., Galea *et al.*, 2002a; 2002b) but also emotional and situational. This, again, may not happen in other disasters, where the prime stressor has better temporal and spatial boundaries. It does characterize, however, the worst of terror threat: spreading uncertainty and fear. It also ensues that intervening in the aftermath of 9/11 was not just *post-traumatic care* – but indeed helping survivors under ongoing threat. In that sense, a person who fearfully avoided subways to lower Manhattan reflected not only his or her own pathological fear, but, in fact, a common apprehension, overcome by some and forbidding for others.

The search for clients

These very particularities have lead to the first question, with which many agencies were faced: *Who is the client?* The first impression that one gets from reading the reports in this volume is that, for quite a time, everyone was searching for a client – with the possible exception of lower Manhattan hospitals and police stations that, for a time, were flooded by those desperately seeking lost relatives – or seeking information about their loved ones' last minutes – or just crying out their grief (a story surprisingly skipped in this section of the book).

Nonetheless, a lot was done. Project Liberty provided face-to-face counseling, education and outreach services to an estimated 1.2 million individuals (Felton *et al.*, this volume), the World Trade Center Worker/Volunteer Mental Health Screening Program has arranged for screening of nearly 5000 workers/volunteers from the World Trade Center (WTC) site, of whom 40% were identified as "cases" and 10% reported significant disability. There were consistent efforts to help affected children (Katz *et al.*, this volume). The New York Consortium for Effective Trauma Treatment provided, and still provides, valuable training for therapists (Foa & Cahill, this volume; Marshall *et al.*, this volume). The Mental Health Association of New York – eventually the only organization to have had prior structure, stature, and routines – could significantly increase its crisis hotline activity, assess distress in different communities, document major changes in outpatient services-utilization, and evaluate the effect of time and anniversary reactions (Draper *et al.*, this volume).

Ongoing help was offered to exposed members of the fire department of New York (FDNY) and Con Edison workers – and the authors have articulated valid principles of addressing institutional cultures whilst providing mental health interventions (Difede *et al.*, this volume).

But the general sense is, still, a hesitant definition of potential clients, at least initially, and than an even more profound question about what to do when a client is finally identified – given the wide array of modes and degrees of exposure and the spectrum of responses and perceived needs. Additionally it seems that with the possible exception of the hotline service, mental health providers in this unique urban disaster were not flooded by help-seeking clients, but rather had to promote help seeking.

This may have implications for future occurrences, the first among which is that needy survivors might preferentially use previously-trusted sources. More information is needed to define the real needs for every level of intervention – given that few of those approached and identified finally "consumed" consulting or treatment services. Only as last resource, and very reluctantly, should one assume a general "barrier" to seeking help or "avoidance" of treatment – which leaves the problem with the client and not with the provider. Reading the chapters in the intervention section gives the impression that many New Yorkers were happy with "softer" modes of assistance, such as telephone conversation, clarification and validation of experience, and minor advice about children and personal fear. Many others have probably turned to lay helpers – the family, the neighbor, the church, and the group of volunteers – and presumably found just enough of what they are looking for. One may never know, therefore, how many "true" cases have skipped an "essentially needed" therapy – or if they needed it at all.

The search for relevant measures

In saturated solution, crystals may suddenly form, and than organize themselves, around incidental irregularities of the matter, such as a grain of dust. Similarly, in novel and complex situations, perception may uncritically organize itself around the first available templates – regardless of those templates being inherently relevant or appropriate.

Posttraumatic stress disorder (PTSD) symptoms – and by extension – symptoms of mental disorders offer such well-rehearsed, available and accessible templates. They, therefore, have been widely used as such to evaluate distress in the aftermath of 9/11. Moreover, studies looking at PTSD symptoms following the Twin Tower collapse yielded significant increase in symptoms – particularly in areas proximal to the disaster (Galea *et al.*, 2003). This has made these symptoms all the more attractive, and was eventually used, at least before the good news about their time-dependent disappearance (Silver *et al.*, 2002), to infer both an epidemic of PTSD and a related, urgent and massive need for treatment.

From a perspective of the terror-prone country of Israel, several analogies might be relevant here. First, the *Diagnostic and Statistical Manual of Mental Disorders, Fourth Edition* (*DSM-IV*) PTSD symptom criteria include behaviors (e.g., avoidance of places and situations) and states of mind (e.g., concern, hypervigilance) that normally occur at the early aftermath of traumatic events and during anticipation of further harm (American Psychiatric Association, 1994; Shalev, 2006; Shalev *et al.*, 2006). These behaviors (e.g., avoiding central places in Jerusalem) are generally proportional to actual (frequency of attacks) or perceived threat – and tend to vanish rapidly when things seem to be going better. A time-dependent decrease in perceived probability of subsequent attacks might, therefore, explain the progressive decline in the prevalence of PTSD-like symptoms in New York City. The idea that treatment provided, or care for the mentally ill has actually contributed to the relatively benign progression of PTSD symptoms in New York City has yet to be proven. There is no data bearing on this important question in this volume's chapters. Thus, we are left without firstly knowing whether PTSD symptoms are, indeed, the essential measure of maladaptive response to mass trauma and secondly without knowing what was the overall yield of interventions provided.

The second lesson from years of exposure to terror in Israel (Bleich *et al.*, 2003; Shalev, 2006) is that terror creates *subsets of highly distressed residents* within affected communities, whilst, at the same time, the majority is surprisingly resilient. Population estimates, therefore, might be misleading as they may both overestimate the prevalence of a disorder initially, and underestimate its impact later, when most of those exposed have ceased to express symptoms, but a minority remains highly distressed.

Along that line, Draper's and colleagues' chapter reports a "lingering devastation of the attacks," as captured by the LifeNet hotline (Draper *et al.*, this volume). They seem to have identified one important feature of post-traumatic morbidity: its persistence and its interaction with subsequent stressors. To an extent, a wish to provide care for all those affected might divert attention from the fewer who have major, "lingering" and progressively deteriorating responses. Later in this chapter I further elaborate on the apparent weakness of *ad hoc* post-disaster efforts relative to stable, community-embedded resources.

The half-full – half-empty glass

Reading of this volume also suggests that most affected New Yorkers – and residents of adjacent areas – showed "some" PTSD symptoms; "a level of" increase in cautious behavior, a bit more cigarettes and alcohol use and some other negative changes. Yet the vocabulary of these reports is somewhat different and requires caution. Wording, such as "dramatic impact on the mental health of millions" may not only misrepresent reality, but also determine illness perception. Whether or not there has been such major impact on mental health (rather than on well being, sense of safety, risk perception, or expressions of distress – all of which may or may not relate to the construct of health) is a matter that the present material does not help to solve.

Similarly, most survivors and witnesses seem to have reported on both half-full and half-empty glasses. Put differently, with the exception of those critically affected by loss, or other components of the event, most people were distressed *and* went on with their lives. Many have "positively" reacted: the number of people who volunteered to help others increased at the aftermath of 9/11. Therefore the prospect of psychological interventions should have equally emphasized the full, or "resilience" part of the reaction and the empty "mental health problems." The same individuals might have experienced both. For mental health professionals, the declared goals of interventions are more than a choice of words. It determines what one looks for and how one plans to intervene.

In practice, however, the choice is far from obvious: Should we advise survivors who expresses some symptoms, report mild to moderate distress and continue to perform quite well that they basically cope well, and can trust their coping to take them to a resolution of the experience, or, conversely, worry about their eventually incubating a chronic mental condition and forcefully invite them to start therapy? Possibly, both the "disease model" and "resiliency models" might have to be combined, since most people experience a mixture of both, and therefore live in a constant tension between reparative and injurious processes. The quality of this inner struggle might ultimately determine the long-term effect of exposure.

But how can one know who does well? In a forthcoming article on resilience during continuous terror (Shalev *et al.*, 2006), we suggest, following others (e.g., Pearlin & Schooler, 1978; Benight & Bandura, 2004) to primarily evaluate *coping efficacy*, as reflected by its effect in four distinct domains: *ability to sustain task performance; controllability of emotions; positive self-perception* and the *capacity to enjoy rewarding interpersonal contacts*. Notwithstanding the specifics of this particular model, the general message here is that one might have to move from counting symptoms – or lack thereof – to evaluating where people are in the continuum of successfully surviving the effect of a potentially traumatic event, and how well they deal with subsequent secondary stressors and with the anticipation of further harm. In so doing we may eventually come to weigh "The cost and benefit of denial" (Lazarus, 1982), or people's need to have a degree of ignorance of their own vulnerability and mortality (Lifton & Olson, 1976) in order to thrive within constraints – which is what life is truly about.

Coming back to those seriously affected, a reading of this volume also suggests that, unfortunately, knowledge driven from DSM-IV criteria and subsequent studies was also used to a half. One wonders, for example, whether a reluctance to clearly *diagnose* acute stress disorder (ASD), an entity that, despite imperfections and limited specificity, *does identify a subgroup at very high risk of chronic PTSD* (e.g., Bryant, 2003). Some of the chapters report that there has been significant reluctance, by survivors, to be tagged by "mental health" labels and use mental health services. I believe that the public's reluctance to be tagged in such way parallels the zeal of professionals to discover and address the eventual "mental health disaster" that was to follow the 9/11 attacks. However, had things been addressed by more seriously considering the disease model *when it applies* (e.g., when diagnostic criteria for ASD are met) then fewer might have been falsely advised that they *were* at risk of developing a terrible disorder (which they somehow knew they weren't) and when severe, unremitting, uncontrollable and inescapable symptoms were identified, surveyors will have more willingly accepted an unambiguous referral for help. Knowledge about high-risk survivors does exist and the capacity to properly identify at least a proportion of them is a pre-requisite for effectively implanting specialized therapies such as CBT (Foa & Cahill, this volume).

Where has 9/11 found psychiatry (and mental health in general)?

During the last 25 years, psychiatry has successfully struggled to develop a reliable classification of mental disorders. Subsequent editions of the DSM-IV have better delineated a set of "Axis I" disorders, among which are PTSD, major depression, phobias, and others. In its search for reliable phenotype, however, psychiatry had to move away from theoretical constructs (which previous classifications had allowed – e.g., by including the construct of neuroses in the classification of mental disorders). As a result, attempts to theorize about psychological processes, whilst still existing (e.g., Pitman, 1988; Foa & Kozak, 1986) did not attain the same widespread recognition and acceptance as DSM symptom criteria.

Additionally, psychiatry, a leading discipline of mental health, has moved away from describing and theorizing about sub-threshold conditions and about the human condition in general. This, again, might have been a reaction to an earlier and overarching theorization, much of which was controversial (e.g., the Freudian theory of obsessive–compulsive disorder; the family communication theories of schizophrenia).

Notwithstanding, psychiatry remained largely without underlying psychology. Psychiatry could reliably recognize, diagnose, and recommend treatment, but could not – and did not care much to define, study, and establish the validity of putative psychological mechanisms that govern living and reactions to life events. This critical gap has not been entirely filled by insights from psychological studies, which hardly made an impact on modern psychiatry. Specifically, in September of 2001 neither psychiatry nor any other body of knowledge had a cohesive, widely accepted and *useful* theory of human response to stress – normal and abnormal. Consequently, the field was left wide open, a state of fact that invited unproven practices to mushroom – since there was no serious conceptual foundation to either accept or refute them.

Furthermore, in the pragmatic world created by DSM-IV, efficacy, as shown in controlled trials, became a golden standard to judge the validity of a "treatment" – regardless of truly understanding the underlying biological or psychological logic. Consequently, standardized procedures acquired special status – and this has immediately led to emphasizing *protocol adherence* by therapists over theoretical understanding and *ad hoc* adaptation of treatment principles to changing realities. An example given concerns the teaching of cognitive behavioral therapies (CBT) – rather than teaching the general principles of therapeutic exposure and cognitive reframing.

Spoken harshly, the 9/11 disaster found psychiatry at the lowest end of its being an a-theoretical discipline, and at the lower end of it's capacity to generate, empirically endorse and systematically create clinicians with advanced understanding of human conditions – including life stress, traumatic stress, and healthy support and recovery. The advice to see a specialist thus became a substitute to the more empowering "here's what you might be able to do" – since the recommendations concerning the latter have not been systematically researched for their effect on the consequences of trauma.

The mental health profession's capacity to react to an event of the magnitude of the 9/11 attacks were, thus, lacking. Firstly, it did not have a clear (and evidence-based) message to the numerous lay helpers – family members, group leaders, and many others – who probably provided most the help throughout the months following the attacks. Second, and most important, the profession was eventually overwhelmed by its incapacity to provide treatment, in the strict sense, to a multitude of potential "clients" who, perhaps, didn't even need professional help. The idea that better training thousands of specialists is the desirable solution to this problem, additionally conveys a disempowering message to a multitude of lay helpers, who actually do the job.

Since this situation is likely to repeat itself in future disasters, a putative conclusion of the material provided calls for *shifting the attention of mental health professionals from phenotypes to principles of recovery and from advanced skills* (which are clearly and essentially needed for those with severe reactions) *to sound post-disaster mental hygiene*, public empowerment and education.

Finally, better appraisal of the context and the unfolding of a major trauma; of ongoing stressors and of the major psychological roles of leaders, ceremonies, rumors, mass media, and other factors, should make the reliance on traditonal formal "therapies" a somewhat detached exercise. Mass trauma, so to speak, does not happen and will not resolve in the quiet consultation room.

Concluding comments

From a perspective of a professional who works in the erratically terror-prone city of Jerusalem, the place on the learning curve of the reported New York experiences is way beyond an initial mixture of trial and error, well into formulating necessary organizational changes, and yet not at the crucial point of revising one's basic understanding of trauma and developing routines and structures.

Several insights are salient, though. First, there is much good will, and many potential partners and contributors when trauma occurs. Help, such as via Project Liberty (Felton *et al.*, this volume), LifeNet (Draper *et al.*, this volume), the Child and Adolescent Trauma Treatment Service (Murray *et al.*, this volume) and other projects was provided pro-bono, and extensively. The interface between these systems of care and the ongoing coverage for mental health care is unclear, and one should hope that disaster mental health care, as a consequence of 9/11 studies will become more better organized, and supported by stable resources.

Second, distress and symptoms are omnipresent – and transient in the majority of cases. This truly calls for redefining and better categorizing interventions into those provided as "first aid" and "help in time" and others that more closely refer to mental disorders and their prevention. To an extent, services provided at the aftermath of 9/11 supplemented and eventually by-passed the existing health care system. This might have been a luxury of a resourceful city, affected by a significant – but not fundamentally ruinous event. Other scenarios, as well as the years-long needs of some survivors of 9/11 may require more central involvement of the existing health care systems – and their training, preparedness, and supply of resources.

Along this line, networks of care with a previous record, and those dedicated to a special group of exposed professionals (Difede *et al.*, this volume) found it somewhat easier to be accepted and used by clients. Additionally, *ad hoc* training is onerous, encounters a degree of resistance (e.g., Cahill *et al.*, this volume; Marshall, this volume), and one wonder how much of it might be retained for the future. One wonders to what extent acquiring and retaining skills in trauma treatment – and particularly in the prevention of severe stress disorder – does not require the opening of operative trauma centers, in which treatment and preventions will be practiced daily, and consequently better assessed, and perfected, such that in the future there will be enough experienced and skilled professionals in emergency rooms, clinics, and hospitals. Trauma, in New York and elsewhere, occurs daily, and the allocation of resources to the prevention of its consequences may both prepare a community for further occurrences, and eventually save numerous survivors from becoming chronically disabled by stress disorders.

Finally, our society may not be able to afford the previous luxury of being risk-averse. If anything, the 9/11 events have brought – or should have brought to an end a naïve illusion that life is essentially uneventful – or at least non-traumatic. One feels embarrassed, in fact, to suggest that as a consequence of the threat of terror *we* should all become risk-savvy – the embarrassment coming from knowing that more New Yorkers than one wishes to enumerate are, by virtue of where they live, risk-savvy, and hardy survivors. There is a lot to be learned from these fellow-citizens.

REFERENCES

American Psychiatric Association (1994). *Diagnostic and Statistical Manual and Mental Disorders, Fourth Edition*. Washington DC: American Psychiatric Press.

Benight, C.C. & Bandura, A. (2004). Social cognitive theory of posttraumatic recovery: the role of perceived self-efficacy. *Behavior Research and Therapy*, **42**(10), 1129–1248.

Bleich, A., Gelkopf, M. & Solomon, Z. (2003). Exposure to terrorism, stress-related mental health symptoms, and coping behaviors among a nationally representative sample in Israel. *Journal of the American Medical Association*, **290**(5), 612–620.

Bryant, R.A. (2003). Early predictors of posttraumatic stress disorder. *Biological Psychiatry*, **53**(9), 789–795.

Cahill, S.P., Hembree, E.A. & Foa, E.B. (this volume). Dissemination of prolonged exposure therapy for posttraumatic stress disorder: successes and challenges. In *9/11: Mental Health In The Wake of Terrorist Attacks*. eds. Y. Neria, R. Gross, R.D. Marshall. Cambridge, UK: Cambridge University Press.

Difede, J., Roberts, J., Jaysinghe, N. & Leck, P. (this volume). Evaluation and treatment of firefighters and utility workers following the World Trade Center attacks. In *9/11: Mental Health in The Wake of Terrorist Attacks*. eds. Y. Neria, R. Gross & R.D. Marshall. Cambridge, UK: Cambridge University Press.

Draper, J., McCleery, G. & Schaedle, R. (this volume). Mental health services support in response to September 11th: the central role of the Mental Health Association of New York City. In *9/11: Mental Health in The Wake of Terrorist Attacks*. eds. Y. Neria, R. Gross & R.D. Marshall. Cambridge, UK: Cambridge University Press.

Felton, C.J., Donahue, S., Lanzara, C.B., Pease, E.A. & Marshall, R.D. (this volume). Project Liberty: Responding to mental health needs after the World Trade Center terrorist attacks. In *9/11: Mental Health in The Wake of Terrorist Attacks*. eds. Y. Neria, R. Gross & R.D. Marshall. Cambridge, UK: Cambridge University Press.

Foa, E.B. & Cahill, S.P. (this volume). Psychological treatments for PTSD: an overview. In *9/11: Mental Health in The Wake of A Terrorist Attacks*. eds. Y. Neria, R. Gross & R.D. Marshall. Cambridge, UK: Cambridge University Press.

Foa, E.B. & Kozak, M.J. (1986). Emotional processing of fear: exposure to corrective information. *Psychological Bulletin*, **99**, 20–35.

Galea, S., Ahern, J., Resnick, H., Kilpatrick, D., Bucuvalas, M., Gold, J. & Vlahov, D. (2002a). Psychological sequelae of the September 11 terrorist attacks in New York City. *New England Journal of Medicine*, **346**, 982–987.

Galea, S., Resnick, H., Ahern, J., Gold, J., Bucuvalas, M., Kilpatrick, D., Stuber, J. & Vlahov, D. (2002b). Posttraumatic stress disorder in Manhattan, New York City, after the September 11th terrorist attacks. *Journal of Urban Health*, **79**, 340–353.

Galea, S., Vlahov, D., Resnick, H., Ahern, J., Susser, E., Gold, J., Bucuvalas, M. & Kilpatrick, D. (2003). Trends of probable post-traumatic stress disorder in New York City after the September 11 terrorist attacks. *American Journal of Epidemiology*, **158**, 514–524.

Katz, C.L., Smith, R., Herbert, R., Levin, S. & Gross, R. (this volume). The World Trade Center Worker/Volunteer Mental Health Screening Program. In *9/11: Mental Health in The Wake of Terrorist Attacks*. eds. Y. Neria, R. Gross & R.D. Marshall. Cambridge, UK: Cambridge University Press.

Lazarus, R. (1982). The costs and benefits of denial. In *The Denial of Stress*. ed. S. Bereznits, New York: International University Press. pp. 1–30.

Lifton, R.J. & Olson, E. (1976). The human meaning of total disaster. *Psychiatry*, **39**, 1–18.

Marshall, R.D. (this volume). Science for the community after 9/11. In *9/11: Mental Health in The Wake of Terrorist Attacks*. eds. Y. Neria, R. Gross & R.D. Marshall. Cambridge, UK: Cambridge University Press.

Murray, L., Rodriguez, J., Hoagwood, K. & Jensen, P. (this volume). In *9/11: Mental Health in The Wake of Terrorist Attacks*. eds. Y. Neria, R. Gross & R.D. Marshall. Cambridge, UK: Cambridge University Press.

National Commission on Terrorist Attacks Upon The United States (2004). *The 9/11 Commission Report*. Washington, DC: U.S. Government Printing Office.

Pearlin, L.I. & Schooler, C. (1978). The structure of coping. *Journal of Health and Social Behavior*, **22**, 337–356.

Pitman, R.K. (1988), Posttraumatic stress disorder, conditioning and network theory. *Psychiatric Annals*, **18**, 182–189.

Shalev, A.Y. The Israeli experience of continuous terrorism (2000–2004). (2006). In *Disasters and Mental Health*, eds. J.J. Lopez-Ibor, G. Christodoulou, M. Maj, N. Sartorious & A. Okasha. London, UK: Wiley & Sons.

Shalev, A.Y., Tuval-Mashiach, R. & Hadar, H. (2004). Posttraumatic stress disorder as a result of mass trauma. *Journal of Clinical Psychiatry*, **65**(Suppl. 1), 4–10.

Shalev, A.Y. Tuval, R., Frenkiel-Fishman, S., Hadar, H. & Eth, S. (2006). Psychological responses to continuous terror: a study of two communities in Israel. *American Journal of Psychiatry*. April; **163**, 667–673.

Silver, R.C., Holman, E.A., McIntosh, D.N., Poulin, M. & Gil-Rivas, V. (2002). Nationwide longitudinal study of psychological responses to September 11. *Journal of the American Medical Association*, **288**, 1235–1244.

35

Learning from 9/11: implications for disaster research and public health

Randall D. Marshall

This volume aims to capture something of the extraordinary breadth and depth of mental health services and research that followed the September 11 attacks – efforts that were often happening simultaneously and in isolation from one another. It is a kind of *documentary* of the post-9/11 mental health responses. We also hope that this book serves as a partial remedy to the fragmentary nature of mental health services and research in the USA, and in particular, after all large-scale disasters. It is multi-disciplinary, such that most readers will encounter perspectives on mental health, community, or disaster theory that are foreign to their professional point of view. Although cooperation and tolerance after disaster are ubiquitous, there are also bitter rivalries and fierce struggles for scarce resources. Disaster can evoke the best, and the worst, in any community. We hope that this book and others like it will help to counteract the often tribalistic rivalry of the disciplines presented herein and encourage efforts to communicate effectively, toward genuine collaboration after future disasters.

The psychological aftermath of 9/11

What sets the post-9/11 epidemiologic work apart from prior disaster studies is its scope and methodology, a methodology that reflects a shift in balancing the often competing needs of scientific rigor and timely implementation. Rapidly implemented large-scale studies like these are extremely difficult to do, but serve a crucial humanitarian purpose in that they can inform program development in the early weeks of a disaster. Epidemiologic research that is implemented months later and published years later has much more limited value to the affected community. More importantly, rapidly implemented studies offer a window into the most volatile, dangerous, and emotionally taxing time frame (that is, immediate post-disaster period) and provide a baseline from which to interpret research that captures later aspects of disaster recovery. It is our view that these priorities should drive most methodologic decisions, which inevitably involve decisions about a certain degree of methodologic compromise in the post-disaster setting (e.g., in order to move quickly, telephone and Internet surveys are necessary with smaller numbers of interviews of validation purposes only rather than face-to-face clinician interviews which have been the gold standard).

The successful utilization of post-9/11 epidemiologic research for services planning in New York and Washington D.C. also has critical implications for funding infrastructure. For example, the present funding mechanisms of the National Institute of Mental Health (NIMH) do not allow rapid (within 4 weeks) implementation of new research that could actually inform services planning. The work described herein relied almost entirely on the generosity of individuals (to undertake projects without funding), then on the commitment of New York institutions like the New York Academy to do their part regardless of funding issues, then on philanthropy, and finally, on government by allowing creative adaptation of existing infrastructures (such as, NIMH studies). We believe that this is a major programmatic deficiency in the USA, in that we are relying at present on serendipity and private enterprise to create the scientific foundation upon which a systematic disaster recovery plan is built.

The readers of this book can observe important, current methodologic controversies in disaster epidemiology, illustrated, for example, by the tensions between the perspectives of the scientists who conducted original 9/11 research, and Dr. North, who conducted research after the Oklahoma City bombing. Dr. North's statement that Dr. Galea and colleagues did not acknowledge the limitations of their work is simply mistaken (North et al., this volume). But the more scientifically important debate concerns criticisms from very traditional viewpoints (e.g., Dr. North) that reflect pre-9/11 disaster science. We argue that these epidemiologic models are fatally flawed because they are too slow, too small scale, and impossible to implement rapidly in order to actually inform services. This chapter also criticizes the 9/11 work for overestimating rates of disorder (North et al., this volume), and this criticism has also been leveled at major national surveys such as the National Comorbidity Study of Kessler and colleagues (1995). In fact, all 9/11 studies were very cautious in their conclusions.

More importantly, it is unlikely that more traditional symptom- and disorder-focused studies of small, highly exposed samples would contribute anything substantially new to the disaster literature. Studies have repeatedly found high rates of mental disorders in highly exposed populations, predicted by vulnerability factors. New research should instead be hypothesis driven and pursue more sophisticated questions that build on these established findings (Norris et al., 2002a, b).

One can observe similar tensions in therapeutics research between efficacy and effectiveness research paradigms. Efficacy research emphasizes highly controlled, labor-intensive, very expensive studies that provide clear answers to a treatment question. They have a place of priority in the early part of a treatment's development. Effectiveness research takes these clear and early findings and attempts to move them into large-scale, real-world, less-controlled conditions. As potentially critical scientific decisions must be made about when, and to what degree, to shift from efficacy to effectiveness methods – for example, when methodologic rigor must be relaxed in order to obtain more generalizable answers to a question – the debate seems to take the form of a clash of cultures. People are arguing about values.

We believe, however, that the new models developed by 9/11 research have moved the field forward, and that a more productive discussion would center on ways to make future disaster- and terrorism-related research even more real-world responsive, hypothesis driven, and multi-disciplinary. These studies without exception demonstrate that rapidly implemented epidemiology is possible after even large-scale disaster, and that it can provide critically important information early in the recovery process that can guide services and intervention planning for government, services institutions, and philanthropy. The 9/11 work actually builds on findings from North and colleagues, and in fact are strikingly consistent with their finding that approximately 30% of those directly exposed will develop chronic posttraumatic stress disorder (PTSD) (North *et al.*, this volume). Likewise, the suggestion that research could have somehow been cleared through a central bureaucracy (North *et al.,* this volume) was floated but quickly rejected soon after 9/11 as both unnecessary and unfeasible in a city as complex as New York, or for that matter, the post-Katrina South.

This work also contributes to our thinking about the definition of trauma itself. It shows, for example, that the pre-9/11 view of how Criterion A trauma is defined is limited and should be reconsidered in light of large-scale events that create an extreme and uncertain threat to the general population and have multiple trauma related after effects (Galea *et al.*, 2005). As discussed with clinical sophistication by Shalev, experts in large-scale disaster appreciate that, after an event like 9/11, traumatic and stressor experiences with mental health consequences are numerous, extended in time over many weeks to months, and can have a cumulative effect such as seen in war veterans or law enforcement personnel (Shalev, this volume).

What is needed from epidemiology is an accurate, scientifically neutral assessment of the negative mental health consequences of disaster so these people can be helped. Dr. North suggests that epidemiologists need to manage or "spin" their results somehow. This idea – that we should put mental health surveys in the "context of resilience" – is peculiar. It is never suggested for other public health threats, for instance. Imagine a New York City report on cases of West Nile virus that concluded by emphasizing how many people are bitten by mosquitoes but do not get the virus (who were "resilient").

There are, of course, constructive criticisms of this work, as of all scientific work. It would have been particularly useful, for example, to follow-up some of the more striking national self-report findings with clinician-based interviews in a subsample, as was done in the National Vietnam Veterans' Readjustment Study (NVVRS) (Kulka *et al.*, 1990). If there are large-scale attacks in the future, we hope that the funding agencies will be farsighted enough to pursue questions that these studies have raised.

Reducing the burden: community response and community recovery

If one searches epidemiologic findings for variables that can be a target of intervention, one finds few are useful. The best predictors across the literature are not amenable to intervention (gender, ethnicity, socioeconomic status) and so are relevant only to academic predictor models and for identifying at-risk populations. Little is known about how to act on these findings to reduce risk. The urgent need for research in this area became painfully clear after 9/11, when millions of dollars were suddenly available specifically for resilence building programs. Dr. Norris points precisely at the problem in her scholarly discussion of the chasm between traditional, narrowly focused symptom-count epidemiology and the services community by raising the question of community effects after disaster (Norris, this volume). Progress in the field will require interdisciplinary models that are as yet underdeveloped. It is notable that the most sweeping and widely discussed consequences of these terrorist attacks – social, economic, and political – cannot be captured scientifically by our current mainstream approaches.

In their commentaries, Dr. Norris (this volume) and Dr. Kaniasty (this volume) offer powerful and original evidence-informed guidelines for both research and intervention based on the deterioration-deterrence model. The chasm between traditional research approaches to disaster and typical services models in the community is in itself evidence of a fractured community.

History may eventually reveal that 9/11 was a unique event in its scope of impact. On the other hand, what appears unique in 9/11 research (relative to previous disaster findings) may emerge as a distinct characteristic of terrorist attacks and threats, in comparison to other kinds of disasters. Two critical differences emerge with complete consistency from all of this work: the striking impact of "indirect" exposure; and the importance of post-event stressors in increasing risk for psychopathology. In essence, it appears that post-event stressors "deplete" the individual's resources for processing the traumatic event, thereby increasing risk for chronic disorder through mechanisms that are poorly understood at present.

As this book goes to press the world is saturated with images of the tragedy, chaos, and violence of Hurricane Katrina. Here we see the principles of Hobfoll's Conservation of Resource (COR) theory played out on US soil (Hobfoll, this volume). We see community members risking their lives to save others, but we also see them armed and ready to kill to protect their resources. We see the breakdown of law and order that occurs when the resources of an entire city have been destroyed, and the availability of basic resources (food, clothing, shelter, and medical care) becomes uncertain.

For any New Yorker, the "keystone" concept described by Fullilove and Saul rings true and powerful (Fullilove & Saul, this volume). The loss of the Towers became a focus for grief and for rage as a symbol of community destruction (Amsel & Marshall, 2003).

The principles of community recovery are illustrated through this section with anecdotes, program descriptions, and testimonials from leaders/authors who were also community members/victims. Long-term follow-up studies of such large-scale community interventions for promoting resilience could potentially make major contributions to the world literature on post-disaster intervention Resilience, currently the "concept du jour" could then have an increasingly solid empirical foundation.

Outreach and intervention in the wake of terrorist attacks

Although this book aims to present formal research efforts in the wake of 9/11, results are not yet available from the handful of such projects around the country. The conspicuous paucity of such intervention projects after 9/11 highlights – once again – that disaster research has been typically focused on the characterization of the problem, rather than its amelioration. At this point in the field, we believe that research resources should be primarily devoted to developing practical and necessarily creative approaches to services research after disaster.

This raises the question of what constitutes "research." The desire to develop responsible and effective programs after 9/11 provoked a new (and hopefully permanent) awareness of the importance of including *evaluation components* in services programs. The absence of any prior public reports describing Federal Emergency Management Agency (FEMA) sponsored programs, for example, was a major impediment to planning evidence-informed programs after 9/11. This deficiency is already being remedied through publication of Project Liberty procedures and results.

At the same time, the naïveté in the mental health community about models of resilience-building community interventions, such as those which FEMA sponsors, and the complete isolation of these two traditions from each other, became a major source of conflict after 9/11. The mental health community was largely unable to understand the rationale for outreach and crisis-counseling programs, perhaps because clinician training and treatment models are rooted in the psychopathology and disease model traditions, rather than health-promoting, community-oriented traditions. There are important distinctions between intervention programs aimed at reducing psychopathology, and programs aimed at reducing community fragmentation and shoring up healthy coping in the general population (e.g., Project Liberty). In fact, Project Liberty was the first FEMA-funded crisis-counseling and education program to incorporate screening and triage functions. Finally, program planners and philanthropic funding institutions were repeatedly confronted with the near-complete absence of research into the nature of resilience, and more importantly, into programs that might actually increase resilience (rather than simply reduce psychopathology).

Lessons for communities confronting large-scale disasters

A core mandate in disaster planning is determining whether there will be a sudden increase in health problems that cannot be served by the community's existing services infrastructure, referred to as its "surge capacity"(Marshall *et al.*, in press). If there is a surge capacity problem, the community will require humanitarian aid in the form of interventions, personnel, and funds for services for these needs to be met. Thus, the core question is this: after large-scale disasters, when a high incidence of new-onset psychologic disorders is likely, how can community capacity be increased to meet the needs of seriously affected disaster victims? The outreach and interventions section of this volume includes a representative set of the types of programs that attempted to meet this mandate in the first 2 years after the attacks. There are lessons to be learned for future large-scale events in every chapter.

In countries with centralized health care systems (e.g., throughout much of Europe, in Israel, and in Canada), surge capacity deficiencies can be partially addressed through policy by shifting resources to make properly trained practitioners more available, improve access to care, and provide public education. In the USA there is no centralization of mental health training, such that policy has a limited role in the short term. Moreover, there is minimal monitoring of training or skill level in practicing clinicians, and no systematic national efforts to implement evidence-based treatments through training. Thus, a major goal after 9/11 was to find efficient alternative ways to rectify the shortage of clinicians with trauma and grief expertise.

Communities cohere and define themselves in many ways that critically influence the way services are sought: geographic, linguistic, professional, socioeconomic, ethnic, and racial characteristics were emphasized in various programs. Availability and acceptability of mental health services vary enormously within communities in the greater New York area. Examples of groups that seemed to require distinctly different kinds of outreach are the following: World Trade Center workers, residents of lower Manhattan, Mandarin-speaking residents, firefighters, utility workers, and children in lower Manhattan schools. Services programs in New York, and in particular the Red Cross programs, focused on vulnerable groups, and these chapters by and large discuss barriers to services and the efforts to overcome these barriers. When funding became available through philanthropy, barriers *other* than financial were revealed including linguistic barriers, shortages of qualified personnel, extreme shortage of high-quality evidence-based trainings, and acceptability to recipients. It is a social reality, supported by considerable research, that health problems in the community are not met simply by making services available. This is the basic justification for public health education campaigns that raise awareness of problems ranging from obesity and hypertension to depression. Breslau's and McNally's dangerously naïve (and incorrect) argument (Breslau & McNally, this volume) – one that also appears in other writings by persons unfamiliar with services issues or research – is that, if persons do not seek services, then they must not have been needed. Even if services had not been sought (in fact they were), it would have demonstrated the failure of services delivery, not the absence of the problem itself.

In fact, as shown by Felton and colleagues (this volume) as well as emerging first-ever publications documenting the results of Project Liberty, services were sought and provided on a massive scale. Project Liberty, which was implemented following FEMA guidelines as a resilience enhancing program using an outreach model, offered psycho-education, support (crisis counseling), and triage to more than 1,000,000 people in more than 12 languages over 2 years. This was a 3-fold increase in service provision by the entire New York State Office of Mental Health compared to the year 2000. Approximately 1/3 of these persons were seeking services for depressive-like symptoms, and 1/3 for PTSD-like symptoms, for a total of more than 600,000 people with possible psychopathology (full and subthreshold) related to 9/11-related problems.

Other programs included the following: (1) The Red Cross paid for mental health treatment for over 10,000 persons with no ability to pay across 46 States (http://www.redcross.org); (2) New York City rolled out a massive program to screen children and provide services throughout its school system of over 1,000,000 children; and (3) 1-800-LIFENET, the crisis counseling and referral service that became the triage service for mental health across the tri-state area, handled 34,000 calls related to 9/11 in 2002, which was more than double the call volume of 2001. This pattern persisted through 2003 (Draper *et al.*, this volume).

LIFENET conducted a study to evaluate the quality of their services, and found indeed that 77% of people had linked to services successfully, and most (89%) reported feeling better 3 months later. The key factor in connecting people in need to services was the partnership between the Project Liberty media campaign and LIFENET, and, later, the increase in service capacity created by Project Liberty and the Red Cross treatment program that paid for 9/11-related services (Draper *et al.*, this volume). Before 9/11, only about 1 in 200 calls were related to PTSD symptoms, whereas for the first 6 months after 9/11, 1:7 calls were related to these symptoms.

Research to date demonstrates the existence of particular vulnerability factors that increase risk for trauma-related disorders after new traumatic experiences. The treatment section of this book, capturing only a few of the mental health programs after 9/11, documents the intelligent and creative use of this research in real-world settings. Many threats to public health are particularly virulent in vulnerable groups (e.g., for a virulent flu strain, the elderly, infants, and other immuno-compromised groups), and rational public health policy must pay special attention to such groups. After 9/11, vulnerability factors were concentrated in the highly exposed, but also in relief workers, volunteers, the poor, the newly unemployed, persons with pre-existing psychiatric problems and disorders, and certain ethnic groups.

There are a number of evidence-based psychosocial approaches to treating all of the disorders known to occur in suddenly increased rates after disaster. This book includes a review of the evidence base for a particularly well-studied treatment for PTSD, prolonged exposure therapy (Foa & Cahill, this volume); a review of the research to date on disseminating this approach to the community (Cahill *et al.*, this volume); and a chapter describing our efforts to disseminate this treatment on a very large scale after 9/11 (Amsel *et al.*, this volume). Our intention in developing this emphasis was to show a continuum of work from laboratory to private office, and not to feed the unfortunate rivalry among therapeutic schools and treatments that continues to plague the mental health field. Similar programs could have and should be developed for other evidence-based psychosocial approaches as well as pharmacologic treatments.

Parents throughout the city were worried about their children's exposure to such a violent and public event and the ensuing chaos. They were right to worry. An estimated 75,000 children grades 4–12 in the New York City school system reported 9/11-related PTSD 6 months after the attacks, and only a minority had received help. Schechter and Coates (this volume) provide a brilliant discussion of state-of-the-art thinking about PTSD-like syndromes in very young children, and discuss the concept of "relational PTSD" that emphasizes the critical role that parents play in exacerbating or mitigating children's reactions as the primary source of a child's feeling of safety (which is the antidote to trauma-related fear). Their theoretical model is particularly important in light of the fact that parental psychopathology, and not the traditional variable of proximity to exposure, was the best predictor of PTSD in children (Hoven *et al.*, 2005). This chapter provides many useful and poignant clinical illustrations of how children were helped using this model.

Another source of confusion in the post-9/11 public discourse has to do with children's vulnerabilities. Are they highly resilient or highly vulnerable? They are both. Schechter and Coates (this volume) clarify this for us by pointing out that children in general show high resilience so long as the disaster leaves the family's functioning intact, but are highly vulnerable when family life is destroyed or disrupted – the extreme form of which is the death of a parent.

The role of the media as vehicle for exposure

In understanding the controversy surrounding two groundbreaking national surveys (Silver *et al.*, this volume; Schlenger *et al.*, 2002), it must be remembered that *Diagnostic and Statistical Manual of Mental Disorders, Fourth Edition* (DSM-IV) is simply a summary of scientific knowledge-to-date, a work-in-progress that should be continually updated by new research findings. This is the answer to arguments that these surveys are to be questioned merely because they do not fit the pre-9/11 meaning of the phrase "trauma exposure." Don Klein has referred to this kind of error as "misplaced concreteness." This point cannot be stressed enough. We cannot develop ways to reduce the impact of fear of terrorism, in its entire spectrum, if we don't acknowledge that it exists.

Research has shown conclusively that media exposure after 9/11 correlated with severity of psychologic reactions, symptoms, and disorder. Concepts from the risk perception literature are particularly useful in understanding these phenomena (Slovic, 1987). The media simultaneously drives anxiety reactions in opposing directions after disaster: providing information about what is happening can reduce anxiety by reducing uncertainty; while (through a different mechanism) increasing negative affect by increasing and reinforcing trauma exposure. Vigilance in the face of uncertain threat is a basic human response, and threat appraisal is characterized by a search for information that will clarify the nature of the threat in order to respond to it.

The psychologic consequences of news-media exposure likely are determined by the threat signal potential of the information. The September 11 attacks are the best-documented instance to date of the potential power of the media to promote widespread horror and fear when the threat potential of the event is uncertain but potentially cataclysmic (e.g., a full-out attack on US soil; additional large-scale attacks on civilians). September 11 differs critically from typical media broadcasts of horrific events in that a very frightening, unfamiliar threat signal (being killed by terrorist attacks on US soil) was being *transmitted through actual, graphic images of destruction and carnage on US soil*. Similar consequences have been documented in Israel through recent research estimating that 9.4% of the population meets criteria for terrorism-related PTSD (Bleich *et al.*, 2003), a relatively high proportion of the entire population. Psychopathology was not predicted by personal exposure to terrorist events – again, additional proof that the causal pathway under extreme and uncertain threat conditions is distinct from that seen in other kinds of trauma and disaster.

The fact that the human consequences of exposure to horror, violence, and sense-less suffering extends to journalists themselves as described in Dr. Newman's research (Newman *et al.*, this volume) is further testament to the importance of pursuing enlightened dialog with media institutions.

Perspectives on 9/11 from outside the affected community

Arieh Shalev is one of the world's leading researchers and theoreticians in the phe-nomenology of PTSD, and in public health issues related to terrorism. True to form, his analysis shows a sophisticated appreciation of both the clinical and the scientific issues involved in trying to understand 9/11 and to develop an ethical and effective response of the programmatic level. He understands the uniqueness of the "exposure" itself, its blurred boundaries, and also appreciates the importance of risk perception in trying to measure overall mental health effects.

He discusses perhaps the most important public health problem in mental health services: the fact that simply making services available in no way guarantees that they will reach persons in need. He also appreciates the fact that 9/11 brought into sharp relief the confusion in the field about how to link the spectrum of responses to trauma with appropriate institutional responses.

Programs might be designed to shore up community cohesion, reduce fear responses by normalizing them, offer opportunities for sense making, provide coun-seling to promote adaptive and resilience-enhancing responses, or treat the minority of persons with identifiable disorder. And, since it is well established that most per-sons in the latter category do not receive services, the most innovative and real-world responsive programs were designed to reduce these barriers, be they financial, stigma-related, institutional (e.g., refusal of insurance companies to provide parity coverage), or patient-related (shame). Finally, Dr. Shalev reminds us of the limita-tions of the mental disorder paradigm, and of the importance of studying the nor-mative process of coping with adversity if we are to ever understand a population's responses to terrorism (Shalev, this volume).

This book includes chapters that are intended to critically examine the findings, concepts, and observations included herein, in the spirit of open discussion. However, in reading the chapter by Breslau and McNally, I was reminded of the National Aeronautics and Space Administration (NASA) official whose job it was to respond to conspiracy theorists who believed the moon landings had actually been elaborately staged. Where does one begin to respond to Breslau and McNally's assertion that there "was no mental health epidemic after 9/11"? (Breslau & McNally, this volume). Galea and Resnick report an approximately 6.0% prevalence of 9/11-related PTSD in the first 6 months, or approximately 810,000 adults (Galea & Resnick, 2005). Even using the most conservative criteria – full PTSD, self-reported functional impairment, and acute distress – PTSD rates in New York City were 2.9%, or approximately 391,500 persons. Using either the lay understanding of the word or the precise definition of epidemic – "prevalent among a people or a community at a special time, and produced by some special causes not generally present in the affected locality (*Oxford English Dictionary*, 2002)" – this is hardly a subtle call.

To list only a few examples of errors and problematic assertions in Breslau's and McNally's opinions: (1) They state there was "no convincing evidence" linking functional impairment and PTSD, which is simply incorrect (see Galea & Resnick 2005, for an extended discussion of this). (2) They make the very basic error of arguing that, because a disorder (acute PTSD) is time limited, it is simply "expectable emotional distress" (Breslau & McNally, this volume). Many psychiatric disorders and medical illnesses are self-limited. Most major depressive episodes are self-limited, but no one argues they are therefore simply "expectable emotional distress." (3) They assert incorrectly that 9/11 studies used unvalidated diagnoses, when all reports include careful evidence of their validity.

It is unfortunate, but this chapter abandons the basic principle that mental health scientists should concern themselves with recognizing and responding to public health needs. The ethical consequences of minimization or outright denial of human suffering after large-scale traumatic events are profound. The post-9/11 debate has become so shrill, it was perhaps inevitable that an event with profound political consequences from the start would become politicized.

Simon Wessely reminds us of basic truisms in psychiatry: distress does not equal symptoms, symptoms do not equal disorder, and disorder is by definition associated with impairment. He and Dr. Shalev also remind us that there is a wide disparity in overall responses to trauma, including both positive and negative. His anecdotal observations about his and others reactions are moving as example of outsider's responses to the attacks (Wessely, this volume). It is notable that Wessely's own group recently conducted a screening in London after the July 7, 2005 bombing of the underground and reported high rates of symptom distress (31%) in spite of the fact that very few Londoners were "directly exposed" to the carnage of this atrocity (Rubin *et al.*, 2005). He concludes by rehashing the widely recognized failure of single session debriefing to reduce or prevent symptoms after trauma. In future planning for acute intervention after disaster much more attention should be devoted to the literature demonstrating successful cognitive–behavioral treatment (CBT) interventions in persons with acute stress disorder (reviewed recently in Bryant, 2005).

In summary, we hope that this book will be a useful guide for future communities after disaster. Equally importantly, we hope that this book will help to keep the many worldwide scientific and services enterprises focused on its ethical mandate to serve the public good after large-scale disaster.

REFERENCES

American Red Cross (http://www.redcross.org).

Amsel, L.V. & Marshall, R.D. (2003). In the wake of terror: the clinical management of subsyndromal psychological sequelae of 9/11 terror attacks. In *September 11: Trauma and Human Bonds*, eds. S. Coates, J. Rosenthal & D. Schechter. New York, NY: The Analytic Press, pp. 75–98.

Amsel, L.V., Neria, Y., Suh, E.J. & Marshall, R.D. (this volume). Mental health community response to 9/11: training therapists to practice evidence-based psychotherapy. In *9/11: Mental Health in the Wake of Terrorist Attacks*, eds. Y. Neria, R. Gross & R.D. Marshall. Cambridge, UK: Cambridge University Press.

Bleich, A., Gelkopf, M. & Solomon, Z. (2003). Exposure to terrorism, stress-related mental health symptoms, and coping behaviors among a nationally representative sample in Israel. *Journal of the American Medical Association*, **290**, 612–620.

Breslau, N. & McNally, R.J. (this volume). The epidemiology of 9/11: the technological advances and conceptual conundrums. In *9/11: Mental Health in the Wake of Terrorist Attacks*, eds. Y. Neria, R. Gross & R.D. Marshall. Cambridge, UK: Cambridge University Press.

Bryant, R.A. (2005). Psychosocial approaches of acute stress reactions. *CNS Spectrums*, **10**, 116–122.

Cahill, S.P., Hembree, E.A. & Foa, E.B. (this volume). Dissemination of prolonged exposure therapy for posttraumatic stress disorder: successes and challenges. In *9/11: Mental Health in the Wake of Terrorist Attacks*, eds. Y. Neria, R. Gross & R.D. Marshall. Cambridge, UK: Cambridge University Press.

Draper, J., McCleery, G. & Schaedle, R. (this volume). Mental health services in response to September 11: the central role of the Mental Health Association of New York City. In *9/11: Mental Health in the Wake of Terrorist Attacks*, eds. Y. Neria, R. Gross & R.D. Marshall. Cambridge, UK: Cambridge University Press.

Felton, C.J., Donahue, S., Barth Lanzara, C., Pease, E.A. & Marshall, R.D. (this volume). Project Liberty: responding to mental health needs after the World Trade Center terrorist attacks. In *9/11: Mental Health in the Wake of Terrorist Attacks*, eds. Y. Neria, R. Gross & R.D. Marshall. Cambridge, UK: Cambridge University Press.

Foa, E.B. & Cahill, S.P. (this volume). Psychological treatments for PTSD: an overview. In *9/11: Mental Health in the Wake of Terrorist Attacks*, eds. Y. Neria, R. Gross & R.D. Marshall. Cambridge, UK: Cambridge University Press.

Fullilove, M.T. & Saul, J. (this volume). Rebuilding communities post-disaster in New York. In *9/11: Mental Health in the Wake of Terrorist Attacks*, eds. Y. Neria, R. Gross & R.D. Marshall. Cambridge, UK: Cambridge University Press.

Galea, S. & Resnick, H. (2005). Posttraumatic stress disorder in the general population after mass terrorist incidents: considerations about the nature of exposure. *CSN Spectrums*, **10**, 107–115.

Galea, S., Nandi, A. & Vlahov, D. (2005). The epidemiology of posttraumatic stress disorder after disasters. *Epidemiological Reviews*, **27**, 78–91.

Hobfoll, S.E. (this volume). Guiding community intervention following terrorist attack. In *9/11: Mental Health in the Wake of Terrorist Attacks*, eds. Y. Neria, R. Gross & R.D. Marshall. Cambridge, UK: Cambridge University Press.

Hoven, C.W., Duarte, C.S., Lucas, C.P., Wu, P., Mandell, D.J., Goodwin, R.D., Cohen, M., Balaban, V., Woodruff, B.A., Bin, F., Musa, G.J., Mei, L., Cantor, P.A., Aber, J.L., Cohen, P. & Susser, E. (2005). Psychopathology among New York city public school children 6 months after September 11. *Archives of General Psychiatry*, **62**, 545–552.

Kaniasty, K. (this volume). Searching for points of convergence: a commentary on prior research on disasters and some community programs initiated in response to September 11, 2001. In *9/11: Mental Health in the Wake of Terrorist Attacks*, eds. Y. Neria, R. Gross & R.D. Marshall. Cambridge, UK: Cambridge University Press.

Kessler, R.C., Sonnega, A., Bromet, E., Hughes, M. & Nelson, C.B. (1995). Posttraumatic stress disorder in the National Comorbidity Survey. *Archives of General Psychiatry*, **52**, 1048–1060.

Kulka, R.A., Schlenger, W.E., Fairbank, J.A., Hough, R.L., Jordan, B.K., Marmar, C.R. & Weiss, D.S. (1990). *Trauma and the Vietnam War generation: Report of findings from the National Vietnam Veterans' Readjustment Study*. New York, NY: Brunner/Mazel.

Marshall, R.D., Amsel, L.V., Neria, Y. & Suh, E.J. (in press). Strategies for dissemination of evidence-based treatments: training clinicians after large-scale disasters. In *Research Methods and Strategies for Studying Mental Health after Disasters and Terrorism*, eds. F. Norris, M. Friedman, P. Watson & J. Hamblen. New York: Guilford Press.

Newman, E., Davis, J. & Kennedy, S.M. (this volume). Journalism and the public during catastrophes. In *9/11: Mental Health in the Wake of Terrorist Attacks*, eds. Y. Neria, R. Gross & R.D. Marshall. Cambridge, UK: Cambridge University Press.

Norris, F.H. (this volume). Community and ecological approaches to understanding and alleviating postdisaster distress. In *9/11: Mental Health in the Wake of Terrorist Attacks*, eds. Y. Neria, R. Gross & R.D. Marshall. Cambridge, UK: Cambridge University Press.

Norris, F.H., Friedman, M.J. & Watson, P.J. (2002a). 60,000 disaster victims speak. Part 1: An empirical review of the empirical literature, 1981–2001. *Psychiatry*, **65**, 207–239.

Norris, F.H., Friedman, M.J. & Watson, P.J. (2002b). 60,000 disaster victims speak. Part II: Summary and implications of disaster mental health research. *Psychiatry*, **65**, 240–260.

North, C.S., Pfefferbaum, B. & Hong, B. (this volume). Historical perspective and future directions in research on psychiatric consequences of terrorism and other disasters. In *9/11: Mental Health in the Wake of Terrorist Attacks*, eds. Y. Neria, R. Gross & R.D. Marshall. Cambridge, UK: Cambridge University Press.

Oxford English Dictionary (2nd ed. on CD-ROM). Oxford University Press, 2002.

Rubin, G.J., Brewin, C.R., Greenberg, N., Simpson, J. & Wessely, S. (2005). Psychological and behavioural reactions to the bombings in London on 7 July 2005: cross sectional survey of a representative sample of Londoners. *British Medical Journal*, **331**(7517): 606.

Schechter, D.S. & Coates, S.W. (this volume). Relationally and developmentally focused interventions with young children and their caregivers in the wake of terrorism and other violent experiences. In *9/11: Mental Health in the Wake of Terrorist Attacks*, eds. Y. Neria, R. Gross & R.D. Marshall. Cambridge, UK: Cambridge University Press.

Schlenger, W.E., Cadell, J.M., Ebert, M., Jordan, A.K., Rourke, K.M., Wilson, D., Thalji, L., Dennis, J.M., Fairbank, J.A. & Kulka, R.A. (2002). Psychological reactions to terrorist attacks: Findings from the National Study of Americans' Reactions to September 11. *Journal of the American Medical Association*, **288**(5), 581–588.

Shalev, A. (this volume). Lessons learned from 9/11: the boundaries of a mental health approach to mass casualty events. In *9/11: Mental Health in the Wake of Terrorist Attacks*, eds. Y. Neria, R. Gross & R.D. Marshall. Cambridge, UK: Cambridge University Press.

Slovic, P. (1987). Perception of risk. *Science*, **236**, 280–285.

Silver, R.C., Holman, E.A., McIntosh, D.N., Poulin, M., Gil-Rivas, V. & Pizarro, J. (this volume). Coping with a national trauma: a nationwide longitudinal study of responses to the terrorist attacks of September 11. In *9/11: Mental Health in the Wake of Terrorist Attacks*, eds Y. Neria, R. Gross & R.D. Marshall. Cambridge, UK: Cambridge University Press.

Wessely, S. (this volume). What mental health professionals should and should not do. In *9/11: Mental Health in the Wake of Terrorist Attacks*, eds. Y. Neria, R. Gross & R.D. Marshall. Cambridge, UK: Cambridge University Press.

Index

acute stress disorder (ASD) 457
　DSM–IV criteria 58
　treatment 479
　　CBT 479–480
acute stress response, during Iraq war 64
adolescents 49, 325, 330
　CATS 275, 378
　community trauma 50
　coping mechanism, type 74
　NYC BOE 89
　and parents, study findings 63–64
adult non-survivors, response 184
adult survivors, public response
　　182–184
alleviating postdisaster distress 149–152
American Psychological Association 210,
　　216, 434
　Task force on Resilience in Response to
　　Terrorism 576
anxiety management training (AMT) 460
appraisal-tendency theory 577–578, 580,
　　584
Arieh Shalev 626
Armed Forces Institute of Pathology
　　(AFIP) 433
Associates in Internal Medicine (AIM)
　　studies 243–244
　design 243
　recruitment 243–244
　sampling 244
avoidance and numbing symptoms 103,
　　348

Barbara Dohrenwend's model 150
Behavioral Health Service 321, 436,
　　437–438
behavioral intention (BI)
　key factors 510–511
binary logistic regression 246
bioethical and legal ramification, of
　　preparedness 599
blamestorming 204
bracket creep 523
bureaucracy management 597–598

call volume
　post 9/11 270
　　broad scale activating agents
　　　290–291
　　media influences 288–290
　　temporal distance, from disaster
　　　291–292
　pre 9/11 284
care delivery model 439–442
caregivers 288, 289, 404, 420, 439
　and child outcome 407–408
　guidelines 412–413
　video feedback, clinician guided
　　417–418
　see also parents
casualty assistance care officer (CACO)
　　432, 558
Center for Occupational and
　　Environmental Medicine (COEM)
　　358, 360–362, 363, 369